ILLUSTRATED DENTAL EMBRYOLOGY, HISTOLOGY, AND ANATOMY

ILLUSTRATED DENTAL EMBRYOLOGY, HISTOLOGY, AND ANATOMY

5TH EDITION

MARGARET J. FEHRENBACH, RDH, MS Primary Author

Oral Biologist and Dental Hygienist; Adjunct Instructor, Bachelor of Applied Science Degree, Dental Hygiene Program, Seattle Central College, Seattle, Washington; Educational Consultant and Dental Science Technical Writer, Seattle, Washington

TRACY POPOWICS, PhD

Associate Professor, Department of Oral Health Sciences, School of Dentistry, University of Washington, Seattle, Washington

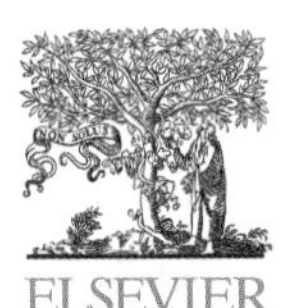

ELSEVIER

Elsevier
3251 Riverport Lane
St. Louis, Missouri 63043

ILLUSTRATED DENTAL EMBRYOLOGY, HISTOLOGY, AND ANATOMY, FIFTH EDITION
ISBN: 978-0-323-61107-7
Copyright © 2020 by Elsevier, Inc. All rights reserved.

No part of this publication may be reproduced or transmitted in any form or by any means, electronic or mechanical, including photocopying, recording, or any information storage and retrieval system, without permission in writing from the publisher. Details on how to seek permission, further information about the Publisher's permissions policies and our arrangements with organizations such as the Copyright Clearance Center and the Copyright Licensing Agency, can be found at our website: www.elsevier.com/permissions.

This book and the individual contributions contained in it are protected under copyright by the Publisher (other than as may be noted herein).

Notice

Practitioners and researchers must always rely on their own experience and knowledge in evaluating and using any information, methods, compounds or experiments described herein. Because of rapid advances in the medical sciences, in particular, independent verification of diagnoses and drug dosages should be made. To the fullest extent of the law, no responsibility is assumed by Elsevier, authors, editors or contributors for any injury and/or damage to persons or property as a matter of products liability, negligence or otherwise, or from any use or operation of any methods, products, instructions, or ideas contained in the material herein.

Previous editions copyrighted 2016, 2011, 2006, 1997 by Saunders, an imprint of Elsevier, Inc.

Library of Congress Control Number: 2019949730

Content Strategist: Joslyn Dumas
Senior Content Development Manager: Luke Held
Senior Content Development Specialist: Kelly Skelton
Publishing Services Manager: Catherine Jackson
Senior Project Manager/Specialist: Carrie Stetz
Design Direction: Paula Catalano

Printed in India

Last digit is the print number: 9 8 7 6 5 4

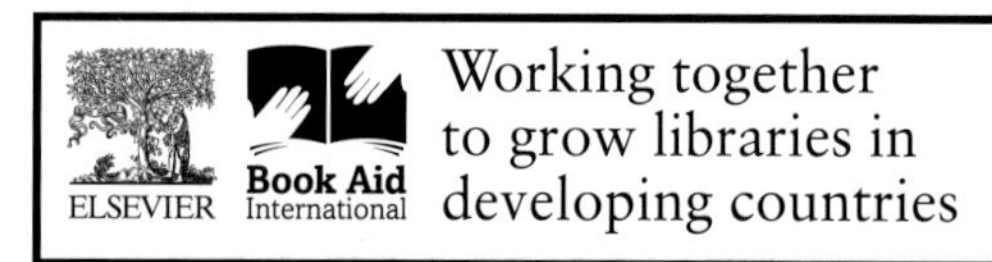

REVIEWERS

Deborah Bush-Munson, CDA, MS
Program Director, Associate Professor
Dental Technologies
St. Louis Community College–Forest Park
St. Louis, Missouri

Tammy S. Clossen, RDH, PHDHP, PhD
Assistant Professor
Dental Hygiene
Pennsylvania College of Technology
Williamsport, Pennsylvania

Jamie Collins, RDH, CDA
Dental Assisting Instructor
Workforce Development
College of Western Idaho
Nampa, Idaho

Sharon Grisanti, RDH, AS, BA, MS
Assistant Professor
Dental Hygiene
Health Education Center
St. Petersburg College
St. Petersburg, Florida

Cathleen Korondi, CDA, RDH, EdD
Professor, Dental Hygiene Program Director
Health Careers
Illinois Central College
Peoria, Illinois

Rina A. Nowka, RDH, MA
Adjunct Clinical Professor
Dental Hygiene
Bergen Community College
Paramus, New Jersey

Danielle Christine Thompson, RDH, BSDH
Adjunct Professor
Dental Hygiene
College of Lake County
Waukegan, Illinois

Christine Kelly Turner, BA(Kin), RDH
Coordinator, Dental Hygiene Program
Health Sciences
Fanshawe College
London, Ontario, Canada

Sandra Michelle Walker, CDA, CPFDA, BS
Department Chair
Dental Assisting
Fayetteville Technical Community College
Fayetteville, North Carolina

PREFACE

OVERVIEW

This textbook provides an extensive background for student dental professionals in the area of oral biology as well as dental professional program graduates who need to take competency examinations or update their background knowledge in this area. The textbook strives to integrate the clinical aspects of dentistry with the basic science information that is key to its successful performance by the dental professional.

The textbook is divided into four units: **Orofacial Structures, Dental Embryology, Dental Histology**, and **Dental Anatomy**. The textbook was organized into units to accommodate differing curriculum; thus, the units do not have to be presented in any specific order. However, the first unit on orofacial structures serves as an outstanding review for the students before further study in oral biology, which is also presented in this textbook.

FEATURES

Each of the four units for this textbook consists of several chapters and each chapter builds on the preceding ones in that unit. Each chapter begins with a Learning Objectives section, which serves as a checkpoint for the students to test their understanding of the chapter's content. In addition, each chapter contains **key terms**, which are in bold when presented for the first time in the textbook along with pronunciations.

The chapters contain figures that incorporate both microscopic and clinical photographs, as well as useful tables and boxes. Most of the photographs are original to this textbook and come from the personal collection of Margaret J. Fehrenbach and the Bernhard Gottlieb Collection (see Acknowledgments). The fine illustrations of the dentitions are original to this textbook, as are most of the other ones in the other areas of oral biology.

Within each chapter are discussions of clinical considerations of the topic covering various treatment situations; these allow for an increased integration of the basic science information into everyday practice for the dental professional. Each chapter contains cross-references to figures and other chapters so that the reader can review or investigate interrelated subjects. The content of this edition incorporates additional input from students and educators as well as the latest information from scientific studies and experts.

The textbook concludes with a bibliography, a complete glossary of key terms using short easy-to-remember phrases with pronunciation guide, and appendixes that contain a review of anatomic nomenclature, units of measurement, permanent tooth measurements, and developmental information for the dentitions.

EVOLVE

A companion **Evolve website** is available for both students and instructors. It can be accessed directly at http://evolve.elsevier.com/Fehrenbach/illustrated.

Instructor Resources

- *Image Collection:* All of the images from the textbook are available electronically and can be downloaded and used in PowerPoint or other classroom lecture formats.
- *Test Bank:* More than 550 objective-style multiple-choice questions are available with accompanying objective mapping, mapping to the CDA and NBDHE test blueprints, Bloom's Taxonomy difficulty levels, rationales, and page/section references for textbook remediation.
- *TEACH Instructor's Resource Manual:* This resource includes detailed lesson plans, PowerPoint lectures courtesy of Margaret J. Fehrenbach with notes that can be individualized for custom presentations, classroom activities, and the answers to the workbook activities.
- *Supplemental Considerations—Additional Material:* Updated information available on topics of interest to specific chapters that build on the core chapter discussion and enrich learning.

Student Resources

- *Practice Quizzes:* Approximately 275 multiple-choice questions are available in an instant-feedback format, with rationales for correct and incorrect answers. Page number references are also included for remediation.
- *Histology Matching Game:* This learning game has drag-and-drop exercises for histologic identification of textbook images.
- *Review and Assessment Questions:* Approximately 650 short-answer questions for discussion, review, and/or assessment.
- *Tooth Identification Exercises:* Matching exercises that correlate a photo of a model permanent tooth with its tooth number and description are available for the students, including instant feedback for self-assessment.

ADDITIONAL RESOURCES

The companion **Workbook for Illustrated Dental Embryology, Histology, and Anatomy** is also available for student use, edited by Margaret J. Fehrenbach. The workbook features activities such as structure identification exercises, glossary exercises, tooth drawing exercises, infection control guidelines for extracted teeth, and review questions. Patient examination procedures for extraoral and intraoral structures, the dentition, and the occlusion have been added to integrate the clinical aspects of dentistry with the basic science information. Case studies are also present for each unit as well as removable flashcards using the original illustrations of the permanent dentition from the textbook.

This textbook is coordinated with the ***Illustrated Anatomy of the Head and Neck*** by Margaret J. Fehrenbach and Susan W. Herring, and it can be considered a companion textbook to complete the curriculum in oral biology. Many of the figures are also presented in the ***Dental Anatomy Coloring Book***, edited by Margaret J. Fehrenbach.

Margaret J. Fehrenbach, RDH, MS
Tracy Popowics, PhD

ACKNOWLEDGMENTS

We would like to thank Private Sector Education Content Director Kristin Wilhelm, Education Content Strategist Joslyn Dumas, Senior Content Development Specialist Kelly Skelton, and Carrie Stetz, Senior Project Manager and Specialist, as well as the rest of the staff at Elsevier, for making this textbook possible.

Most of the elegant microscopic sections that are original to this textbook are from the Bernhard Gottlieb Collection, courtesy of James E. McIntosh, PhD, Professor Emeritus, Department of Biomedical Sciences, Baylor College of Dentistry, Dallas, Texas. Bernhard Gottlieb was a Viennese physician and dentist (1886–1950) who taught at Baylor College and authored hundreds of scientific articles and four textbooks. Most importantly, he is responsible for the beginnings of oral histology. He is also acknowledged to be the first dental professional to integrate basic science information with clinical dental treatment. We are proud to continue his legacy in this manner.

Finally, we would like to thank our dear families, colleagues, and students.

Margaret J. Fehrenbach
Tracy Popowics

CONTENTS

1

Face and Neck Regions

Additional resources and practice exercises are provided on the companion Evolve website for this book: http://evolve.elsevier.com/Fehrenbach/illustrated.

LEARNING OBJECTIVES

1. Define and pronounce the key terms in this chapter.
2. Locate and identify the regions and associated surface landmarks of the face on a diagram and a patient.
3. Locate and identify the regions and associated surface landmarks of the neck on a diagram and a patient.
4. Integrate the clinical considerations for the surface anatomy of the face and neck into patient examination and care.

FACE AND NECK

Dental professionals must be comfortably familiar with the surface anatomy of the face and neck as discussed in this introduction to **Unit 1** to provide comprehensive dental care. The superficial features of the face and neck provide essential landmarks for many of the deeper anatomic structures.

Examination of these accessible features on a patient, both by visualization and palpation, can give information about the health of deeper tissue. A certain degree of variation in surface features can be considered within a normal range. However, a change in a surface feature in a patient may signal a condition of clinical significance and must be noted in the patient record as well as correctly followed up by the examining dental professional. Thus, the variations among individuals are not what should be noted but the changes in a particular individual.

Some of these surface changes in the features of the face and neck may be due to underlying developmental disturbances. Knowledge of the surface features of the face and neck additionally helps dental professionals to understand the associated developmental pattern. **Unit 2** describes the development of the face and neck and associated developmental disturbances. However, other visible surface changes may be due to underlying associated histologic tissue changes.

In **Unit 3,** the histology of the face and neck is correlated with its visible surface features. Thus, dental professionals need to study face and neck surface structures before continuing further in the study of dental embryology and histology as well as dental anatomy as presented in **Unit 4**.

In this textbook, the illustrations of the face and neck as well as any structures associated with them, are oriented to show the head in anatomic position (see **Appendix A**), unless otherwise noted. This is the same position as if the patient in a clinical setting is viewed straight on while sitting upright in the dental chair.

FACE REGIONS

Both the face and neck surfaces are divided into regions as is the head itself. Within each region are certain surface landmarks. It is important to practice finding these landmarks in each region using a personal mirror while referring to this textbook as well as the **Workbook for Illustrated Dental Embryology, Histology, and Anatomy** in order to improve your skills of examination. Later, locating them on peers and then on patients in a clinical setting will add a real-world level of competence.

The **regions of the face** include the frontal, orbital, nasal, infraorbital, zygomatic, buccal, oral, and mental regions (Fig. 1.1). **Lymph nodes (limf)** are located in certain areas of the face and head and when palpable should be noted in the patient record (Fig. 1.2, also see Fig. 11.16).

Frontal, Orbital, and Nasal Regions

The **frontal region** (**fruhn**-tl) of the face includes the forehead and the area above the eyes (Fig. 1.3). In the **orbital region** (**awr**-bi-tl) of the face, the eyeball and all its supporting structures are contained in the **orbit** (**awr**-bit) of the skull, which is the bony eye socket.

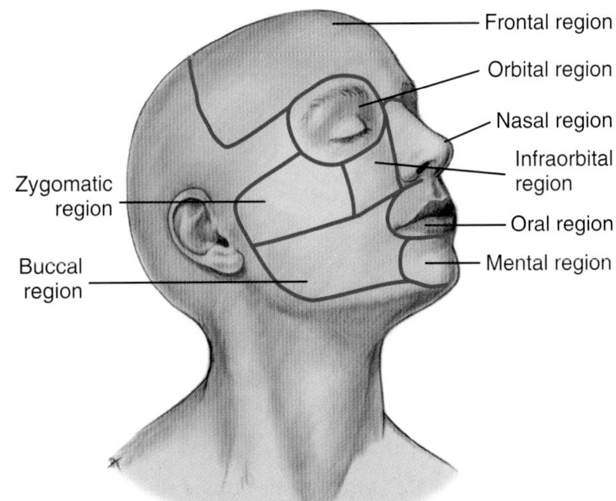

Fig. 1.1 Regions of the face include the frontal, orbital, infraorbital, nasal, zygomatic, buccal, oral, and mental. (Modified from Fehrenbach MJ, Herring SW. *Illustrated Anatomy of the Head and Neck*. 5th ed. St. Louis: Elsevier; 2017.)

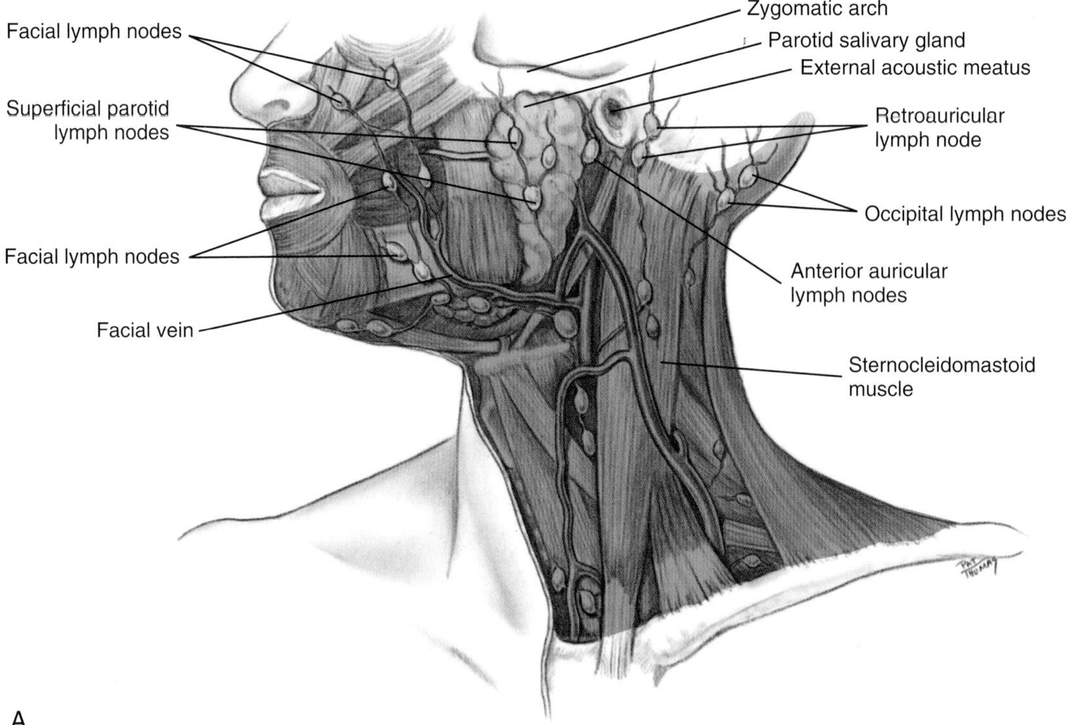

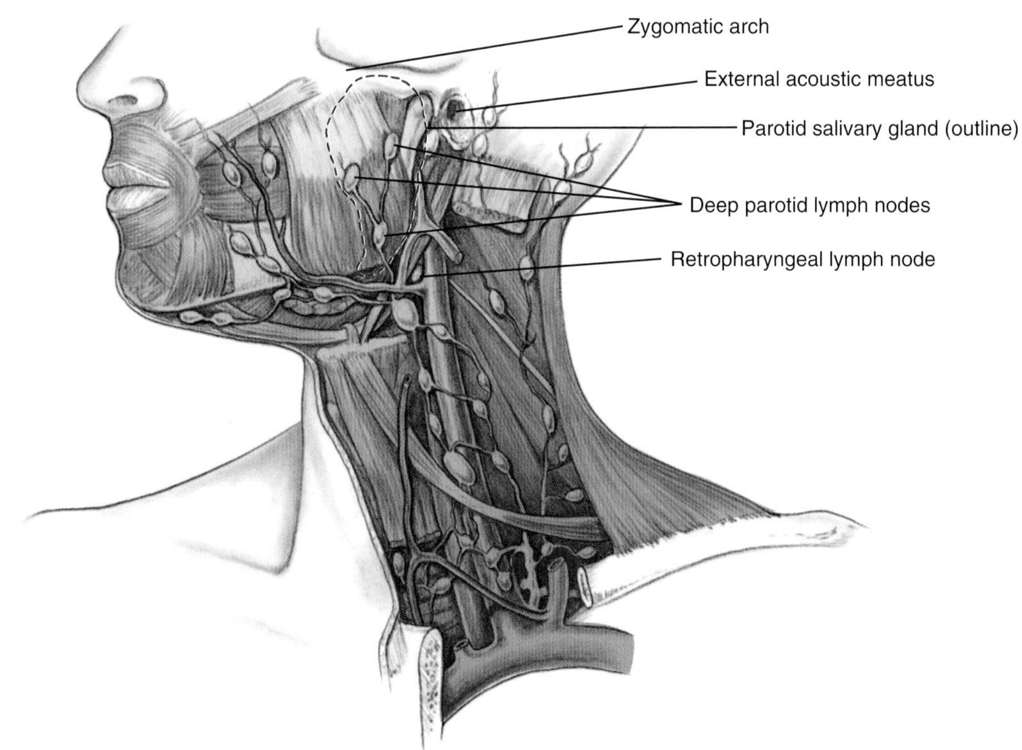

Fig. 1.2 Lymph Nodes of the Head. **A,** Superficial nodes. **B,** Deep nodes. (From Fehrenbach MJ, Herring SW. *Illustrated Anatomy of the Head and Neck.* 5th ed. St. Louis: Elsevier; 2017.)

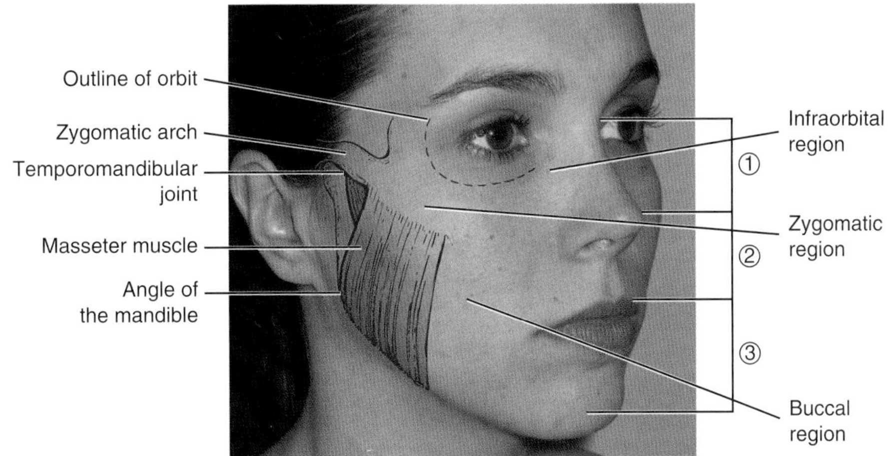

Fig. 1.3 Landmarks of the frontal, orbital, infraorbital, zygomatic, buccal, and mental regions as well as the three divisions of the vertical dimension of the face (see also Fig. 1.10). (From Fehrenbach MJ, Herring SW. *Illustrated Anatomy of the Head and Neck*. 5th ed. St. Louis: Elsevier; 2017.)

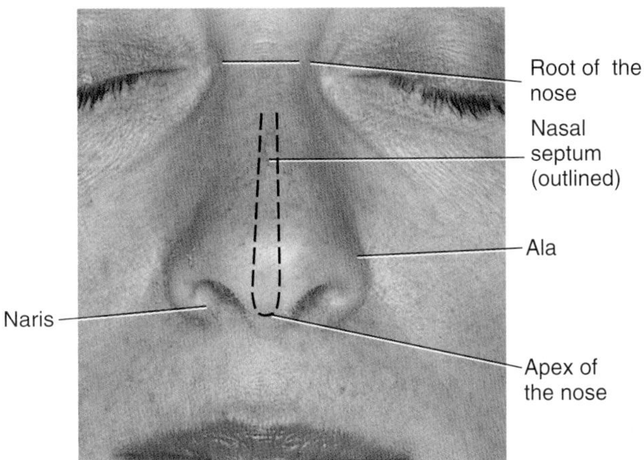

Fig. 1.4 Landmarks of the nasal region with the nasal septum highlighted *(dashed lines)*. (From Fehrenbach MJ, Herring SW. *Illustrated Anatomy of the Head and Neck*. 5th ed. St. Louis: Elsevier; 2017.)

The main feature of the **nasal region** (**ney**-zuhl) of the face is the **external nose** (Fig. 1.4). The **root of the nose** is located between the eyes and the tip is the **apex of the nose** (**ey**-peks). Inferior to the apex on each side of the nose is a nostril or **naris** (**nair**-iz) (plural, **nares** [**nair**-eez]). The nares are separated by the midline **nasal septum** (**sep**-tuhm). The nares are also bounded laterally by winglike cartilaginous structures, each **ala** (**ey**-luh) (plural, **alae** [**ey**-lee]) of the nose.

Infraorbital and Zygomatic Regions

The **infraorbital region** (in-fruh-**awr**-bi-tl) of the face is located inferior to the orbital region and lateral to the nasal region (see Fig. 1.3). Farther laterally is the **zygomatic region** (zahy-guh-**mat**-ik), which overlies the bony support for the cheek, the **zygomatic arch**. The zygomatic arch extends from just below the lateral margin of the eye toward the middle part of the external ear.

Inferior to the zygomatic arch and just anterior to the external ear is the **temporomandibular joint (TMJ)** (tem-puh-roh-man-**dib**-yuh-ler). This is the location where the upper skull forms a joint with the lower jaw (see Fig. 19.1). The movements of the joint occur when the mouth is opened and closed using the lower jaw or the lower jaw is moved to the right or left. To palpate the lower jaw moving at the TMJ on a patient, a finger is gently placed into the external ear canal during movement.

Buccal Region

The **buccal region (buhk**-uhl) of the face is composed of the soft tissue of the cheek (see Fig. 1.3). The cheek forms the side of the face and is a broad area of the face between the nose, mouth, and ear. Most of the upper cheek is fleshy, formed by a mass of mostly fat and muscles. One of these muscles forming the cheek is the strong **masseter muscle** (mass-**seh**-ter/mass-**see**-ter), which is palpated when a patient clenches the teeth together (see Fig. 19.8, *A*). The sharp angle of the lower jaw inferior to the earlobe is the **angle of the mandible** (**man**-duh-buhl). The **parotid salivary gland** (puh-**rot**-id **sal**-uh-ver-ee) has a small part that can be palpated on a patient in the buccal region as well as in the zygomatic region (Fig. 1.5, see Fig. 11.7). Thus the parotid is located irregularly from the zygomatic arch down to the posterior border of the lower jaw.

Oral Region

The **oral region** of the face has many structures within it, such as the lips and oral cavity (Fig. 1.6, see Figs. 2.2 and 2.11). The upper and lower lips are fleshy folds that mark the gateway of the oral cavity proper. With relation to the oral cavity, however, each lip begins as the vermilion border and includes only those areas that are redder in color with variations as to tone. This redder color is the result of blood vessels being seen through a translucent mucous membrane, rather than from inherent reddish pigmentation. This is easily demonstrated by blanching the lip with pressure. Thus the **vermilion zone** (ver-**mil**-yuhn) of each lip has a darker reddish appearance than the surrounding skin, with the lips outlined from the surrounding skin by a transition zone, the **mucocutaneous junction** (myoo-koh-kyoo-**tey**-nee-us) at the **vermilion border.** Between the vermilion zone and the inner oral cavity is the intermediate zone.

On the midline of the upper lip extending downward from the nasal septum is a vertical groove, the **philtrum** (**fil**-truhm). The philtrum terminates in a thicker area of the midline of the upper lip, the **tubercle of the upper lip** (**too**-ber-kuhl). Underlying the upper lip is the upper jaw or **maxilla** (mak-**sil**-uh) (Fig. 1.7, *A*). The bone underlying the lower lip is the lower jaw or **mandible** (Fig. 1.7, *B*). For more information on the jaws, see a detailed discussion in **Chapter 2.** The upper and lower lips meet at each corner of the mouth or the **labial commissure** (**ley**-bee-uhl **kom**-uh-shoor).

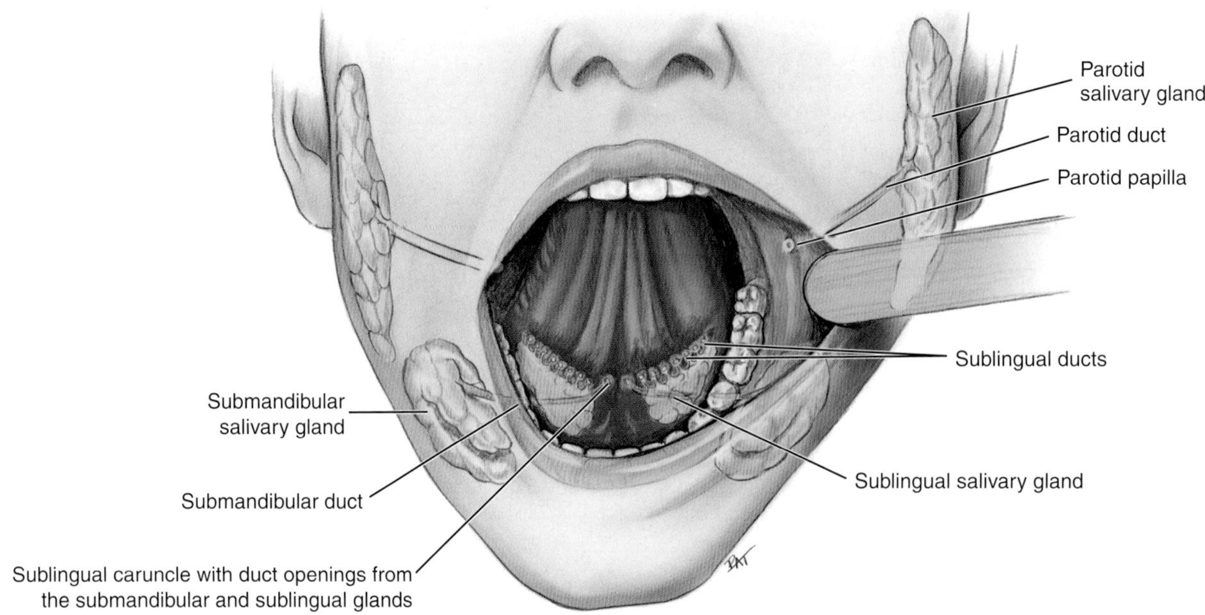

Fig. 1.5 Major Salivary Glands. (From Fehrenbach MJ, Herring SW. *Illustrated Anatomy of the Head and Neck*. 5th ed. St. Louis: Elsevier; 2017.)

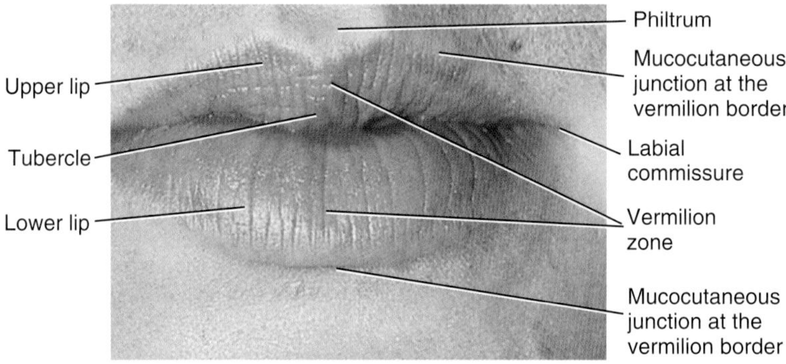

Fig. 1.6 Upper and Lower Lips with the Vermilion Zones and Mucocutaneous Junctions at the Vermilion Borders. (From Fehrenbach MJ, Herring SW. *Illustrated Anatomy of the Head and Neck*. 5th ed. St. Louis: Elsevier; 2017.)

Clinical Considerations with Lips

Disruption of the vermilion zone may make it hard to determine the exact location of its mucocutaneous junction at the vermilion border between the lips and the surrounding skin (Fig. 1.8). These changes may be due to scar tissue from past traumatic incidents, developmental disturbances, or cellular changes in the tissue, such as those that occur with solar damage. These changes may also represent a more serious condition, such as cancer; however, this can be verified only with tissue biopsy and microscopic examination. If disruption is initially only from solar damage, protection of the lips (especially the lower lip) with sunscreen is important because sun exposure increases the risk of cancerous changes. The risk of cancerous changes with the lips can be increased with chronic alcohol and tobacco use.

If disruption of the vermilion zone and its mucocutaneous junction at the vermilion border has been caused by a traumatic incident, noting it in the patient record is important given that the rest of the oral cavity may be affected. If this change is part of a past medical-dental history of a cleft lip, this also needs to be noted (see Fig. 4.8).

Mental Region

The chin is the major feature of the **mental region** (**men**-tl) of the face. The bone underlying the mental region is the mandible or lower jaw. The midline of the mandible is marked by the **mandibular symphysis** (man-**dib**-yuh-ler **sim**-fuh-sis) (see Fig. 4.5).

On the lateral aspect of the mandible, the stout flat plate of the **mandibular ramus** (**rey**-muhs) (plural, **rami** [**rey**-mahy]) extends superiorly and posteriorly from the body of the mandible on each side (see Fig. 1.7, *B* and Fig. 1.9). At the anterior border of the ramus is a thin sharp margin that terminates in the **coronoid process** (**kawr**-uh-noid). The main part of the anterior border of the ramus forms a concave forward curve, the **coronoid notch**.

The posterior border of the ramus is thickened and extends from the angle of the mandible to a projection, the **mandibular condyle** (**kon**-dahyl) with its neck. The articulating surface of the condyle is the head of mandibular condyle within the TMJ. Between the coronoid process and the condyle is a depression, the **mandibular notch**.

Clinical Considerations with Facial Esthetics

The face can be divided vertically into thirds and this perspective is considered the **vertical dimension of the face** (see Fig. 1.3). A discussion of vertical dimension allows a comparison of the three divisions of the face for functional and esthetic purposes using the **Golden Proportions**, which is a set of guidelines (Fig. 1.10 and see Fig. 1.3). Loss of height in the lower third, which contains the teeth and jaws, can occur in certain circumstances causing pronounced changes in the functions as well as esthetics of the orofacial structures (see Fig. 14.22).

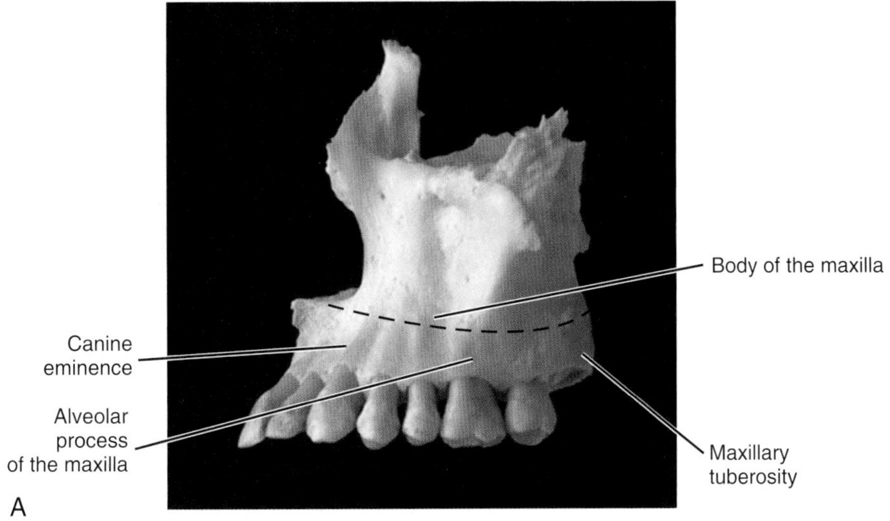

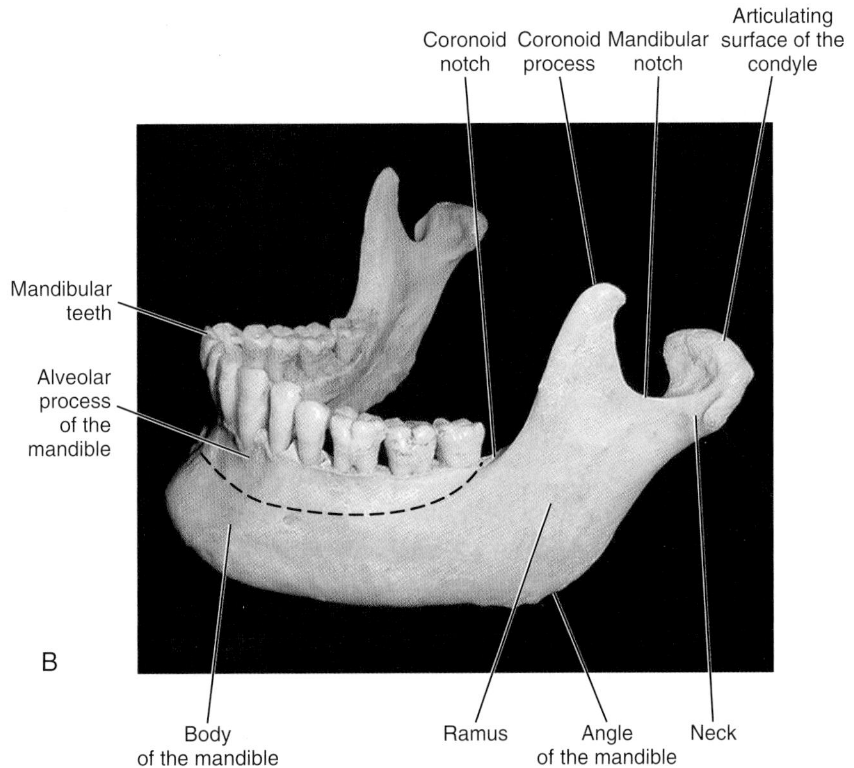

Fig. 1.7 Landmarks of the maxilla **(A)** and mandible **(B)**. (From Fehrenbach MJ, Herring SW. *Illustrated Anatomy of the Head and Neck*. 5th ed. St. Louis: Elsevier; 2017.)

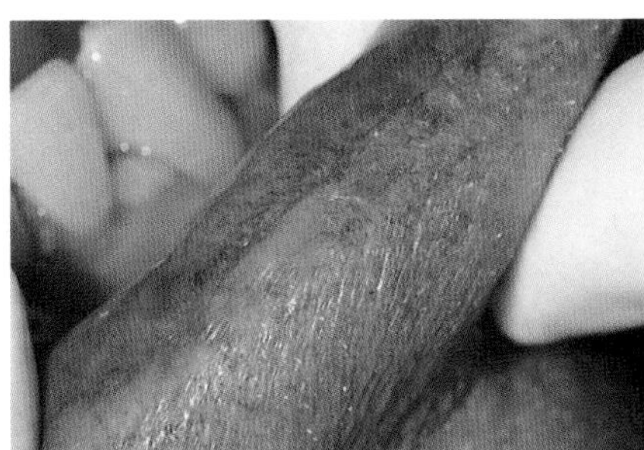

Fig. 1.8 Disruption of vermilion zone and its mucocutaneous junction at the vermilion border on the lower lip due to solar damage. (Courtesy of Margaret J. Fehrenbach, RDH, MS.)

NECK REGIONS

The **regions of the neck** extend from the skull and lower jaw down to the clavicles and sternum (Fig. 1.11). Lymph nodes are located in certain areas of the neck and, when palpable on a patient, should be noted in the patient record (Fig. 1.12). The regions of the neck can be divided further into different cervical triangles using the large bones and muscles located in the area.

The large strap muscle, the **sternocleidomastoid muscle (SCM)** (stur-noh-klahy-duh-**mas**-toid), is easily palpated on each side of the neck of a patient (see Fig. 1.11), with its borders dividing the neck into further regions. At the anterior midline is the **hyoid bone** (**hahy**-oid), which is suspended in the neck. Many muscles attach to the hyoid bone,

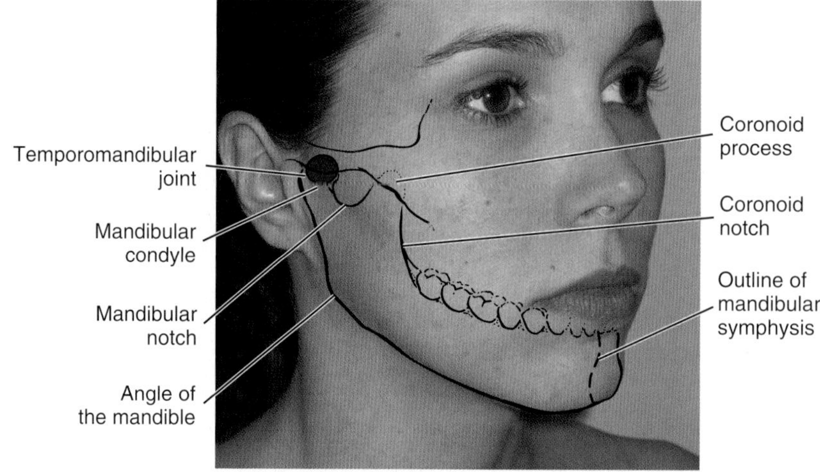

Fig. 1.9 Landmarks of the Mandible Integrated with Overlying Facial Features. (From Fehrenbach MJ, Herring SW. *Illustrated Anatomy of the Head and Neck*. 5th ed. St. Louis: Elsevier; 2017.)

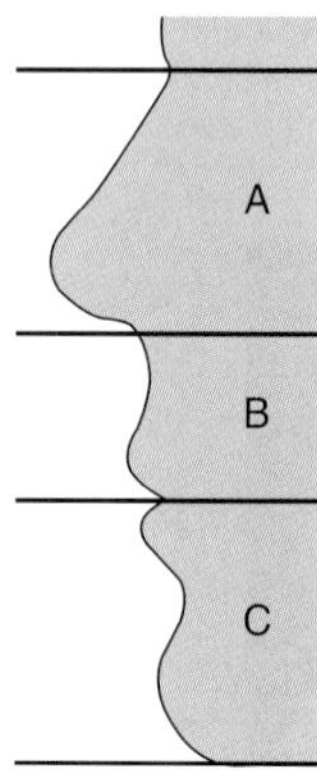

Fig. 1.10 Golden Proportions of the Face with its Three Divisions Illustrating the Considerations of Vertical Facial Dimension. Nasal height *(A)* is related to maxillary height *(B)* as 1.000:0.618; sum of nasal height and maxillary height *(A + B)* are related to mandibular height *(C)* as 1.618:1.000; mandibular height *(C)* is related to maxillary height *(B)* as 1.000:0.618; orofacial height *(B + C)* is related to nasal height *(A)* as 1.618:1.000. Note that each ratio is 1.618, which is integral to these guidelines. These guidelines can also be used when considering the esthetics of the related smile. See also Figure 1.3.

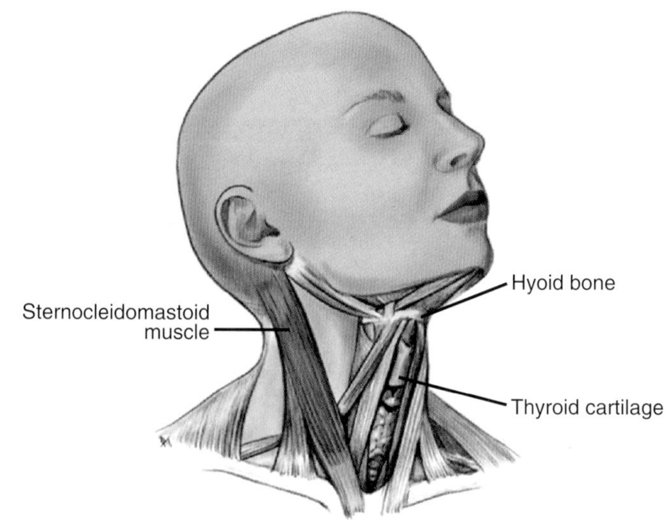

Fig. 1.11 Landmarks of the Neck Region. (From Fehrenbach MJ, Herring SW. *Illustrated Anatomy of the Head and Neck*. 5th ed. St. Louis: Elsevier; 2017.)

which controls the position of the base of the tongue. Also found in the anterior midline and inferior to the hyoid bone is the **thyroid cartilage** (**thahy**-roid **kahr**-ti-lij) that is the prominence of the **larynx** (**lar**-ingks), which is considered the "voice box." The vocal cords as ligaments of the larynx are attached to the posterior surface of the thyroid cartilage.

The **thyroid gland**, an endocrine gland, can also be palpated on a patient within the midline cervical area (Fig. 1.13 and see **Chapter 11**). Thus the thyroid gland is located inferior to the thyroid cartilage, at the junction of the larynx and the trachea. The **parathyroid glands** (pahr-uh-**thahy**-roid) are also endocrine glands that are located close to or within the posterior aspect of each side of the thyroid gland but cannot be palpated in a patient. The **submandibular salivary gland** (sub-man-**dib**-yuh-ler) and the **sublingual salivary gland** (sub-**ling**-gwuhl) can also be palpated in a patient in the neck region (see Fig. 1.5 and Fig.11.7).

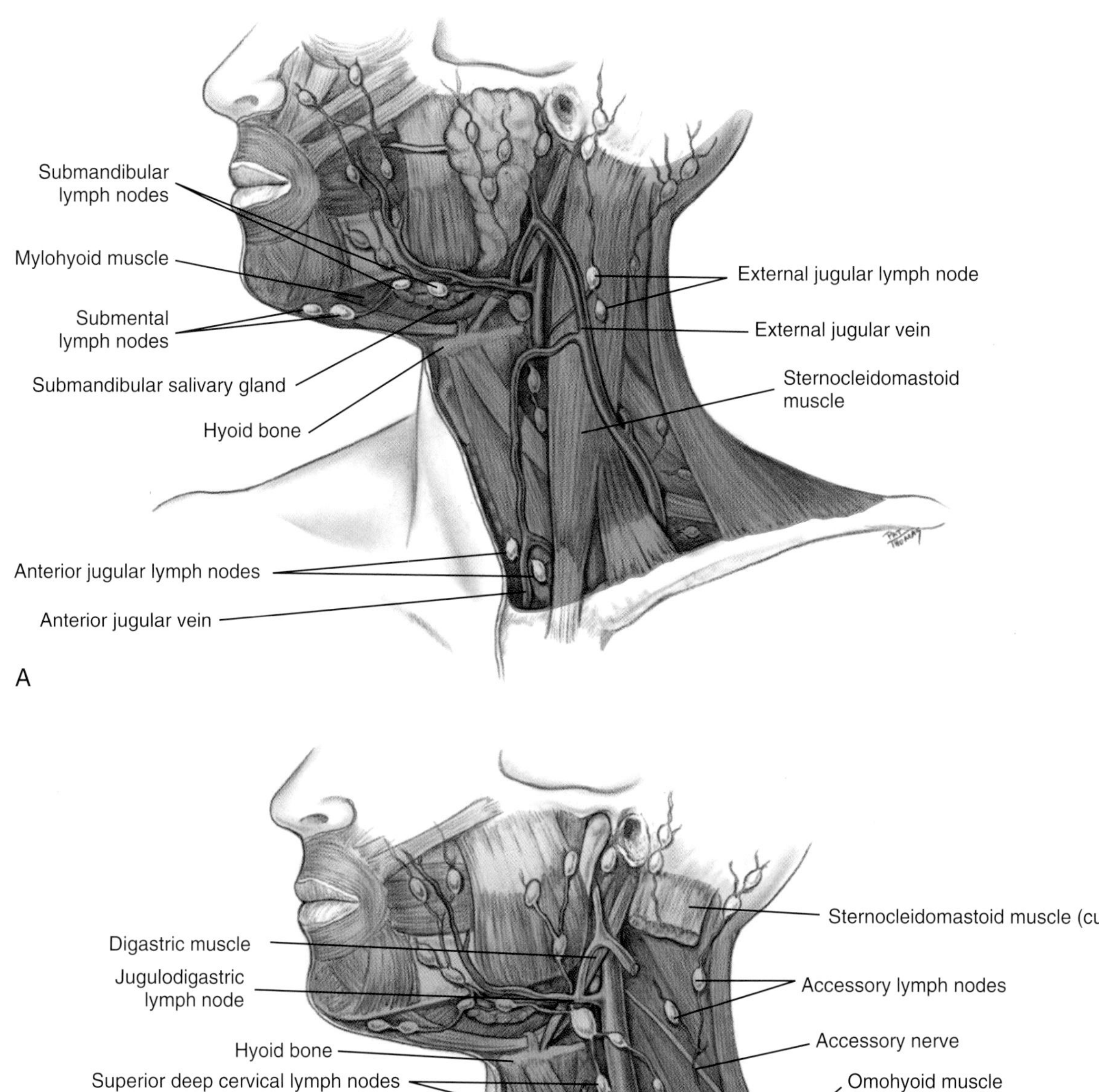

Fig. 1.12 Lymph Nodes of the Neck. **A,** Superficial cervical nodes. **B,** Deep cervical nodes. (From Fehrenbach MJ, Herring SW. *Illustrated Anatomy of the Head and Neck*. 5th ed. St. Louis: Elsevier; 2017.)

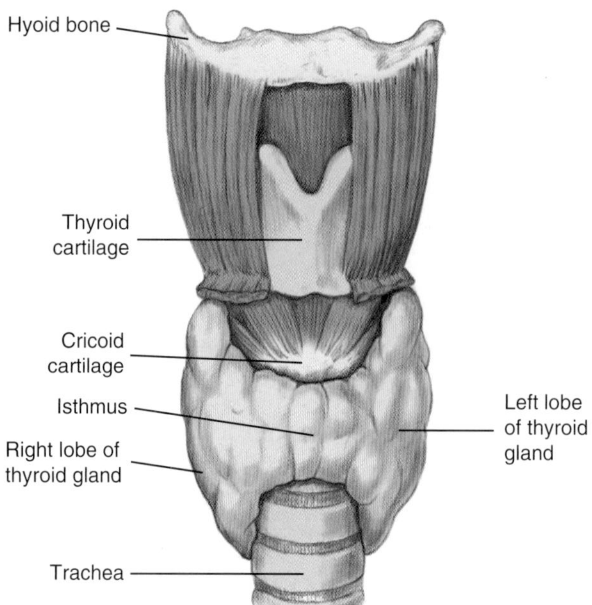

Fig. 1.13 Thyroid Gland. (From Fehrenbach MJ, Herring SW. *Illustrated Anatomy of the Head and Neck*. 5th ed. St. Louis: Elsevier; 2017.)

2

Oral Cavity and Pharynx

Additional resources and practice exercises are provided on the companion Evolve website for this book: http://evolve.elsevier.com/Fehrenbach/illustrated.

LEARNING OBJECTIVES

1. Define and pronounce the key terms in this chapter.
2. Locate and identify the divisions and associated surface landmarks of the oral cavity on a diagram and a patient.
3. Integrate the clinical considerations for the surface anatomy of the oral cavity into patient examination and care.
4. Outline the divisions of the pharynx and identify them on a diagram.
5. Integrate the study of surface anatomy of the visible divisions of the pharynx into patient examination and care.

ORAL CAVITY PROPERTIES

A dental professional must be totally committed to improving the overall health of every patient. In order to accomplish this, dental professionals must be particularly knowledgeable about their main area of focus, the oral cavity as well as the adjacent throat or pharynx and its health. To visualize this area of focus successfully, it is important to know the boundaries, terminology, and divisions of the oral cavity as well as the pharynx as discussed in this second chapter of **Unit 1**. Later, **Unit 2** describes the development of oral tissue and associated developmental disturbances. Following that, **Unit 3** describes the underlying histology of orofacial tissue that gives each tissue its characteristic surface features. Even later, **Unit 4** discusses dental anatomy.

A certain degree of variation can be possible in the oral cavity and visible divisions of the pharynx. However, a change in any tissue or associated structure in a patient may signal a condition of clinical significance and must be noted in the patient record as well as correctly followed up by the examining dental professional. Thus, it is not the variations among individuals that should be noted but the changes in a particular individual.

In this textbook, the illustrations of the oral cavity and pharynx, as well as any structures associated with them, are oriented to show the head in anatomic position (see **Appendix A**), unless otherwise noted. This is the same as if the patient in a clinical setting is viewed straight on while sitting upright in the dental chair.

ORAL CAVITY DIVISIONS

The oral cavity is divided into the vestibules, jaws with alveolar processes, teeth, and oral cavity proper. Within each part of the oral cavity are certain surface landmarks. It is important to practice finding these surface landmarks in the oral cavity using a personal mirror while referring to this textbook as well as the **Workbook for Illustrated Dental Embryology, Histology, and Anatomy** in order to improve skills of examination. Later, locating them on peers and then on patients in a clinical setting adds a real-world level of competence.

An understanding of the divisions of the oral cavity is aided by knowing its boundaries; many structures of the face and oral cavity mark the boundaries of the oral cavity (Fig. 2.1). The lips of the face mark the anterior boundary of the oral cavity and the throat (or pharynx) is the posterior boundary. The cheeks of the face mark the lateral boundaries and the roof of the mouth or palate marks the superior boundary. The floor of the mouth is the inferior border of the oral cavity.

In addition, many oral structures are identified with orientational terms based on their relationship to other orofacial structures, such as the facial surface, lips, cheek, tongue, and palate (see Fig. 2.1). Those structures closest to the facial surface are **facial**. Those facial structures closest to the lips are **labial (ley-bee-uhl)**. Those facial structures close to the inner cheek are **buccal** (**buhk**-uhl). Those structures closest to the tongue are **lingual** (**ling**-gwuhl). Those lingual structures closest to the palate are **palatal** (**pal**-uh-tl).

Oral Vestibules

The upper and lower horseshoe-shaped spaces in the oral cavity between the lips and cheeks anteriorly and laterally and the teeth and their soft tissue medially and posteriorly are considered the **vestibules (ves-tuh-byoolz)**, having both a maxillary and mandibular vestibule (Fig. 2.2). These oral vestibules are lined by a mucous membrane or **oral mucosa**

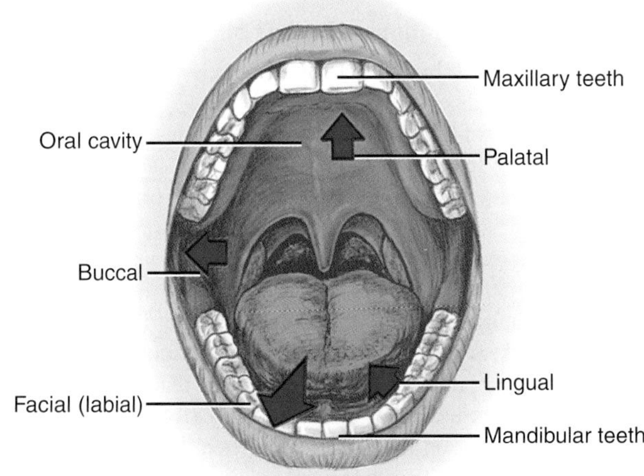

Fig. 2.1 Oral cavity and the jaws with the designation *(arrows)* of the orientational terms *facial, labial, buccal, palatal,* and *lingual.* (From Fehrenbach MJ, Herring SW. *Illustrated Anatomy of the Head and Neck.* 5th ed. St. Louis: Elsevier; 2017.)

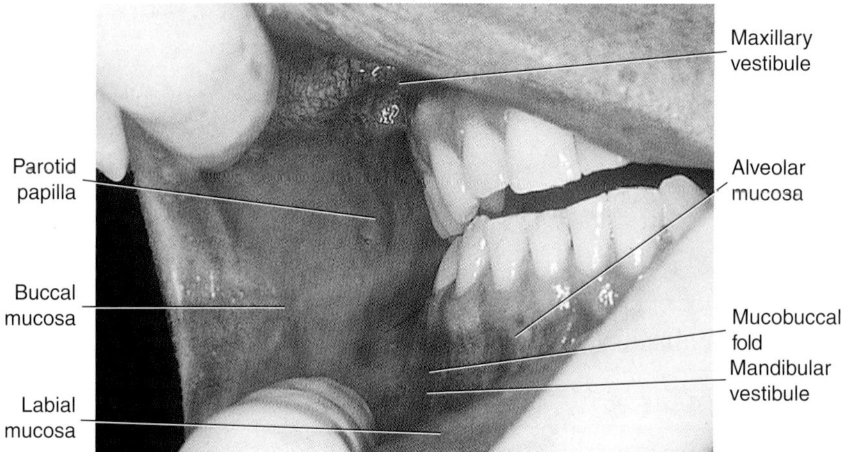

Fig. 2.2 Vestibules of the Oral Cavity with its Landmarks. (From Fehrenbach MJ, Herring SW. *Illustrated Anatomy of the Head and Neck*. 5th ed. St. Louis: Elsevier; 2017.)

(myoo-**koh**-suh). The inner parts of the lips are lined by a pinkish **labial mucosa**. The labial mucosa is continuous with the equally pinkish **buccal mucosa** that lines the inner cheek. However, both the labial and buccal mucosa may vary in coloration, as do other regions of the oral mucosa, in individuals with pigmented skin (see Fig. 9.23).

The buccal mucosa covers a dense pad of underlying fat tissue at the posterior part of each vestibule, the **buccal fat pad**. The buccal fat pad acts as a protective cushion during **mastication** (mass-ti-**keyt**-shuhn) or chewing. On the inner part of the buccal mucosa, just opposite the maxillary second molar, is a small elevation of tissue, the **parotid papilla** (puh-**rot**-id puh-**pil**-uh) (plural, **papillae** [puh-**pil**-ee]). The parotid papilla protects the opening of the **parotid duct** (or Stensen duct) of the parotid salivary gland (see Figs. 1.5 and 11.7).

Deep within each vestibule is the **vestibular fornix** (veh-**stib**-yuh-ler **fawr**-niks), where the pinkish labial mucosa or buccal mucosa meets the redder **alveolar mucosa** (al-**vee**-uh-ler myoo-**koh**-suh) at the **mucobuccal fold** (myoo-koh-**buhk**-uhl). The **labial frenum** (**free**-nuhm) (plural, **frena** [**free**-nuh]) is a fold of tissue located at the midline between the labial mucosa and the alveolar mucosa on the upper and lower dental arches (see Fig 2.9).

 Clinical Considerations with Oral Mucosa

On the surface of the labial and buccal mucosa is a common variation, **Fordyce spots** (**for**-dice) (or granules) (Fig. 2.3, *A*). These are visible as small yellowish elevations on the oral mucosa. They represent deeper deposits of sebum from trapped or misplaced sebaceous gland tissue, usually associated with hair follicles in other regions but not here. Most of the population has these harmless small bumps; however, they become more prominent with age due to thinning of the overlying tissue.

Another variation noted on the buccal mucosa is the **linea alba** (**lin**-ee-uh **ahl**-buh) (see Fig. 2.3, *B*). This is a white ridge of calloused tissue (or hyperkeratinization) that extends horizontally at the level where the maxillary and mandibular teeth come together and occlude (considered the occlusal plane); similar ridges of white tissue can sometimes be present on the tongue perimeter. An excess amount of this whitened ridge on either the buccal mucosa or tongue can be associated with certain oral parafunctional habits (see Fig. 9.7).

Jaws, Alveolar Processes, and Teeth

The jaws, the maxilla and mandible, are deep to the lips and within the oral cavity (Fig. 2.4 and see Fig. 1.7). The maxilla consists of two maxillary bones that become sutured together at the midline during development. The maxilla has a nonmovable articulation with many facial and skull bones and each maxillary bone includes a body and four processes. Each **body of the maxilla** (mak-**sil**-uh) is superior to the teeth and contains the **maxillary sinus** (**mak**-suh-ler-ee **sahy**-nuhs). In contrast, the mandible is a single bone with a movable articulation with the temporal bones at each temporomandibular joint (TMJ). The heavy horizontal part of the lower jaw inferior to the teeth is the **body of the mandible**.

The **alveolar process** or alveolar bone is the bony extension for both the maxilla and mandible that contain each tooth socket or **alveolus** (al-**vee**-uh-luhs) (plural, **alveoli** [al-**vee**-uh-lahy]) (see Fig. 14.14). All the teeth are attached to the bony surface of the alveoli by the fibrous **periodontal ligament (PDL)** (per-ee-oh-**don**-tl), which allows slight tooth movement within the alveolus while still supporting the tooth.

Each of the mature and fully erupted teeth consists of both the **crown** and the **root(s)** (Figs. 2.5 and 2.6). The crown of the tooth is composed of the extremely hard outer **enamel** (ih-**nam**-uhl) layer and the moderately hard inner **dentin** (**den**-tin) layer overlying the **pulp** of the tooth. The pulp is the soft innermost layer in the tooth. The dentin layer continues to cover the soft tissue of the pulp of the tooth in the root(s), but the outermost layer of the root(s) is composed of **cementum** (si-**men**-tuhm). The bonelike cementum is the part of the tooth that attaches to the PDL, which then attaches to the alveolus of bone, holding the tooth in its socket.

Dental Arches

The alveolar processes with the teeth in the alveoli are also considered **dental arches**, of which there are two: the **maxillary arch** and the **mandibular arch** (see Fig. 2.4). The teeth in the maxillary arch are the **maxillary teeth** and the teeth in the mandibular arch are the **mandibular teeth**.

Just distal to the last tooth of the maxillary arch is a tissue-covered elevation of the bone, the **maxillary tuberosity** (too-buh-**ros**-i-tee) (see Fig. 2.11). Similarly, on the lower jaw is a dense pad of tissue located just distal to the last tooth of the mandibular arch, the **retromolar pad** (reh-troh-**moh**-ler). The tooth types in both arches of the teeth of children or **primary teeth** include **incisors** (in-**sahy**-zuhrz), **canines** (**kahy**-nahyz), and **molars** (**moh**-lerz). Adult teeth or **permanent teeth** also include all the same tooth types as the primary teeth as well as **premolars** (pree-**moh**-luhrz).

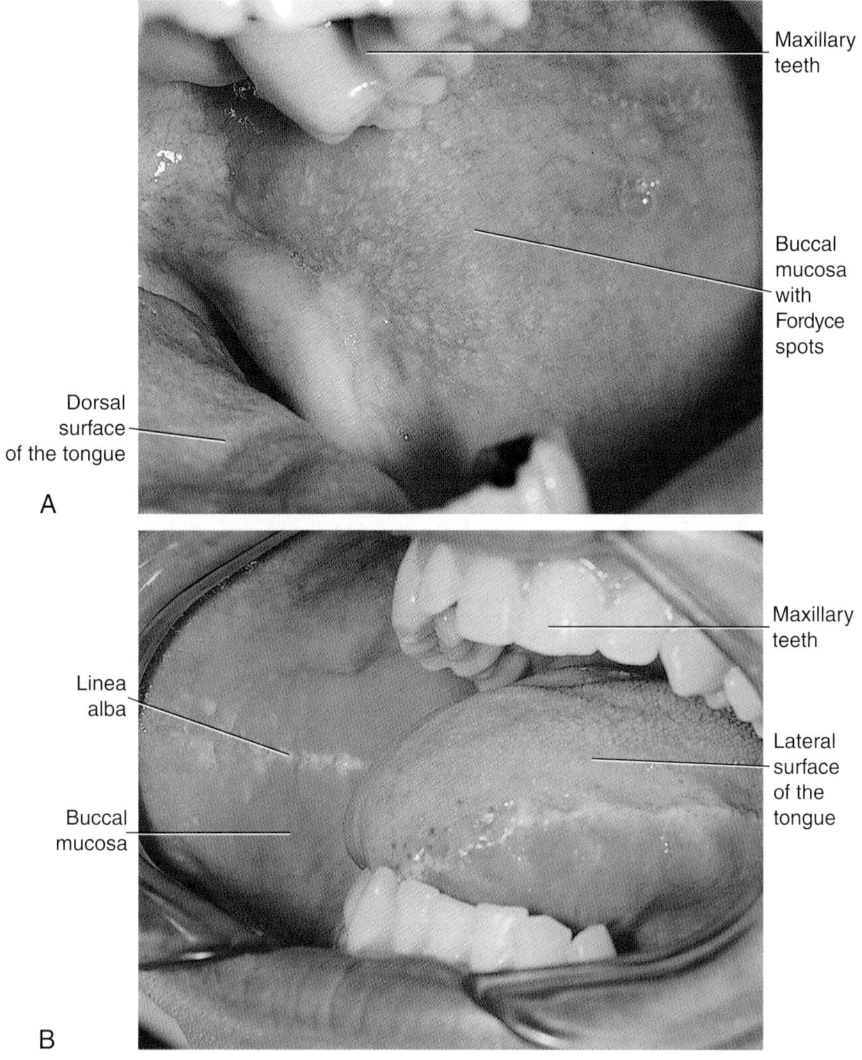

Fig. 2.3 Buccal Mucosa and Labial Mucosa with its Variations. **A,** With Fordyce spots visible as small yellowish elevations. **B,** With the linea alba visible as a white ridge of hyperkeratinization that extends horizontally at the level where the teeth occlude, with a similar white ridge on the lateral surface of the tongue. (Courtesy of Margaret J. Fehrenbach, RDH, MS.)

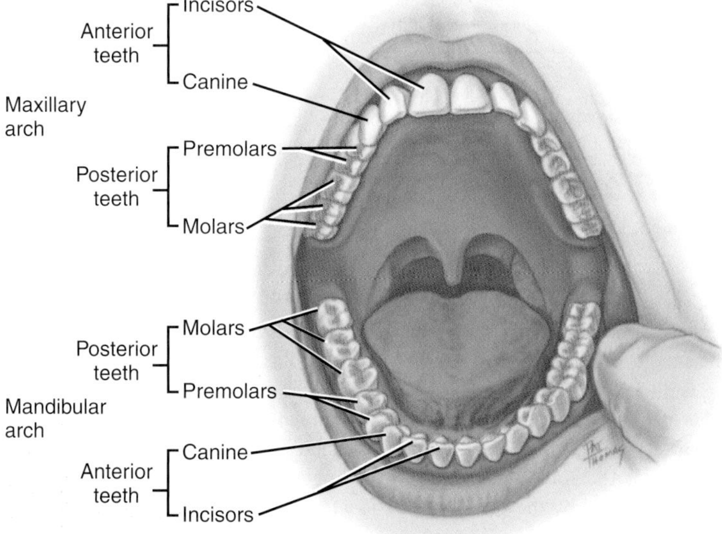

Fig. 2.4 Diagram of the Adult Dental Arches, Each with its Permanent Teeth and its Landmarks.

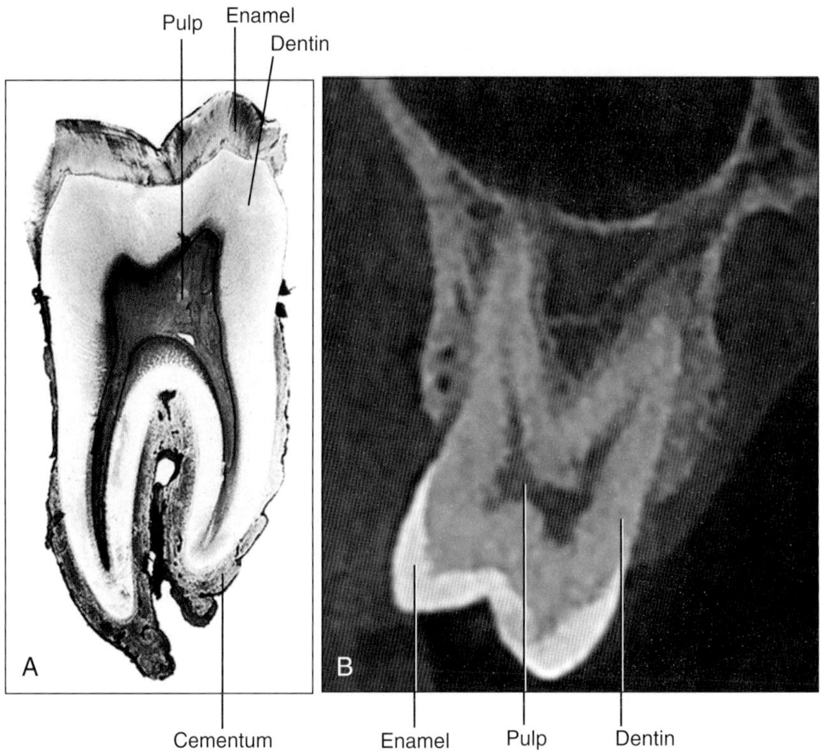

Fig. 2.5 Distribution of the Various Tissue Types of the Tooth. **A,** Gross specimen of tooth cross-sectioned. **B,** Radiograph of tooth. (From Nanci A. *Ten Cate's Oral Histology.* 9th ed. St. Louis: Elsevier; 2018.)

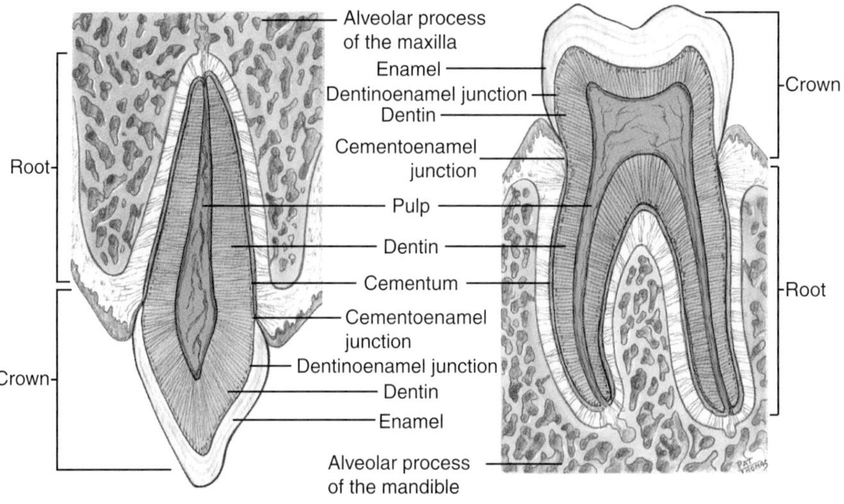

Fig. 2.6 Diagram of an alveolar process of both a single-rooted tooth and a multirooted tooth showing the crown and root as well as associated tissue types.

The teeth in the front of the mouth, the incisors and canines, are considered **anterior teeth.** The teeth located toward the back of the mouth, the molars and premolars if present, are considered **posterior teeth.** The permanent maxillary anterior teeth are supplied by the anterior superior alveolar artery, with the permanent maxillary posterior teeth by the posterior superior alveolar artery; all of the permanent mandibular teeth are supplied by branches of the inferior alveolar artery. Additionally, the maxillary teeth are drained by the posterior superior alveolar vein, with mandibular teeth drained by the inferior alveolar vein. Later **Unit 4** discusses the dental anatomy of each tooth of both dentitions, primary and permanent.

Clinical Considerations with Alveolar Process

A less than common variation present usually on the facial surface of the alveolar process of the maxillary arch is **exostoses** (ek-os-**stoh**-seez). They are localized developmental growths of bone covered in oral mucosa with a possible hereditary etiology and which may be associated with occlusal trauma (Fig. 2.7, see **Chapter 20**). They may be single or multiple lesions and unilateral or bilateral raised hard areas located in the premolar to molar region covered by oral mucosa. They appear on radiographs as radiopaque (light) areas. They may interfere with radiographic analysis as well as restorative and periodontal therapy and thus must be noted in the patient record.

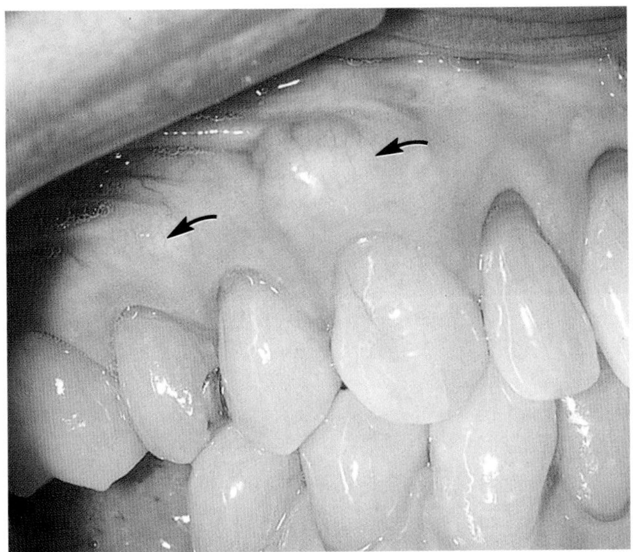

Fig. 2.7 Variation of exostoses *(arrows)* on the facial surface of the maxillary arch. (Courtesy of Margaret J. Fehrenbach, RDH, MS.)

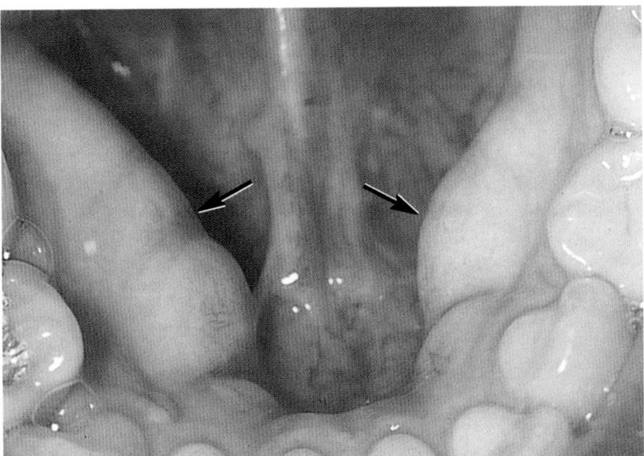

Fig. 2.8 Variation of bilateral mandibular tori *(arrows)* on the lingual surface of the mandibular arch. (Courtesy of Margaret J. Fehrenbach, RDH, MS.)

Another similar variation present on the lingual surface of the mandibular arch is the **mandibular torus** (**tohr**-uhs) (plural, **tori** [**tohr**-ahy]) (Fig. 2.8). Each torus is a developmental growth of bone with a possible hereditary etiology similar to exostoses and may also be associated with grinding, which is considered *bruxism*. They are usually present bilaterally in the area of the premolars and can appear as lobulated or nodular raised areas with clefting or even contact each other over the midline.

Mandibular tori are covered in oral mucosa and vary in size. They are slow growing and asymptomatic lesions, which may be seen on radiographs as radiopaque (light) masses. They may interfere with speech, oral hygiene procedures, radiographic film placement and analysis, as well as prosthetic therapy of the mandibular alveolar process. The patient may require reassurance of their background and they must be noted in the patient record.

Gingival Tissue

Surrounding the maxillary and mandibular teeth in the alveoli and covering the alveolar processes are the soft tissue gums or **gingiva** (jin-**jahy**-vuh) or more accurately but not usually by the dental community using the plural term, **gingivae** (jin-**juh**-vee), which are composed of a firm pink oral mucosa (Fig. 2.9). The gingival tissue that tightly adheres to the alveolar process surrounding the roots of the teeth is the **attached gingiva**; this includes the maxillary tuberosity and retromolar pad. The line of demarcation between the firmer and pinker attached gingiva and the movable and redder alveolar mucosa that lines the vestibules is the scallop-shaped **mucogingival junction** (myoo-koh-**jin**-juh-vuhl).

At the gingival margin of each tooth is the **marginal gingiva** (**mahr**-juh-nahl) (or free gingiva), which forms a cuff above the neck of the tooth (Fig. 2.10). The **free gingival groove** (jin-**juh**-vuhl) separates the marginal gingiva from the attached gingiva. This outer groove varies in depth according to the area of the oral cavity; the groove is especially prominent on mandibular anterior teeth and premolars. At the most coronal part of the marginal gingiva is the **free gingival crest.**

The **interdental gingiva** (in-ter-**den**-tl) is the gingival tissue between adjacent teeth adjoining the attached gingiva, with each individual extension being an **interdental papilla**. The attached gingiva may have areas of **melanin pigmentation** (**mel**-uh-nin), especially at the base of each interdental papillae (see Fig. 9.23). The circular inner

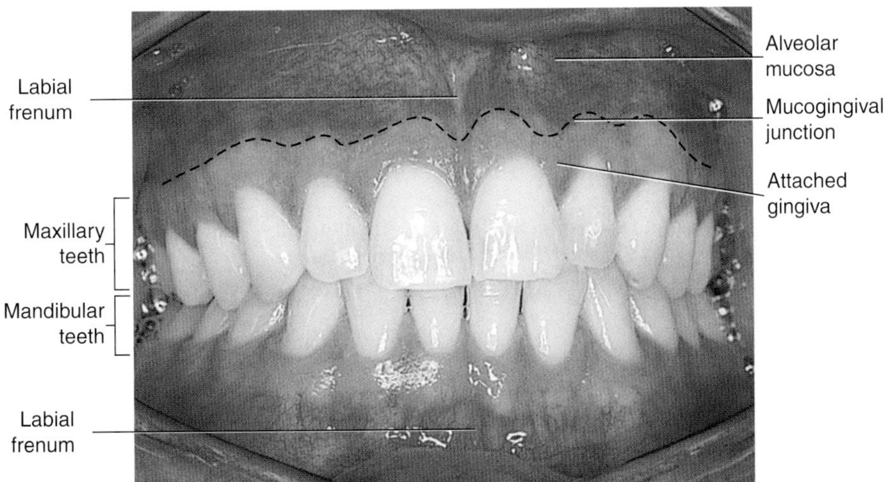

Fig. 2.9 Gingival tissue and its landmarks on the maxillary arch, with the mucogingival junction highlighted *(dashed line)*. (From Fehrenbach MJ, Herring SW. *Illustrated Anatomy of the Head and Neck.* 5th ed. St. Louis: Elsevier; 2017.)

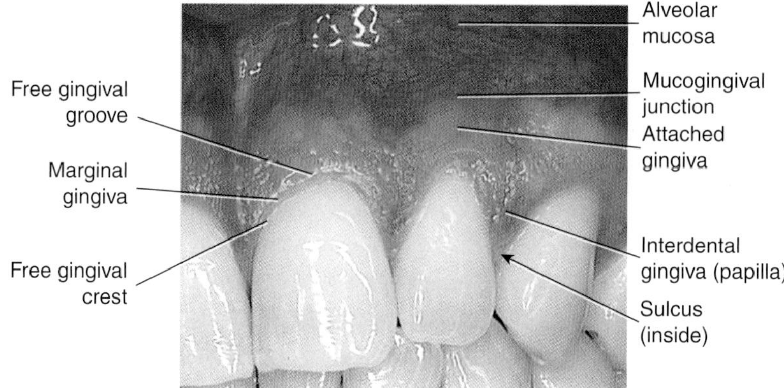

Fig. 2.10 Close-up of the gingival tissue and its landmarks, with the location of the gingival sulcus noted *(arrow)*. (From Fehrenbach MJ, Herring SW. *Illustrated Anatomy of the Head and Neck*. 5th ed. St. Louis: Elsevier; 2017.)

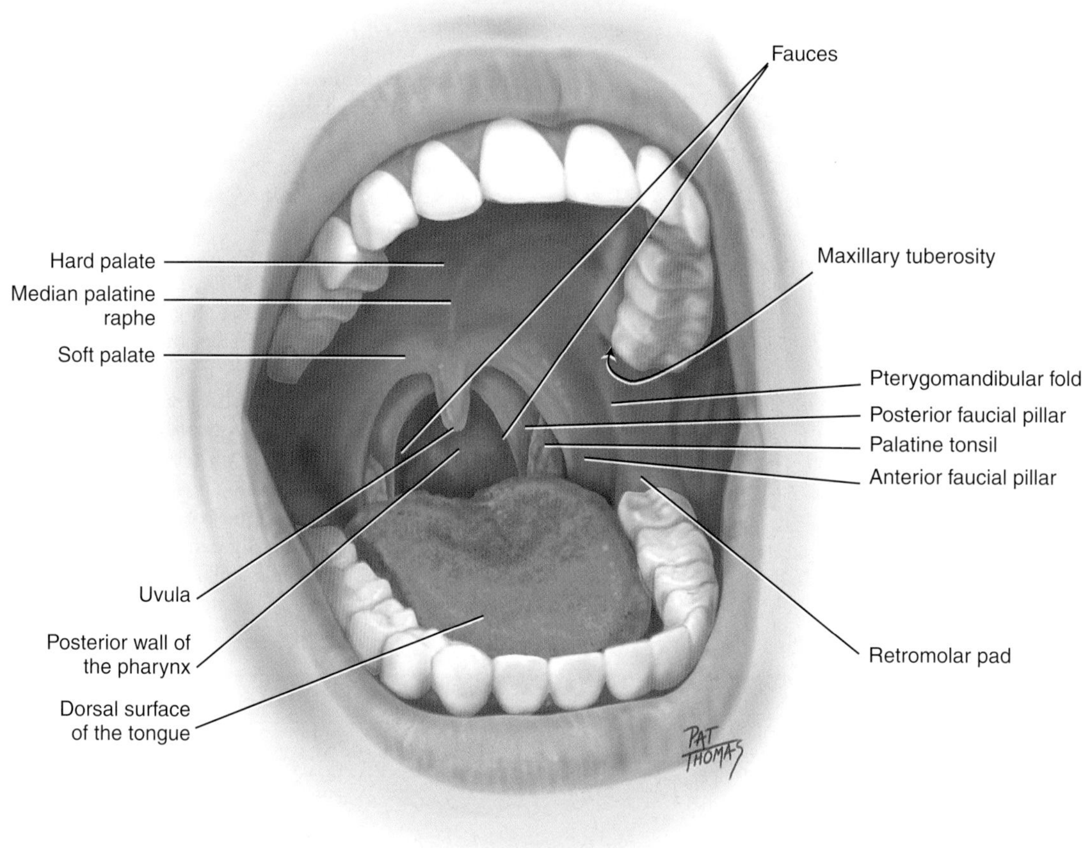

Fig. 2.11 Oral Cavity Proper and the Landmarks that Form its Boundaries. (From Fehrenbach MJ, Herring SW. *Illustrated Anatomy of the Head and Neck*. 5th ed. St. Louis: Elsevier; 2017.)

surface of the gingival tissue of each tooth faces an equally rounded space, the **gingival sulcus** (**suhl**-kuhs).

Oral Cavity Proper

The inside of the mouth is known as the **oral cavity proper** (Fig. 2.11). The space of the oral cavity is enclosed anteriorly by both the maxillary arch and mandibular arch. Posteriorly, the opening from the oral cavity proper into the pharynx or throat is the **fauces** (**faw**-seez).

The fauces are formed laterally on each side by the **anterior faucial pillar** (**faw**-shuhl) and the **posterior faucial pillar**. The **palatine tonsils** (**pal**-uh-tahyn **ton**-suhlz) are located between these folds of tissue created by underlying muscles and are what patients consider their "tonsils," which can become enlarged when involved with

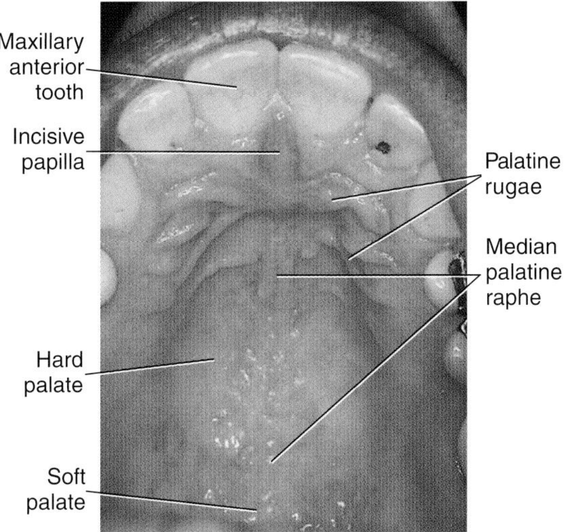

Fig. 2.12 Palate and its Landmarks. (From Fehrenbach MJ, Herring SW. *Illustrated Anatomy of the Head and Neck*. 5th ed. St. Louis: Elsevier; 2017.)

inflammation (see Fig. 11.18). Included within the oral cavity proper are the palate, tongue, and floor of the mouth.

Palate

Within the oral cavity proper is the roof of the mouth or **palate** (**pal**-it). The palate separates the oral cavity from the nasal cavity. The bony whiter anterior arched part is the **hard palate** (Fig. 2.12, see Fig. 5.5). The hard palate shows the absence of a mucogingival junction on the palatal aspect. Instead, the mucosa of the palatal attached gingiva blends imperceptibly with the mucosa of the hard palate.

A small bulge of tissue at the most anterior part of the hard palate that is lingual to the anterior teeth is the **incisive papilla** (in-**sahy**-ziv). Directly posterior to this papilla are **palatine rugae** (**pal**-uh-tahyn **roo**-gee/jee), which are firm irregular ridges of tissue radiating from the incisive papilla.

The yellower, looser, and softer posterior part of the palate is the **soft palate** (see Fig. 2.11). A midline muscular structure, the **uvula** (**yoo**-vyuh-luh) of the palate, hangs down from the posterior margin of the soft palate. The midline ridge of tissue that runs full length of the palate from the incisive papilla to the uvula is the **median palatine raphe** (**mee**-dee-uhn **ray**-fee), which overlies the bony fusion of the palate.

The **pterygomandibular fold** (ter-i-goh-man-**dib**-yuh-ler) also extends from the junction of hard and soft palates down to the mandible, just posterior the most distal mandibular tooth, and stretches when the mouth is opened wider. This fold covers a deeper fibrous structure and separates the cheek from the throat or pharynx.

Clinical Considerations with Palate

A less than common variation noted on the midline of the hard palate is the **palatal torus,** which is similar to the mandibular torus in presentation and etiology (Fig. 2.13). The torus can interfere if prosthetic therapy of the maxillary alveolar process is considered. It needs to be noted in the patient record and patients may need to be reassured as to its background. More serious pathology of the palate, such as a history of cleft palate, also needs to be noted because of its impact on dental care (see Fig. 5.6).

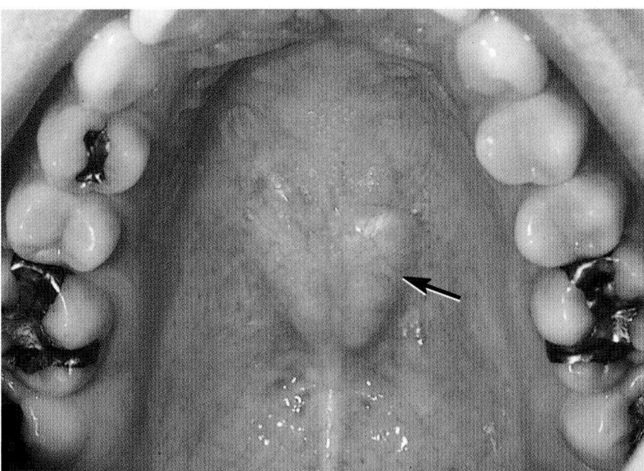

Fig. 2.13 Variation of the palatal torus *(arrow)* on the midline of the hard palate. (Courtesy of Margaret J. Fehrenbach, RDH, MS.)

Tongue

The **tongue** is a prominent feature of the oral cavity proper (Fig. 2.14). The posterior one-third of the tongue is the *pharyngeal part* or **base of the tongue.** The base of the tongue attaches to the floor of the mouth. The base of the tongue does not lie within the oral cavity proper but within the oral part of the throat (discussed later in the chapter). The anterior two-thirds of the tongue is the *oral part* or **body of the tongue**, which lies within the oral cavity proper. The tip of the tongue is the **apex of the tongue**. Separating the tongue into a posterior one-third and an anterior two-thirds is important as the two have different innervation, structure, and embryonic development.

The top or **dorsal surface of the tongue** (**dawr**-suhl) has a midline depression, the **median lingual sulcus**, corresponding to the position of a midline fibrous structure deeper in the tongue and fusion tissue area. Certain surfaces of the tongue have small elevated structures of specialized mucosa, the **lingual papillae**, some of which are associated with taste buds (see Figs. 9.16 to 9.20). Taste buds are the specialized organs of taste.

The slender threadlike whitish lingual papillae are the **filiform lingual papillae** (**fil**-uh-fawrm), which give the dorsal surface its velvety texture. The reddish small mushroom-shaped dots on the dorsal surface are the **fungiform lingual papillae** (**fuhn**-juh-fawrm/**fuhn**-guh-fawrn). Farther posteriorly on the dorsal surface of the tongue and more difficult to see clinically is an inverted V-shaped groove, the **sulcus terminalis** (tur-**muh**-nal-is). The sulcus terminalis is the visible division that separates the base from the body of the tongue, demarcating a line of fusion of tissue during the tongue's development.

The 10 to 14 larger mushroom-shaped lingual papillae, the **circumvallate lingual papillae** (sur-kuhm-**val**-eyt) line up along the anterior side of the sulcus terminalis on the body. Where the sulcus terminalis points backward toward the throat is a small pitlike depression, the **foramen cecum** (fuh-**rey**-muhn **see**-kuhm). Even farther posteriorly on the dorsal surface of the base of the tongue is an irregular mass of tissue, the **lingual tonsil** (see **Chapter 11**).

The side or **lateral surface of the tongue** has vertical ridges, the **foliate lingual papillae** (foh-lee-eyt) (Fig. 2.15).

The underside or **ventral surface of the tongue** has large visible blood vessels, the deep lingual veins, which pass close to the surface (Fig. 2.16). Lateral to each deep lingual vein is the **plica fimbriata**

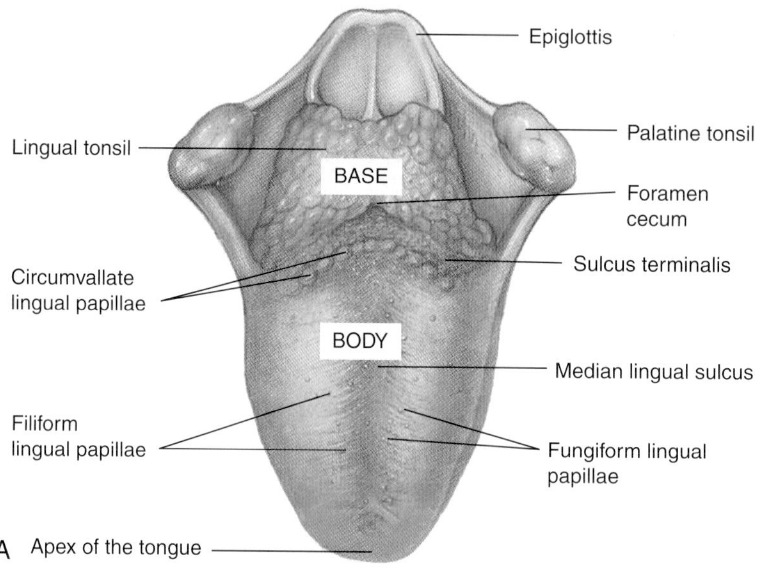

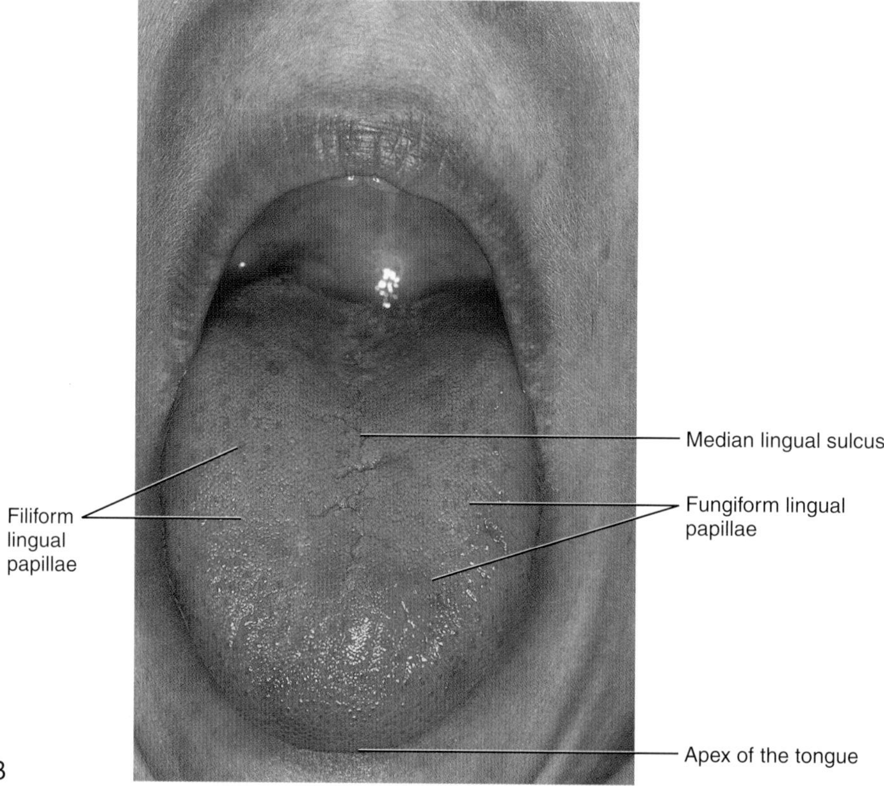

Fig. 2.14 Dorsal Surface of the Tongue with its Landmarks. **A,** Diagram. **B,** Clinical view. (From Fehrenbach MJ, Herring SW. *Illustrated Anatomy of the Head and Neck*. 5th ed. St. Louis: Elsevier; 2017.)

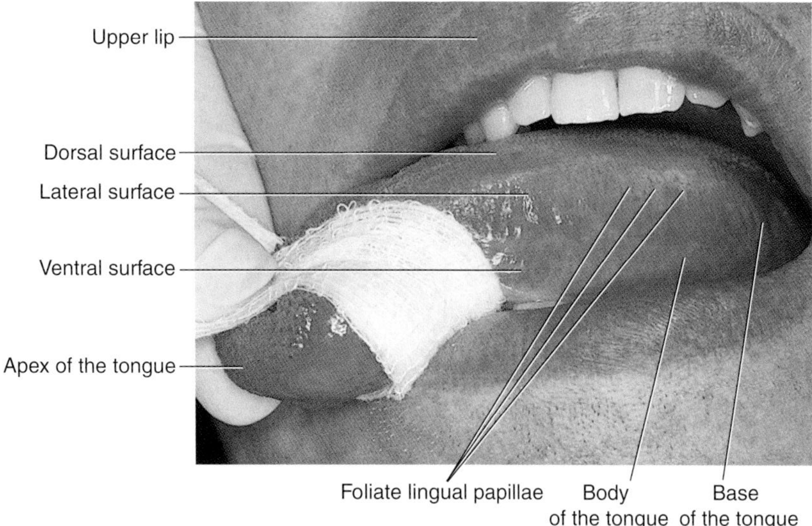

Fig. 2.15 Lateral Surface of the Tongue with its Landmarks. (From Fehrenbach MJ, Herring SW. *Illustrated Anatomy of the Head and Neck.* 5th ed. St. Louis: Elsevier; 2017.)

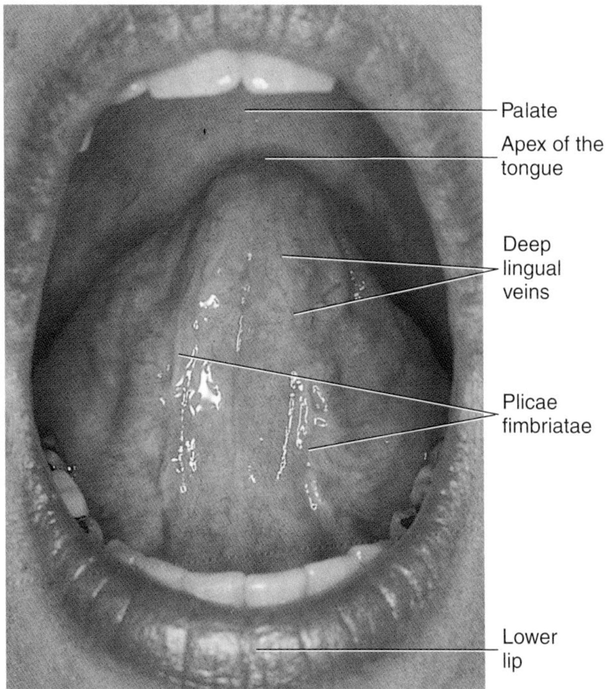

Fig. 2.16 Ventral Surface of the Tongue with its Landmarks. (From Fehrenbach MJ, Herring SW. *Illustrated Anatomy of the Head and Neck.* 5th ed. St. Louis: Elsevier; 2017.)

(**plahy**-kuh fim-bree-**ahy**-tuh) (plural, **plicae fimbriatae** [**plahy**-kee fim-bree-**ahy**-tee]) with its fringelike projections.

Floor of the Mouth

The **floor of the mouth** is located in the oral cavity proper, inferior to the ventral surface of the tongue (Fig. 2.17). The **lingual frenum** is an anterior midline fold of tissue between the ventral surface of the tongue and the floor of the mouth.

A ridge of tissue on each side of the floor of the mouth, the **sublingual fold**, joins in a V-shaped configuration extending from the lingual frenum to the base of the tongue (see Figs. 1.5 and 11.7). The small papilla or **sublingual caruncle** (**kar**-uhng-uhl) at the anterior end of each sublingual fold contains openings of the **submandibular duct** and **sublingual duct** (or Wharton duct and Bartholin duct, respectively) from both the sublingual as well as the submandibular salivary gland. The sublingual folds represent the underlying sublingual salivary gland and also contain openings of its sublingual duct.

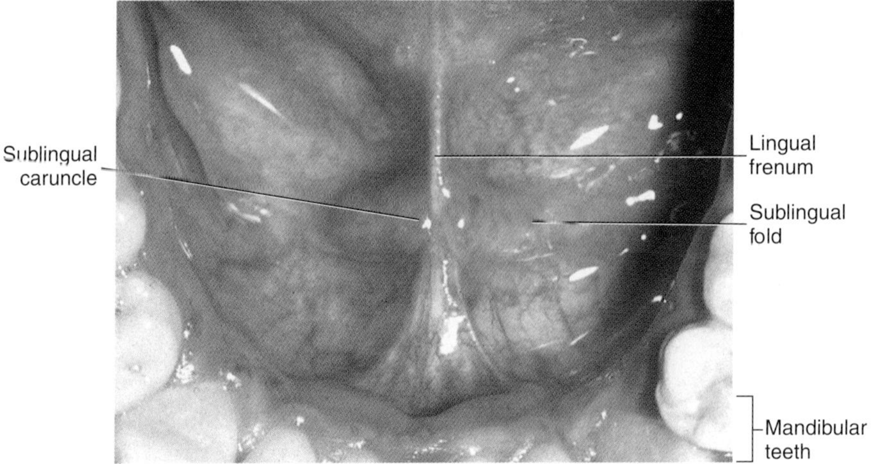

Fig. 2.17 Floor of the Mouth with its Landmarks. (From Fehrenbach MJ, Herring SW. *Illustrated Anatomy of the Head and Neck.* 5th ed. St. Louis: Elsevier; 2017.)

PHARYNGEAL DIVISIONS

The oral cavity proper provides the entrance into the deeper structure of the throat or **pharynx** (**far**-ingks). The pharynx is a muscular tube that has both respiratory and digestive system functions. It has three divisions, the nasopharynx, oropharynx, and laryngopharynx (Fig. 2.18).

The division of the pharynx that is superior to the level of the soft palate is the **nasopharynx** (ney-zoh-**far**-ingks), which is continuous with the nasal cavity. Only part of the nasopharynx is visible during an intraoral examination by a dental professional (see Fig. 2.11).

The division that is between the soft palate and the opening of the larynx is the **oropharynx** (ohr-oh-**far**-ingks). The oropharynx is considered the oral part of the pharynx and is visible in most cases to the dental professional. The fauces, discussed earlier, mark the boundary between the oropharynx and the oral cavity proper.

Finally, the **laryngopharynx** (luh-ring-goh-**far**-ingks) is the more inferior division of the pharynx, close to the laryngeal opening. To examine the more extensive parts of the nasopharynx, as well as the laryngopharynx or even the oropharynx in some patients, special diagnostic tools are needed.

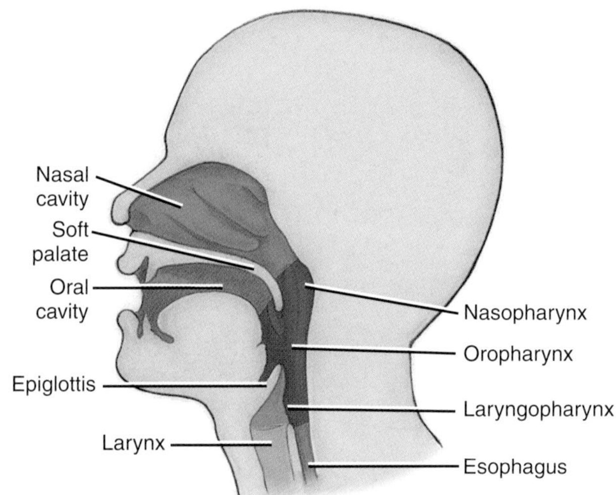

Fig. 2.18 Midsagittal Section of the Head with the Divisions of the Pharynx and Associated Regions. (From Fehrenbach MJ, Herring SW. *Illustrated Anatomy of the Head and Neck.* 5th ed. St. Louis: Elsevier; 2017.)

3

Prenatal Development

Additional resources and practice exercises are provided on the companion Evolve website for this book: http://evolve.elsevier.com/Fehrenbach/illustrated.

LEARNING OBJECTIVES

1. Define and pronounce the key terms in this chapter.
2. Outline the preimplantation period, including the major events that occur during this first week of prenatal development.
3. Integrate a study of the preimplantation period of prenatal development into the development of the orofacial structures and the clinical considerations due to developmental disturbances associated with these structures.
4. Outline the second week of prenatal development during the embryonic period, including the major events that occur.
5. Outline the third week of prenatal development during the embryonic period, including the major events that occur.
6. Outline the fourth week of prenatal development during the embryonic period, including the major events that occur.
7. Integrate the study of the embryonic period of prenatal development into orofacial development and the clinical considerations due to developmental disturbances associated with these structures.
8. Outline the fetal period of prenatal development, including the major events that occur after the eighth week until birth within this period.
9. Identify the structures present during prenatal development on a diagram.
10. Integrate the study of the fetal period of prenatal development into orofacial development and the clinical considerations due to developmental disturbances associated with these structures.

PRENATAL DEVELOPMENT

Dental professionals need to have a clear understanding of the major events of prenatal development in order to understand the development of the structures of the face, neck, and oral cavity and the underlying relationships among these structures. **Embryology** (em-bree-**ol**-uh-jee) is the study of prenatal development and is introduced in this first chapter of **Unit 2**.

Prenatal development (pree-**neyt**-l) begins with the start of pregnancy and continues until the birth of the child. The 9 months of gestation are usually divided into 3-month time spans or trimesters. In contrast, prenatal development consists of three distinct successive periods, the preimplantation period, embryonic period, and fetal period (Table 3.1) with varying time spans. The preimplantation period and the embryonic period make up the first trimester of the pregnancy and the fetal period constitutes the last two trimesters.

Each of the structures of the face, neck, and oral cavity has a **primordium** (prahy-**mawr**-dee-uhm), the earliest recognizable stage of development in an organ or tissue during prenatal development. This information about the embryologic background of a structure also helps in the appreciation of any clinical considerations that may occur in these structures due to developmental disturbances.

Clinical Considerations for Prenatal Development

Developmental disturbances that involve the orofacial structures as well as other parts of the body can include **congenital malformations** (kuhn-**jen**-i-tuhl mal-fawr-**mey**-shuhns) or birth defects, which are evident at birth. Most of these occur during both the preimplantation period and the embryonic period and thus involve the first trimester of the pregnancy (discussed later in this chapter). Such malformations occur in 3 out of 100 cases and are one of the leading causes of infant death. This does not include anatomic variants, which are common, such as variation in the lesser details of a bone's shape. **Amniocentesis** (am-nee-oh-sen-**tee**-sis) or amniotic fluid test (AFT) is a prenatal diagnostic procedure to detect chromosomal abnormalities where the amniotic fluid and its fetal cells are grown after removal for microscopic study of the chromosomes as well as sampled for determination of other fetal complications. Pregnant women now have the option of getting a new type of prenatal genetic test, one that does not pose any risk and can be performed very early in the pregnancy. This **noninvasive prenatal testing (NIPT)** is a cell-free fetal DNA test that involves a simple blood draw from the pregnant woman.

Malformations can be due to genetic factors, such as chromosome abnormalities or environmental agents and factors. These environmental agents and factors involved in causing malformations can include infections, drugs, and radiation and are considered to be **teratogens** (ter-**rat**-uh-juhnz) (Table 3.2). Women of reproductive age should avoid teratogens to protect the developing infant from possible congenital malformations (discussed later in this chapter).

Malformations in the face, neck, and oral cavity range from a serious cleft in the face or palatal region to small deficiencies of the soft palate or developing cysts underneath an otherwise intact oral mucosa. Dental professionals should remember that any orofacial congenital malformations discovered when examining a patient are usually understandable and traceable to a specific time in the embryologic development of the individual. Thus, the dental professional must initially understand the development of an individual's orofacial region including its sequential process to later understand any associated pathology present.

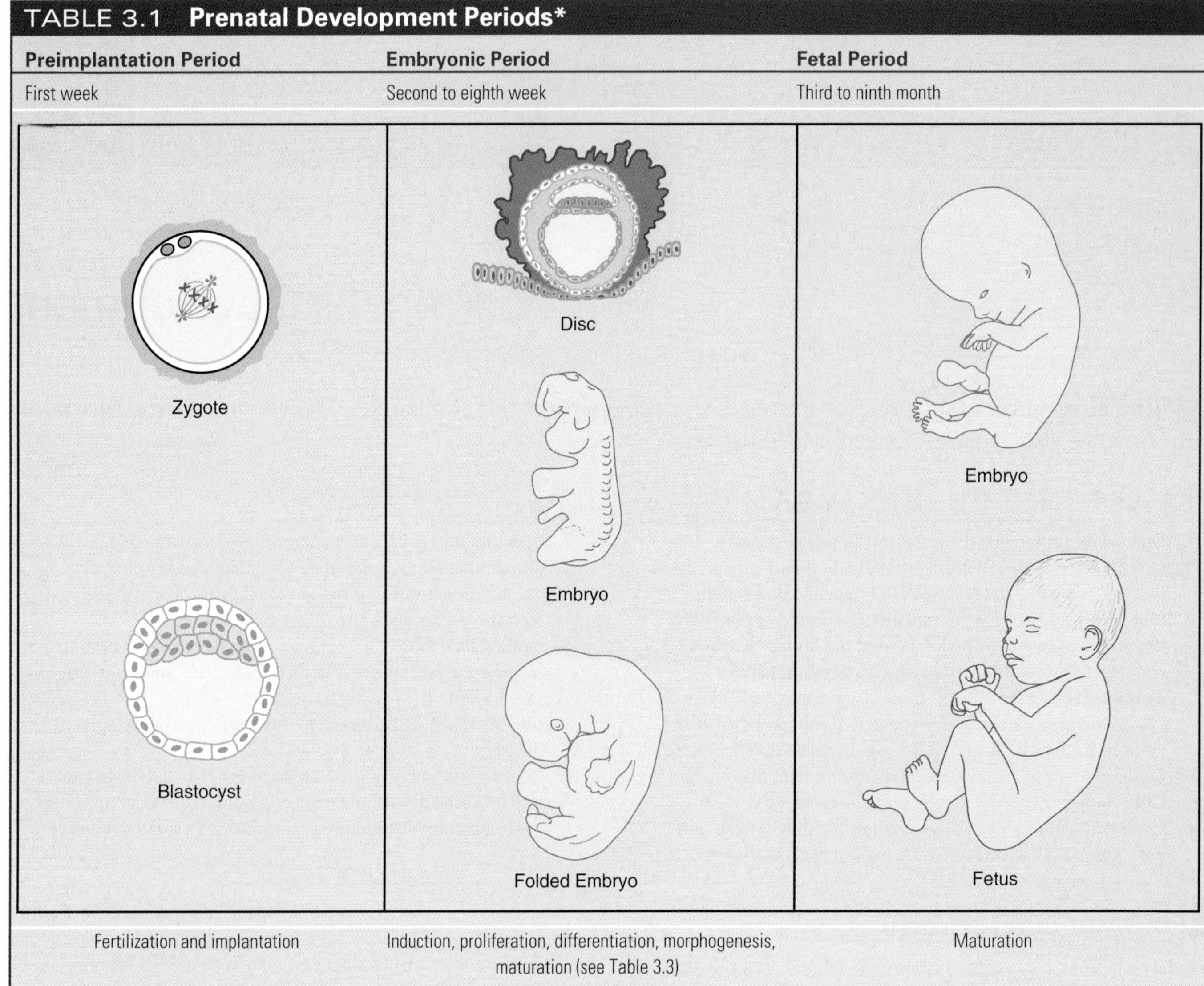

TABLE 3.1 Prenatal Development Periods*

Preimplantation Period	Embryonic Period	Fetal Period
First week	Second to eighth week	Third to ninth month
Zygote; Blastocyst	Disc; Embryo; Folded Embryo	Embryo; Fetus
Fertilization and implantation	Induction, proliferation, differentiation, morphogenesis, maturation (see Table 3.3)	Maturation

*The structure size is not accurate; instead is it just used for general information.

TABLE 3.2 Known Teratogens Involved in Congenital Malformations

Teratogen	Description
Drugs	Ethanol, tetracycline, phenytoin sodium, lithium, methotrexate, aminopterin, diethylstilbestrol, warfarin, thalidomide, isotretinoin (retinoic acid), androgens, progesterone
Chemicals	Methylmercury, polychlorinated biphenyls
Infections	Rubella virus, syphilis spirochete, herpes simplex virus, human immunodeficiency virus
Radiation	High levels of ionizing type*

*The American Dental Association recommends the use of dosimeters and work practice controls for pregnant dental staff who work with radiographic equipment. Studies of pregnant patients receiving dental care have affirmed the safety of dental treatment including the administration of radiographs when using the protective controls. The American College of Obstetricians and Gynecologists (2017) reaffirmed its opinion: "Patients often need reassurance that prevention, diagnosis, and treatment of oral conditions, including dental x-rays (with shielding of the abdomen and thyroid) … [are] safe during pregnancy."

PREIMPLANTATION PERIOD

The first period of prenatal development, the **preimplantation period** (pree-im-plan-**tey**-shuhn), takes place during the first week after conception (see Table 3.1). At the beginning of the first week, conception takes place where a woman's **ovum** (**oh**-vuhm) is penetrated by and united with a man's **sperm** during **fertilization** (fur-tl-uh-**zey**-shuhn) (Fig. 3.1). This union of the ovum and sperm subsequently forms a fertilized egg or **zygote** (**zahy**-goht).

During fertilization, the final stages of **meiosis** (mahy-**oh**-sis) occur in the ovum. The result of this process is the joining of the ovum's chromosomes with those of the sperm (see Chapter 7). This joining of chromosomes from both biologic parents forms a new individual with "shuffled" chromosomes. To allow this formation of a new individual the sperm and ovum are joined resulting in the proper number of chromosomes, which is the diploid number of 46. If both these cells, sperm and ovum, instead carried the full complement of chromosomes fertilization would result in a zygote with *two times* the proper number, resulting in severe congenital malformations and prenatal death (see later discussion).

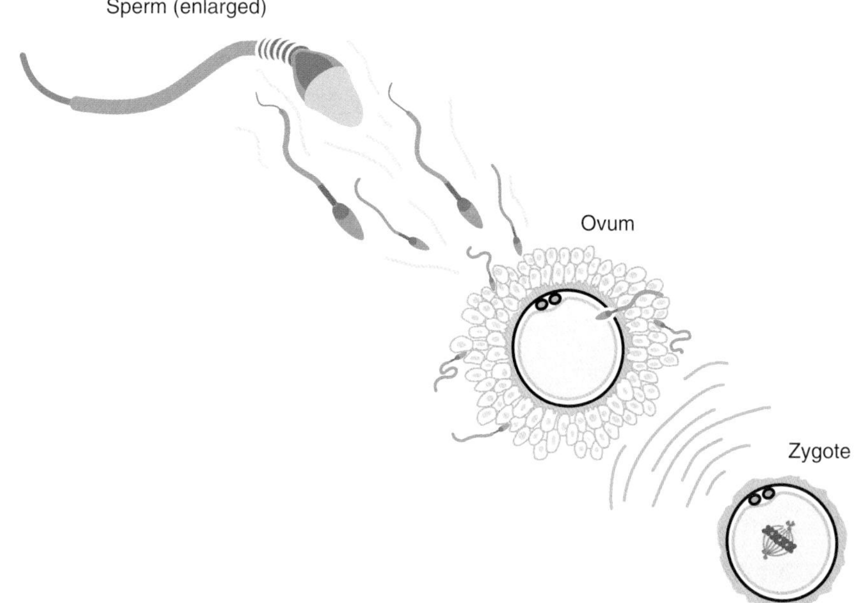

Fig. 3.1 Sperm fertilizes the ovum and unites with it to form the zygote after the process of meiosis and during the first week of prenatal development. Both the chromosomes of the ovum and sperm are involved in the process.

This situation of excess chromosomes is avoided with meiosis because during their development in the gonads, this process enables the ovum and sperm to reduce by one-half the usual number of chromosomes to haploid number of 23. Thus the zygote has received half its chromosomes from the woman and half from the man, with the resultant genetic material a reflection of both biologic parents.

The photographic analysis of a person's chromosomes is done by orderly arrangement of the pairs in a **karyotype** (**kar**-ee-uh-tahyp), with the sex known by the presence of either having *XX* chromosomes for a woman or *XY* for a man (Fig. 3.2).

After fertilization, the zygote then undergoes mitosis or individual cell division that splits it into more and more cells due to **cleavage** (**klee**-vij) (see Table 7.2). After initial cleavage, the solid ball of cells becomes a *morula*. Because of the ongoing process of mitosis and secretion of fluid by the cells within the morula, the zygote now becomes a **blastocyst** (**blas**-toh-sist) (or blastula) (Fig. 3.3). The rest of the first week is characterized by further mitotic cleavage in which the blastocyst splits into smaller and more numerous cells as it undergoes successive cell divisions by mitosis.

Thus mitosis is a process that takes place during tissue growth or regeneration, which is different from meiosis that takes place during fertilization as discussed (see Table 7.2). Mitosis that occurs during cell division is the self-duplication of the chromosomes of the parent cell and their equal distribution to two daughter cells. The result is that the daughter cells have the same chromosome number and hereditary potential as the parent cells. As it grows by cleavage, the blastocyst travels from the site where fertilization took place to the uterus.

By the end of the first week, the blastocyst stops traveling and undergoes **implantation** (im-plan-**tey**-shuhn) and thus becomes embedded in the prepared endometrium, the innermost lining of the uterus on its back wall. After a week of cleavage, the blastocyst consists of a layer of peripheral cells, the **trophoblast layer** (**trof**-oh-blast) and a small inner mass of embryonic cells or **embryoblast layer** (**em**-bree-oh-blast) (Fig. 3.4). The trophoblast layer later gives

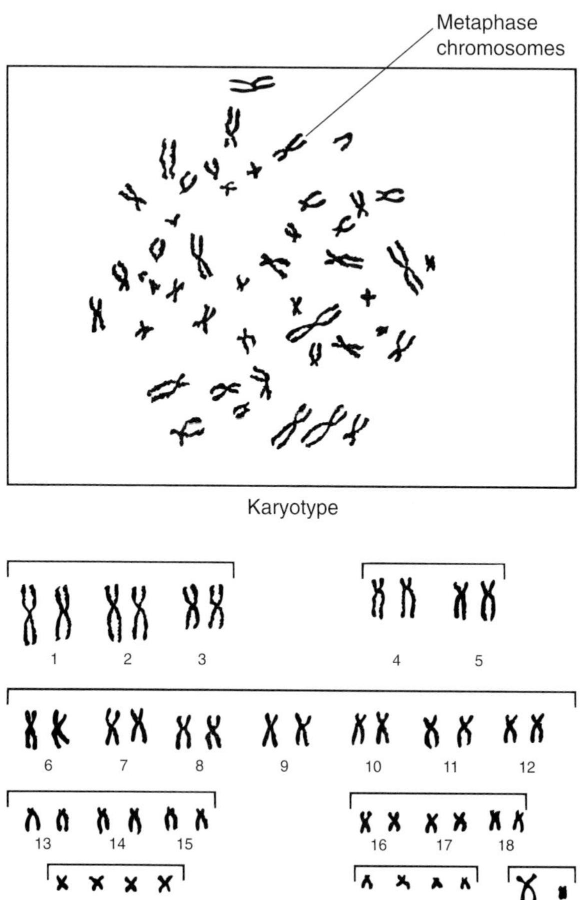

Fig. 3.2 Example of a karyotype demonstrating a photographic analysis of the chromosomes with its orderly arrangement of the pairs. This karyotype is of a man since it has both *X* and *Y chromosomes* because the presence of the *Y* determines maleness.

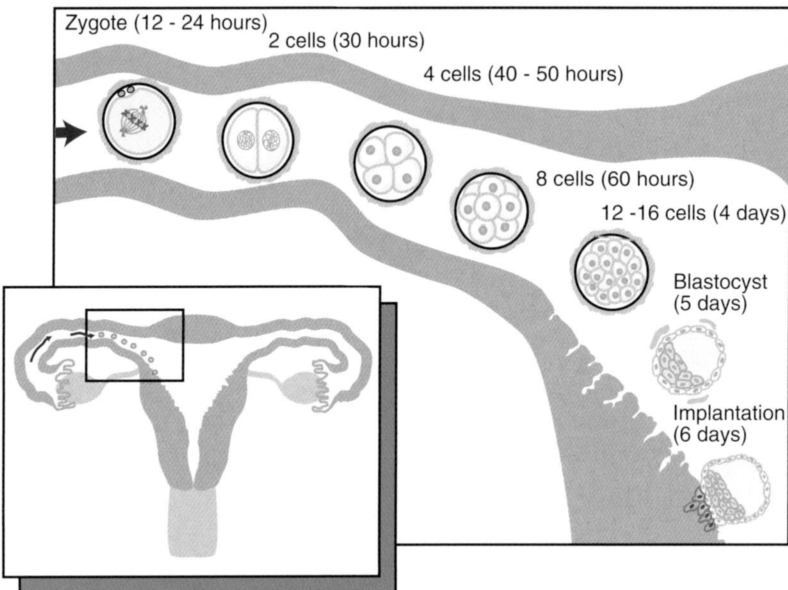

Fig. 3.3 Zygote undergoing mitotic cleavage to form a blastocyst that travels to become implanted in the endometrium of the uterus.

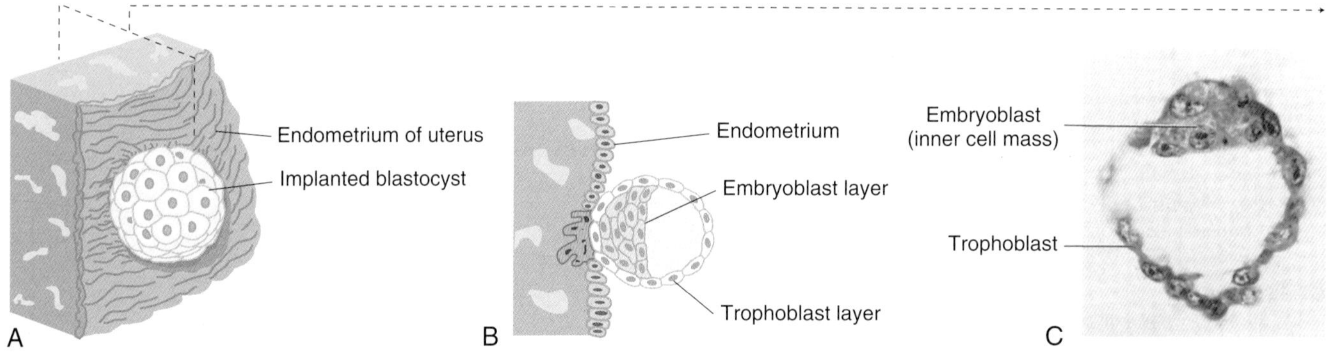

Fig. 3.4 Blastocyst. **A,** Embryoblast layer and trophoblast layer. **B,** Cross section. **C,** Photomicrograph of sections of blastocysts recovered from the endometrium of the uterus at 4 days. (**C,** From Hertig AT, Rock J, Adams EC. A description of 34 human ova within the first seventeen days of development. *Am J Anat.* 1956;98:435.)

rise to important prenatal support tissue. The embryoblast layer later gives rise to the embryo during the prenatal period that follows the embryonic period.

Clinical Considerations for Preimplantation Period

If any disturbances occur in the basic process of meiosis during fertilization, major congenital malformations result from the chromosomal abnormality, which occur in 1 out of 10 cases. An example of this is **Down syndrome** (**sin**-drohm) or *trisomy 21* where an extra chromosome number 21 is present after meiotic division (Fig. 3.5). A **syndrome** is a group of specific signs and symptoms. This syndrome presents with certain orofacial features that include a flat broad face with widely spaced eyes, flat-bridged nose, epicanthic folds, oblique eyelid fissures, furrowed lower lip, tongue fissures, lingual papillae hypertrophy, and various levels of intellectual disability. An arched palate and weak tongue muscles lead to an open mouth position with protrusion of the tongue of usual size and articulated speech is often difficult. It may also involve delayed tooth eruption, fewer teeth present with microdontia, and increased levels of periodontal disease.

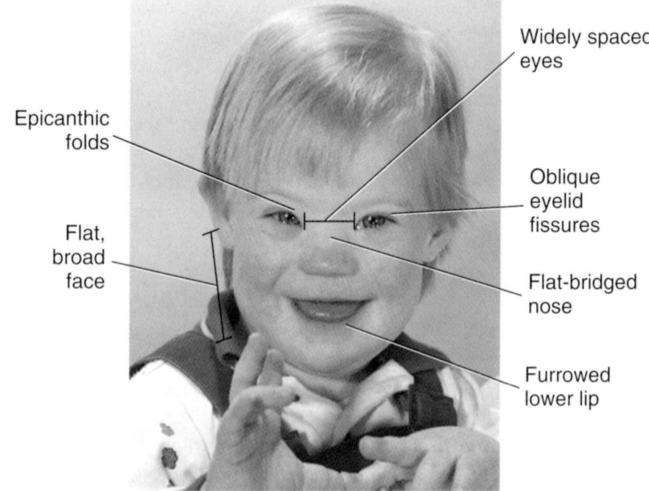

Fig. 3.5 Down syndrome from an extra chromosome number 21 presents with noted orofacial features as well as various levels of intellectual disability. (From Zitelli BJ, Davis HW. *Atlas of Pediatric Physical Diagnosis.* 7th ed, St. Louis: Elsevier; 2018.)

TABLE 3.3 Developmental Processes

Process	Description
Induction	Action of one group of cells on another that leads to establishment of developmental pathway in responding tissue
Proliferation	Controlled cellular growth and accumulation of byproducts
Differentiation	Change in identical embryonic cells to become distinct structurally and functionally
Morphogenesis	Development of specific tissue structure or differing form due to embryonic cell migration or proliferation and inductive interactions
Maturation	Attainment of adult function and size due to proliferation, differentiation, morphogenesis

Implantation of the zygote may also occur outside the uterus with an **ectopic pregnancy** (ek-**top**-ik), most occurring within the fallopian tube. This disturbance has several causes but is usually associated with factors that delay or prevent transport of the dividing zygote to the uterus, such as scarred uterine tubes due to pelvic inflammatory disease. In the past, ectopic pregnancies ruptured causing loss of the embryo and threatening the life of the pregnant woman but now they are successfully treated with medication.

EMBRYONIC PERIOD

The second period of prenatal development, the **embryonic period** (em-bree-**on**-ik), extends from the beginning of the second week to the end of the eighth week (see Table 3.1). Certain physiologic processes or spatial and temporal events of *patterning* occur during this period, which are considered key to the further development (Table 3.3). These physiologic processes include induction, proliferation, differentiation, morphogenesis, and maturation (discussed next). These processes cause the structure of the implanted blastocyst to become, with further development, an **embryo** (**em**-bree-oh). These physiologic processes also allow the teeth and associated orofacial structures as well as other organ structures to develop in the embryo (see Table 6.1).

The first physiologic process involved during prenatal development is the process of **induction** (in-**dunk**-shuhn), which is the action of one group of cells on another that leads to the establishment of the developmental pathway in the responding tissue. Over time, the populations of embryonic cells vary in the competence of their response to induction. Just what triggers cells to develop into structures from cellular interactions is only beginning to be understood, but many developmental disturbances can result from a failure of induction, leading to a further failure of initiation of certain embryologic structures. Induction can also occur in the later stages of development when the structure just increases in size, but these time periods do not seem to be as sensitive.

Another type of physiologic process that follows induction as well as the other processes is the dramatic process of **proliferation** (pruh-lif-uh-**rey**-shuhn), which is controlled levels of cellular growth present during most of prenatal development. Later, migration of these proliferated cells also occurs. Finally, growth also occurs as a result of an accumulation of cellular byproducts.

Growth may be by **appositional growth** (ap-uh-**zish**-uhn-uhl), in which tissue enlarges by the addition of layers on the outside of a structure. In contrast, growth may be by **interstitial growth** (in-ter-**stish**-uhl), which occurs from deep within a tissue type or organ. Hard tissue growth (such as mature bone or hard dental tissue) is usually appositional, whereas soft tissue (such as skin or gingival tissue) increases by interstitial growth. Some tissue types (such as cartilage and immature bone tissue) use both types of growth to attain their final mature size.

It is important to note that growth is not just an increase in overall size, like a balloon being blown up, but it involves differential rates for the different internal tissue types and organs. An example of this varied rate of growth is tooth eruption in a child, which occurs over many years, allowing for the associated growth of the jaws that surround and support the teeth.

In the process of **differentiation** (dif-uh-ren-shee-**ay**-shuhn), a change occurs in the embryonic cells, which are identical genetically but later become quite distinct structurally and functionally. Thus cells that perform specialized functions are formed by differentiation during the embryonic period. Although these functions are minimal at this time, the beginnings of all major tissue types, organs, and organ systems are formed during this period from these specialized cells.

Differentiation occurs at various rates in the embryo. Many parts of the embryo are affected, including the cells, tissue types, organs, and systems. Various terms describe each one of these types of differentiation, and it is important to note the specific delineation between each of them. **Cytodifferentiation** (sy-toh-dif-uh-ren-shee-**ay**-shuhn) is the development of different cell types. **Histodifferentiation** (his-toh-dif-uh-ren-shee-**ay**-shuhn) is the development of different histologic tissue types within a structure. **Morphodifferentiation** (mawr-fuh-dif-uh-ren-shee-**ay**-shuhn) is the development of the differing **morphology** (mawr-**fol**-uh-jee), which makes up its structure or shape for each organ or system.

During the embryonic period, the complexity of the structure and function of these cells increases. This is accomplished by **morphogenesis** (mawr-fuh-**jen**-uh-sis), which is the process of development of specific tissue structure or shape. Morphogenesis occurs due to the migration or proliferation of embryonic cells, which is followed by the inductive interactions of those cells. As previously mentioned, induction continues to occur throughout the embryonic period as a result of the new varieties of cells interacting with each other, producing an increasingly complex organism.

Finally, the physiologic process of **maturation** (mach-uh-**rey**-shuhn) of the tissue types and organs begins during the embryologic period and continues later during the fetal period. It is important to note that the physiologic process of maturation of the individual tissue types and organs also involves the processes of proliferation, differentiation, and morphogenesis. Thus, maturation is not the attainment of just the correct adult size but also the correct adult structure and function of tissue types and organs.

An embryo is recognizable by the eighth week of prenatal development, which is the end of the embryonic period. This chapter discusses only the major events of the second, third, and fourth weeks of the embryonic period. The remaining weeks of prenatal development that are pertinent to dental professionals are addressed in **Chapters 4 and 5**, which then describe the more detailed development of the orofacial structures.

SECOND WEEK

During the second week of prenatal development within the embryonic period, the implanted blastocyst grows by increased proliferation of the embryonic cells, with differentiation also occurring resulting in changes in cellular morphogenesis; every ridge, bump, and recess now indicates these increased levels of cellular differentiation. This increased number of embryonic cells creates the **embryonic cell layers** (or germ layers) within the blastocyst. A **bilaminar embryonic disc**

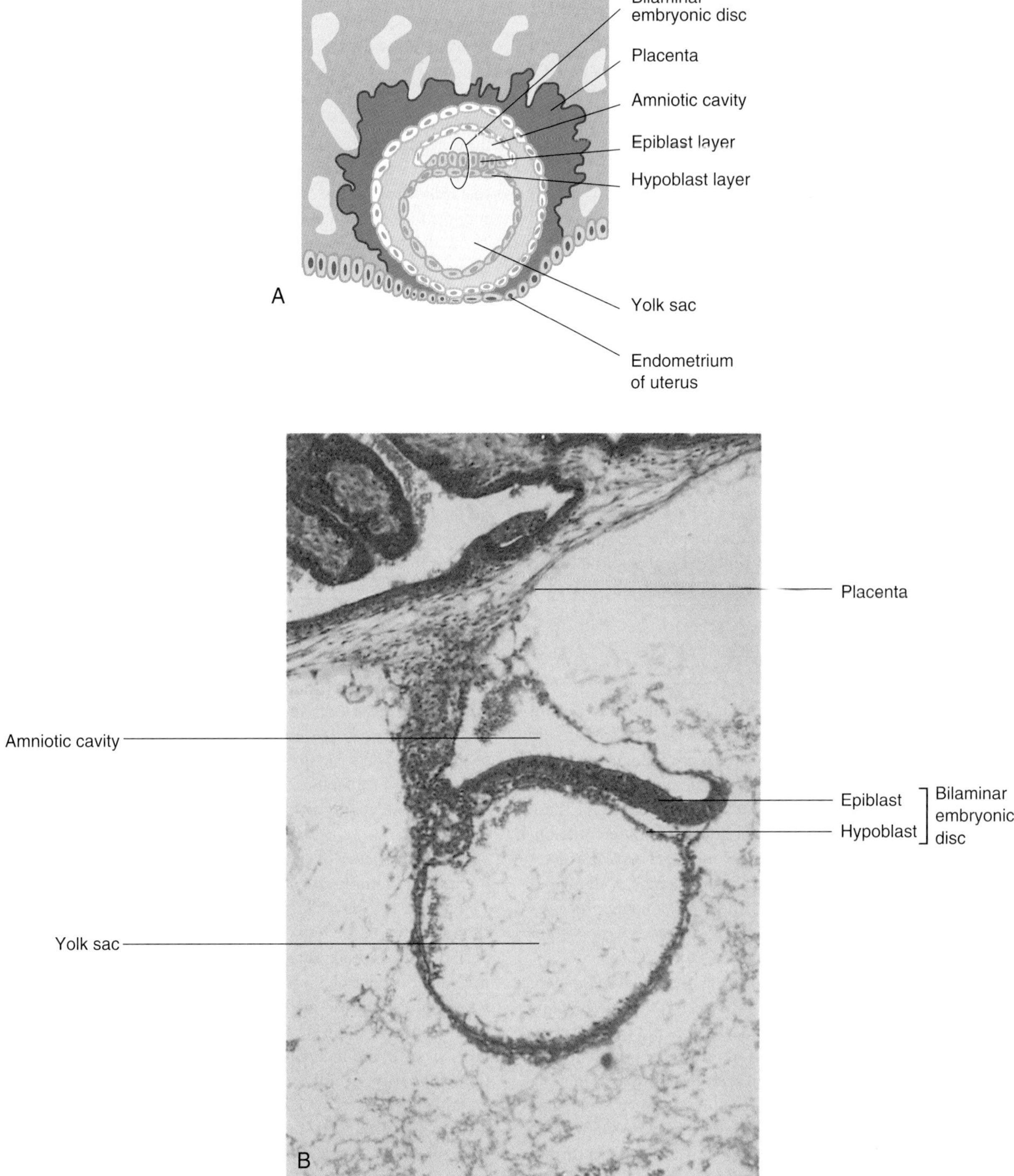

Fig. 3.6 Cross Section of the Blastocyst Forming the Bilaminar Embryonic Disc. **A,** Epiblast layer and hypoblast layer surrounded by the amniotic cavity and yolk sac. **B,** Photomicrograph of longitudinal section of an embedded 14-day embryo. (**B,** From Nishimura H, ed. *Atlas of Human Prenatal Histology.* Tokyo: Igaku-Shoin; 1983.)

(bahy-**lam**-uh-nuhr) is eventually developed from the blastocyst and appears as a three-dimensional but flattened circular plate of bilayered cells (Fig. 3.6).

The bilaminar embryonic disc (or disk) has both a superior and inferior layer. The superior **epiblast layer** (**ep**-uh-blast) is composed of high columnar cells, and the inferior **hypoblast layer** (**hahy**-puh-blast) is composed of small cuboidal cells. After its creation, the disc is suspended in the endometrium lining the uterus between two fluid-filled cavities, the **amniotic cavity** (am-nee-**ot**-ik), which faces the epiblast layer, and the **yolk sac**, which faces the hypoblast layer and serves as initial nourishment for the disc. The bilaminar embryonic disc later develops into the embryo as prenatal development continues.

Even later, the **placenta** (pluh-**sen**-tuh), a prenatal organ that joins the pregnant woman and developing embryo, develops from the interactions of the trophoblast layer and endometrial tissue. The formation of the placenta and the developing umbilical circulation permit

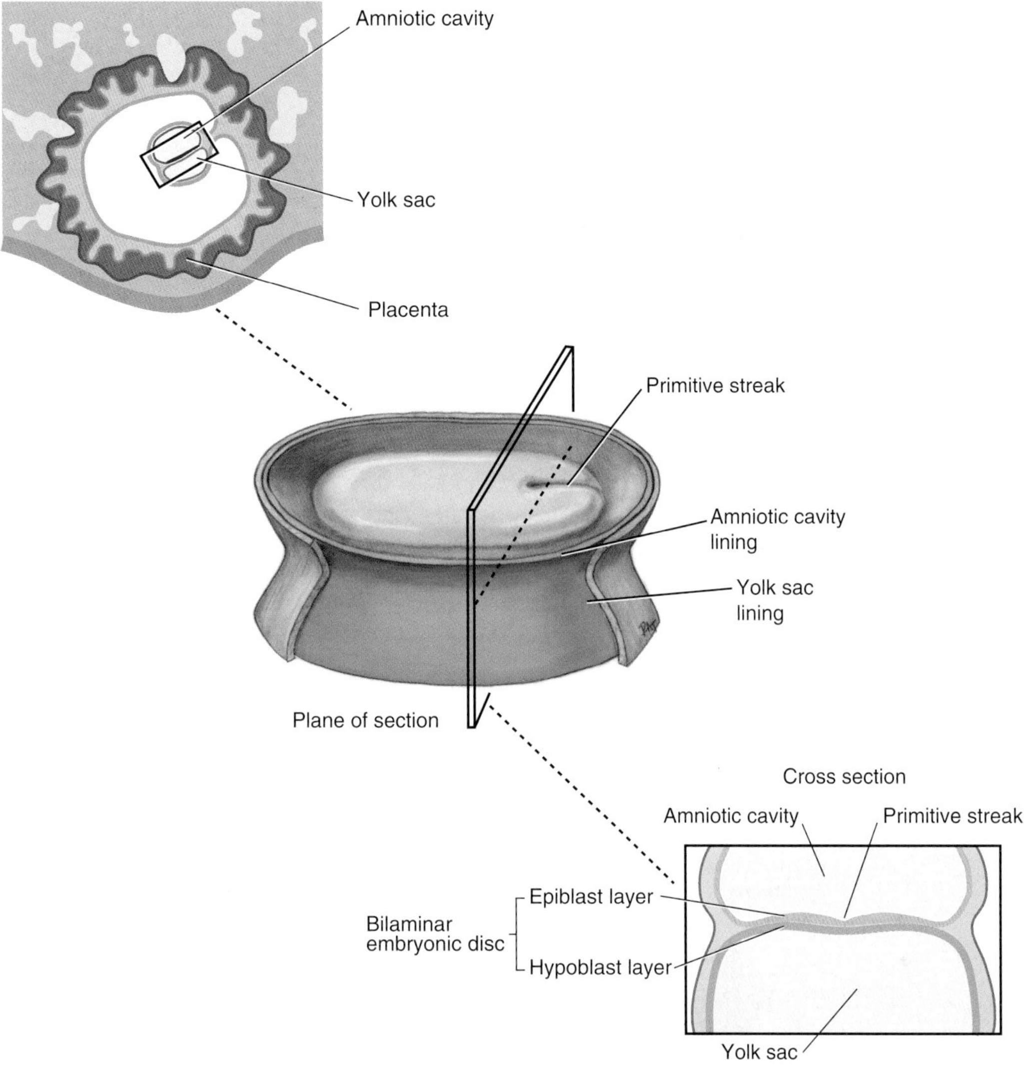

Fig. 3.7 Bilaminar embryonic disc with primitive streak resulting in bilateral symmetry.

selective exchange of soluble bloodborne substances between them. This includes oxygen and carbon dioxide as well as nutritional and hormonal substances.

THIRD WEEK

During the beginning of the third week of prenatal development within the embryonic period, the **primitive streak** forms within the bilaminar disc (Fig. 3.7). This furrowed rod-shaped thickening in the middle of the disc results from an increased proliferation of cells in the midline area. The primitive streak causes the disc to have **bilateral symmetry** (**sim**-uh-tree), with a right half and left half; most of the further development of each half of the embryo mirrors the other half. If looked at from a superior view, the embryo would resemble the shape of a sole of a shoe with the head end wider than the tail end and with a slightly narrowed middle.

In addition, during the beginning of the third week some cells from the epiblast layer move or migrate toward the hypoblast layer only in the area of the primitive streak (Fig. 3.8). These migratory cells locate in the middle between the epiblast and hypoblast layers and become **mesoderm** (**mez**-uh-durm), an embryonic connective tissue as well as embryonic **endoderm** (**en**-doh-durm). Mesodermal cells have the potential to proliferate and differentiate into diverse types of connective tissue, forming cells such as fibroblasts, chondroblasts, and osteoblasts (see Chapter 8).

With three layers present, the bilaminar embryonic disc has thickened into a **trilaminar embryonic disc** (trahy-**lam**-i-nahr) (Fig. 3.9). Thus the trilaminar embryonic disc has three embryonic cell layers. With the creation of the new embryonic cell layers of mesoderm and embryonic endoderm, the epiblast layer is now considered **ectoderm** (**ek**-tuh-durm). At the same time, the hypoblast layer has been displaced by the cells migrating into the primitive streak and now becomes extra-embryonic endoderm.

Within the trilaminar embryonic disc, each embryonic cell layer is distinct from the others and thus gives rise to specific tissue (Table 3.4, see Table 8.1). The ectoderm gives rise to the skin epidermis, the central nervous system (CNS), and other structures. The mesoderm gives rise to connective tissue, such as skin dermis, cartilage, bone, blood, muscle, and other associated tissue. The endoderm gives rise to the respiratory epithelium and cells of glands.

Mesoderm and associated tissue are found in all areas of the future embryo except at certain embryonic membranes at both ends of the embryo and the pharyngeal pouches (discussed later in this chapter). In these areas without mesoderm present both the ectoderm and endoderm fuse together, thereby preventing the migration of mesoderm between them.

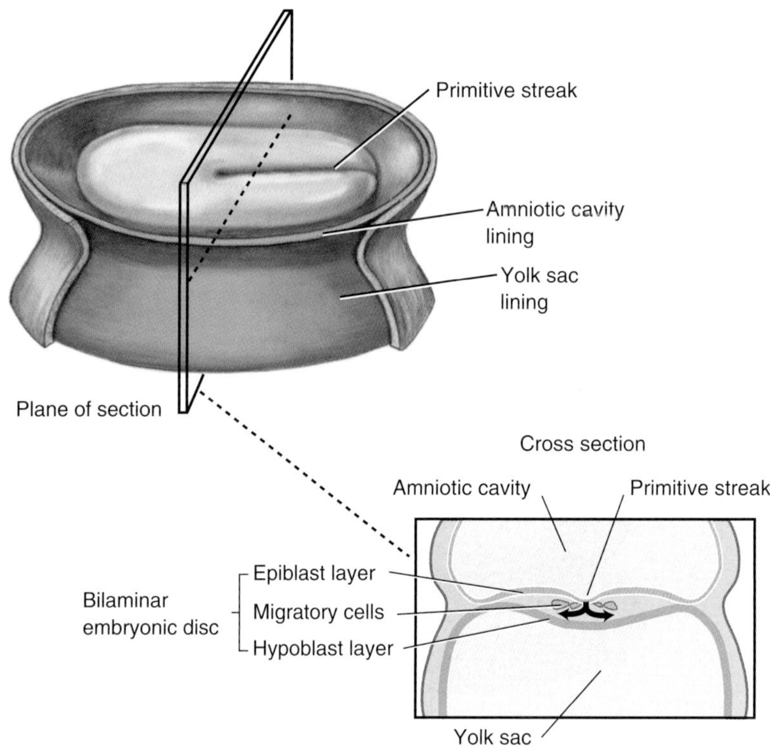

Fig. 3.8 Bilaminar embryonic disc with migration of the epiblast layer cells toward the hypoblast layer to form the new mesoderm layer.

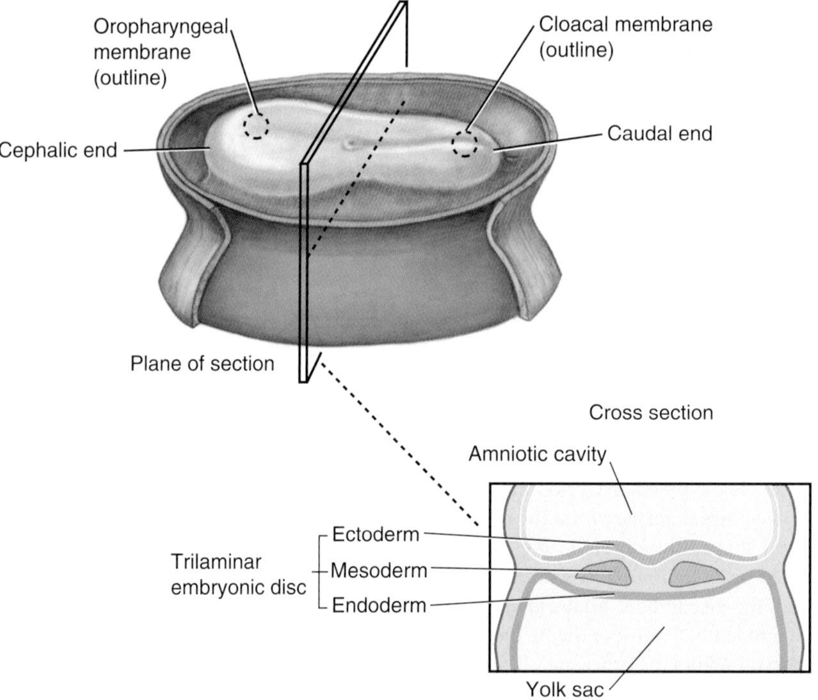

Fig. 3.9 After the formation of the middle layer of mesoderm, the resulting trilaminar embryonic disc consists of the ectoderm, mesoderm, and endoderm. The cephalic and caudal ends of the disc are associated with the oropharyngeal and cloacal membranes *(dashed circles)*.

Because the trilaminar embryonic disc has undergone so much growth during the past 3 weeks, certain anatomic structures of the disc become apparent. The disc now has a **cephalic end** (suh-**fal**-ik) or *head end.* At the cephalic end the oropharyngeal membrane forms, which consists of only ectoderm externally and endoderm internally, without any intermediate mesoderm. This membrane is the location of the future primitive mouth or stomodeum of the embryo and thus the beginning of the digestive tract (see Fig. 4.1). The disc also has a **caudal end** (**kawd**-l) or *tail end* (see Fig. 3.9). At the caudal end the cloacal membrane forms, which is the location of the future anus or terminal end of the digestive tract.

TABLE 3.4 Development of Embryonic Cell Layers

	Ectoderm	Mesoderm	Endoderm	Neural Crest Cells*
Origin	Epiblast layer	Migrating cells from epiblast layer	Migrating cells from epiblast layer	Migrating neuroectoderm
Histologic features	Columnar	Varies	Cuboidal	Varies
Future structures	Epidermis; sensory epithelium of eyes, ears, nose, nervous system, neural crest cells; mammary and cutaneous glands	Dermis, muscle, bone, lymphatics, blood cells and bone marrow, cartilage, reproductive and excretory organs	Respiratory and digestive system linings, liver, pancreatic cells	Components of nervous system pigment cells, connective tissue proper, cartilage, bone, certain dental tissue

*Neural crest cells from neuroectoderm are included, but they are not present in embryonic disc until later part of third week; neural crest cells are considered to be *fourth embryonic cell layer* by embryologists.

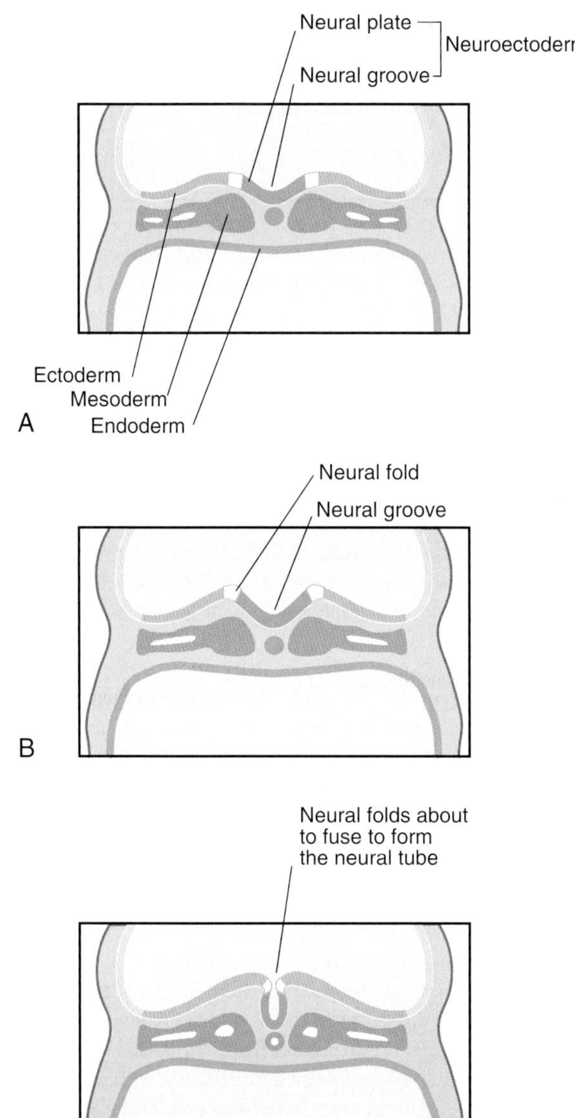

Fig. 3.10 Central Nervous System of the Embryo Beginning to Form. **A,** Formation of the neuroectoderm from the ectoderm within the neural plate that thickens to form the neural groove. **B,** Neural groove deepens to become surrounded by the neural folds. **C,** Neural folds meet and fuse, forming the neural tube.

During the latter part of the third week, the CNS begins to develop in the embryo (Fig. 3.10). Many steps occur during this week to form the beginnings of the spinal cord and brain (see Table 8.7). First, a specialized group of cells differentiates from the ectoderm and is now considered **neuroectoderm** (noor-oh-**ek**-toh-durm). These cells are localized to the **neural plate** (**noor**-uhl) of the embryo, which is a central band of cells that extends the length of the embryo, from the cephalic end to the caudal end. This plate undergoes further growth and thickening, which cause it to deepen and invaginate inward forming the **neural groove**.

Near the end of the third week, the neural groove deepens further and is surrounded by the **neural folds**. As further growth of the neuroectoderm occurs, the **neural tube** is formed during the fourth week by the neural folds undergoing **fusion** (**fyoo**-zhunh) at the most superior part. The neural tube forms the future spinal cord as well as other neural tissue of the CNS (see Table 3.4).

Other areas of the embryo also undergo fusion during the third week and in subsequent weeks as the embryo develops, but the process occurs differently depending on the structures involved. In the case of the neural tube (and also the palate as discussed in Chapter 5), the process of fusion, as the term implies, causes the joining of two separate surfaces on the embryo (Fig. 3.11). However, in the case of facial fusion, the process of fusion can also include the elimination of a groove between two adjacent processes appearing as swellings on the same surface of the embryo. In these latter cases, merging of underlying tissue and cell migration into the groove produces the joining of the facial processes (see Figs. 4.3 and 4.4).

In addition, during the third week another specialized group of cells, the **neural crest cells (NCCs)**, develop from neuroectoderm (Fig. 3.12). These cells migrate from the crests of the neural folds and then join the mesoderm to form **mesenchyme** (**mez**-eng-kahym). The mesenchyme is involved in the development of many face and neck structures, such as with the pharyngeal or branchial arches, because they differentiate to form most of the connective tissue of the head (see Chapter 4).

On reaching their predetermined destinations, the NCCs undergo differentiation into diverse cell types that are, in part, specified by local environmental influences. Embryologists consider the NCCs to be a *fourth embryonic cell layer* (see Table 3.4). In future development, these cells become involved in the formation of components of the nervous system, melanocyte pigment cells, connective tissue proper, cartilage, bone, and certain dental tissue by becoming a specialized type of mesenchyme, ectomesenchyme, such as with the formation of the pulp, dentin, cementum, alveolar process, and periodontal

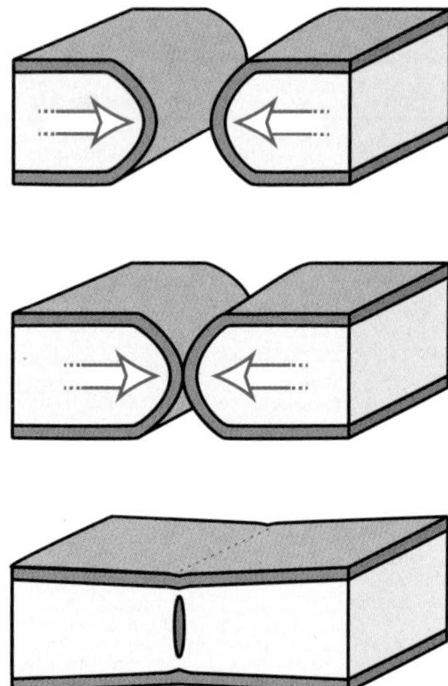

Fig. 3.11 Process of fusion that can have the joining of swellings or tissue from *different* surfaces of the embryo, which occurs with the neural tube, upper lip, and palate. This is unlike the fusion with the joining of swellings or tissue on the *same* surface of the embryo that occurs on the face (see Fig. 4.4).

ligament (see Fig. 6.1). Thus, NCCs are essential in formation of most oral and dental tissue, except for the enamel and certain types of cementum, as well as the development of the face and neck (see Chapters 4, 5, and 6).

By the end of the third week, the mesoderm additionally differentiates and begins to divide on each side of the tube into 38-paired cuboidal segments of mesoderm forming the **somites** (**soh**-mahyts) (Fig. 3.13). The somites later appear as distinct elevations on the surface of the sides of the embryo and continue to develop in the following weeks of prenatal development, giving rise to most of the skeletal structures of the head, neck, and trunk, as well as the associated muscles and dermis of the skin.

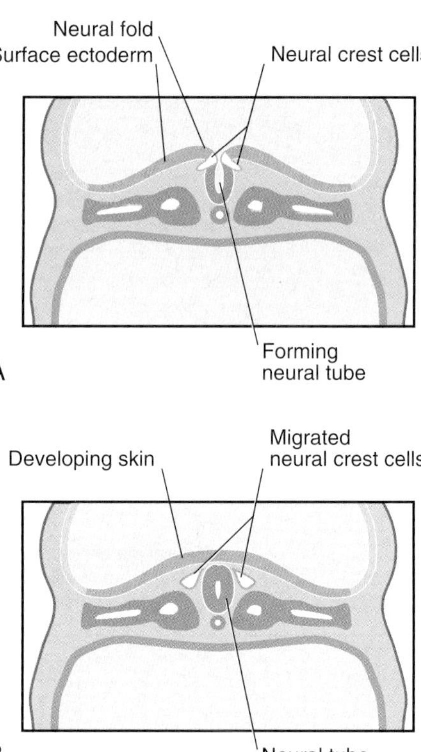

Fig. 3.12 Neural crest cells from the neural folds **(A)** will migrate and join with the mesoderm to form the mesenchyme **(B)** to affect tissue development.

FOURTH WEEK

During the fourth week of prenatal development within the embryonic period the trilaminar embryonic disc undergoes anterior (or cephalic) and lateral **embryonic folding**, which places forming tissue types into their proper positions for further embryonic development as well as producing a tubular embryo (Fig. 3.14). This folding results from extensive proliferation of the ectoderm and differentiation of basic tissue and occurs mostly at the cephalic end, where the brain will form. This cephalic tissue grows beyond the oropharyngeal membrane to overhang the developing heart.

Folding due to increased growth occurs not only at the cephalic end but also at the caudal end and at the sides of the embryo simultaneously. As a result of this folding, the positions of the embryonic cell layers take on a more recognizable placement for the further development of the embryo.

Thus, after folding of the disc, the endoderm lies inside the ectoderm, with mesoderm filling in the areas between these two layers. This movement of the embryonic cell layers forms one long and hollow tube lined by endoderm from the cephalic end to the caudal end of the embryo—specifically, from the **oropharyngeal membrane** (ohr-oh-fuh-**rin**-jeez-uhl) to the **cloacal membrane** (kloh-**ey**-kuhl). This tube is the future digestive tract and is separated into three major regions, the foregut, midgut, and hindgut.

The anterior part of this tube is the **foregut** (**fawr**-guht), which forms the primitive pharynx or primitive throat and includes a part of the primitive yolk sac as it becomes enclosed with folding (see Fig. 4.10). The two more posterior parts, the **midgut** (**mid**-guht) and **hindgut** (**haynd**-guht), respectively, go on to form the rest of the mature pharynx, as well as the remainder of the digestive tract (see Fig. 2.18). During development of the digestive tract, four pairs of pharyngeal pouches will form from evaginations on the lateral walls lining the pharynx (see Fig. 4.11).

Finally, during the fourth week the face and neck begin to develop, with the primitive eyes, ears, nose, oral cavity, and jaw areas. The development of the face and neck is discussed in Chapter 4, and the development of the associated oral cavity is described in Chapters 5 and 6.

Clinical Considerations for Embryonic Period

Because the beginnings of all essential external and internal structures are formed during the embryonic period, this is considered the most critical period of prenatal development. Thus, developmental disturbances occurring during this period may give rise to major congenital malformations of the embryo (as discussed earlier).

One syndrome that can occur within this period is **ectodermal dysplasia** (ek-tuh-**durm**-uhl dis-**pley**-zhuh), which involves the abnormal development of one or more structures from ectoderm (Fig. 3.15). This syndrome has a hereditary etiology and presents with abnormalities of the teeth, skin, hair, nails, eyes, facial structure, and glands because these are derived from ectoderm or associated tissue. There may be partial or complete anodontia, the absence of some or all teeth in each dentition and the teeth that are present for either dentition frequently have developmental disturbances (see Chapter 6). Partial or full dentures are used for both functional and esthetic purposes but need to

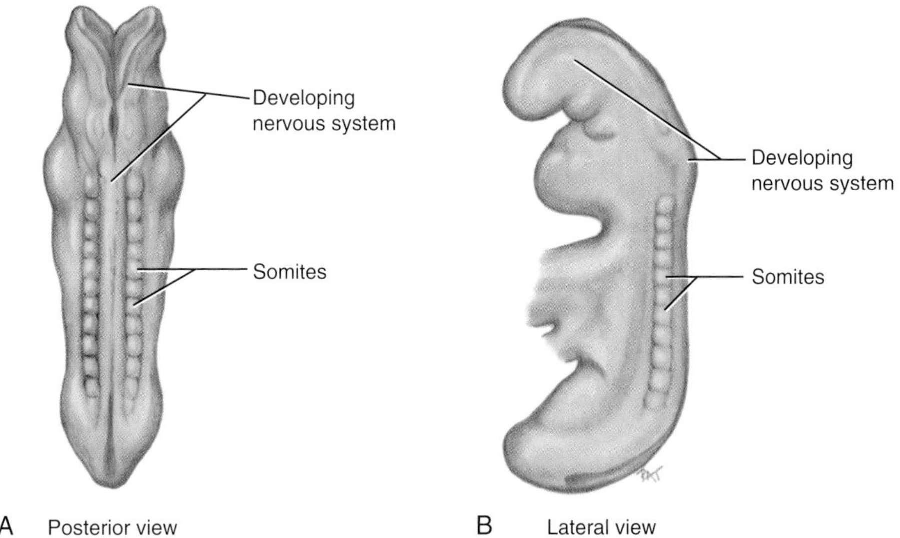

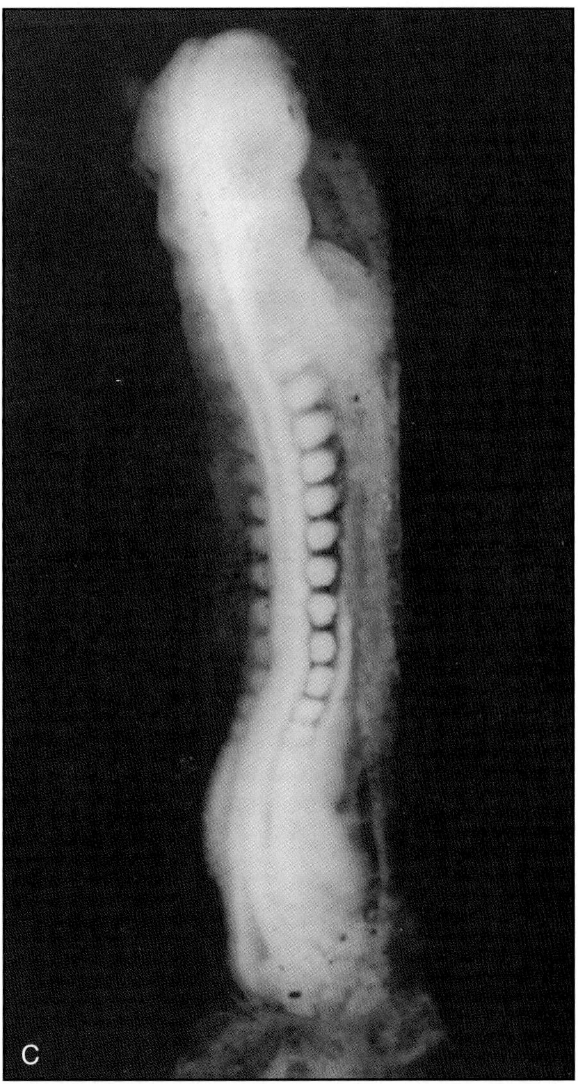

Fig. 3.13 Differentiated Mesoderm Gives Rise to the Somites. **A** and **B,** Somites are located on both the sides of the developing nervous system. **C,** Oblique view of 13-somite embryo at around 24 days. (**C,** From Moore KL, Persaud TVN, Shiota K. *Color Atlas of Clinical Embryology*. 2nd ed. Philadelphia: Saunders; 2000.)

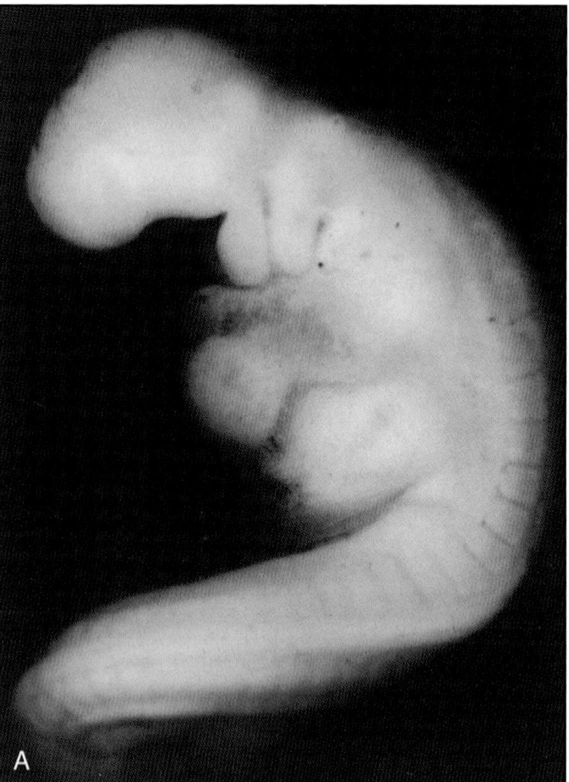

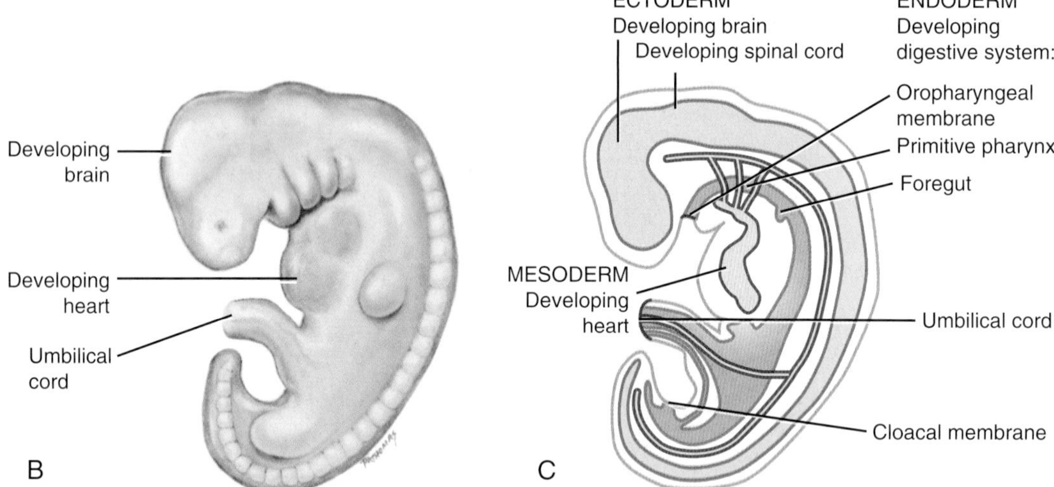

Fig. 3.14 Trilaminar Embryonic Disc Has Folded into the Embryo. A and **B,** Disc now has undergone embryonic folding as a result of extensive growth of the ectoderm, and there is development of the brain with spinal cord, heart, and digestive tract. **C,** With the folding, the endoderm is now inside the ectoderm, with the mesoderm filling in the areas between the two tissue types, except at the two embryonic membranes as shown on cross section. (**A,** From Nishimura H, Semba R, Tanimura T, Tanaka O. *Prenatal Development of the Human With Special Reference To Craniofacial Structures: An Atlas*. Washington, DC: National Institutes of Health; 1977.)

be reconstructed periodically as the jaws continue to grow; implants may be considered after growth halts if bone levels of each remaining alveolar process are adequate.

If there is failure of migration of the NCCs to the facial region, **Treacher Collins syndrome** (**TCS**) (**tree**-chuhr **kol**-uhz) or mandibulofacial dysostosis develops in the embryo (Fig. 3.16). This results in failure of specific areas of orofacial development, presenting with downward slanting eyes, underdeveloped zygomatic bone, drooping lateral lower eyelids, and conductive hearing loss, with malformed or absent ears as well as dental developmental disturbances, such as anodontia with absent teeth, enamel dysplasia with abnormal mineralization, and micrognathia with its small lower jaw.

In addition, if teratogens are present during the active differentiation of a tissue type or organ, after crossing from pregnant woman by way of the placenta, this can raise the incidence of congenital malformations. An example of an infective teratogen for the embryo is the virus causing **rubella** (roo-**bell**-uh), which can result in cataracts,

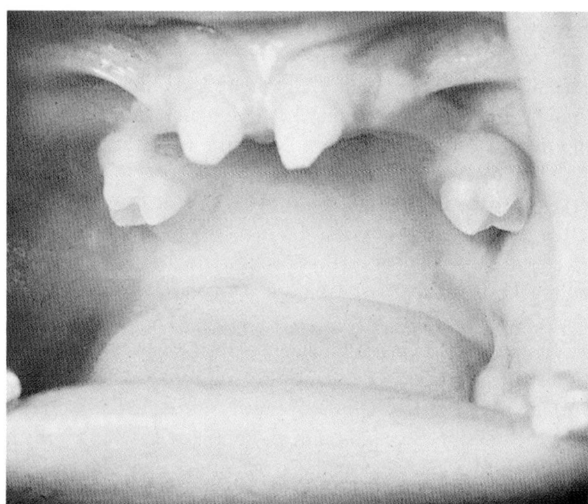

Fig. 3.15 Ectodermal dysplasia is marked by the abnormal development of ectodermal structures resulting in certain facial features and an absence of teeth or anodontia (partial in this case). (Courtesy of Margaret J. Fehrenbach, RDH, MS.)

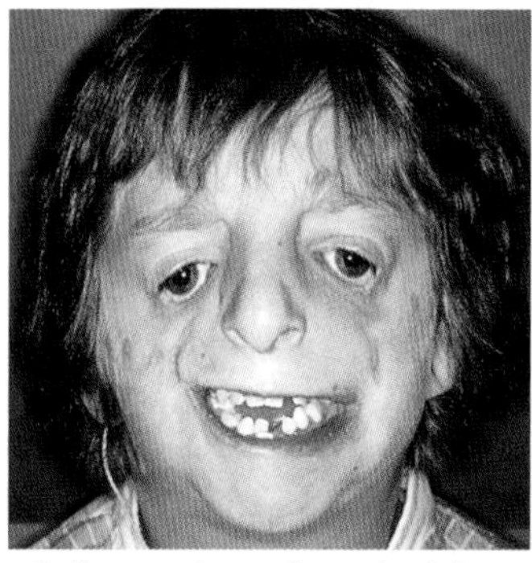

Fig. 3.16 Treacher Collins syndrome from the failure of migration of the neural crest cells to the facial region in the embryo presents with areas without complete orofacial development, having marked features, including micrognathia (or small lower jaw). (Courtesy of L.B. Kaban, MD, DMD.)

cardiac defects, and deafness. Another infective teratogen is the *Treponema pallidum* bacterial spirochete causing **syphilis** (**sif**-uh-lis) because it produces defects in the incisors (Hutchinson incisor) and molars (mulberry molar), as well as blindness, deafness, and may also involve paralysis if not treated (Fig. 3.17) (see Chapters 16 and 17).

An example of the result of a teratogenic drug effect during the embryonic period is **fetal alcohol syndrome (FAS)** (**feet**-l) (Fig. 3.18). High levels of ethanol ingested by a pregnant woman such as with alcoholic drinks cross the placenta and can result in prenatal and postnatal growth deficiency, intellectual disabilities, and other facial disturbances, such as small head circumference, low nasal bridge, short nose, small midface, widely spaced eyes with epicanthic folds and eyelid fissures, indistinct philtrum, and thin upper lip. Oral changes, such as crowding of the dentition, mouth breathing, anterior open bite, and associated gingivitis, may occur possibly because of an increased finger sucking habit. However, the effects of ethanol on prenatal development can include much more than those set defining criteria and prenatal exposure to ethanol can potentially impact development at almost any point in the pregnancy from embryonic through fetal development. No safe amount of ethanol or safe time for ingestion is known at this time.

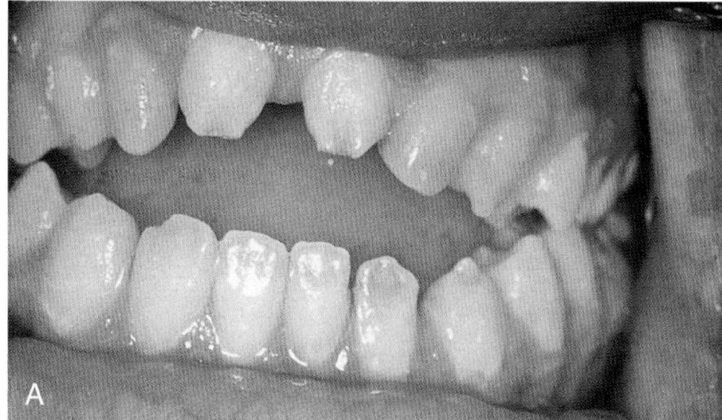

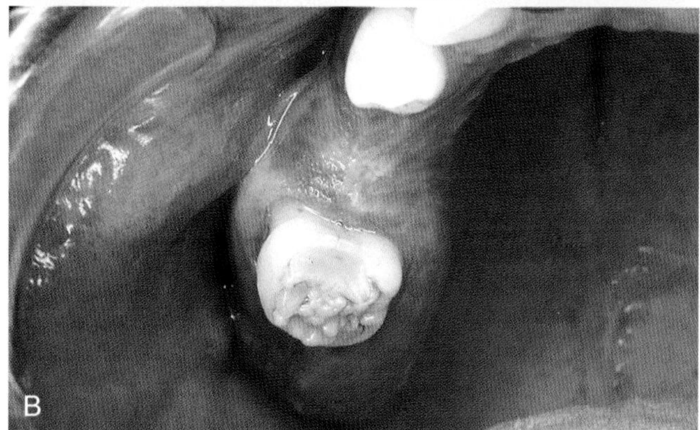

Fig. 3.17 Dental Anomalies from Syphilis as an Infective Teratogen. A, Hutchinson incisors. **B,** Mulberry molar. (Courtesy of George Blozis, DDS, MS.)

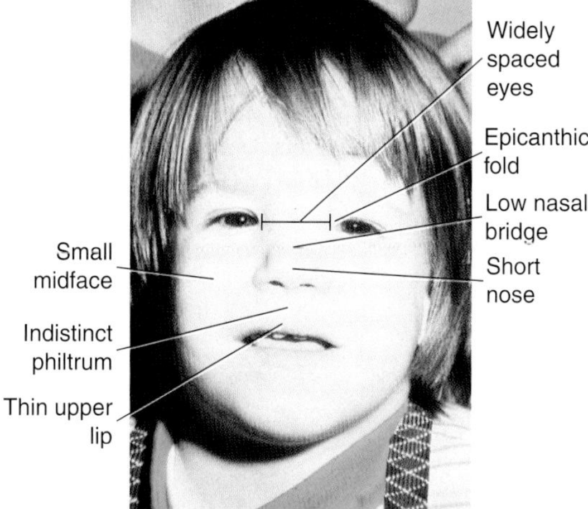

Fig. 3.18 Fetal alcohol syndrome presents with noted orofacial features and various levels of intellectual disability. This syndrome is caused by the pregnant women's excessive use of ethanol during the embryonic period. (From Streissguth AP, Landesman-Dwyer S, Martin JC, et al. Teratogenic effects of alcohol in humans and laboratory animals. *Science*. 1980;209:353-361.)

Direct exposure to high levels of radiation can act as an environmental teratogen during the embryonic period. Radiation may injure embryonic cells, resulting in cell death, chromosome injury, and delay of mental and physical growth. The severity of embryonic damage is associated with the absorbed dose, the dose rate, and the state of embryonic or fetal development at the time of exposure.

However, congenital abnormalities have not been directly linked to a diagnostic level of radiation, such as that used in the dental setting.

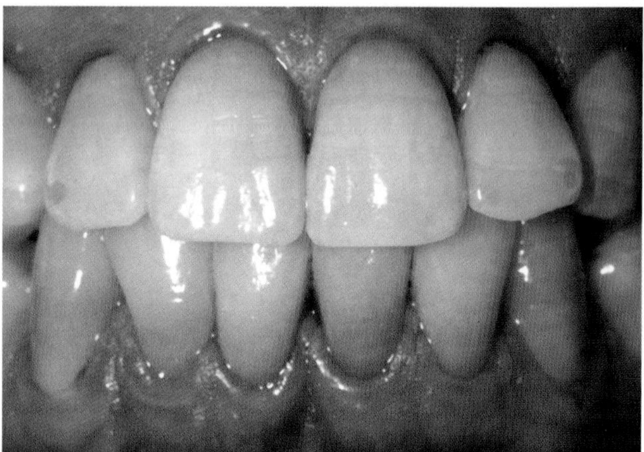

Fig. 3.19 Facial view of the permanent teeth with moderate to slight yellow and brown tetracycline stain caused by the ingestion of the drug by a child during the time of development of the permanent dentition. In many cases, extensive vital whitening (or bleaching) may also be effective to help even out the tooth color. (Courtesy of Margaret J. Fehrenbach, RDH, MS.)

Scattered radiation from a radiographic examination of the oral cavity administers a dose of only a few millirads to a pregnant woman, which is not known to be teratogenic to an embryo. Nevertheless, even this small dose should be avoided during pregnancy unless an emergency situation requires it; the correct dosage and timing of radiographs as well as protective precautions should be used with all patients at all times as well as with the administering dental professionals.

Failure of fusion of the neural tube results in neural tube defects of the tissue overlying the spinal cord, such as the meninges, vertebral arches, muscles, and skin. One type of neural tube defect is **spina bifida** (**spa-hy**-nuh **bif**-i-duh), characterized by defects in the vertebral arches and various degrees of disability. Nutritional and environmental factors can also have an important role as teratogens in causing neural tube defects; folic acid supplements are now being recommended during pregnancy to help prevent this defect as well as cleft lip and cleft palate (see Figs. 4.8 and 5.6).

FETAL PERIOD

The final period of prenatal development, the **fetal period**, follows the embryonic period (see Table 3.1). It encompasses the beginning of the ninth week or third month continuing to the ninth month, with the maturation of existing structures occurring as the embryo enlarges to become a **fetus** (**fee**-tuhs). This process involves not only the physiologic process of maturation of the individual tissue types and organs but also further proliferation, differentiation, and morphogenesis, as discussed before with the development of the embryo.

Although developmental changes with the fetus are not as dramatic as those that occur during the embryonic period, they are important because they allow the newly formed tissue types and organs to function. Even though the embryo has been breathing since the third week of prenatal development, by the end of the fourth month the fetal heartbeat and fetal movements are also present.

Clinical Considerations for Fetal Period

Systemic tetracycline antibiotic therapy of the pregnant woman can act as a teratogenic drug during the fetal period. This sometimes life-saving therapy can result in **tetracycline stain** (te-truh-**sahy**-kleen) with the child's primary teeth that are developing at that time. This intrinsic yellow to yellow-brown discoloration within the teeth can occur in varying degrees as the antibiotic becomes chemically bound to the dentin for the life of the tooth. This stain is easily visible because of the transparency of overlying enamel.

The adult's permanent teeth may also be affected, similarly to the primary teeth, if the drug is given to a child during their development (Fig. 3.19). If the permanent teeth are involved, treatment may require full-coverage crowns or veneers to improve the appearance of the teeth, although, in some cases, extensive vital tooth whitening may even out the discoloration. Thus this type of antibiotic therapy should be avoided whenever possible when treating pregnant women and children. Studies also show that overuse of amoxicillin in children with ear and respiratory infections may be involved in pitting and intrinsic stain in the permanent tooth enamel, resulting in enamel dysplasia (see Box 6.1, O, P).

4

Face and Neck Development

Additional resources and practice exercises are provided on the companion Evolve website for this book: http://evolve.elsevier.com/Fehrenbach/illustrated.

LEARNING OBJECTIVES

1. Define and pronounce the key terms in this chapter.
2. Outline the events that occur during facial development, describing each step in its formation.
3. Identify the structures present during facial development on a diagram.
4. Integrate the study of the facial development into understanding the observed orofacial structures and the clinical considerations due to developmental disturbances of these structures.
5. Outline the events that occur during neck development, describing each step in its formation.
6. Identify the structures present during neck development on a diagram.
7. Integrate the study of neck development into understanding the observed orofacial structures and the clinical considerations due to developmental disturbances of these structures.

FACIAL DEVELOPMENT

Dental professionals must have a clear understanding about the development of the face to further relate the underlying structural relationships to any developmental disturbances that may be present.

The face and its associated tissue begin to form during the fourth week of prenatal development within the embryonic period (Fig. 4.1 and Box 4.1). During this time, the rapidly growing brain of the embryo bulges over the oropharyngeal membrane and developing heart (Fig. 4.2). The area of the future face is now squeezed between the developing brain and heart with the formation of the three embryonic layers and resultant embryonic folding (see Fig. 3.14).

All three embryonic layers are involved in facial development, the ectoderm, mesoderm, and endoderm (Table 4.1). Early development of the face is also dominated by the proliferation and migration of ectomesenchyme, which is derived from neural crest cells (NCCs) (see **Chapter 3** for more discussion).

Facial development includes the formation of the primitive mouth, mandibular arch, maxillary process, frontonasal process, and nose. Facial development depends on the five major facial processes (or prominences) that form during the fourth week and surround the primitive mouth of the embryo, the single frontonasal process and paired maxillary and mandibular processes (Fig. 4.3). Thus these facial processes become the centers of growth for the face. The adult face is divided into thirds: upper face, midface, and lower face. These divisions of the face also roughly correspond to the three centers of facial growth during prenatal development. In summary, the upper face is derived from the frontonasal process, the midface from the maxillary processes, and the lower face from the mandibular processes.

The facial development that starts in the fourth week will be completed later in the twelfth week within the fetal period. The face changes shape considerably as it grows from being an embryo to forming into a fetus. Thus overall facial proportions develop during the later fetal period. It is important to note that the development of the associated oral structures is occurring at the same time as discussed in **Chapters 5 and 6**.

Most of the facial structures develop by fusion of swellings or tissue on the *same* surface of the embryo (Fig. 4.4). A cleft or furrow is initially located between these adjacent swellings due to proliferation, differentiation, and morphogenesis (see Table 3.3). However, with most facial fusion, these furrows are usually eliminated as the underlying mesenchyme migrates into the furrow, making the embryonic facial surface smooth. This migration takes place because adjacent mesenchyme grows and merges beneath the external ectoderm during the maturation of the structure. In some cases, a slight groove or line may remain on the facial surface showing where the fusion of the swellings took place.

Differing from this type of fusion that takes place on the facial surface is the type of fusion that occurs during development of the upper lip and palate (see Fig. 3.11). In contrast to most facial fusion, both upper lip and palatal fusion involve the fusion of swellings or tissue from *different* surfaces of the embryo, such as that which occurs with the fusion of the neural tube (see Fig. 3.10, *C*).

The overall growth of the face is in both an inferior and anterior direction in relationship to the cranial base. The growth of the upper face is initially the most rapid, in keeping with its association with the rapidly developing brain. Subsequently, the forehead ceases to grow significantly after age 12. In contrast, the midface and lower face grow more slowly over a prolonged period of time and finally cease to grow late in puberty. Much later, the eruption of the permanent third molars, which occurs at approximately 17 to 21 years of age, marks the end of the major growth of the lower two-thirds of the face. The underlying facial bones, also developing at this time, depend on centers of bone formation by intramembranous ossification (see Fig. 8.12).

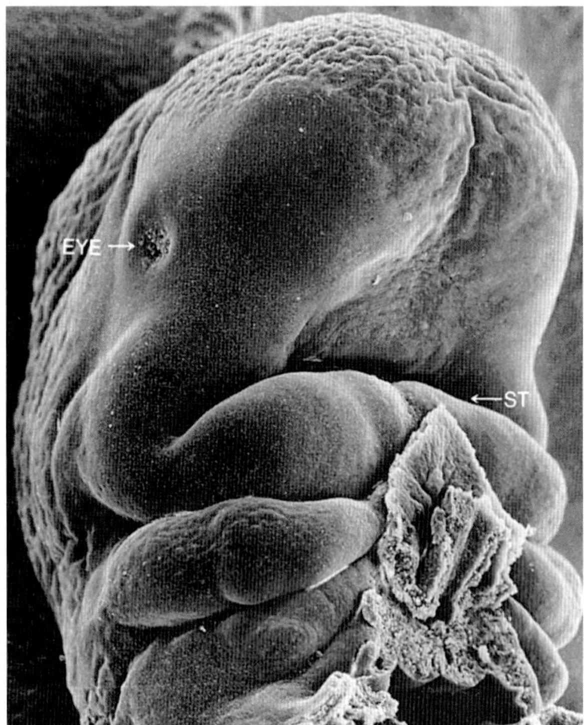

Fig. 4.1 Scanning electron micrograph of the embryo at the fourth week, showing the developing face with its stomodeum *(ST)* and lens placode for the eye as well as the developing brain (nearby anterior placed developing heart has been cut away to display the pharyngeal or branchial arches). (Courtesy of K.V. Hinrichsen, MD, Medizinische Fakultät, Institut für Anatomie, Ruhr-Universität Bochum, Bochum.)

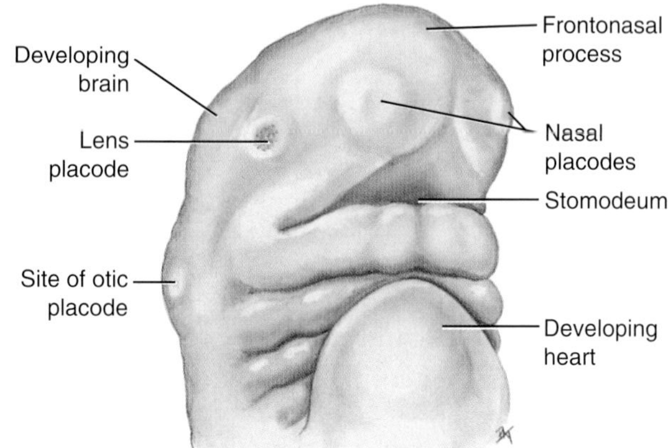

Fig. 4.2 Embryo at the fourth week of prenatal development showing the developing brain, the forming face from the growth of the frontonasal process with its stomodeum and placodes, and the developing heart.

BOX 4.1 Facial Development Within the Fourth Week of Prenatal Development

Developmental Events Overview (Not in Precise Order of Occurrence)

- Disintegration of the oropharyngeal membrane of stomodeum enlarges the primitive mouth, allowing access to the primitive pharynx
- Mandibular processes fuse to form the mandibular arch that then fuses to form the mandible and lower lip
- Frontonasal process forms and gives rise to the nasal placodes, nasal pits, medial and lateral nasal processes, and intermaxillary segment to form the nose and primary palate
- Maxillary process forms from the mandibular arch on each side of the stomodeum
- Maxillary processes fuse with each medial nasal process to form upper lip and with each mandibular arch to form the labial commissures

TABLE 4.1 Embryonic Orofacial Development

Embryonic Structures	Origin	Future Structures
Stomodeum	Ectodermal depression enlarged by disintegration of oropharyngeal membrane	Oral cavity proper
First pharyngeal or branchial arch (or *mandibular arch*)	Fused mandibular processes and neural crest cells	Lower lip, lower face, mandible with associated tissue (other arch derivatives shown in Table 4.2)
Maxillary process(es)	Superior and anterior swelling(s) from mandibular arch and neural crest cells	Midface, upper lip sides, cheeks, secondary palate, posterior part of maxilla with associated tissue, zygomatic bones, part of temporal bones
Frontonasal process	Ectodermal tissue and neural crest cells	Medial and lateral nasal processes
Nasal pits	Nasal placodes	Nasal cavities
Medial nasal process(es)	Frontonasal process medial to nasal pits	Middle of nose, philtrum region, intermaxillary segment
Intermaxillary segment	Fused medial nasal processes	Anterior part of maxilla with associated tissue, primary palate, nasal septum
Lateral nasal process(es)	Frontonasal process lateral to nasal pits	Nasal alae

STOMODEUM AND ORAL CAVITY FORMATION

At the beginning of the fourth week, the primitive mouth has become the **stomodeum** (stoh-muh-**dee**-uhm), which initially appeared as a shallow depression in the embryonic surface ectoderm at its cephalic end (see Figs. 4.1 and 4.2). At this time, the stomodeum is limited in depth by the oropharyngeal membrane (see Fig. 3.14). This temporary membrane, consisting of external ectoderm overlying endoderm, was formed during the third week of prenatal development. The membrane also separates the stomodeum from the primitive pharynx. The primitive pharynx is the cranial part of the foregut, which is the beginning of the future digestive tract.

The first event in the development of the face during the latter part of the fourth week of prenatal development is disintegration of the oropharyngeal membrane (Fig. 4.5). With this disintegration of the membrane, the primitive mouth is increased in depth and enlarges in width across the surface of the midface. Access now occurs through the stomodeum between the internal primitive pharynx and the outside fluids of the amniotic cavity that surrounds the embryo. In future development, the stomodeum will give rise to the oral cavity, which will be lined by oral epithelium, derived from ectoderm as a

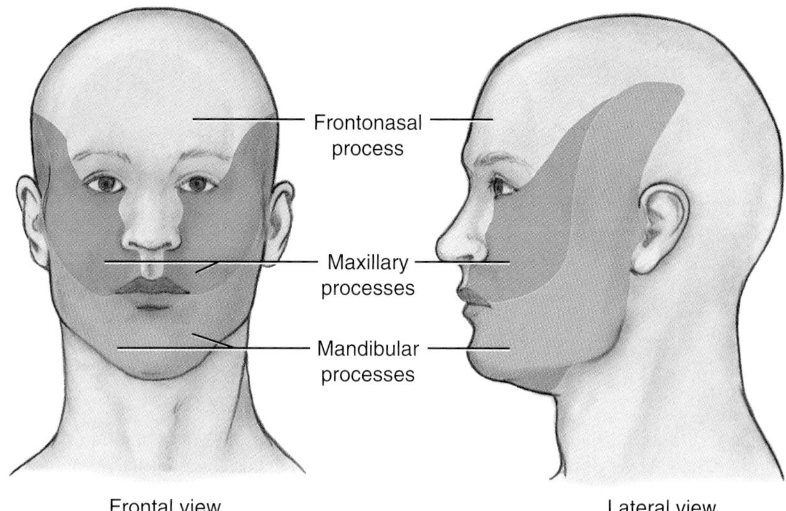

Fig. 4.3 Adult face with its embryonic derivatives of the five facial processes, the single frontonasal process, and paired maxillary and mandibular processes.

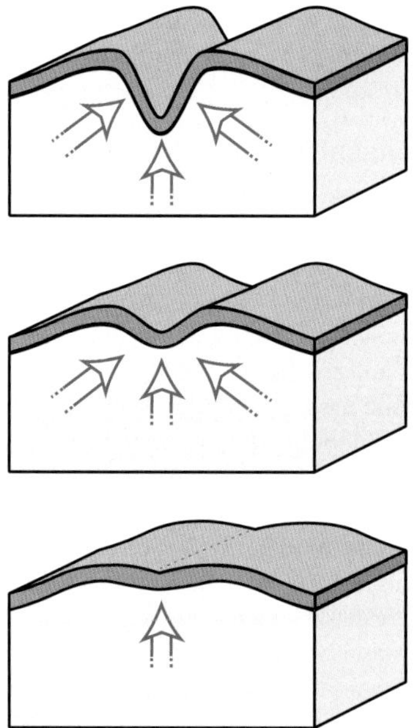

Fig. 4.4 Facial fusion can involve the elimination of a furrow between two adjacent swellings of tissue on the *same* surface of the embryo. This fusion process differs from that of the neural tube, upper lip, and palatal fusion, which is the fusion of two separate structures from two *different* surfaces (see Fig. 3.11).

result of embryonic folding. Additionally, the oral epithelium derived from both ectoderm and associated underlying mesodermal tissue will give rise to the teeth and associated tissue types as discussed in **Chapter 6** (see Fig. 6.1).

MANDIBULAR ARCH AND LOWER FACE FORMATION

After formation of the stomodeum but still within the fourth week, two bulges of tissue appear inferior to the primitive mouth, the two **mandibular processes** (see Fig. 4.5). These processes consist of a core of mesenchyme formed in part by NCCs that migrated to the facial region to join with the mesoderm; they are covered externally by ectoderm and internally by endoderm.

These paired mandibular processes then fuse at the midline to form the **mandibular arch,** the developmental form of the future lower dental arch, the mandible. After fusion, the mandibular arch then extends as a band of tissue found inferior to the stomodeum and between the developing brain and heart. In the midline, on the surface of the mature bony mandible, is the mandibular symphysis indicating where the mandible is formed by fusion of right and left mandibular processes (see Fig. 1.9). The mandibular arch and its associated tissue are the first parts of the face to form after the stomodeum, separating it from the developing cardiac bulge.

The mandibular arch is also considered the *first branchial (or pharyngeal) arch* (discussed later in this chapter). Thus this tissue depends on NCCs for its formation as do all the other more inferior five branchial (or pharyngeal) arches. During the growth of the mandibular arch, **Meckel cartilage** (**mek**-uhl **kahr**-ti-lij) forms within each side of the arch (see Fig. 5.3, *A* and *B*). Most of this cartilage disappears as the bony mandible forms by intramembranous ossification lateral to and in close association with the cartilage; yet, it also contributes a small part to the mandible (see **Chapters 5 and 8**).

In future development, the developing mandibular arch directly gives rise to the lower face, including the lower lip. Thus the mandibular arch will also give rise not only to the mandible but additionally its mandibular teeth and associated tissue. The mandible of the embryo initially appears underdeveloped, however, it achieves its characteristic mature prominent form as it develops further during the fetal period (see Figs. 4.5 and 4.3, respectively).

The mesoderm of the mandibular arch forms the muscles of mastication (masseter, temporalis, and pterygoids) as well as some palatal muscles and suprahyoid muscles (see Fig. 19.8). Because these muscles are derived from the mandibular arch, they are innervated by the nerve of the first arch, the trigeminal nerve or fifth cranial nerve (see Table 13.3). The mandibular arch is also involved in the formation of the tongue (see Fig. 5.9).

During the fifth to sixth week, primitive muscle cells from the mesoderm in the mandibular arch begin to differentiate. These primitive muscle cells become oriented to the site of origin and insertion of the masticatory muscles that they will form. By the seventh week, the mandibular muscle mass has grown larger and its cells have begun to migrate into the areas where they will begin to differentiate into the four muscles of mastication as discussed. Muscle cell migration occurs before bone formation in the facial area.

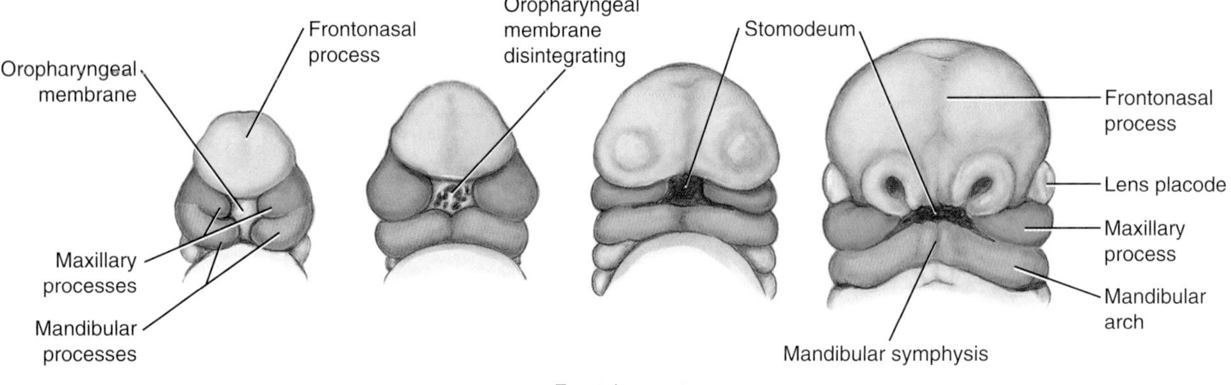

Fig. 4.5 During the third to fourth week, disintegration of the oropharyngeal membrane enlarges the stomodeum of the embryo and allows access between the primitive mouth and the primitive pharynx. The frontonasal process also enlarges, helping to form the nasal region. Mandibular processes give rise to the maxillary processes and then fuse together at the mandibular symphysis, forming the mandibular arch inferior to the enlarged stomodeum.

By the tenth week, the mandibular muscle masses have become well organized bilaterally into the four muscles of mastication. Nerve branches from the trigeminal nerve are incorporated early in these muscle masses. The muscle cells of the masseter and medial pterygoid muscles have formed a vertical sling that inserts into the site that will form the angle of the mandible. The temporalis muscle cells have differentiated in the temporal fossa and are inserting into the developing coronoid process. The lateral pterygoid muscle cells, which arise from the infratemporal fossa, extend horizontally into the mandibular condyle and disc of the temporomandibular joint.

FRONTONASAL PROCESS AND UPPER FACE FORMATION

During the fourth week, the **frontonasal process** (fruhn-toh-**ney**-zuhl) also forms as a bulge of tissue but at the most cephalic end of the embryo, which is the cranial boundary of the stomodeum (see Fig. 4.2). In future development, the frontonasal process gives rise to the upper face, which includes the forehead, bridge of the nose, primary palate, nasal septum, and all structures associated with the medial nasal processes.

Placode Development

On the embryo are placodes, which are rounded areas of specialized thickened ectoderm found at the location of developing structures. The facial area of the embryo has two **lens placodes** (**plak**-ohdz), which are initially located fishlike on each side of the frontonasal process (see Figs. 4.1 and 4.2). Later in development, these lens placodes migrate medially from their lateral positions and form the future eyes and associated tissue.

The two **otic placodes** (**oh**-tik) are even more laterally and posteriorly placed and form pits that create the future internal ear and the associated tissue as they appear to rise to their mature position as a result of their relative growth. Parts of the nearby branchial or pharyngeal apparatus of the embryonic neck later form the external and middle ear (discussed later in this chapter).

In addition to the lens and otic placodes, the two **nasal placodes** (**ney**-zuhl) form in the anterior part of the frontonasal process just superior to the stomodeum during the fourth week (see Fig. 4.2). These button-like structures form as bilateral ectodermal thickenings that later develop into olfactory epithelium located in the mature nose for the sensation of smell. In **Chapter 6,** there will be discussion of the orally placed dental placodes from which the tooth germs are produced.

Nose and Paranasal Sinus Formation

During the fourth week, the tissue around the nasal placodes on the frontonasal process undergoes growth, thus starting the development of the nasal region and the nose. The placodes then become submerged forming a depression in the center of each placode, the **nasal pits** (or olfactory pits) (Fig. 4.6). These nasal pits later develop into the nasal cavity (Fig. 4.7, *A*, and see Fig. 11.19).

Deepening of the nasal pits produces a nasal sac that grows internally toward the developing brain. At first, the nasal sacs are separated from the stomodeum by the **oronasal membrane** (ohr-oh-**ney**-zuhl). This temporary membrane disintegrates, bringing the nasal and oral cavities into communication in the area of the primitive choanae, posterior to the developing primary palate. At the same time, the superior, middle, and inferior nasal conchae are developing on the lateral walls of the developing nasal cavities.

Some of the paranasal sinuses develop later during the fetal period and others develop after birth. All form as outgrowths of the walls of the nasal cavities and become air-filled extensions of the nasal cavities in the adjacent bones, such as in the maxilla and the frontal bone (see Fig. 11.21).

The middle part of the tissue growing around the nasal placodes appears as two crescent-shaped swellings located between the nasal pits. These are the **medial nasal processes** (**mee**-dee-uhl) (see Fig. 4.6). In future development, the medial nasal processes will fuse together externally to form the middle part of the nose from the root of the nose to the apex of the nose as well as the tubercle of the upper lip and philtrum (see Figs. 1.4 and 1.6).

The paired medial nasal processes also fuse internally and grow inferiorly on the inside of the stomodeum, forming the **intermaxillary segment** (in-ter-**mak**-suh-ler-ee) (or premaxillary segment) by the end of the seventh week of prenatal development (see Fig. 4.7, *B* and *C* and see Fig. 5.1). The intermaxillary segment is involved in the formation of certain maxillary teeth (incisors) and associated structures, such as the primary palate and nasal septum.

On the outer part of the nasal pits are two other crescent-shaped swellings, the **lateral nasal processes** (see Fig. 4.6). In future development, the lateral nasal processes form the alae of the nose, and the

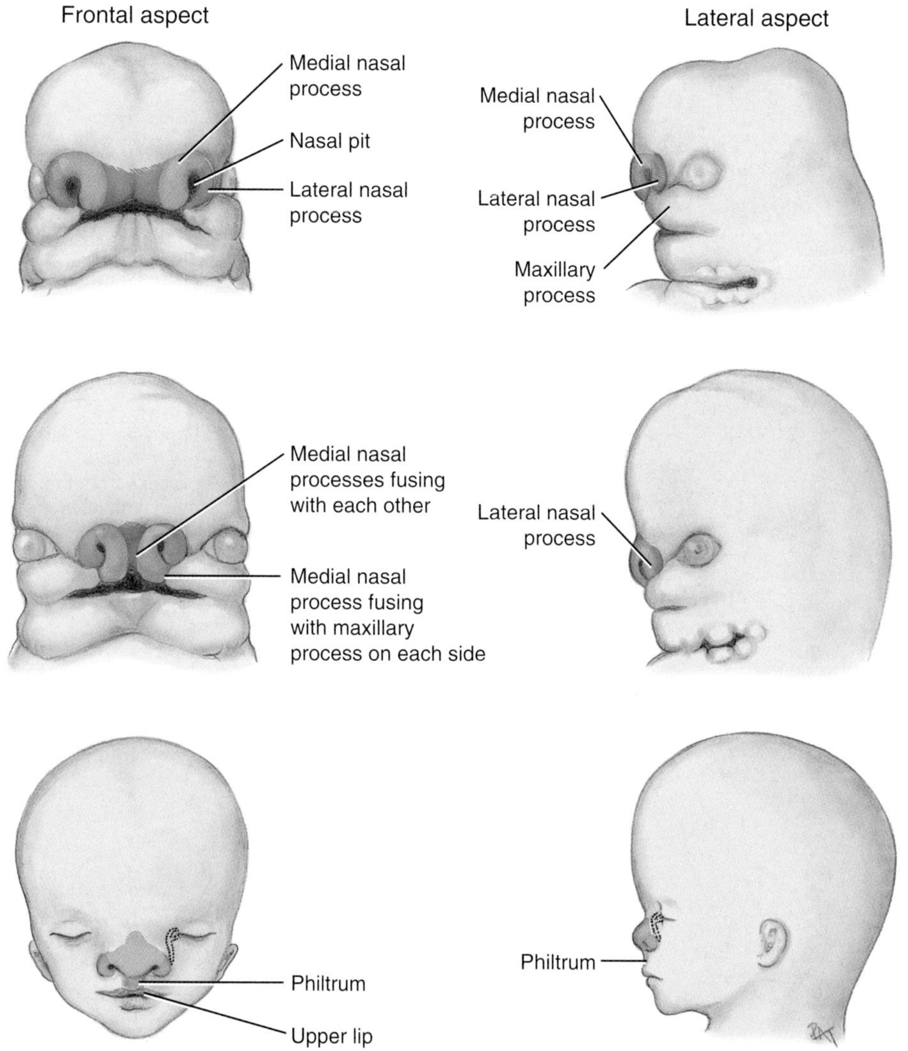

Fig. 4.6 Development of the nose from the fusion of the medial and lateral nasal processes; also showing the formation of the upper lip from the medial process fusing with the maxillary process on each side of the stomodeum.

fusion of the lateral nasal, maxillary, and medial nasal processes forms the nares (see Fig. 1.4). The embryonic nose remains visually flat, however, until the fetal period when facial development is completed, allowing for a more mature elevated appearance.

MAXILLARY PROCESS AND MIDFACE FORMATION

During the fourth week of prenatal development within the embryonic period, a tissue swelling forms from increased growth of the mandibular arch on each side of the stomodeum, the **maxillary process**. Subsequently, each maxillary process will grow superiorly and anteriorly around the stomodeum (see Fig. 4.5). Because it is formed from the mandibular arch, the maxillary process is also formed from mesenchyme provided by NCCs that joined with the mesoderm.

In future development, the maxillary processes will form the midface. This includes the sides of the upper lip, cheeks, secondary palate, and posterior part of the maxilla with its canines, certain posterior teeth, and associated tissue. This tissue also forms the zygomatic bones and parts of the temporal bones.

UPPER AND LOWER LIP FORMATION

During the start of the sixth week of prenatal development, the upper lip begins formation when each maxillary process fuses with each medial nasal process on both sides of the stomodeum, which are brought into proximity by proliferation of the NCC-derived mesenchyme (see Figs. 4.6 and 4.7 *A*),. Thus the maxillary processes contribute to the sides of the upper lip and the two medial nasal processes contribute to the midline philtrum (see Fig. 1.6).

This fusion of these processes to form the upper lip is similar to the fusion of the neural tube and palate because it takes place between two processes on *different* surfaces on each side of the face (see Fig. 3.11). The maxillary and medial nasal processes grow toward one another and fusion initially occurs at the ectodermal surfaces where the processes contact one another. The fused ectodermal tissue is temporarily trapped between the joining processes and later disappears so that the mesenchyme is continuous across the fused medial nasal and maxillary processes.

Fusion of these processes to form the upper lip is completed during the end of the seventh week of prenatal development when the grooves between the processes are obliterated. The maxillary processes on each

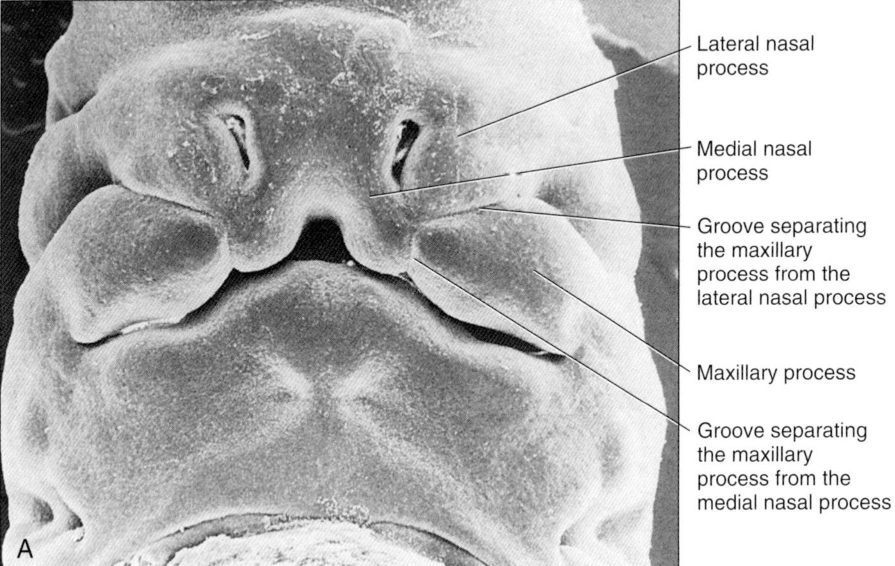

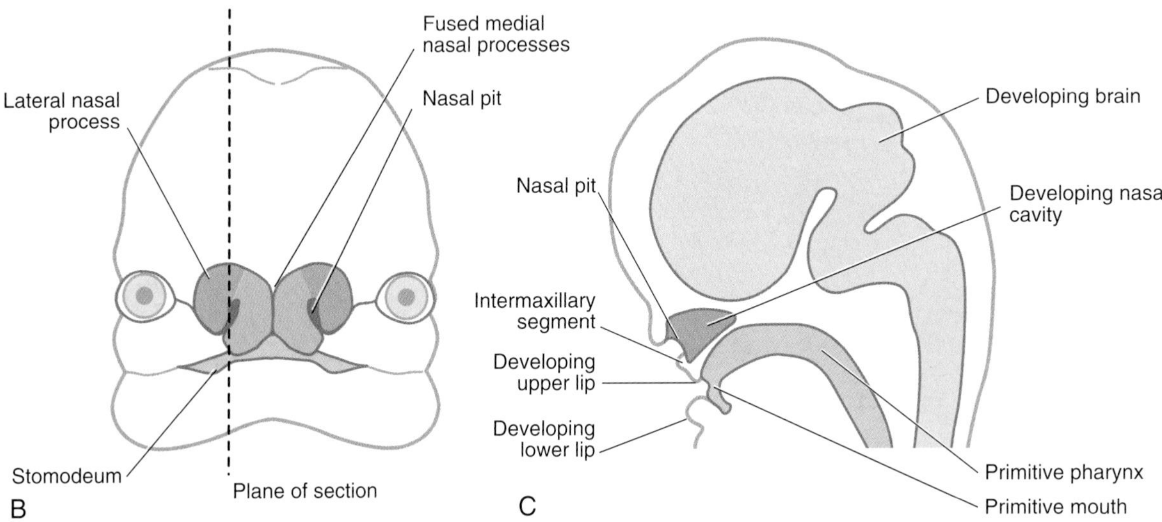

Fig. 4.7 Embryo at 6 Weeks. **A,** Photograph of forming upper and lower lip. **B** and **C,** Sagittal sections of the head showing the development of the intermaxillary segment from the fusion of medial nasal processes on the inside of the stomodeum. (**A,** Courtesy of K.K. Sulik, PhD.)

side of the developing face partially fuse with the mandibular arch on each side to create each labial commissure, with the mandibular arch already forming the lower lip.

 Clinical Considerations for Upper Lip Development

Failure of fusion of the maxillary process with the medial nasal process can result in **cleft lip (kleft)**, with varying degrees of disfigurement and disability present in the upper lip (Figs. 4.8 and 4.9). The ectodermal tissue trapped within the fusing processes may also fail to disappear. Thus the mesenchyme is prevented from growing together across the two processes. This somewhat common disturbance may be hereditary or associated with environmental factors. It also may be isolated or associated with other developmental abnormalities, such as cleft palate (see Fig. 5.6, *C* to *E*). Cleft lip occurs in about 1 in 1000 cases (about 1%). The cleft results from a failure of the mesenchyme to grow beneath the ectoderm to obliterate any grooves between these processes or even a deficiency or absence of mesenchyme in the area.

These clefts of the lip can be located at one side or both sides of the upper lip; thus it may be unilateral or bilateral and may also vary from a notch in the vermilion zone of the upper lip (with an incomplete cleft) to more severe cases (with a complete cleft) that extend into the floor of the naris and through the alveolar process of the maxilla.

Cleft lip is more common and more severe in men and it is also more commonly unilateral and on the left side. It can complicate nursing and feeding of the child as well as present challenges with speech development and facial appearance and it may also increase oronasal infection levels. It is treated by oral and plastic surgery, with dental intervention; however, speech and hearing therapy may also be needed.

CERVICAL DEVELOPMENT

The development of the neck parallels the development of the face over time, beginning during the fourth week of prenatal development within the embryonic period and completed during the fetal period

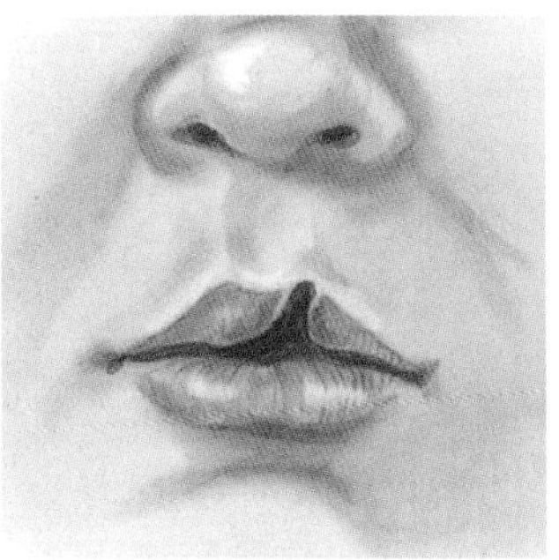

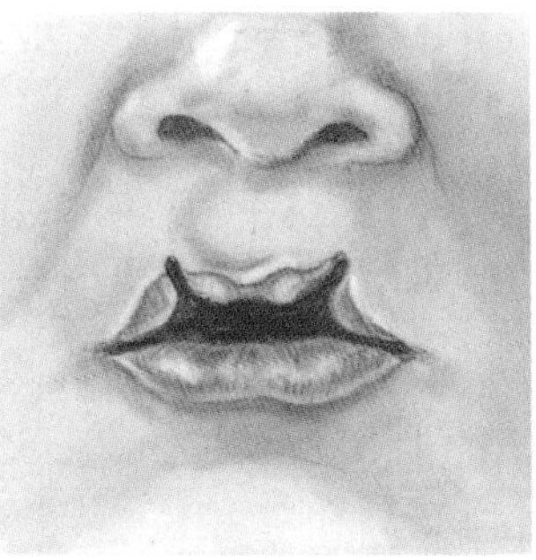

Unilateral cleft lip Bilateral cleft lip

Fig. 4.8 Two main types of cleft lip deformities, unilateral and bilateral clefts.

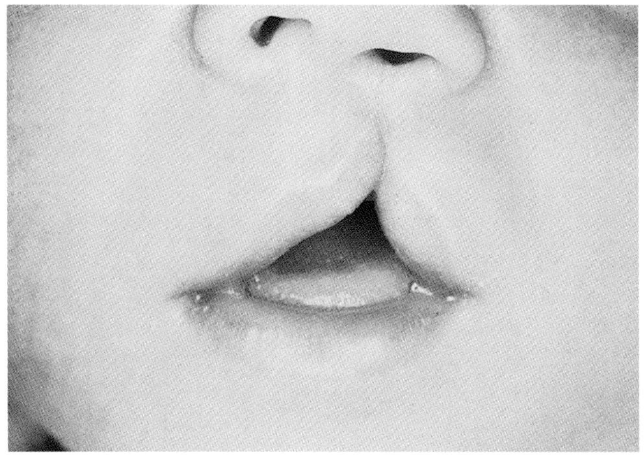

Fig. 4.9 Unilateral cleft lip that is located at the side of the midline of the oral cavity where the facial processes failed to fuse. (Courtesy of Margaret J. Fehrenbach, RDH, MS.)

(Fig. 4.10, *A*). The neck and its associated tissue develop from the primitive pharynx and the branchial (or pharyngeal) apparatus, which will be discussed in the next sections. Dental professionals must understand the development of the neck to relate its underlying structural relationships to any developmental disturbances that may be present.

PRIMITIVE PHARYNX FORMATION

The beginnings of the hollow tube of the embryo are derived from the anterior part of the foregut and will form the **primitive pharynx,** which is the future oral part of the pharynx or oropharynx (see Fig. 4.10, *B* and see Fig. 2.18). The foregut is originally derived from the endoderm embryonic cell layer (see Fig 3.14). The primitive pharynx widens cranially where it joins the primitive mouth or later the stomodeum and narrows caudally as it joins the esophagus. The endoderm of the pharynx lines the internal parts of the branchial (or pharyngeal) arches and passes into balloon-like areas of the pharyngeal pouches (discussed later in this chapter). However, this same endoderm does not come to line the oral cavity proper or nasal cavity. Instead, the oral cavity proper and nasal cavity are both lined by ectoderm as a result of embryonic folding.

The caudal part of the primitive pharynx forms the esophagus, which leads to the stomach. A ventral outgrowth forms the laryngopharynx, larynx, and trachea and ends in the superior part of the developing lungs. The developing thyroid gland is also an anterior outpouching or *evagination* from the ventral wall of the pharynx (see Fig. 11.14).

APPARATUS FORMATION

Discussed earlier, the **branchial apparatus** (**brang**-kee-uhl ap-uh-**rat**-uhs) or pharyngeal apparatus consists of arches, grooves and membranes, as well as pouches. There is a concerted effort by the medical profession that needs to be adopted also by the dental profession to move away from the use of the term *branchial* that refers to gills and use instead the term *pharyngeal* since our bodies do not have gills but do have a nearby pharynx.

During the fourth week of prenatal development, stacked bilateral swellings of tissue appear inferior to the stomodeum and include the mandibular arch. These are the pharyngeal or **branchial arches**, with the mandibular arch being the first pharyngeal or branchial arch and the other more inferior arches numbered in craniocaudal sequence (Fig. 4.11 and see Fig. 4.10, *A*). These pharyngeal or branchial arches consist of a total of six pairs of U-shaped bars of which the central core consists of mesenchyme derived from mesoderm invaded by NCCs, now referred to as *ectomesenchyme*. This neural-derived mesenchyme condenses to form a bar of cartilage in each arch. The pharyngeal or branchial arches are also covered externally by ectoderm and lined internally by endoderm that supports the lateral walls of the primitive pharynx. The oropharyngeal membrane divides the first arch into the stomodeum that is lined by ectoderm and the pharynx that is lined by endoderm.

The pharyngeal or branchial arches are located bilaterally in series along the anterior-posterior axis of the embryo and bend to support the lateral walls of the developing pharynx. It is important to note that the **fifth branchial arch** or pharyngeal arch is often so rudimentary that often it is absent or it may be included within the fourth branchial arch or pharyngeal arch. The pharyngeal or branchial arches will give rise to important structures of the face and neck (Table 4.2).

Each paired pharyngeal or branchial arch has its own developing cartilage, nerve, vascular, and muscular components within each mesenchymal core. The first two pairs of arches develop to the greatest extent of all the arches and are also the only ones specifically named. In general, these first two pairs of arches form the midface and lower face, respectively, and the lower four pairs of arches are involved in the formation of the structures of the neck.

The **first branchial arch** or pharyngeal arch, which is also known as the mandibular arch and its associated tissue were described earlier and include Meckel cartilage. Forming within the **second branchial arch** or pharyngeal arch, which is also known as the **hyoid arch,** is cartilage similar to that of the mandibular arch, **Reichert cartilage** (**ri**-kert). Most of it disappears during development; however, parts of it are responsible for a middle ear bone, a process of the temporal bone, and parts of the hyoid bone.

Additionally, the perichondrium surrounding Reichert cartilage gives rise to the ligament of the hyoid bone. The mesoderm of the hyoid arches helps form the muscles of facial expression, the middle ear muscles, and a suprahyoid muscle. Because these muscles are derived from the hyoid arches, these structures are all innervated by the nerve of the second arches, which is the facial nerve or seventh cranial nerve. The hyoid arches along with the third and fourth branchial or pharyngeal arches are also involved in formation of the tongue (see Fig. 5.9).

During the seventh week, the muscle cells from the mesoderm of the hyoid arches have begun to differentiate. These muscle cells then begin to migrate over the mandibular muscle masses. By the tenth week, the muscle cells have migrated superiorly all over the face, forming a thin sheet of muscle masses. Both superficial and deep groups of muscle fibers eventually develop from these muscle masses and become attached to the newly differentiating bones of the facial skeleton as the muscles of facial expression. The nerve from the facial nerve is incorporated early in these muscle masses.

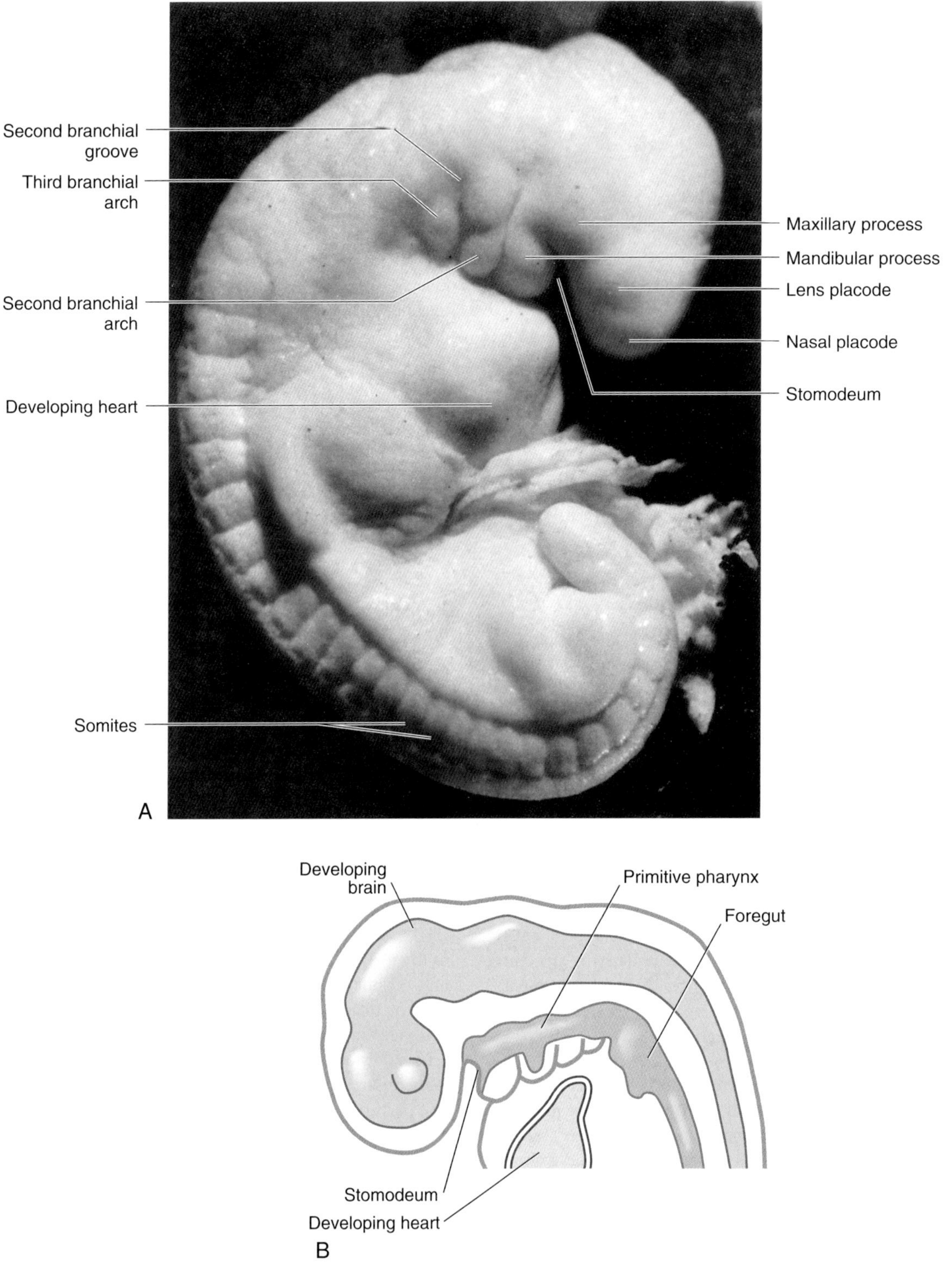

Fig. 4.10 Embryo During the Fourth Week of Prenatal Development. A, Photograph. **B,** Diagram. Internally, the foregut gives rise to the primitive pharynx, which will form the oropharynx. **(A,** Courtesy of K.V. Hinrichsen, MD, Medizinische Fakultät, Institut für Anatomie, Ruhr-Universität Bochum, Bochum.)

The **third branchial arch** or pharyngeal arch has an unnamed cartilage associated with it. This cartilage will be responsible for the formation of parts of the hyoid bone. The only muscle to be derived from the mesoderm of each third arch is a pharyngeal muscle. Each pair of arches is innervated by the glossopharyngeal nerve or ninth cranial nerve.

Both the **fourth branchial arch** or pharyngeal arch and the **sixth branchial arch** or pharyngeal arch also have unnamed cartilage associated with them. These arches fuse and participate in the formation of most of the laryngeal cartilages. The mesoderm of these arches is associated with the muscles of the larynx and pharynx. These structures are innervated by the ninth and tenth cranial nerves, although

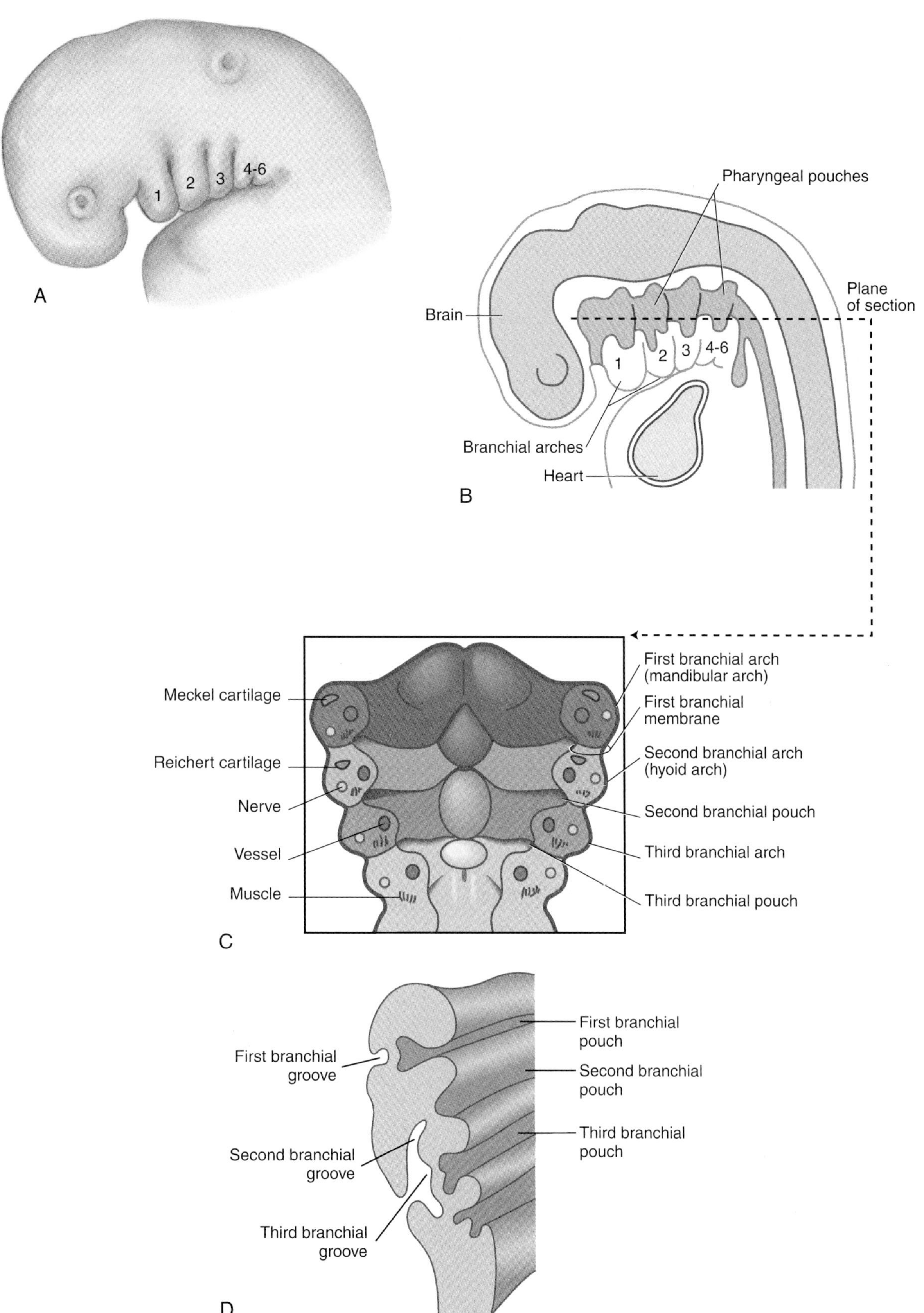

Fig. 4.11 Embryo During the Fourth Week of Prenatal Development. **A** to **D,** Diagrams of two sections with the six pharyngeal or branchial arches highlighted along with corresponding grooves and pouches.

TABLE 4.2 Arches and Derivative Structures

Arches	Future Nerves and Muscles	Future Skeletal Structures and Ligaments
First arches (or *mandibular arches*)	Trigeminal nerve, muscles of mastication, mylohyoid and anterior belly of digastric, tensor tympani, tensor veli palatini muscles	Malleus and incus of middle ear, including anterior ligament of the malleus, sphenomandibular ligament, and parts of sphenoid bone (see also Table 4.1)
Second arches (or *hyoid arches*)	Facial nerve, stapedius muscle, muscles of facial expression, posterior belly of digastric muscle, stylohyoid muscle	Stapes and parts of malleus and incus of middle ear, stylohyoid ligament, styloid process of temporal bone, lesser cornu of hyoid bone, upper part of body of hyoid bone
Third arches	Glossopharyngeal nerve, stylopharyngeal muscle	Greater cornu of hyoid bone, lower part of body of hyoid bone
Fourth through sixth arches	Superior laryngeal branch and recurrent laryngeal branch of vagus nerve, levator veli palatini muscles, pharyngeal constrictors, intrinsic muscles of larynx	Laryngeal cartilages

the nerves of these arches are branches of the vagus nerve or tenth cranial nerve.

The sensory innervation of the mucosa of the oral cavity, pharynx, and larynx also reflects the development of the pharyngeal or branchial arches. In summary, each pharyngeal or branchial arch is associated with a particular cranial nerve: for first arch it is the trigeminal or fifth cranial nerve; for the second cranial arch it is the facial or seventh cranial nerve; for the third arch it is the glossopharyngeal or ninth cranial nerve; for the fourth and sixth arches it is the vagus or tenth cranial nerve. In addition to supplying muscles, these cranial nerves also supply the sensory innervation to the mucosa in the area of the corresponding arch.

As a result, the oral cavity and the anterior two-thirds of the tongue formed from the first arch come to be supplied by the trigeminal nerves (see **Chapter 5**). The maxillary nerve supplies the structures formed in association with the maxillary process such as the nasal cavity and palate, while the more caudal regions are supplied by the mandibular nerve, the nerves of the mandibular processes.

The posterior one-third of the tongue and oropharynx receive their nerve supply from the glossopharyngeal nerves and the interior of the larynx with the laryngopharynx are supplied by the vagus nerves.

However, the facial nerve, the nerve of the second arch, does not supply the nasal or oral cavities or that of the pharynx with general sensory or motor innervation. It is thought that, around the time that the tuberculum impar and the copula fuse within the developing tongue, the tissue associated with the second arch are excluded from the interior of the primitive pharynx so that not any of mucosa is supplied by the facial nerve. An exception is the special sensory innervation of the anterior two-thirds of the tongue and the hard and soft palates, corresponding with taste. It important to note that the mucosa nerve supply is a complex subject and not easily mapped out even though some textbooks try.

TABLE 4.3 Pharyngeal Pouches and Derivative Structures

Pouches	Future Structures
First pouches	Tympanic membrane (with first branchial or pharyngeal groove), tympanic cavity, mastoid antrum, auditory (pharyngotympanic) tube
Second pouches	Crypts and lymphatic nodules of palatine tonsils
Third and fourth pouches	Parathyroid and thymus glands

Between neighboring arches, external grooves are noted on each side of the embryo. These are the pharyngeal or **branchial grooves** (see Fig. 4.11). Only the first groove, which is located between the first and second arches at approximately the same level as the first pharyngeal pouches, gives rise to a definitive mature structure of the head and neck (discussed later in this chapter).

To accomplish this the first groove becomes deeper to the extent that the ectoderm of the groove contacts the endoderm of the pharyngeal pouches. At this time, only a thin double-layered membrane, the first pharyngeal or branchial membrane, separates the groove from the pouches, although mesenchyme later separates these two layers. This membrane, with its three layers, develops into the tympanic membrane (or eardrum). Thus the first groove forms the external acoustic meatus. Other membranes appear in the bottom of each of the four grooves, although in contrast, they are only temporary structures.

By the end of the seventh week, the last four grooves are obliterated as a result of a sudden spurt of growth experienced by the pair of hyoid arches, which grow in an inferior direction and eventually form the neck. This obliteration of grooves gives the mature neck a smooth surface contour.

At the same time, four well-defined pairs of **pharyngeal pouches** (fuh-**rin**-jee-uhl) develop as endodermal evaginations from the lateral walls lining the pharynx (see Fig. 4.11). The pouches develop as balloon-like structures in a craniocaudal sequence between the arches. The fifth pharyngeal pouches are absent or rudimentary. Many structures of the face and neck are developed from the pharyngeal pouches (Table 4.3).

The first pharyngeal pouches form between the first and second branchial or pharyngeal arches and become the auditory (pharyngotympanic) tubes. The palatine tonsils are derived from the lining of the second pharyngeal pouches and also from the pharyngeal walls. The parathyroid glands and thymus gland are derived from the lining of the third and fourth pharyngeal pouches. Additionally, a part of the thymus gland is of ectodermal origin.

The processes concerning growth and development of the thymus gland are not complete with birth. The thymus is a relatively large lymphatic organ during the perinatal period and then later starts to diminish in relative size during puberty. By adulthood, the thymus located at the superior part of the breastbone is often scarcely recognizable; however, it still is functioning by secreting thymic hormones and by maturing T-cell lymphocytes (see Fig. 8.16).

Clinical Considerations for Branchial (or Pharyngeal) Apparatus Development

Most congenital malformations in the neck originate during transformation of the pharyngeal or branchial apparatus into its mature derivatives. Some of these are a result of the persistence of parts of the apparatus that usually disappear during development of the neck and its associated tissue.

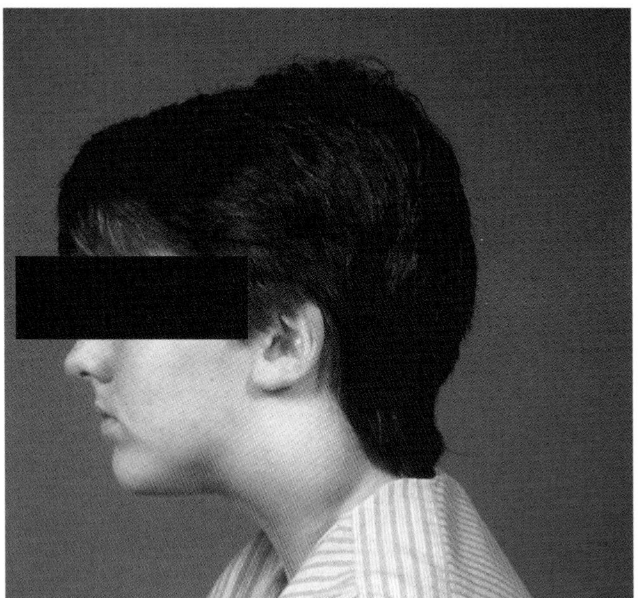

Fig. 4.12 A branchial cleft cyst from the second arch, which is associated with a slowly enlarging and painless swelling on the lateral surface of the neck. These large cysts often lie free in the neck just inferior to the angle of the mandible, but they may develop anywhere along the anterior border of the sternocleidomastoid muscle such as in this case. (Courtesy of Pierre Soucy, MD, Division of Paediatric Surgery, Children's Hospital of Eastern Ontario, Ottawa, Canada.)

The second pharyngeal or branchial grooves occasionally do not become obliterated and thus parts remain to form a **branchial cleft cyst** (Fig. 4.12). These cleft cysts may drain through pathologic sinuses along the neck but may also remain free in the lateral neck tissue just inferior to the angle of the mandible and anywhere along the anterior border of the sternocleidomastoid muscle. These cysts do not become apparent until they produce a slowly enlarging painless swelling that may be associated with small pits and skin tags that may involve fluid drainage from a sinus tract. The cyst is treated by surgical excision or, more recently, sclerotherapy.

5

Orofacial Development

Additional resources and practice exercises are provided on the companion Evolve website for this book: http://evolve.elsevier.com/Fehrenbach/illustrated.

LEARNING OBJECTIVES

1. Define and pronounce the key terms in this chapter.
2. Outline the events that occur during palatal development, describing each step of its formation.
3. Identify the structures present during palatal development on a diagram.
4. Integrate the study of palatal development into understanding the present structure and the clinical considerations due to developmental disturbances involved in palatal development.
5. Outline the events that occur during nasal cavity and nasal septum development.
6. Identify the structures present during nasal cavity and nasal septum development on a diagram.
7. Integrate the study of nasal cavity and nasal septum development into understanding the present structure.
8. Outline the events that occur during the tongue development, describing each step of its formation.
9. Identify the structures present during tongue development on a diagram.
10. Integrate the study of tongue development into understanding the present structure and the clinical considerations due to developmental disturbances involved in tongue development.

FURTHER OROFACIAL DEVELOPMENT

This chapter continues with embryonic orofacial development, starting from where the sequence left off with the development of the stomodeum, face, and neck in **Chapter 4** (see Figs. 4.1 and 4.2 and also Box 4.1). Thus this chapter discusses the development of the associated orofacial structures, including the palate, nasal septum, nasal cavity, and tongue, with tooth development being discussed in **Chapter 6**. The orofacial structures discussed in this chapter develop during the fourth week to the twelfth week of prenatal development, spanning the later part of the embryonic period and early part of the fetal period. However, the development of other orofacial structures (such as the jaws, temporomandibular joint, and salivary glands) is discussed with their associated histology in later chapters.

Dental professionals must have a clear understanding about the development of the oral structures to relate to their present structure as well as to any developmental disturbances that may be present.

PALATAL DEVELOPMENT

The formation of the palate, initially in the embryo and later in the fetus, takes place over several weeks of prenatal development (Table 5.1). The formation of the palate starts during the fifth week of prenatal development within the embryonic period from two separate embryonic structures, the primary palate and secondary palate. The final palate is then completed later during the twelfth week within the fetal period. The palate is developed in three consecutive stages, the formation of the primary palate, formation of the secondary palate, and completion of the final palate.

The completion of the final palate involves the fusion of swellings or tissue from *different* surfaces of the embryo to meet and join, similar to that of the fusion of the neural tube and the components of the upper lip (see Fig. 3.11). In contrast, most of the other structures of the orofacial region develop by the joining of swellings or tissue on the *same* surface of the embryo, which leads to the elimination of furrows between the facial processes (see Fig. 4.4).

PRIMARY PALATE FORMATION

During the fifth week of prenatal development and still within the embryonic period, the intermaxillary segment forms (Fig. 5.1, *A*). The intermaxillary segment arises as a result of fusion of the two medial nasal processes internally within the embryo (see Fig. 4.7). The intermaxillary segment is an internal wedge-shaped mass that extends inferiorly and deep to the nasal pits on the inside of the stomodeum. It initially serves as a partial floor of the nasal cavity and the nasal septum.

The intermaxillary segment also gives rise to the **primary palate** (or primitive palate). At this time, the primary palate also serves as only a partial separation between the developing oral cavity proper and the nasal cavity (see Fig. 5.1, *B*). In future development, the primary palate will form the premaxillary part of the maxilla, which is the anterior one-third of the hard palate. This smaller part of the hard palate is located anterior to the incisive foramen and will contain certain maxillary anterior teeth (incisors) (see Fig. 2.12). The formation of the primary palate completes the first stage of palate development.

SECONDARY PALATE FORMATION

During the sixth week of prenatal development, within the embryonic period, the bilateral maxillary processes give rise to two **palatal shelves** (or lateral palatine processes) (Figs. 5.2, 5.3, *A-B,* and 5.4). These shelves grow inferiorly and deep on the inside of the stomodeum in a vertical direction, along both sides of the developing tongue. The tongue is forming on the floor of the primitive pharynx at this time and as it grows, it initially fills the common nasal and oral cavity (tongue development is discussed later in this chapter).

As the developing tongue muscles begin to function, the tongue contracts and moves out of the way of these developing palatal shelves; thus the tongue avoids being an obstacle to the future fusion of the palatal shelves by moving both anteriorly and inferiorly. This process is aided by the growth of the lower jaw primordium. The movement of the tongue makes it now confined solely to the oral cavity proper and out of the developing nasal cavity, which is completed around the eighth week of prenatal development.

Because of unknown shelf-elevating forces the palatal shelves, after growing in a vertical direction, "flip" up in a superior direction within a few hours of the movement of the tongue. Thus the shelves move into a horizontal position, which is now superior to the developing tongue. Next, the two palatal shelves elongate and move medially toward each other meeting to join and then fusing to form the **secondary palate**.

The secondary palate will give rise to the posterior two-thirds of the hard palate, which contains certain maxillary anterior teeth (canines) and posterior teeth, all located posterior to the incisive foramen (Fig. 5.5). The secondary palate also gives rise to the soft palate and its uvula. The median palatine raphe within the mucosa lining and the associated deeper median palatine suture on the adult bone indicate the line of fusion of the palatal shelves. The formation of the secondary palate is completed during the second stage of palate development.

TABLE 5.1 Palatal Development

Time Period	Palatal Structures Involved
Fifth to sixth week	Primary palate: Intermaxillary segment from fused medial nasal processes
Sixth to twelfth week	Secondary palate: Fused palatal shelves from maxillary processes
Twelfth week	Final palate: Fusion of all three processes

PALATE COMPLETION

To complete the palate, the posterior part of the primary palate meets the secondary palate due to increased growth and these structures gradually fuse in an anterior to posterior direction (see Figs. 5.2, 5.3, *A-B,* and 5.4). When these three processes completely fuse, they form the final palate including the hard and soft palate, during the twelfth week of prenatal development. Now, the mature oral cavity becomes completely separated from the nasal cavity, which has begun to undergo development of its nasal septum (discussed next).

Bone formation (or ossification) has already begun in the anterior hard palate by the time palatal fusion is completed (see **Chapter 8**). In contrast in the more posterior soft palate, mesenchyme from the first and second pharyngeal or branchial arches migrates into the area to form the palatal muscles that will be involved in swallowing and speech (discussed later in this chapter).

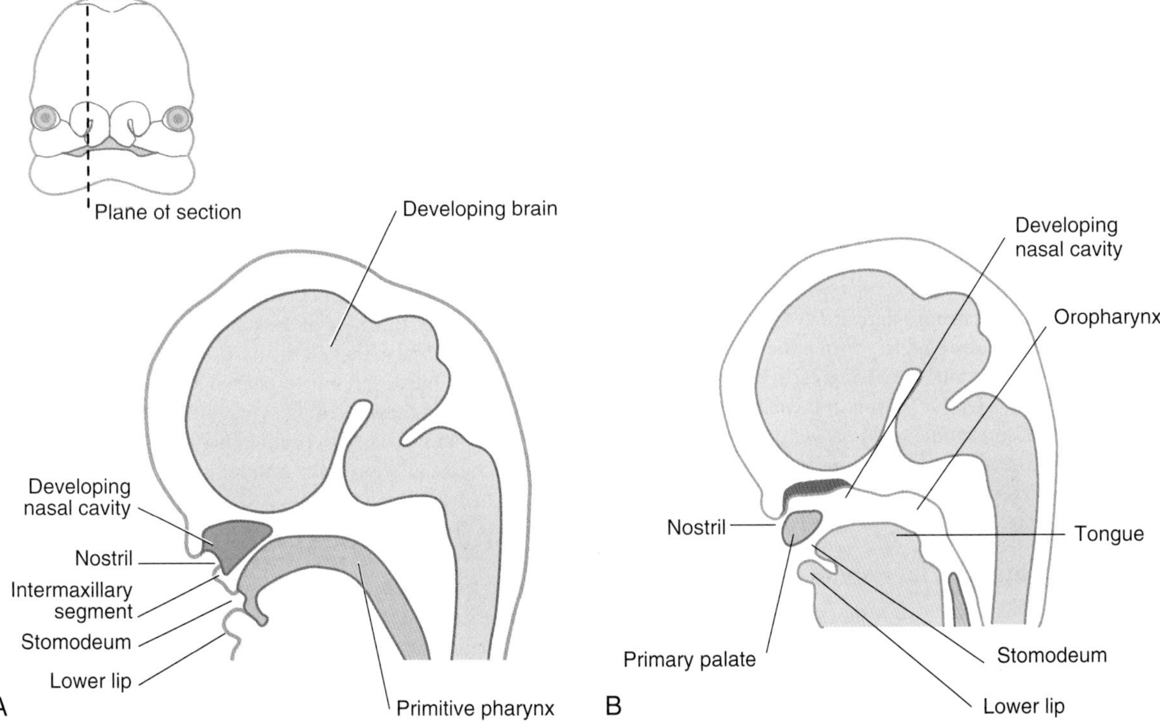

Fig. 5.1 Sagittal Sections of the Head Showing the Intermaxillary Segment. A, Formation of the intermaxillary segment from the fusion of the two medial nasal processes on the inside of the stomodeum of the embryo. **B,** Intermaxillary segment forms into the primary palate, which serves as a partial separation between the developing oral and nasal cavities.

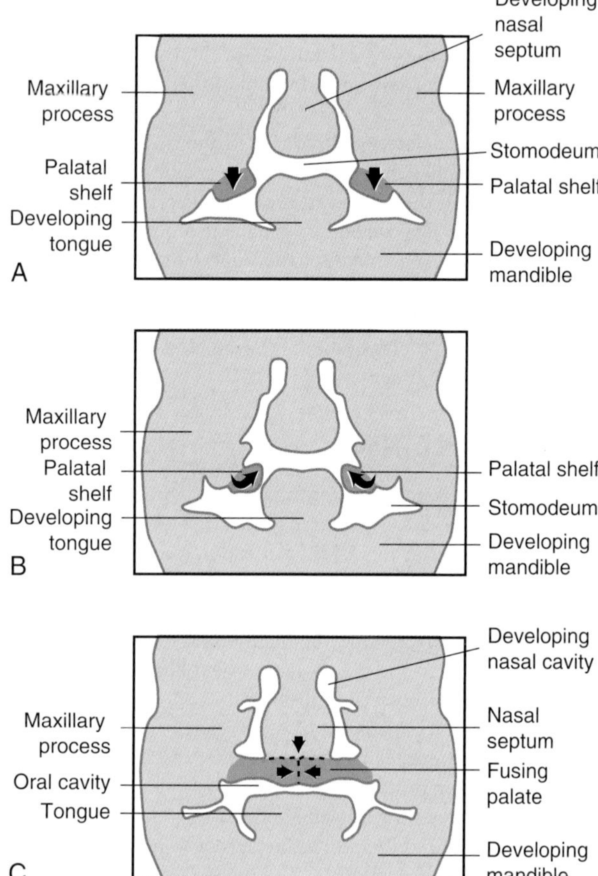

Fig. 5.2 Developing Palate is Highlighted in a Coronal Section Through the Developing Head. A, Palatal shelves formation from the maxillary process deep on the inside of the stomodeum. The growing shelves are vertical *(arrows)* and the position of the developing tongue is between the shelves. **B,** Palatal shelves grow in a horizontal direction toward each other after "flipping" in a superior direction *(arrows)* to form the secondary palate. **C,** Fusion of the three processes *(arrows)* to complete the final palate in the fetus, the primary palate with two palatal shelves to form the secondary palate.

The small paired nasopalatine canals persist after development near the median plane of the mature palate at the site of the junction of the primary palate and the secondary palate (see Fig. 5.5, *A-B*). These canals are represented in the mature hard palate by the incisive foramen beneath the surface incisive papilla, which is the common opening for the bilateral nasopalatine canals. An irregular suture extends from the incisive foramen to the alveolar process of the maxilla between the maxillary lateral incisor and canine teeth on each side. It demarcates where the primary and secondary palates fused. This bony fusion is completed within the first year of birth, with the overlying epithelium already fused by that time.

Clinical Considerations for Palatal Development

Failure of fusion of the palatal shelves with the primary palate and/or with each other results in **cleft palate** with varying degrees of disability (Fig. 5.6). This somewhat common disturbance may be hereditary or associated with environmental factors. Cleft palate occurs 1 or 2 in 1000 cases (about 1%). It may also be isolated or associated with other abnormalities, such as cleft lip (Fig. 5.7); however, it may involve only the soft palate or may extend through to the hard palate. Isolated forms of cleft palate are less common than cleft lip but are more common in women, unlike cleft lip, which is more common in men.

Complications with cleft palate can include difficulty with nursing or feeding the child, increased oronasal infections, and challenges with speech development and appearance. Treatment includes oral and plastic surgery with dental intervention; however, speech and hearing therapy may also be necessary. **Cleft uvula** is the least complicated form of cleft palate (Fig. 5.8). However, it may still cause **velopharyngeal insufficiency (VPI)** (vee-loh-fuh-**rin**-jee-uhl in-suh-**fish**-uhn-see), a disorder that prevents the *velum* or soft palate from closing against the posterior pharyngeal wall during speech in order to close off the nasal cavity, which is needed for the production of most of speech sounds. It can also occur with a history of other forms of cleft palate, irregular adenoids/adenoidectomy, cervical spine anomalies, or oral/pharyngeal tumor removal.

NASAL CAVITY AND SEPTUM DEVELOPMENT

The nasal cavity forms in the same time frame as the palate, from the fifth to twelfth week of prenatal development. It will later serve as part of the respiratory system (see Fig. 11.19). The future nasal septum of the nasal cavity is also developing when the palate is forming. The structure of the nasal septum, similar to the primary palate, is a growth from the fused medial nasal processes (see Figs. 5.2, 5.3, *A-B,* and 5.4). The tissue types that form the nasal septum will grow inferiorly and deep to the medial nasal processes and superior to the stomodeum.

The vertical nasal septum then fuses with the horizontally oriented final palate after it forms. This fusion begins in the ninth week and is completed by the twelfth week. With the formation of the nasal septum and final palate, the paired nasal cavity and the single oral cavity in the fetus become completely separate. The nasal cavity and the oral cavity also undergo development of different types of mucosa, such as respiratory mucosa and oral mucosa, respectively (see **Chapters 9 and 11**).

The developing nasal septum has considerable influence on determining the final orofacial form. It transmits septal growth "pull and thrust" to facial bones, such as the maxilla as it expands its vertical length, which is a dramatic sevenfold amount between the tenth week of prenatal development and subsequent birth.

TONGUE DEVELOPMENT

The tongue develops during the fourth to eighth weeks of prenatal development (Table 5.2). It develops from independent swellings located internally on the floor of the primitive pharynx that were formed by the first four pharyngeal or branchial arches (see Table 4.2).

Specifically, the body of the tongue develops from the first pharyngeal or branchial arch, and the base of the tongue originates later from the second, third, and fourth pharyngeal or branchial arches. The furrows between these swellings are eliminated by fusion similar to that on the facial surface with proliferation, migration, and merging of the mesenchyme inferior to the ectoderm into the furrows (see Fig. 4.4).

BODY OF TONGUE FORMATION

During the fourth week of prenatal development, within the embryonic period, the tongue begins its development. The tongue development begins as a triangular median swelling, the **tuberculum impar** (too-**ber**-kuh-luhm **im**-pahr) (or median tongue bud) (Fig. 5.9, *A-B*). The single tuberculum impar is located in the midline and is formed on the mandibular arch, which is considered the first pharyngeal or branchial arch, at the floor of the primitive pharynx within the embryo's conjoined nasal and oral cavities (see Fig. 4.11).

Later, two oval **lateral lingual swellings** (or distal tongue buds) develop on each side of the tuberculum impar (see Fig. 5.9, *A-B*). It is

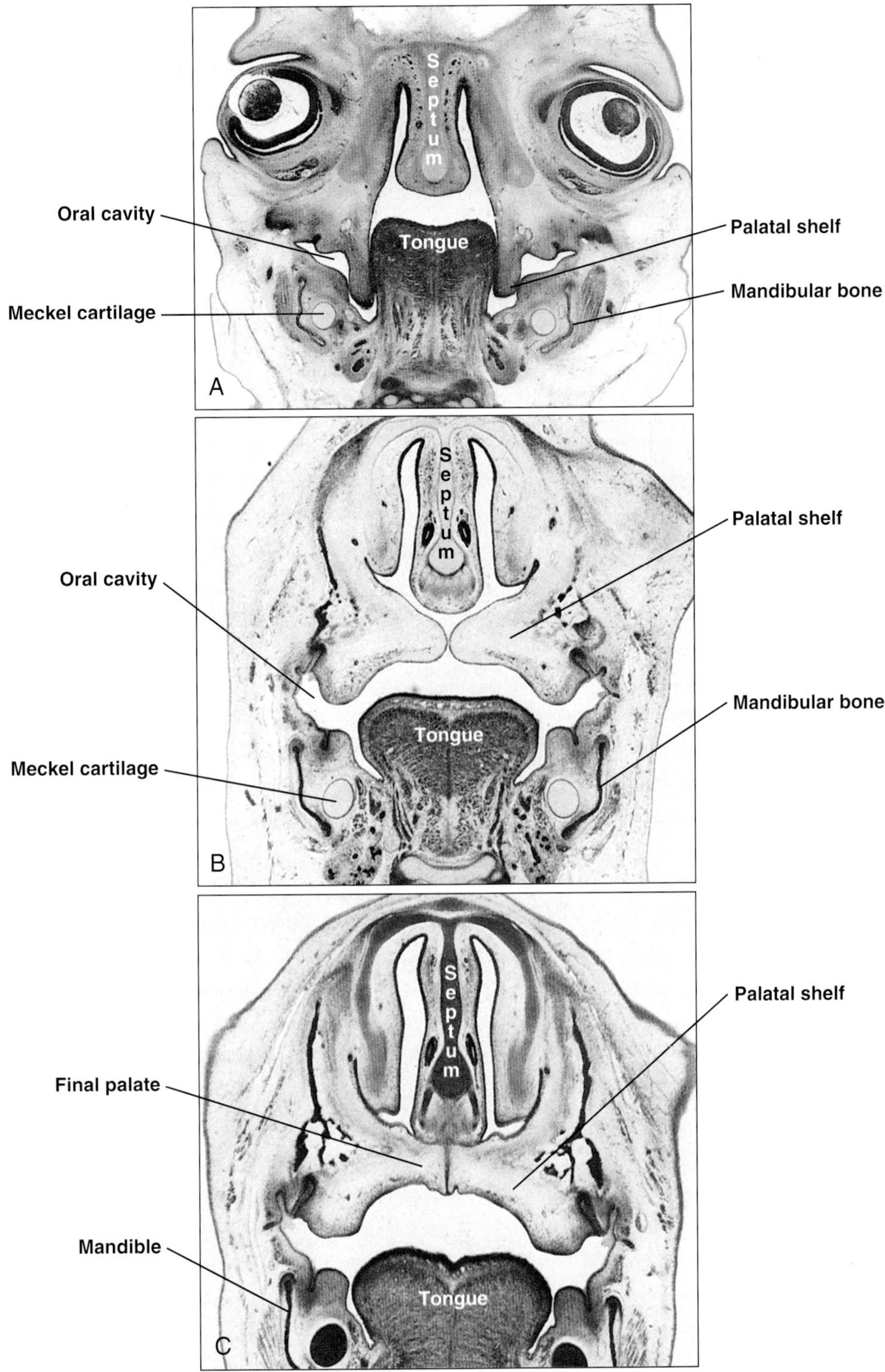

Fig. 5.3 Photomicrographs of the coronal section through the developing head showing the palatal shelves during the formation of the secondary palate at the seventh week (**A**) and then the ninth week (**B** and **C**). Note the position of the tongue, forming palate, and nasal septum (with its nasal cavity), which changes over time. The palatal shelves have moved into a horizontal position superior to the tongue and now a final palate will be fully completed with fusion and the nasal and oral cavities will be separate. The teeth in the future dental arches *(arrows)*, mandibular bone, and Meckel cartilage are also developing during this same time period. (From Nanci A. *Ten Cate's Oral Histology*. 9th ed. St. Louis: Elsevier; 2018 and adapted from Diewert VM. A morphometric analysis of craniofacial growth and changes in spatial relations during secondary palatal development in human embryos and fetuses. *Am J Anat*. 1983;167:495.)

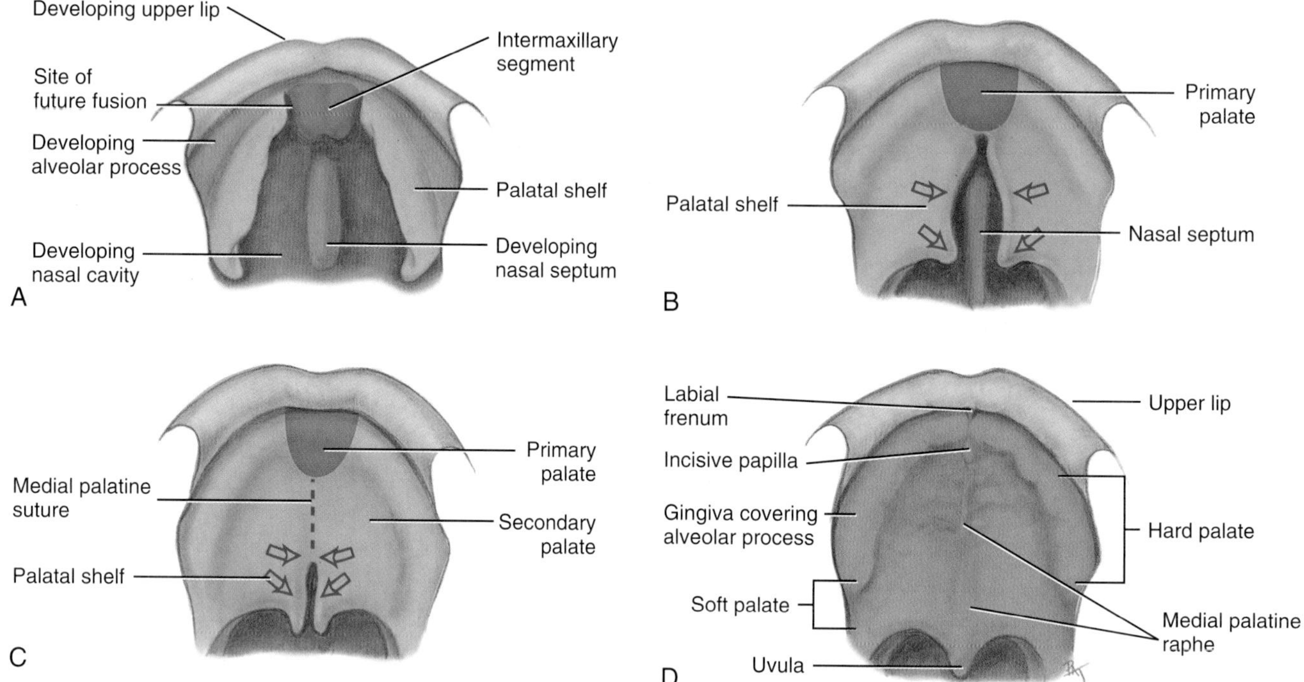

Fig. 5.4 Development of the Palate and Nasal Septum from an Inferior View. Early stages of development of both the palate with its palatal shelves and the intermaxillary segment **(A)**, formation of primary palate **(B)**, nasal septum fusion with the final palate **(C)** in order to separate the nasal and oral cavities completely **(D)**. Note that growth of the palatal shelves is indicated by *arrows* in **B** and **C** with their fusion from anterior to posterior.

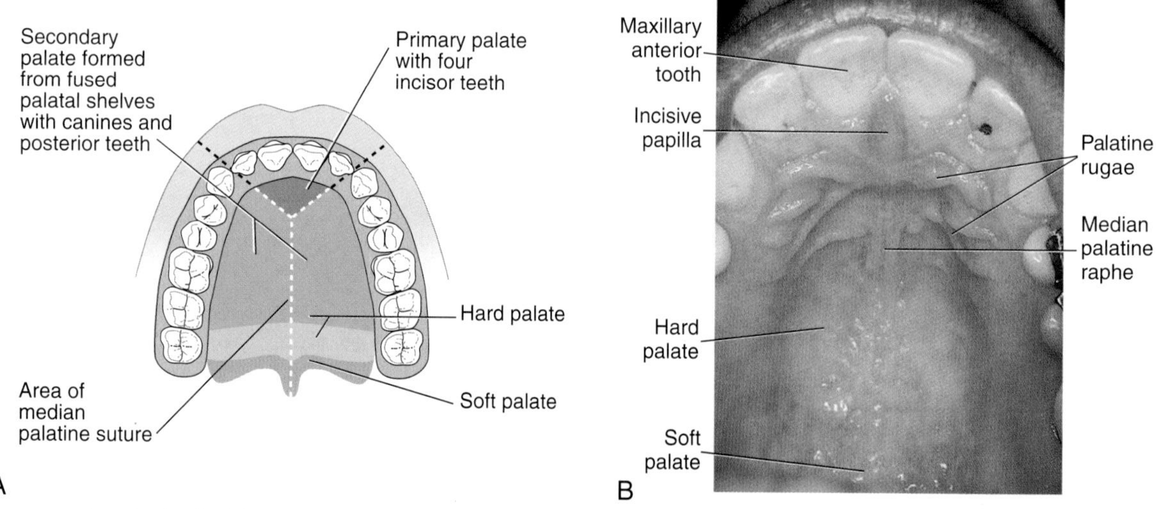

Fig. 5.5 Adult Palate with its Derivative Developmental Structures, Such as the Permanent Teeth. A, Diagram with suture areas highlighted *(dashed lines)*. **B,** Mature palate with associated embryologic landmarks. (**B,** Courtesy of Margaret J. Fehrenbach, RDH, MS.)

important to note that these anterior swellings are from the further growth of mesenchyme of the mandibular arch. The paired lateral lingual swellings grow in size and merge with each other.

Then the two fused swellings overgrow and encompass the disappearing tuberculum impar to form the anterior two-thirds of the mature tongue, the body of the tongue, which lies within the oral cavity proper. The median lingual sulcus is a superficial demarcation of the line of fusion of the two lateral lingual swellings as well as of a deeper fibrous structure (see Fig. 2.14). Thus the tuberculum impar itself does not form any recognizable part of the mature tongue. Around the

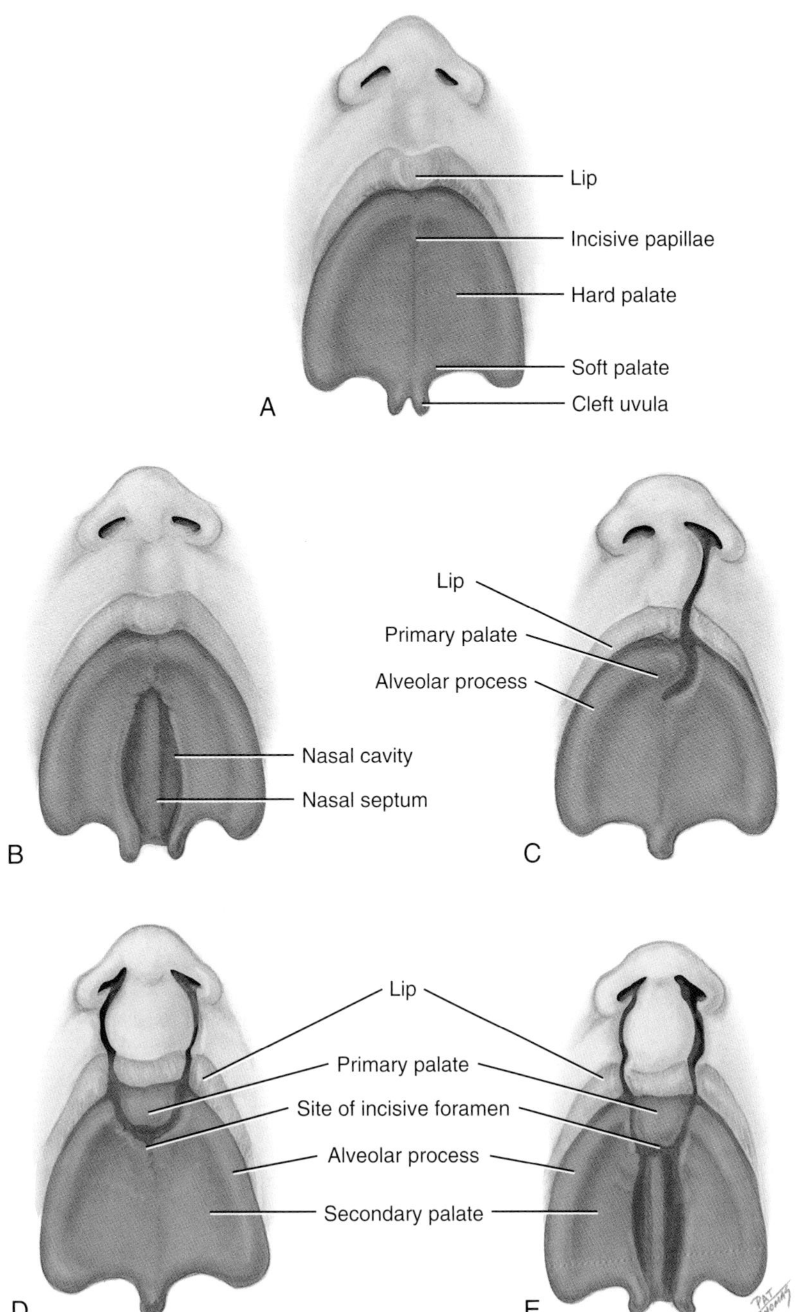

Fig. 5.6 Various Degrees of Cleft Palate. **A,** Cleft uvula. **B,** Bilateral cleft of the posterior palate. **C,** Complete unilateral cleft of the lip and alveolar process of the maxilla with a unilateral cleft of the primary palate. **D,** Complete bilateral cleft of the lip and alveolar process with bilateral cleft of the primary palate. **E,** Complete bilateral cleft of the lip and alveolar process with complete bilateral cleft of both the primary and secondary palates.

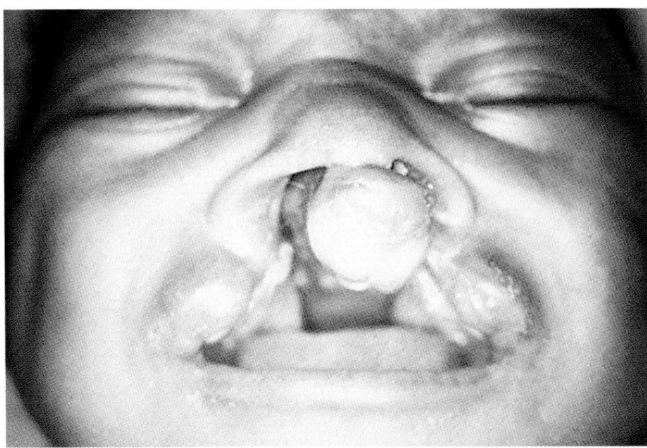

Fig. 5.7 Complete bilateral cleft of the lip and alveolar process with complete bilateral cleft of both the primary and secondary palates with nasal cavity involvement. (Courtesy of Margaret J. Fehrenbach, RDH, MS.)

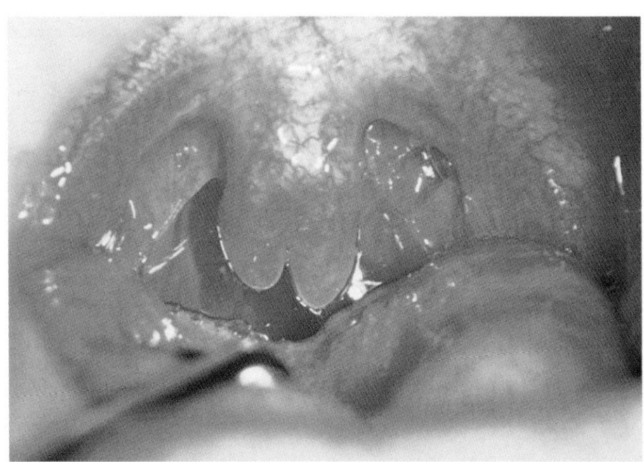

Fig. 5.8 Cleft uvula, which is the least complicated form of cleft palate. (Courtesy of Margaret J. Fehrenbach, RDH, MS.)

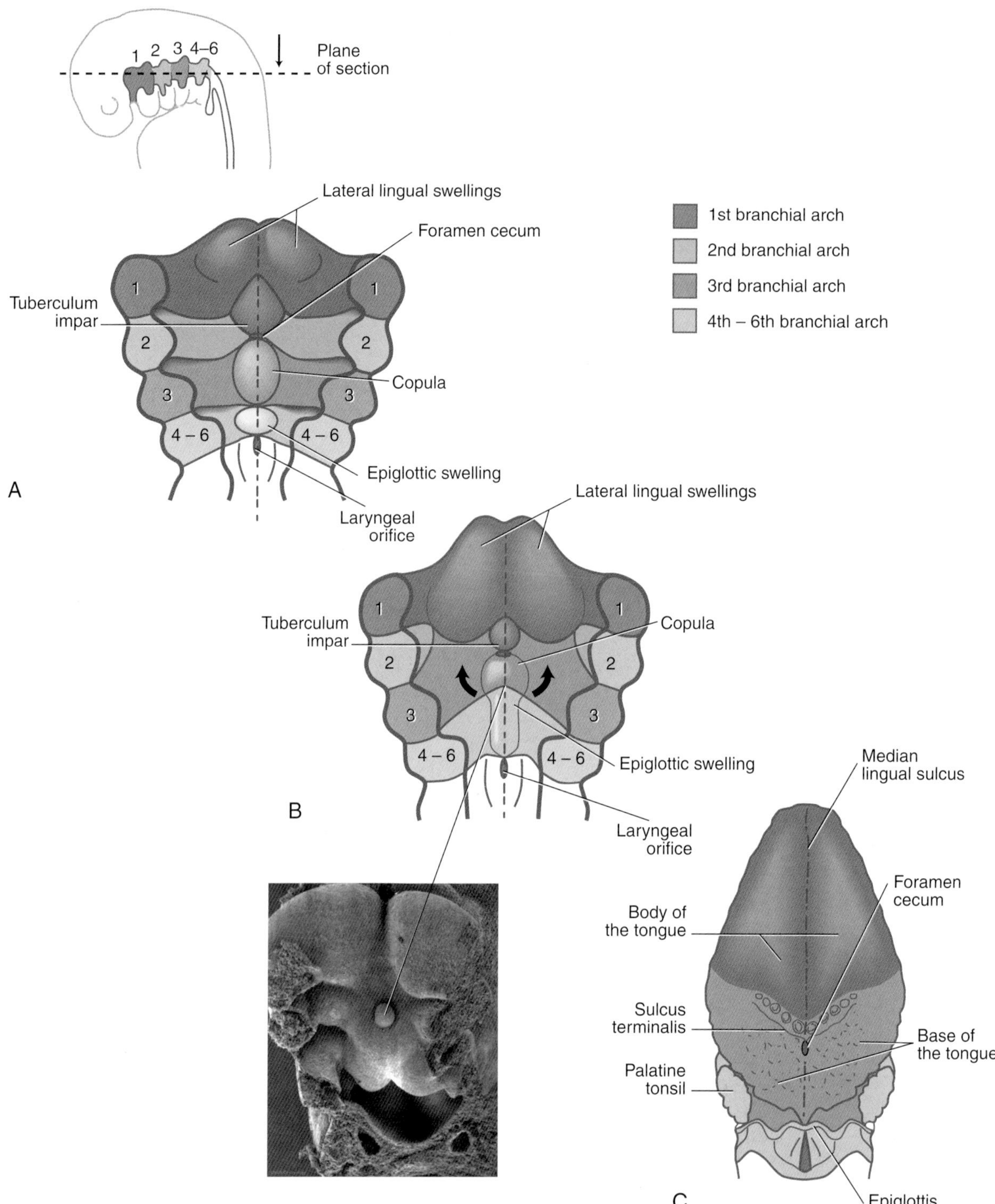

Fig. 5.9 Diagram of the Development of the Tongue with Derivations from the Pharyngeal or Branchial Arches Highlighted. **A,** Tuberculum impar and lateral lingual swellings forming the body of the tongue. **B,** Copula and its involvement forming the base of the tongue *(arrows)* along with a scanning electron microgram of the head region showing internal detail of pharyngeal arches forming the tongue. **C,** Final fusion of the anterior swellings and the posterior swellings to complete the tongue. (**B,** Scan courtesy of Mark Hill, BSc, PhD, UNSW Embryology, Sydney, Australia.)

TABLE 5.2 Tongue Development

Time Period	Tongue Structures Involved
Fourth to eighth weeks	Body: Tuberculum impar and lateral lingual swellings appear
	Base: Copula overgrowing second pharyngeal or branchial arches
Eighth week	Completed tongue: Merging of anterior swellings of body and copula of base

lingual swellings, the cells degenerate forming a sulcus, which frees the body of the tongue from the floor of the mouth, except for the attachment of the midline lingual frenum (see Fig. 2.17).

BASE OF TONGUE FORMATION

Immediately posterior to these fused anterior swellings, the **copula** (**kop**-yuh-luh) becomes evident (see Fig. 5.9, *B*). The single midline copula is mostly formed from the fusion of the mesenchyme of the third and parts of the fourth pharyngeal or branchial arch. The copula gradually overgrows the hyoid arch, which is considered the second pharyngeal or branchial arch. This overgrowth will form the posterior one-third of the mature tongue, the base of the tongue.

Even farther posterior to the copula is the projection of a third median swelling, the **epiglottic swelling** (ep-i-**glot**-ik), which develops from the mesenchyme of the posterior parts of the fourth pharyngeal or branchial arches (see Fig. 5.9, *B*). This swelling marks the development of the most posterior region of the tongue and site of the future epiglottis.

COMPLETION OF TONGUE FORMATION

As the tongue develops still further, the copula of the tongue base after overgrowing the second arch merges with the anterior swellings of the first arch of the tongue body during the eighth week of prenatal development (see Fig. 5.9, *C*). This fusion is superficially demarcated by the sulcus terminalis on the mature dorsal surface of the tongue, which is an inverted V-shaped groove marking the border between the base of the tongue and its body (see Fig. 2.14).

The sulcus terminalis points backward toward the oropharynx at a small pit-like depression, the foramen cecum, which is the beginning of the thyroglossal duct. This duct shows the origin of the thyroid gland and the migration pathway of the thyroid gland into the neck region. It forms an open connection between the initial area of thyroid gland development and its final location. This duct later closes off and becomes obliterated before birth unless it undergoes cystic transformation (see Fig. 11.14). However, no similar anatomic landmark is found between the base of the tongue and the epiglottic region after development.

By the end of the eighth week, the tongue has completed the fusion of these swellings. The tongue then contracts and moves anteriorly and inferiorly to avoid becoming an obstacle to the developing palatal shelves. However, the entire tongue is in the oral cavity proper at birth; its base and epiglottic region later descend into the oropharynx by 4 years of age, while the body remains in the oral cavity proper. Thus the tongue moves out of the pharynx into its proper place in the oral cavity proper. The tongue usually doubles in length, breadth, and thickness between birth and puberty, which is when it reaches its maximum size.

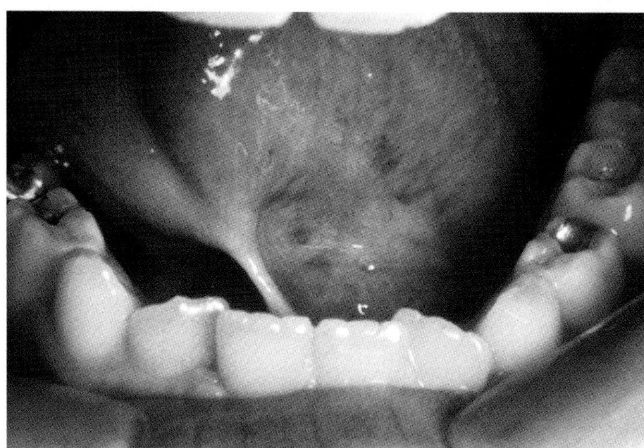

Fig. 5.10 Ankyloglossia resulting from a short attachment of the lingual frenum that extends to the tongue apex. (Courtesy of Margaret J. Fehrenbach, RDH, MS.)

The intrinsic muscles of the tongue are believed to originate from the mesoderm of the occipital somites and not from the pharyngeal or branchial arches (see Fig. 3.13). Primitive muscle cells from these somites migrate into the developing tongue, taking their motor nerve supply from the hypoglossal nerve or twelfth cranial nerve. Reviewing the discussion in this part of the chapter explains how the single structure of the tongue is innervated by various cranial nerves (V, VII, IX, X, and XII). This is because the tongue develops from the first four pairs of pharyngeal or branchial arches, each with its own cranial nerve and the occipital somites. See **Chapter 4** for further discussion of the development of the innervation of the mucosa of the oral cavity, pharynx, and larynx.

The lingual papillae, small elevated structures of specialized mucosa on the dorsal surface, appear toward the end of the eighth week (see Figs. 2.14 and 9.16 to 9.20). The circumvallate and foliate lingual papillae appear first, close to the terminal branches of the glossopharyngeal nerve or ninth cranial nerve. The fungiform lingual papillae appear later, near the terminations of the chorda tympani branches of the facial nerve or seventh cranial nerve. Finally, the filiform lingual papillae develop during the early fetal period, which comprises the tenth to eleventh weeks.

The taste buds involved in taste sensation and that are associated with certain lingual papillae (circumvallate, foliate, and fungiform) develop during the eleventh to thirteenth weeks by inductive interaction between the epithelial cells of the tongue and invading nerve cells from the chorda tympani of the facial nerve or seventh cranial nerve as well as the glossopharyngeal nerve or ninth cranial nerve.

Clinical Considerations for Tongue Development

Abnormalities of the tongue are uncommon. However, one type that is more common than others is **ankyloglossia** (ang-kuh-lo-**glaw**-see-uh), sometimes described as "tongue-tied," which results from a short attachment of the lingual frenum that extends to the tongue apex (Fig. 5.10). This restricts the movement of the tongue to varying degrees and may be associated with other craniofacial abnormalities.

However, the tight lingual frenum usually stretches with time and use (see Fig. 2.17). If it has not adjusted over time and with movement is still not functional, orofacial myofunctional therapy (OMT) may be attempted before surgically cutting the lingual frenum is considered (see **Chapter 20**).

6

Tooth Development and Eruption

Additional resources and practice exercises are provided on the companion Evolve website for this book: http://evolve.elsevier.com/Fehrenbach/illustrated.

LEARNING OBJECTIVES

1. Define and pronounce the key terms in this chapter.
2. Outline the five stages of tooth development.
3. Integrate the study of tooth development into understanding the present tooth anatomy and the clinical considerations due to developmental disturbances.
4. Outline the process of root development.
5. Integrate the study of root development into understanding the present tooth anatomy and the clinical considerations due to developmental disturbances.
6. Discuss periodontal ligament and alveolar process development.
7. Identify the structures present during tooth crown and root development as well as the periodontal ligament and alveolar process development on a diagram.
8. Outline the events that occur during tooth eruption.
9. Identify the structures present during tooth eruption on a diagram.
10. Integrate the study of tooth eruption into understanding the present tooth anatomy and the clinical considerations due to developmental disturbances.

TOOTH DEVELOPMENT

Odontogenesis (oh-don-tuh-**jen**-uh-sis) is the process of tooth development. Dental professionals must have a clear understanding of the stages of odontogenesis and the physiologic basis of each stage. Developmental disturbances can occur within each stage of odontogenesis, affecting the physiologic processes taking place. These developmental disturbances can have ramifications that may affect the dental care of a patient.

The term **dentition** (den-**tish**-uhn) is used to describe the natural teeth in the jaws (see **Chapter 15**). There are two dentitions, the primary dentition and the permanent dentition. The **primary dentition** of a child develops during the prenatal period and consists of 20 teeth, which erupt and are later shed (or exfoliated) (see **Chapter 18**). As the primary teeth are shed and the jaws grow and mature, the **permanent dentition** consisting of as many as 32 teeth gradually erupts and replaces the primary dentition (see **Chapters 16 and 17**). Overlapping between the primary and permanent dentition is a transitional time period in a preteen presenting with a mixed dentition, having some teeth from both dentitions (see Figs. 15.4 and 18.17).

This chapter initially focuses on the development of the primary dentition and then its eruption and shedding. The final discussion centers on the eruption of the permanent dentition. The process of development for both dentitions is similar; only the associated time frame for each is different. The overall general dental anatomy associated with both these dentitions as well as dentition periods is discussed further in **Chapter 15**.

Odontogenesis takes place in stages, which occur in a sequential fashion for both dentitions (Table 6.1). Odontogenesis is a continuous process until completed having no clear-cut beginning or end point between stages. However, these stages are used to help focus on the different events in odontogenesis and are based on overall the shape of the developing structures. After initiation of odontogenesis, the initial identifiable stages in tooth development include the bud stage, the cap stage, and the bell stage. Odontogenesis then progresses to the apposition stage with the formation of the partially mineralized dental tissue types, such as enamel, dentin, and cementum, and then finally to the maturation stage for these structures through continued mineralization (Table 6.2).

During these stages of odontogenesis, many physiologic processes occur. In many ways, these parallel the processes that occur in the formation of other embryonic structures, such as the face. These physiologic processes include induction, proliferation, differentiation, morphogenesis, and maturation (see Table 3.3). Except for the induction processes between cells, many of these processes overlap but still are also mostly continuous during odontogenesis. However, one individual process does tend to be predominant, specially marking each stage of odontogenesis (see Table 6.1).

The molecular aspect of tooth development is interesting in that it shares many similarities with development of a number of other organs (e.g., lung and kidney) and that of the limbs. Interestingly, many of these pathways result from *epithelial-mesenchymal interactions* in which essentially the same molecular mediators are implicated.

In the past, the study of odontogenesis included a discussion of *developmental lobes* that were thought to be growth centers during tooth development. These parts of the crown of the tooth are both microscopically and clinically visible by the presence of associated depressions. Whether there may be any justification for including them in a discussion of tooth formation remains controversial; developmental lobes may simply be evidence of the tooth form only. For completeness, information concerning developmental lobes is included in this textbook in **Unit 4**.

Not all the teeth in each dentition begin to develop at the same time across each arch of the jaws. The initial teeth for both dentitions develop in the mandibular anterior region, followed later by the maxillary anterior region, and then development progresses posteriorly in

TABLE 6.1 Tooth Development Stages

Stage and Time Span*	Microscopic Structure	Main Processes	Histologic Features
Initiation stage at sixth to seventh week		Induction	Ectoderm lining stomodeum gives rise to oral epithelium and then to dental lamina with its dental placodes; adjacent to deeper ectomesenchyme, which is derived from neural crest cells. Both tissue types are separated by basement membrane
Bud stage at eighth week		Proliferation	Growth of dental placode into bud shape that penetrates growing ectomesenchyme
Cap stage at ninth to tenth week		Proliferation, differentiation, morphogenesis	Formation of tooth germ as enamel organ forms into cap shape that surrounds inside mass of dental papilla, with outside mass of dental sac, both from ectomesenchyme
Bell stage at eleventh to twelfth week		Proliferation, differentiation, morphogenesis	Differentiation of enamel organ into bell shape with four cell types and dental papilla into two cell types
Apposition stage at various times		Induction, proliferation	Dental tissue types secreted in successive layers as matrix
Maturation stage at various times		Maturation	Dental tissue types fully mineralize to mature form

*Note that these are approximate prenatal time spans for the development of the primary dentition.

both jaws. This posterior progression of odontogenesis allows time for both the upper and lower jaws to grow to accommodate the increased number of primary teeth, the larger primary molars, and then finally the overall larger permanent teeth.

The primary dentition develops during both the embryonic period and fetal period of prenatal development. Most of the permanent dentition is formed during the fetal period. Tooth development continues for years after birth, especially considering the later formation of the permanent second and third molars (see **Unit 4** and **Appendix D** for tooth development timelines). Thus, the teeth have the longest developmental period of any set of organs in the body.

TABLE 6.2 Dental Hard Tissue

	Enamel	Dentin	Cementum	Alveolar Process
Embryologic background	Enamel organ	Dental papilla	Dental sac	Dental sac
Tissue source or type	Epithelium	Connective tissue	Connective tissue	Connective tissue
Formative cells	Ameloblasts	Odontoblasts	Cementoblasts	Osteoblasts
Incremental lines	Lines of Retzius	Imbrication lines of von Ebner	Arrest and reversal lines	Arrest and reversal lines
Mature cells	None, all lost within reduced enamel epithelium with eruption	None within, only dentinal tubules with processes found instead in pulp	Cementocytes	Osteocytes
Resorptive cells	None per se; cells secrete proteinases	Odontoclasts	Odontoclasts	Osteoclasts
Inorganic material levels (approximate)	96%	70%	65%	60%
Organic material and water levels (approximate)	1% organic, 3% water	20% organic, 10% water	23% organic, 12% water	25% organic, 15% water
Regeneration after eruption	None; only may undergo remineral-ization	Possible	Possible	Possible
Vascularity	None	None	None	Present
Innervation	None	Possibly present within dentinal tubule, found instead in pulp	None	Present

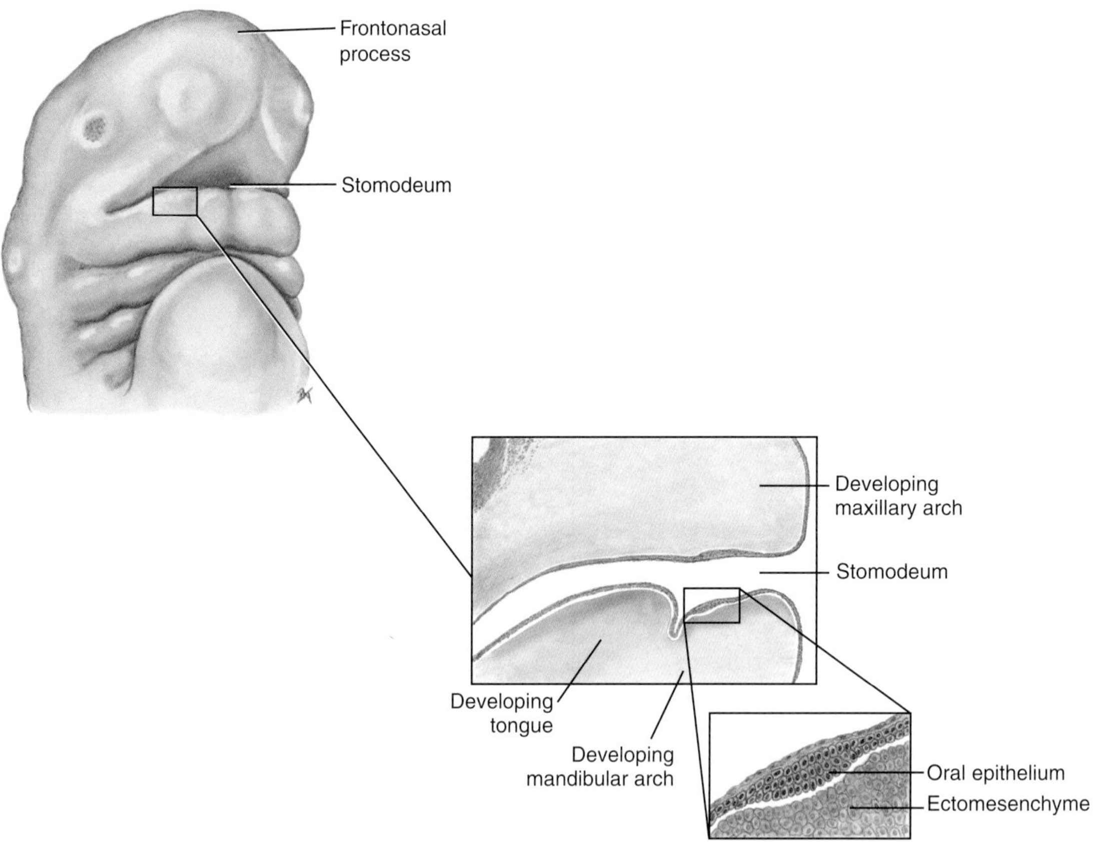

Fig. 6.1 Initiation stage of odontogenesis of the primary teeth on cross section within the developing mandibular arch. The stomodeum is now lined by oral epithelium, with the deeper ectomesenchyme derived from neural crest cells. A similar situation is occurring in the maxillary arch.

INITIATION STAGE

Odontogenesis of the primary dentition begins between the sixth and seventh week of prenatal development, during the embryonic period (Fig. 6.1). This first stage of tooth development, known as the **initiation stage**, involves the physiologic process of induction, which is an active interaction between the embryologic tissue types. Studies show that ectodermal tissue must influence the mesenchymal tissue in order to initiate odontogenesis, but the exact mechanisms are unknown at this time. Tooth initiation involves an initial signal from the ectoderm to the mesenchyme. The mesenchyme responds by reciprocally inducing the ectoderm to continue the developmental progression.

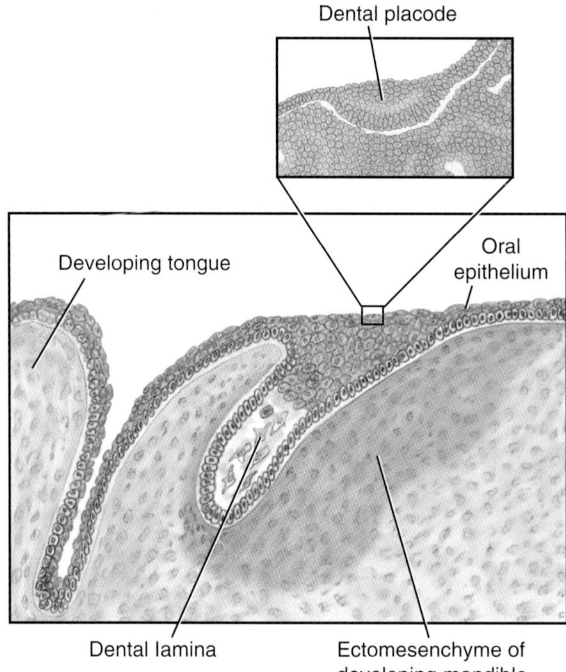

Fig. 6.2 Development of the dental lamina from the oral epithelium lining the mandibular arch. In addition, within the dental lamina, the dental placodes are forming where primary teeth will later form during the initiation stage, which is surrounded by ectomesenchyme. A similar situation is also occurring in the maxillary arch.

At the beginning of the sixth week, the stomodeum of the embryo (or primitive mouth) is lined by ectoderm (see **Chapter 4**). The outer part of the ectoderm gives rise to **oral epithelium** (ep-uh-**thee**-lee-um) (plural, **epithelia** [ep-uh-**thee**-lee-uh]). The oral epithelium initially consists of two horseshoe-shaped bands of tissue at the surface of the stomodeum, one band for each future dental arch. At the same time, deep to the forming oral epithelium there is a type of mesenchyme known as **ectomesenchyme** (ek-toh-**mes**-eng-kahym), which is derived from neural crest cells (NCCs) that have migrated to the region (see Fig. 6.1).

Dental professionals need to consider the importance of NCCs. In addition to assisting in the formation of the cranial sensory ganglia, they also differentiate to form most of the connective tissue of the head. Embryonic connective tissue for most of the rest of the body is derived from mesoderm and is known as *mesenchyme,* whereas in the head it is ectomesenchyme, reflecting its origin from neuroectoderm (see **Chapters 3 and 4**). The proper migration of NCCs is essential for the development of the head and neck as well as the teeth. All the tissue of the mature tooth (except enamel and certain types of cementum) and its supporting periodontium are directly derived from NCCs and any complication in the formation of these influencing cells prevents proper dental development (see Fig. 3.16 of Treacher Collins syndrome [TCS]).

An important acellular structure that separates the oral epithelium and the ectomesenchyme within the stomodeum is the basement membrane. The basement membrane involved here is similar to the one separating all epithelium and connective tissue (see Fig. 8.4).

During the latter part of the seventh week, the oral epithelium grows deeper, penetrating the ectomesenchyme and is induced to produce an adjoining layer, the **dental lamina** (**lam**-uh-nah) (Fig. 6.2). This growth occurs in each of the developing jaws where the two future curved dental arches of the primary dentition will form. The dental lamina begins to form initially in the midline for both arches and progresses posteriorly. The underlying ectomesenchyme also begins to undergo changes.

At this time there are also **dental placodes** forming within each dental lamina, which resemble morphologically, as well as in their molecular regulation, the placodes found during the development of other ectodermal organs, such as the lens, otic, and nasal placodes (see **Chapter 4**). Each dental placode consist of plate-like thickened epithelium associated with an underlying neural crest derived mesenchyme or neuroectoderm. They function as the first signaling centers of the tooth (the enamel knot discussed later is the second). There is a molecular crosstalk dialogue between oral ectoderm and odontogenic mesenchyme during tooth development.

Clinical Considerations with Initiation Stage Disturbances

Lack of initiation within the dental placode within the dental lamina results in the absence of a single tooth or multiple teeth (partial) or an entire dentition (complete), producing **anodontia** (an-uh-**don**-shee-uh) (or hypodontia) (Box 6.1, *A-B*). However, partial anodontia is more common and most commonly occurs with the permanent third molar, maxillary lateral incisor, and mandibular second premolar (listed in order of occurrence). Anodontia can be associated with the syndrome of ectodermal dysplasia because many components of the tooth germ are indirectly or directly of ectodermal origin (see Fig. 3.15).

Anodontia can also result from endocrine dysfunction, systemic disease, and exposure to excess radiation, such as that in radiation therapy used with cancer treatment. These cases may have disruption of occlusion, along with esthetic complications. Patients may need tooth replacement in the form of partial or full dentures, bridges, and/or implants. If severe, it can result in complete disruption of the development of the jaws.

In contrast, abnormal initiation may result in the development of one or more extra teeth, which are considered **supernumerary teeth** (soo-per-**noo**-muh-rer-ee) (or hyperdontia) (see Box 6.1, *C-D*). These extra teeth are initiated from persisting dental placodes within the dental lamina and have a hereditary etiology. Certain regions of both dentitions have an increased risk of having supernumerary teeth (listed in order of occurrence), such as between the maxillary central incisors (or mesiodens, see **Chapter 16**), distal to the maxillary third molars (or distomolar, a "fourth molar"), and in the premolar region (or perimolar) of both dental arches (see **Chapter 17**). They are smaller tooth forms than are usually present and most are accidentally discovered on radiographic examination. These extra teeth may be either erupted or nonerupted, and in both cases may cause dentition displacement, crowding, and delayed eruption to the adjacent teeth as well as occlusal disruption. Thus removal by surgery is often necessary and/or orthodontic therapy.

Smaller-than-normal placodes lead to missing and microdontic teeth, whereas larger placodes induce supernumerary and macrodontic teeth. However, all of the data so far show that there is no single gene that is directly connected with odontogenesis or the lack of any specific tooth. Instead, tooth initiation and morphogenesis occur by an orchestration of numerous genetic and epigenetic factors. At the same time, most of the developmental defects in teeth usually occur as a result of mutations in genes encoding signaling molecules and transcription factors.

BOX 6.1 Common Dental Developmental Disturbances with Involved Developmental Stage*

Initiation Stage

Disturbance: Anodontia, partial or complete

Description: Absence of permanent or primary teeth commonly includes permanent third molar, maxillary lateral incisor **(A)**, second premolar **(B)** with partial anodontia

Etiologic factors: Hereditary, endocrine dysfunction, systemic disease, excess radiation exposure prevents tooth germ(s) formation

Clinical ramifications: Disruption of occlusion and esthetic complications treated by prosthetic replacement with partial or full dentures, bridges, and/or implants

Absent permanent maxillary lateral incisor

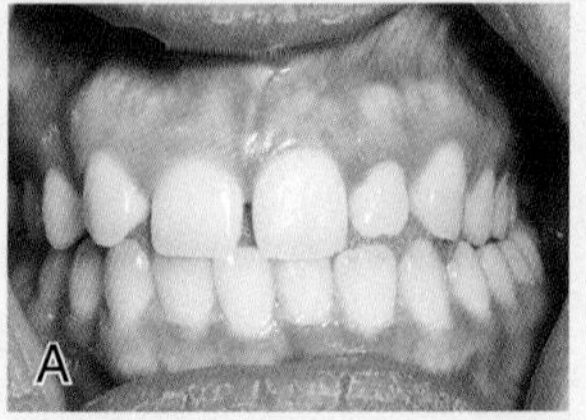

Absent permanent mandibular second premolar with retained primary mandibular second molar

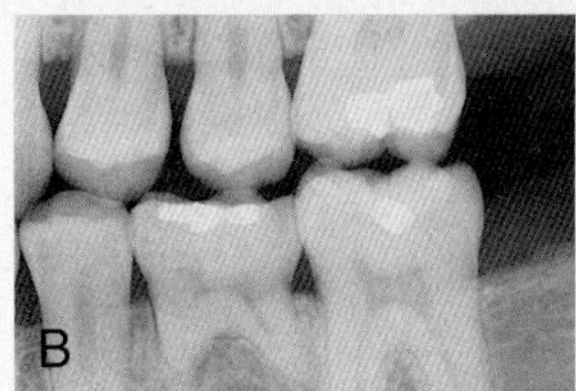

Disturbance: Supernumerary tooth or teeth

Description: Development of one or more extra teeth commonly noted between permanent maxillary central incisors (mesiodens—**C, D**), distal to third molars (distomolar), and premolar region (perimolar)

Etiologic factors: Hereditary with extra tooth germ(s) formation from persisting dental placodes within the dental lamina

Clinical ramifications: Crowding, failure of eruption, and disruption of occlusion treated by surgical removal if needed and/or orthodontic therapy

Mesiodens between maxillary central incisors

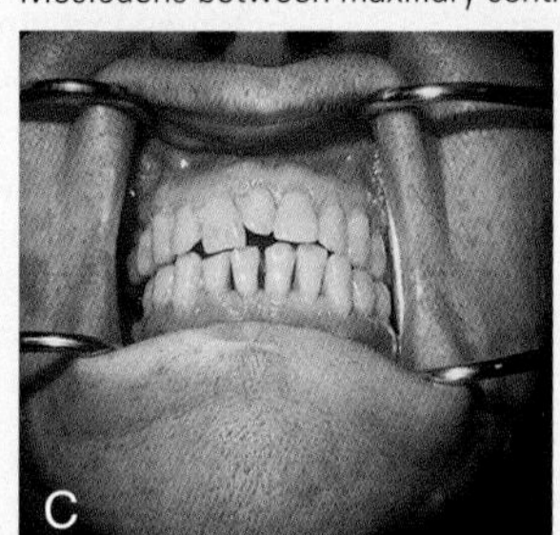

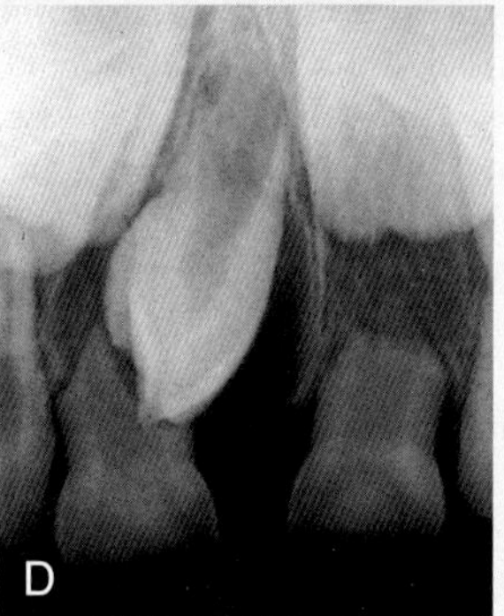

Bud Stage

Disturbance: Microdontia or macrodontia, partial or complete

Description: Abnormally small or large teeth commonly affecting permanent maxillary lateral incisor **(E)** and third molar with partial microdontia **(F)**

Etiologic factors: Hereditary with partial; endocrine dysfunction with complete

Clinical ramifications: Esthetic and spacing complications treated with full restorative crown on microdontic tooth (lateral incisor) and/or possibly extraction (third molar)

Peg lateral

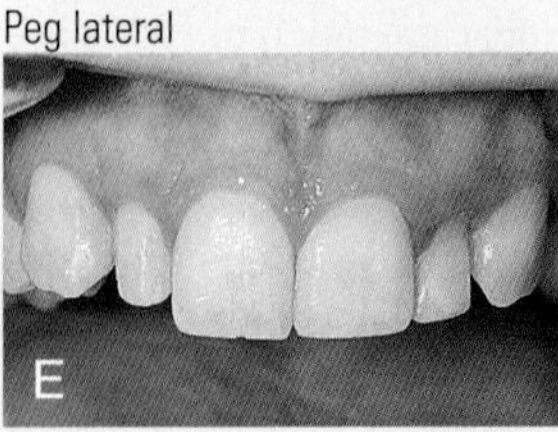

Peg molar

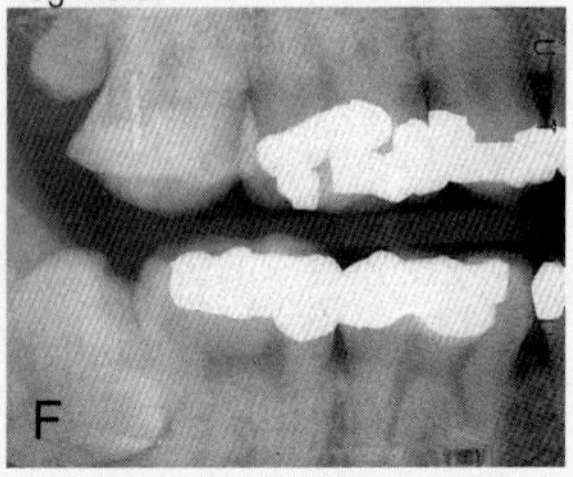

F

BOX 6.1 Common Dental Developmental Disturbances with Involved Developmental Stage*—cont'd

Cap Stage

Disturbance: Dens in dente **(G, H)**
Description: Enamel organ invaginates into dental papilla commonly affecting permanent maxillary lateral incisor
Etiologic factors: Hereditary
Clinical ramifications: Deep lingual pit that may need endodontic therapy

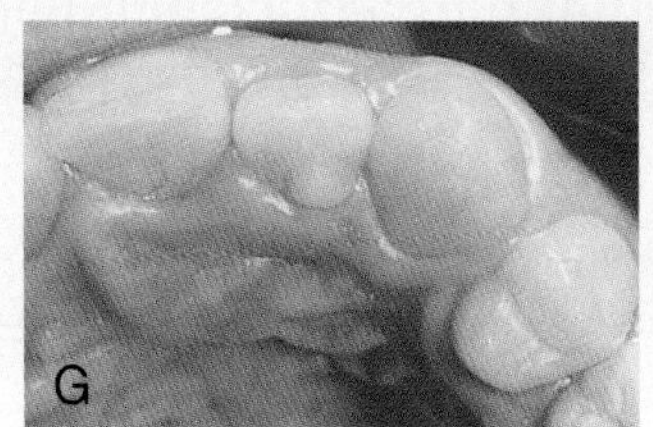

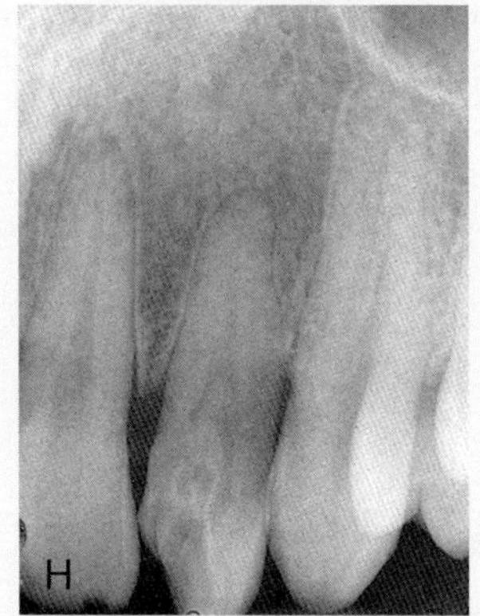

Disturbance: Gemination **(I, J)**
Description: Tooth germ tries to divide and develops large single-rooted tooth with one pulp cavity and "twinning" commonly affecting crown of anteriors with correct number in primary or permanent dentition
Etiologic factors: Hereditary
Clinical ramifications: Esthetic and spacing complications treated by orthodontic therapy

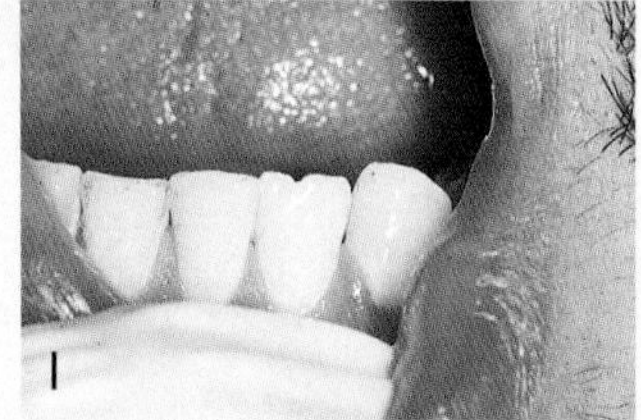

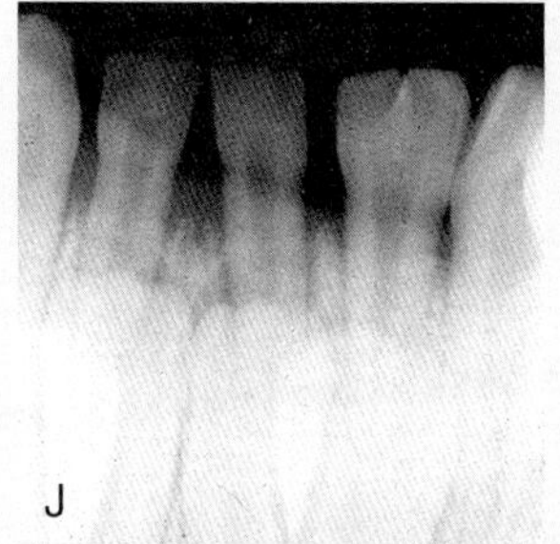

Disturbance: Fusion **(K, L)**
Description: Union of two adjacent tooth germs that result in large tooth with two pulp cavities with one less tooth in dentition commonly affecting anteriors and within primary dentition *(arrow)*
Etiologic factors: Pressure
Clinical ramifications: Esthetic and spacing complications treated by orthodontic therapy

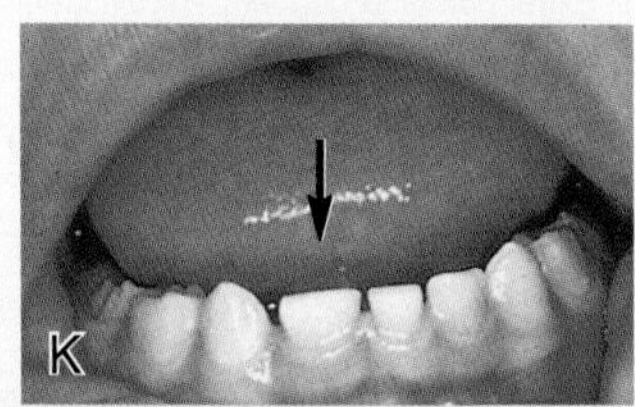

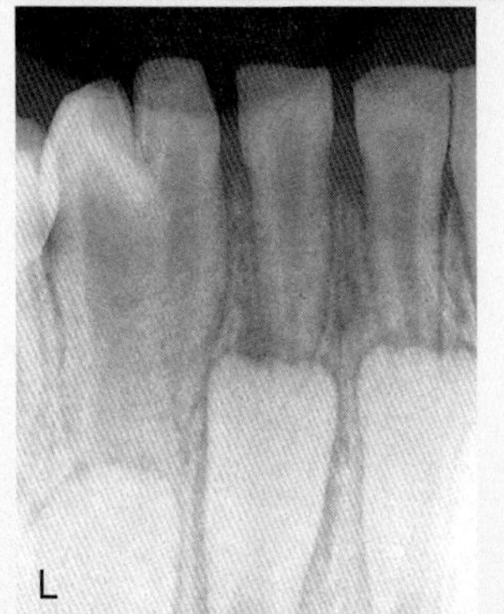

Continued

BOX 6.1 Common Dental Developmental Disturbances with Involved Developmental Stage*—cont'd

Cap Stage

Disturbance: Tubercle **(M, N)**
Description: Small, rounded enamel extensions forming extra cusps commonly noted on permanent posteriors occlusal surface or anteriors lingual surface
Etiologic factors: Trauma, pressure, or metabolic disease affecting enamel organ
Clinical ramifications: Occlusal complications

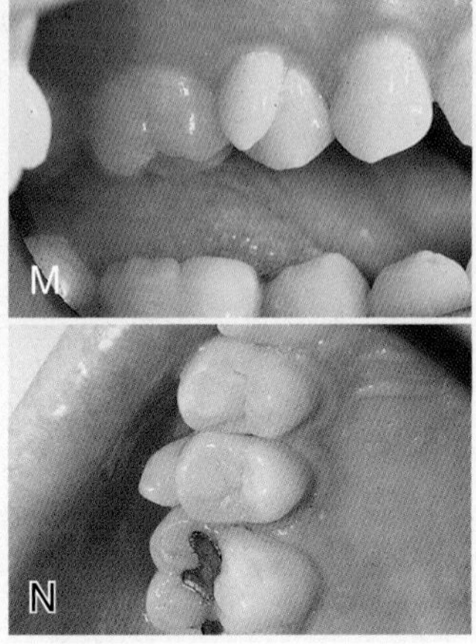

Apposition and Maturation Stage

Disturbance: Enamel dysplasia
Description: Faulty enamel development from interference involving ameloblasts resulting in enamel pitting (enamel hypoplasia, **O**) and/or intrinsic color changes (enamel hypocalcification, **P**) with possible changes in enamel thickness
Etiologic factors: Local or systemic from traumatic birth, systemic infections, nutritional deficiencies, or dental fluorosis
Clinical ramifications: Esthetic and function complications

Enamel hypoplasia (with disclosing solution)

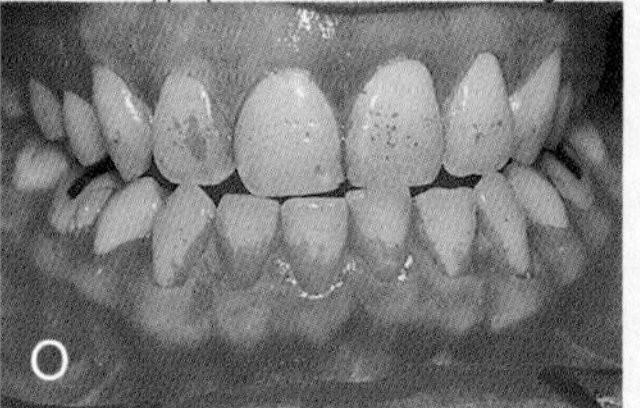

Enamel hypocalcification *(arrows)*

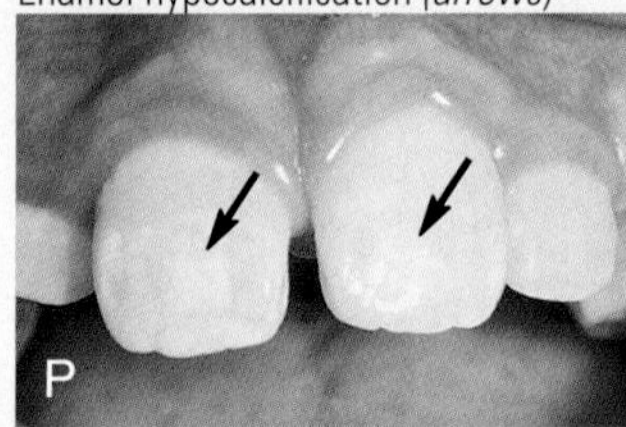

Disturbance: Concrescence **(Q)**
Description: Union of root structure of two or more teeth by cementum commonly affecting permanent maxillary molars
Etiologic factors: Traumatic injury or crowding of teeth
Clinical ramifications: Extraction or endodontic complications

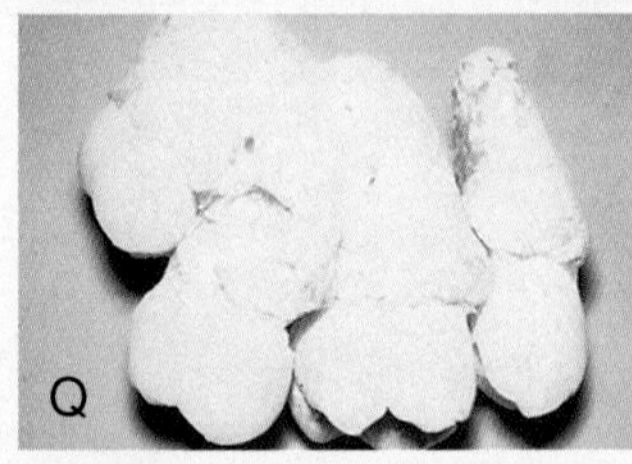

Disturbance: Enamel pearl **(R, S)**
Description: Enamel sphere on root *(arrow)*
Etiologic factors: Displacement of ameloblasts to root surface
Clinical ramifications: Commonly confused as calculus deposit on root and may prevent effective homecare

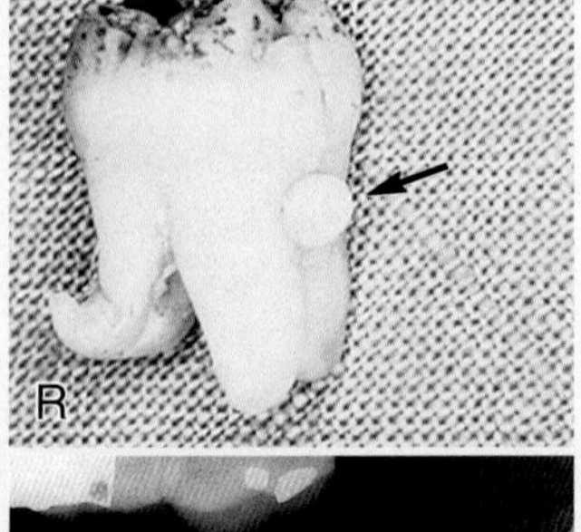

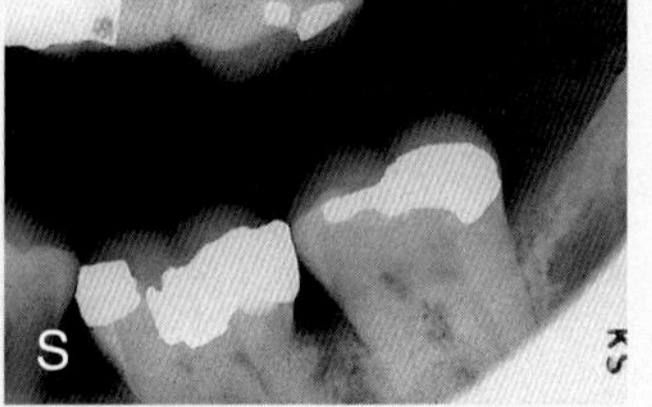

* Figures courtesy of Margaret J. Fehrenbach, RDH, MS.

BUD STAGE

The second stage of odontogenesis is considered the **bud stage** and occurs at the beginning of the eighth week of prenatal development for the primary dentition (Figs. 6.3 and 6.4). This stage is named for an extensive proliferation of the dental placodes into buds, with these three-dimensional oval masses penetrating into the surrounding ectomesenchyme. At the end of the proliferation process involving the dental placodes of the primary dentition, both the future maxillary arch and the future mandibular arch will each have 10 buds. The underlying ectomesenchyme also undergoes adjacent proliferation. However, a basement membrane remains between the bud and the surrounding growing and condensing ectomesenchyme.

Each of these buds from a dental placode, together with the surrounding ectomesenchyme, will develop into a tooth germ with its associated supporting tissue during the next stage. Thus, all the teeth and their associated tissue types develop from both ectoderm and the mesenchymal tissue, ectomesenchyme, the latter of which is derived from NCCs. These two distinct tissue types interact at all stages of odontogenesis, supporting the concept of induction.

However, only proliferation of these two tissue types occurs during this stage; no structural change occurs in the cells of either the dental placodes or ectomesenchyme as later occurs with differentiation and morphogenesis of these tissue types. In regions where teeth will not be developing, the dental lamina remains uniformly thickened because it lines the stomodeum but does not produce buds. Later, this non-tooth-producing part of the dental lamina disintegrates as the developing oral mucosa comes to line the maturing oral cavity.

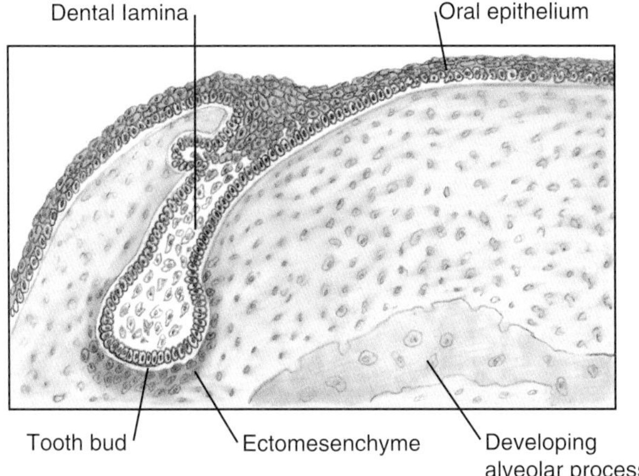

Fig. 6.3 Bud stage, which involves extensive proliferation of each of the dental placodes into the ectomesenchyme in the form of buds, together creating the future tooth germs.

Clinical Considerations with Bud Stage Disturbances

Abnormal proliferation of the tooth bud can cause a single tooth or multiple teeth (partial) or an entire dentition (complete) to be larger or smaller in form than usual. Abnormally large teeth result in **macrodontia** (mak-ruh-**don**-shuh); abnormally small teeth result in **microdontia** (mahy-kruh-**don**-shuh) (see Box 6.1, *E-F*). Individual teeth can sometimes appear larger than usual as a result of splitting of the enamel organ or fusion of two adjacent tooth germs; however, this is not a true case of *partial macrodontia* (discussed later in this chapter).

In contrast, the dentition can appear smaller by being within a large set of jaws, which is considered *relative microdontia*. With true partial microdontia, hereditary factors are involved and the teeth that are commonly affected are the permanent maxillary lateral incisor (known as a peg lateral; see **Chapter 16**) and the permanent third molar (known as a peg molar; see Fig. 17.50). This can lead to esthetic and spacing complications that are treated with full restorative crowns on partial microdontic teeth (with the lateral incisor) and/or extraction (as with the third molar).

A case of *complete microdontia* of either dentition rarely occurs but can be associated with hypopituitarism or Down syndrome (see Fig. 3.5). In contrast, systemic conditions such as childhood hyperpituitarism (or gigantism) can produce *complete macrodontia*.

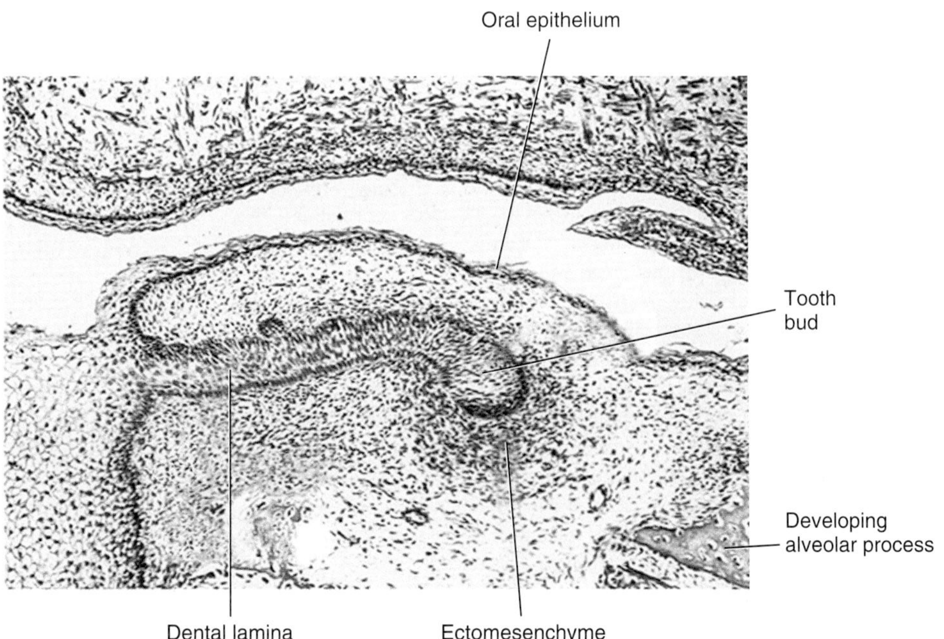

Fig. 6.4 Photomicrograph of the bud stage, which involves extensive proliferation of the each of the dental placodes into the ectomesenchyme in the form of buds, together creating the future tooth germs. (From Nanci A. *Ten Cate's Oral Histology*. 9th ed. St. Louis: Elsevier; 2018.)

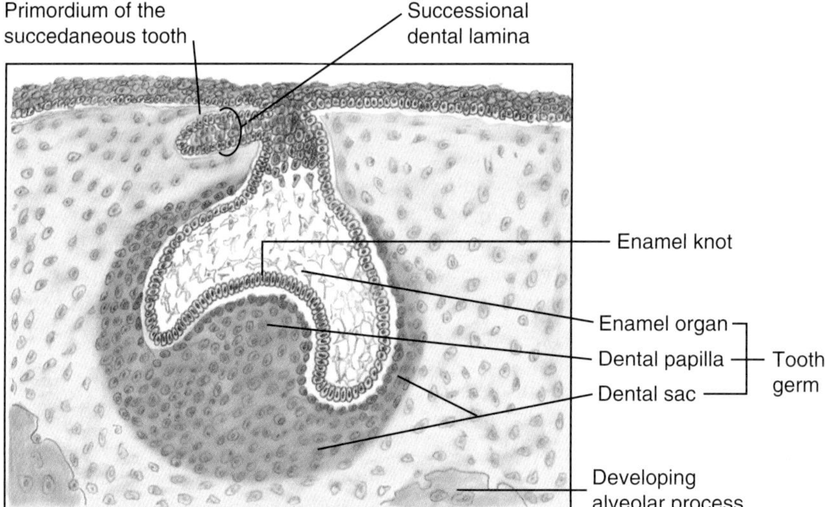

Fig. 6.5 Cap stage, which involves proliferation and differentiation to form the tooth germ, the primordium of a primary tooth. The tooth germ at this time consists of the enamel organ, dental papilla, and dental sac. The primordium of the permanent succedaneous tooth from the growth of the successional dental lamina *(circle)* is located lingual to the primary tooth germ and is in the bud stage.

CAP STAGE

The third stage of odontogenesis is considered the **cap stage** and occurs for the primary dentition between the ninth and tenth week of prenatal development, during the fetal period (Figs. 6.5 and 6.6). The physiologic process of proliferation continues during this stage, but the tooth bud from the dental placode does *not* grow into a large sphere surrounded by ectomesenchyme. Instead, there is unequal growth in different parts of the tooth bud, leading to formation of a three-dimensional cap shape overlying the ectomesenchyme that is still attached superiorly to the dental lamina.

Thus not only does proliferation characterize this stage, but various levels of differentiation are also occurring, including the more specific processes of cytodifferentiation, histodifferentiation, and morphodifferentiation. Additionally, during this stage a primordium of the tooth (or tooth germ) forms, containing each of the primordial types of tissue necessary to develop the future tooth. Therefore, the predominant physiologic process during the cap stage is one of morphogenesis.

From these combined physiologic processes, a depression results in the deepest part of each tooth bud of a dental placode, forming the cap shape of the **enamel organ** (see Figs. 6.5 and 6.6). It is important to note that the enamel organ was originally derived from ectoderm, making enamel an ectodermal product. In future development, the enamel organ will produce enamel on the outer surface of the crown of the tooth. The innermost margin of the cap shape of the enamel organ orchestrates the future crown form of the tooth, such as cusps. This specifically occurs through nondividing cells in the **enamel knot** present in the region of the developing posterior teeth, the second signaling center of tooth development.

A part of the ectomesenchyme deep to the buds has now condensed into a mass within the concavity of the cap of the enamel organ. This inner mass of ectomesenchyme is now considered the **dental papilla** (see Figs. 6.5 and 6.6). The dental papilla will produce the future dentin and pulp for the inner part of the tooth. It is important to note that the dental papilla is originally derived from ectomesenchyme, which is derived from NCCs. Thus dentin and pulp are of mesenchymal origin. However, a basement membrane still exists as before, but now it is between the enamel organ and the dental papilla, being the site of the future dentinoenamel junction.

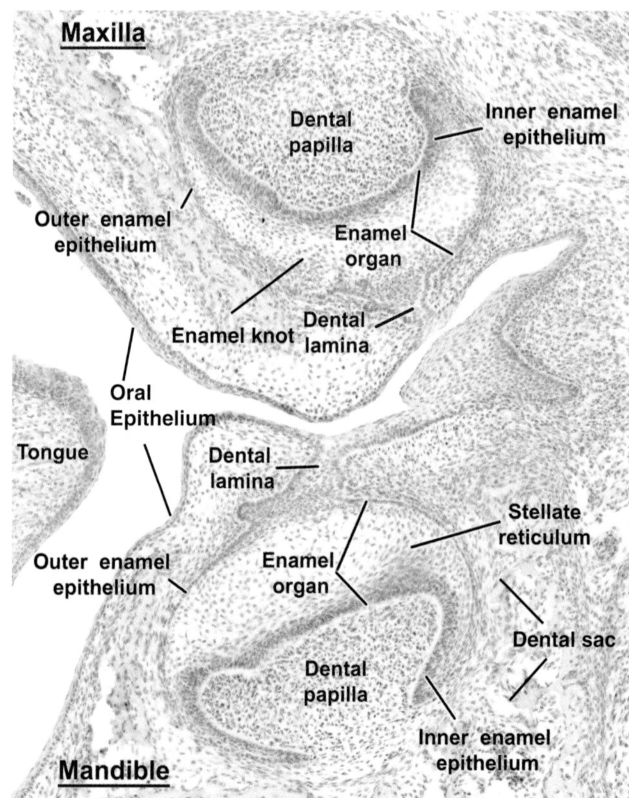

Fig. 6.6 Photomicrograph of the cap stage on both the future maxillary and mandibular arch. Note the formation of the enamel organ from the dental placode as well as the adjacent dental papilla and dental sac from the ectomesenchyme. The enamel organ sits over a mass of ectomesenchymal cells, the dental papilla, which is the future pulp. The oral epithelium is lining the outer part of the stomodeum and intramembranous bone development is also occurring underneath the designation for each of the jaws. (Courtesy of Y. Zhang.)

TABLE 6.3 Tooth Germ During Cap Stage

Component	Histologic Features	Future Dental Tissue
Enamel organ	Formation of tooth bud in cap shape with deep central depression	Enamel
Dental papilla	Condensed mass of ectomesenchyme within concavity of enamel organ	Dentin and pulp
Dental sac	Condensed mass of ectomesenchyme surrounding outside of enamel organ	Cementum, periodontal ligament, alveolar process

The remaining ectomesenchyme surrounding the outside of the cap of the enamel organ condenses into the **dental sac** (or dental follicle). In future development, the capsule-like dental sac will produce the periodontium, which are the supporting tissue types of the tooth that includes cementum, periodontal ligament, and alveolar process. It is important to note that the dental sac is originally derived from ectomesenchyme; thus this supporting dental tissue is of mesenchymal origin. A similar basement membrane also separates the enamel organ and dental sac.

At the end of the cap stage, these three embryologic structures, the enamel organ, dental papilla, and dental sac, are now considered together to be the **tooth germ**, which is the primordium of the tooth (Table 6.3). These initial 10 tooth germs housed within each of the two developing dental arches develop into the primary dentition after each tissue type undergoes differentiation.

Already at the tenth week of prenatal development, during the cap stage for each primary tooth, initiation is occurring for the anterior teeth of the permanent dentition and then later for the premolars of the permanent dentition. Each primordium for these initially formed permanent teeth appears as a lingual extension of the associated dental placodes into the ectomesenchyme in relationship to the developing primary tooth germs. Its site of origin is the **successional dental lamina** (suhk-**sesh**-shuhn-uhl) (see Fig. 6.26). The successional dental lamina is associated with the dental stalk, a short epithelial connection between the tooth germ and the oral epithelium.

Permanent teeth formed with primary predecessors are considered to be **succedaneous** (suhk-si-**dey**-nee-us) and include the anterior teeth and premolars, which replace the primary anterior teeth and molars, respectively. The crown of each permanent succedaneous tooth will erupt lingual to the root(s) of its primary predecessor if the primary tooth has not been fully shed.

In contrast, the permanent molars are **nonsuccedaneous** (nohn-suhk-si-**dey**-nee-us) and have no primary predecessors. Instead, the six permanent molars per dental arch develop much later than both the anterior teeth and premolars from a posterior extension of the dental lamina distal to the dental lamina of the primary second molar, with its associated ectomesenchyme for each of the four quadrants of the oral cavity (see Fig. 6.26).

Clinical Considerations with Cap Stage Disturbances

During the cap stage, the enamel organ may abnormally invaginate by growth into the dental papilla, resulting in **dens in dente** (**denz in den**-tehy) or dens invaginatus (see Box 6.1, *G-H*). The teeth most commonly affected are the permanent maxillary incisors, especially the lateral incisor and may be associated with hereditary factors (see **Chapter 16**). The invagination produces an enamel-lined pocket extending from the lingual surface. This usually leaves the tooth with a deep lingual pit where the invagination occurs and may appear as a "tooth within a tooth" on radiographic examination. This lingual pit may lead to pulpal exposure and pathology with subsequent endodontic therapy; therefore early detection is important. Application of sealant or a restoration in the opening of the invagination is the recommended treatment to prevent pulpal involvement.

If the condition of dens in dente is detected before complete eruption of the tooth, the removal of gingival tissue to facilitate cavity preparation and restoration may be indicated. The advisability of performing endodontic procedures on such a tooth with pulpal degeneration depends on its pulp morphology and the restorability of the crown.

Another disturbance that can occur during the cap stage is **gemination** (jem-uh-**ney**-shuhn) (see Box 6.1, *I-J*). This disturbance occurs as the single tooth germ tries unsuccessfully to divide into two tooth germs by invagination occurring during the proliferation stage of the growth cycle of the tooth, which then results notably in a large single-rooted tooth with a common enlarged pulp cavity. The tooth exhibits "twinning" in the crown, resulting in a broader falsely macrodontic tooth, similar to fusion (discussed next). However, when this is verified by radiographic examination, it shows only one pulp cavity, with the correct number of teeth within either dentition with this disturbance.

The appearance of splitting can be detected as a cleft with varying depths in the incisal surface or it may manifest as two adjoining crowns. It usually occurs in the anterior teeth in either dentition but mostly within the primary dentition, shows hereditary factors, and can create complications in esthetics and spacing that can be treated by orthodontic therapy in the permanent dentition along with reduction of the mesiodistal width of the tooth to allow development of the occlusion by periodic disking.

Another disturbance that can occur during the cap stage is **fusion** (see Box 6.1, *K-L*). This results from the union of two adjacent tooth germs, which may result from pressure in the region which leads to a broader falsely macrodontic tooth similar to gemination. However, when it is verified by radiographic examination, it shows two separate and distinct pulp cavities with the resulting enamel, dentin, and pulp united.

Fusion usually occurs only in the crown of the tooth, but it can involve both the crown and root and notably each arch of the dentition with this disturbance has one less tooth. It occurs more commonly with the anterior teeth and usually within the primary dentition. It can present complications in esthetics and spacing that can be treated by orthodontic therapy. Also dental caries may develop in the line of fusion of the crowns, necessitating the placement of a restoration. Another frequent finding in fusion of primary teeth is the congenital absence of one of the corresponding permanent teeth.

Teeth may also have **tubercles** (**too**-ber-kuhls) that appear as small rounded enamel extensions forming extra cusps (see Box 6.1, *M-N*; also **Chapters 16 and 17**). They are mostly noted on the occlusal surface of permanent molars, especially the third molars, and may also be present as a lingual extension on the cingulum on permanent maxillary anterior teeth, especially lateral incisors and canines but can be found on any tooth in both dentitions. This disturbance may be due to trauma, pressure, or metabolic disease that affects the enamel organ as it forms the crown and may present occlusal complications.

BELL STAGE

The fourth stage of odontogenesis is considered the **bell stage** (Figs. 6.7 and 6.8), which occurs for the primary dentition between the eleventh and twelfth week of prenatal development. It is characterized by continuation of the ongoing processes of proliferation, differentiation, and morphogenesis. However, differentiation on all levels occurs to

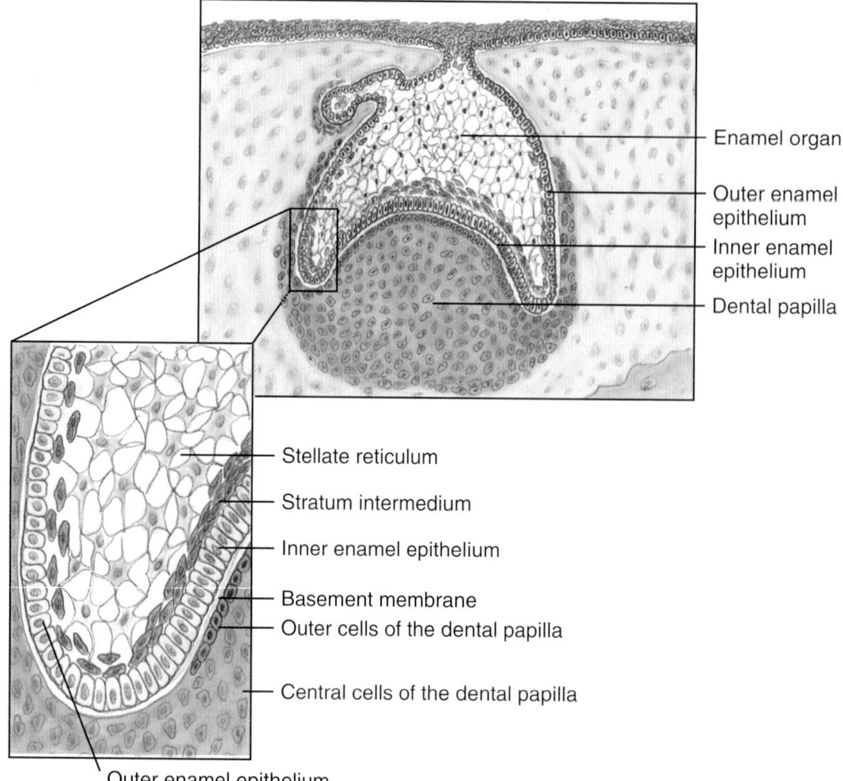

Fig. 6.7 Transitioning from the cap stage to the bell stage, the latter of which will exhibit differentiation of the tooth germ to its furthest extent. Both the enamel organ and dental papilla have begun to be differentiated into various layers in preparation for the appositional growth of enamel and dentin, respectively.

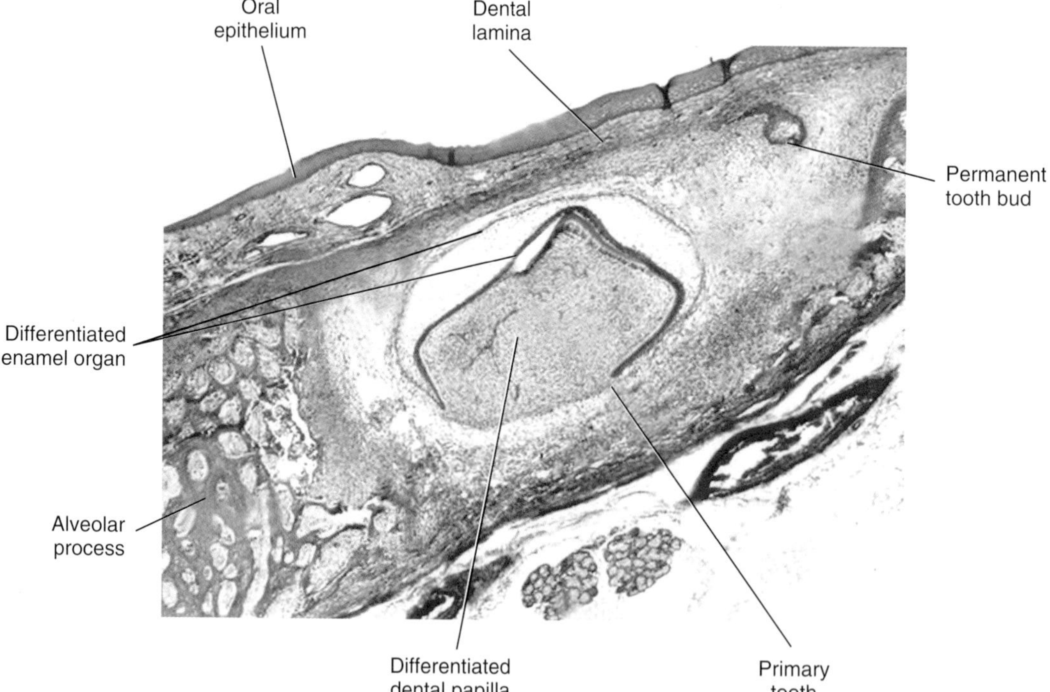

Fig. 6.8 Photomicrograph of the bell stage of the primary tooth, which exhibits differentiation of the tooth germ to its furthest extent. Both enamel organ and dental papilla have differentiated into various layers in preparation for the appositional growth of enamel and dentin, respectively. (From CD-ROM from Nanci A. *Ten Cate's Oral Histology*. 6th ed. St. Louis: Elsevier; 2003.)

TABLE 6.4 **Bell Stage Structures (From Outer to Inner)**

Cell Layers	Histologic Features	Role in Tooth Formation
Dental sac	Increasing amount of collagen fibers forming around enamel organ	Will differentiate into cementum, periodontal ligament, alveolar process
Outer enamel epithelium	Outer cuboidal cells of enamel organ	Serves as protective barrier for enamel organ
Stellate reticulum	More outer star-shaped cells in many layers, forming network within enamel organ	Supports production of enamel matrix
Stratum intermedium	More inner compressed layer of flat to cuboidal cells	Supports production of enamel matrix
Inner enamel epithelium	Innermost tall columnar cells of enamel organ	Will differentiate into ameloblasts that form enamel matrix
Outer cells of dental papilla	Outer layer of cells of dental papilla nearest inner enamel epithelium of enamel organ. Basement membrane is between outer layer and inner enamel epithelium	Will differentiate into odontoblasts that form dentin matrix
Central cells of dental papilla	Central cell mass of dental papilla	Will differentiate into pulp tissue

its furthest extent and as a result, four different types of cells are now found within the enamel organ (Table 6.4). These cell types include the outer enamel epithelium, stellate reticulum, stratum intermedium, and inner enamel epithelium (from outer to inner).

Thus the cap shape of the enamel organ, evident during the last stage, now assumes a three-dimensional bell shape as the undersurface of the cap deepens. During this stage, the tooth crown assumes its final shape through morphodifferentiation and the cells that will be producing the hard tissue of the crown (both the ameloblasts and odontoblasts) undergo further histodifferentiation.

The outer cuboidal cells of the enamel organ are the **outer enamel epithelium (OEE)**. The OEE serves as a protective barrier and nutritional supply for the rest of the enamel organ during enamel production. The innermost tall columnar cells of the enamel organ are the **inner enamel epithelium (IEE)**. In future development, the IEE will differentiate by phases into enamel-secreting cells (ameloblasts). However, a basement membrane still remains between the IEE and the adjacent dental papilla.

The cells of IEE will exert an organizing influence on the underlying mesenchymal cells in the dental papilla, which later differentiate into odontoblasts. At the same time, the cells of the OEE organize a network of capillaries that will bring nutrition to the ameloblasts. In preparation to formation of enamel, at the end of bell stage, the formerly smooth surface of the OEE is laid in folds. Between the folds, adjacent mesenchyme of the dental sac forms papillae that contain capillary loops and thus provide nutritional supply for the intense metabolic activity of the avascular enamel organ. Over time, the cells of the OEE then become flat, develop microvilli, and show increased mitochondria.

Between the OEE and IEE are the two innermost layers or *dental core*, the **stellate reticulum** (**stel**-eyt ri-**tik**-yuh-luhm) and **stratum intermedium** (**strat**-uhm in-ter-**meed**-ee-uhm). The stellate reticulum consists of star-shaped cells in many layers, forming a network. The stellate reticulum undergoes shrinkage as the intercellular fluid is utilized for nutrition and the space is then utilized by the forming enamel. The stratum intermedium is made up of a compressed layer of flat to cuboidal cells. The stratum intermedium cells show high alkaline phosphatase enzyme activity that is important for enamel mineralization. Both of these two intermediately placed layers of the enamel organ help support the future production of enamel.

Within the bell stage, the dental lamina is disintegrating, so the tooth now continues its development divorced from the oral epithelium. The crown pattern of the tooth has been established by folding of the IEE. This folding has reduced the amount of stellate reticulum over the future cusp tip. Dentin and enamel have begun to form at the crest of the folded IEE. The folding that occurs as the crown develops results from intrinsic growth caused by differential rates of mitotic division within the IEE. The cessation of mitotic division within cells of the IEE that correspond with future cusp tips is what determines the shape of a tooth. When the tooth germ is growing rapidly during the cap-to-bell stage, cell division occurs throughout the IEE. As development continues, division ceases at a particular point because the cells of the IEE are beginning to differentiate and assume their eventual function of producing enamel.

The point at which IEE cell differentiation first occurs represents the site of future cusp development. Because the IEE is constrained between the cervical loop and cusp tip, continued cell proliferation causes it to buckle and form a cuspal outline. Eventually differentiation of IEE and papilla cells sweeps down along the cusp slopes and is followed by the deposition of dentin and enamel first at the cusp tip. These two matrices are deposited face to face, thereby defining the DEJ. The occurrence of a second zone of cell differentiation within the IEE leads to the formation of a second cusp, a third zone leads to a third cusp, and so on until the final cuspal pattern of the tooth is determined. As discussed previously, these zones are determined by molecular signals in the primary and secondary enamel knot.

It is also during the bell stage of development that the dental lamina breaks down and the enamel organ loses connection with the oral epithelium. At the same time, the dental lamina between tooth germs also degenerates. Remnants of the dental lamina may remain in the adult mucosa as clumps of resting cells, the epithelial pearls (discussed later in this chapter).

At the same time, the dental papilla within the concavity of the enamel organ also undergoes extensive histodifferentiation so that it now consists of two types of tissue in layers, the **outer cells of the dental papilla** and **central cells of the dental papilla** (see Table 6.4). In future development, the outer cells of the dental papilla will differentiate into dentin-secreting cells (or odontoblasts), whereas the central cells of the dental papilla become the primordium of the pulp. The outermost placed dental sac increases only its amount of collagen fibers at this time and thus undergoes histodifferentiation into its mature dental tissue types of cementum, periodontal ligament, and alveolar process later than that of both the enamel organ and dental papilla.

APPOSITION AND MATURATION STAGES

The final stages of odontogenesis include the **apposition stage** (ap-uh-**zish**-uhn) (or secretory stage) during which the enamel, dentin, and cementum are secreted in successive layers upon those already present. These hard dental tissue types are initially secreted as a **matrix**

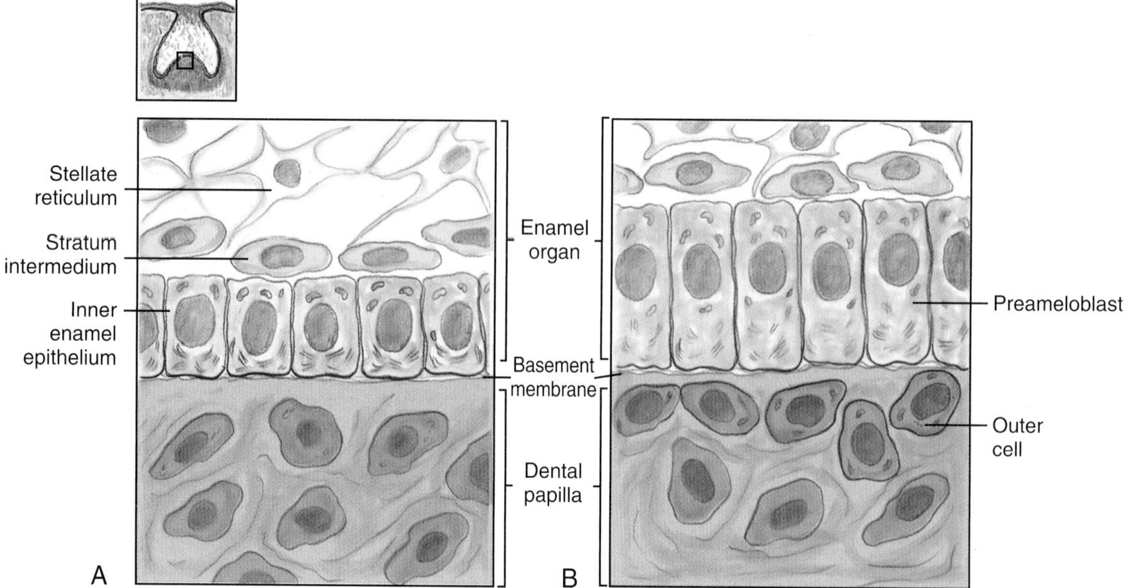

Fig. 6.9 Close-up view of inner enamel epithelium of the enamel organ differentiating into the preameloblasts, the future cells that will form into ameloblasts and secrete enamel matrix. **A,** Inner enamel epithelium, with the central nuclei, line up along the basement membrane. **B,** Inner enamel epithelium that has elongated and repolarized the nuclei to become preameloblasts. The outer cells of the dental papilla are also lined up on the opposite side of the basement membrane.

(plural, **matrices**) (**mey**-triks, **mey**-tri-seez), which is an extracellular substance or surrounding medium that in this case is partially mineralized. However, the matrix produced at this time serves as a framework for later full mineralization to the tissue type's expected level. This level of mineralization varies between enamel being the hardest, with dentin the next hardest, and finally to cementum, which has a similar hardness to bone tissue.

During the apposition stage, the process of induction continues to occur between the ectodermal tissue of the enamel organ and mesenchymal tissue of the dental papilla and dental sac; specifically, these are examples of the biologic concept of *reciprocal induction*. Acting not only as a boundary between the two tissue types, the basement membrane conveys communications between the cells of the enamel organ, the dental papilla, and the dental sac, allowing for these important tissue interactions. Studies show that these interactions are necessary for the production of enamel, dentin, and cementum by the proliferation of cellular byproducts.

The final stage of odontogenesis, the **maturation stage**, is reached when the matrices of the hard dental tissue types subsequently fully mineralize to their correct levels. It is important to note that the period of time for these two final stages varies according to the tooth involved but overall involves the same chronology as the initiation of odontogenesis.

The maturation through mineralization of each type of matrix occurs later and is a different process for both enamel and dentin. However, the cell bodies of odontoblasts will remain within adjoining pulp attached by the odontoblastic processes. In contrast, the cell bodies of the ameloblasts (now in maturation stage) will be involved first in the final phases of the mineralization process and active tooth eruption but will later be lost after tooth eruption (see later discussion). These specific steps of the stages will be discussed within the chapters that discuss that mature enamel (see **Chapter 12**) and mature dentin (see **Chapter 13**). The results of the maturation of each hard dental tissue are noted in Table 6.2; importantly, this table should be again consulted during the histologic study of each hard dental tissue in **Unit 3**.

Coronal Enamel and Dentin Production

The next part of the chapter will be mostly focused first on the production of enamel and coronal dentin with the development of the crown of the tooth discussed (maturation of each tooth tissue and its histology are discussed in **Chapters 12 and 13**, respectively). The process is a complicated dance production between producing cells and their respective matrices. This follows the same timeline as tooth development, given that development begins in the crown and then proceeds to the root, which is evident on most periapical or panoramic radiographs of a mixed dentition (see Fig. 6.27, *A*). Root development with root dentin and cementum formation is discussed later in this chapter.

Preameloblast Formation

The events in the production of enamel and coronal dentin include the formation over time of first preameloblasts, then odontoblasts with dentin matrix production, and finally ameloblasts with enamel matrix production as well as the dentinoenamel junction from the basement membrane (see Table 6.4).

After the formation of the IEE in the bell-shaped enamel organ, these innermost cells grow even more columnar as they elongate and differentiate into **preameloblasts** (pree-**am**-uh-loh-blastz) (Fig. 6.9), lining up alongside the basement membrane. During this differentiation process, the nucleus in each cell moves away from the center of the cell to the position farthest away from the basement membrane that separates the enamel organ from the dental papilla. This movement of the nuclei in each IEE cell occurs during cellular **repolarization** (re-poh-ler-uh-**zey**-shuhn) and studies show its importance in the change of the IEE cells into preameloblasts. In addition, the majority of each cell's organelles become situated in the cell body distal to the nucleus.

In future development, the preameloblasts will induce dental papilla cells to differentiate into dentin-forming cells (or odontoblasts)

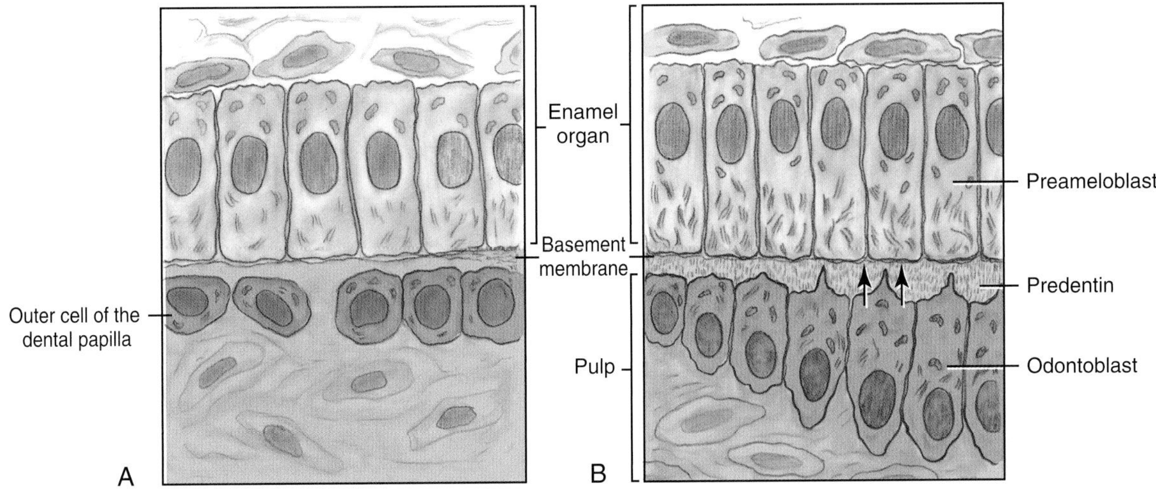

Fig. 6.10 Close-up view of the outer cells of the dental papilla, which are induced to differentiate into the odontoblasts and form predentin upon the formation of preameloblasts from the inner enamel epithelium. **A,** Outer cells of the dental papilla line up along the basement membrane with repolarization of the nuclei to become odontoblasts. **B,** Odontoblasts start dentinogenesis, the appositional growth of predentin on their side of the basement membrane *(arrows)*.

and then will themselves differentiate into cells that secrete enamel (or ameloblasts). Thus these initial changes to the cells occur within a presecretory stage with distinct phases where IEE is formed during the bell stage of tooth development (morphogenic phase) and then become preameloblasts (during differentiation phase), which much later become ameloblasts (during secretory stage, discussed later). These changes reflect the overall life cycle events of these complex cells involved in enamel production.

Odontoblast and Dentin Matrix Formation

After the IEE differentiates into preameloblasts, the outer cells of the dental papilla are induced to differentiate into **odontoblasts** (oh-**don**-tuh-blastz) by the newly stepped-up preameloblasts (Figs. 6.10 and 6.11). During this time, these cells also undergo cellular repolarization, which results in their nuclei moving from the center of the cell to a position in the cell farthest from the separating basement membrane. These repolarized cells also start to line up adjacent to the basement membrane in a mirror-image orientation on the opposite side from the already orderly preameloblasts.

After the differentiation and repolarization, the odontoblasts begin **dentinogenesis** (den-tin-noh-**jen**-uh-sis), the appositional growth of dentin matrix or **predentin**, laying it down on their side of the now disintegrating basement membrane. Thus the odontoblasts start their synthetic and secretory activity usually before enamel matrix production begins. This timing difference in production explains why the dentin layer in any location in a developing tooth is slightly thicker than the corresponding layer of enamel matrix.

Ameloblast and Enamel Matrix Formation

After the differentiation of odontoblasts from the outer cells of the dental papilla and their formation of predentin, the basement membrane between the preameloblasts and the odontoblasts disintegrates. This disintegration of the basement membrane allows the preameloblasts to contact the newly formed predentin, which induces the preameloblasts to differentiate into **ameloblasts** (**am**-uh-loh-blastz). The cellular changes in these cells show extensive Golgi complex surrounded by increased levels of rough endoplasmic reticulum, reflecting the intense synthetic and secretory activity going on.

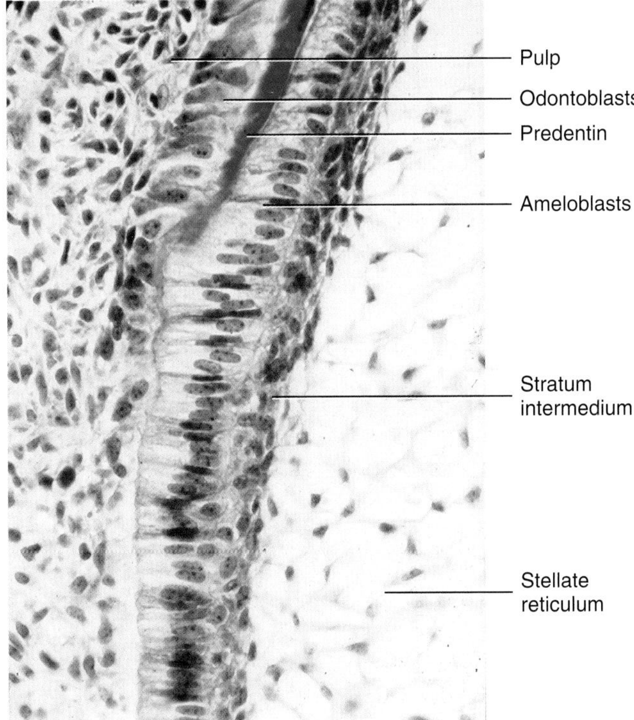

Fig. 6.11 Photomicrograph of the formation of predentin from the odontoblasts that then encloses the forming pulp from the central cells of the dental papilla. The enamel organ has its layers on the other side of the basement membrane that includes only the ameloblasts, stratum intermedium, and stellate reticulum in this view. (From Nanci A. *Ten Cate's Oral Histology*. 9th ed. St. Louis: Elsevier; 2018.)

After differentiation, the ameloblasts begin **amelogenesis** (am-uh-loh-**jen**-uh-sis), the appositional growth of **enamel matrix**, laying it down on their side of the now disintegrating basement membrane (Figs. 6.12, 6.13, 6.14, and 6.15). The enamel matrix is directly secreted from **Tomes process** (**tomes**), an angled distal part of each ameloblast that faces the fully disintegrated basement membrane, as there is group movement of the ameloblasts away from the basement membrane.

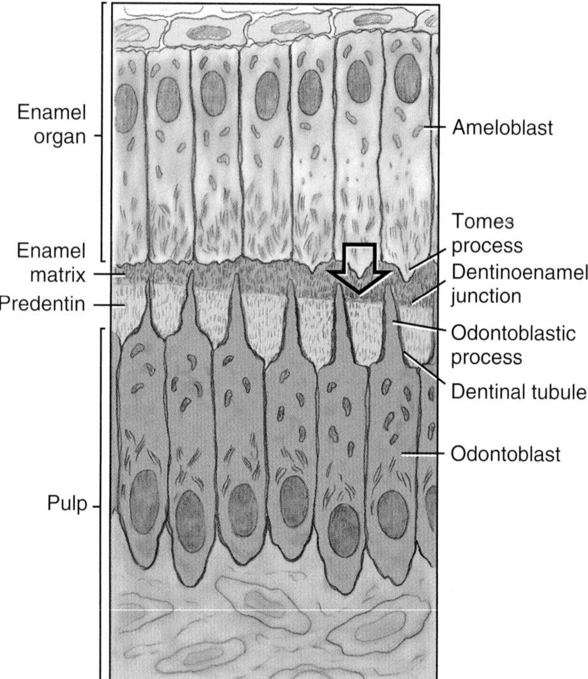

Fig. 6.12 Preameloblasts being induced to differentiate into ameloblasts and beginning amelogenesis from Tomes process *(under large arrow)* with the appositional growth of enamel matrix on their side of the basement membrane. Later, this membrane will disintegrate and mineralize to form the dentinoenamel junction. The predentin is thicker than the enamel matrix because the odontoblasts differentiate and start matrix production usually before the production by the ameloblasts. The predentin forms around the dentinal tubules that contain the odontoblastic process attached to the odontoblasts.

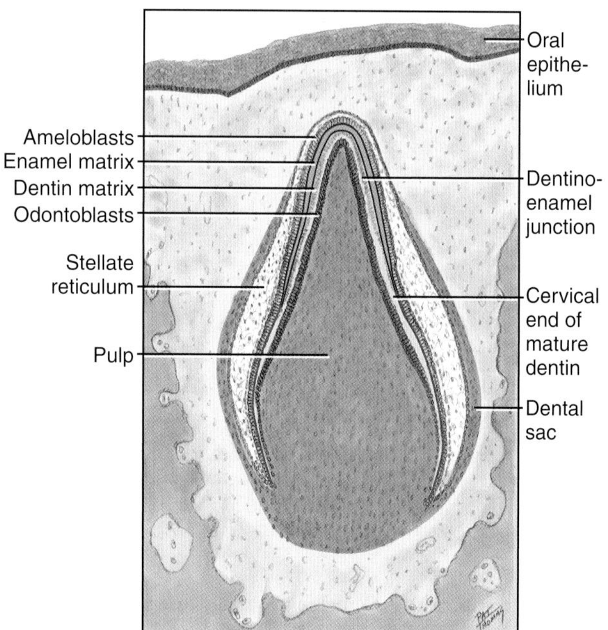

Fig. 6.13 Apposition Stage Demonstrating Both Enamel and Dentin Matrix Formation.

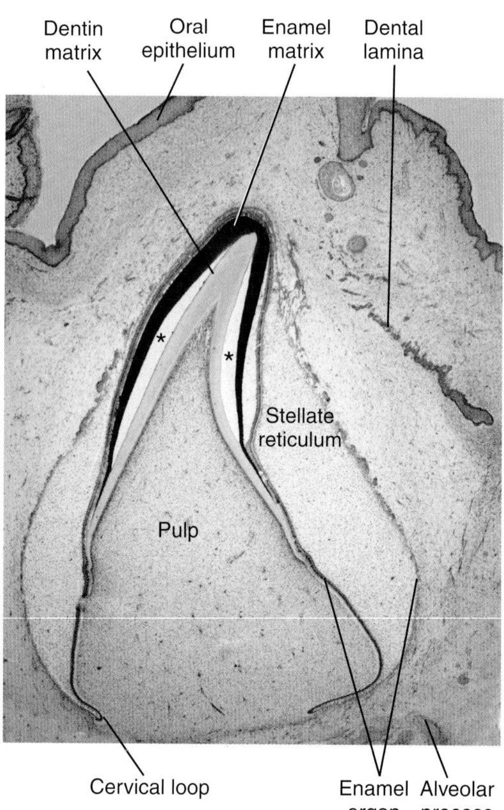

Fig. 6.14 Photomicrograph stage of tooth development. Dentin matrix and enamel matrix have begun to form at the crest of the folded inner enamel epithelium. The dental lamina is disintegrating so the tooth now continues its development divorced from the oral epithelium. The crown pattern of the tooth has been established by folding of the inner enamel epithelium. This folding has reduced the amount of stellate reticulum over the future cusp tip. The space indicated by asterisks is an artifact. (Courtesy of B. Kablar.)

Dentinoenamel Junction Formation

With the newly formed enamel matrix in contact with the predentin, mineralization of the disintegrated basement membrane now occurs, forming the **dentinoenamel junction (DEJ)** (den-tih-noh-ih-**nam**-uhl), the inner junction between the dentin and enamel tissue. Continued appositional growth of both types of dental matrix now becomes regular and rhythmic as the cellular bodies of both the odontoblasts and ameloblasts initially retreat away from the DEJ, forming their perspective tissue types.

However, the odontoblasts, unlike the ameloblasts, will leave attached cellular extensions in the length of the predentin **odontoblastic process** (oh-**don**-tuh-blast-ik) as they move away from the DEJ. Each odontoblastic process is contained in a mineralized cylinder, the **dentinal tubule**.

Clinical Considerations with Apposition Stage and Maturation Stage Disturbances

Certain factors may interfere with the metabolic processes of the ameloblasts, resulting in **enamel dysplasia** (dis-**pley**-zhuh), which is the faulty development of enamel (see Box 6.1, *O-P*). Many different types are possible and have either a local or a systemic etiology. *Local enamel dysplasia* may result from trauma or infection occurring to a small group of ameloblasts. *Systemic enamel dysplasia* involves larger numbers of ameloblasts and may result from

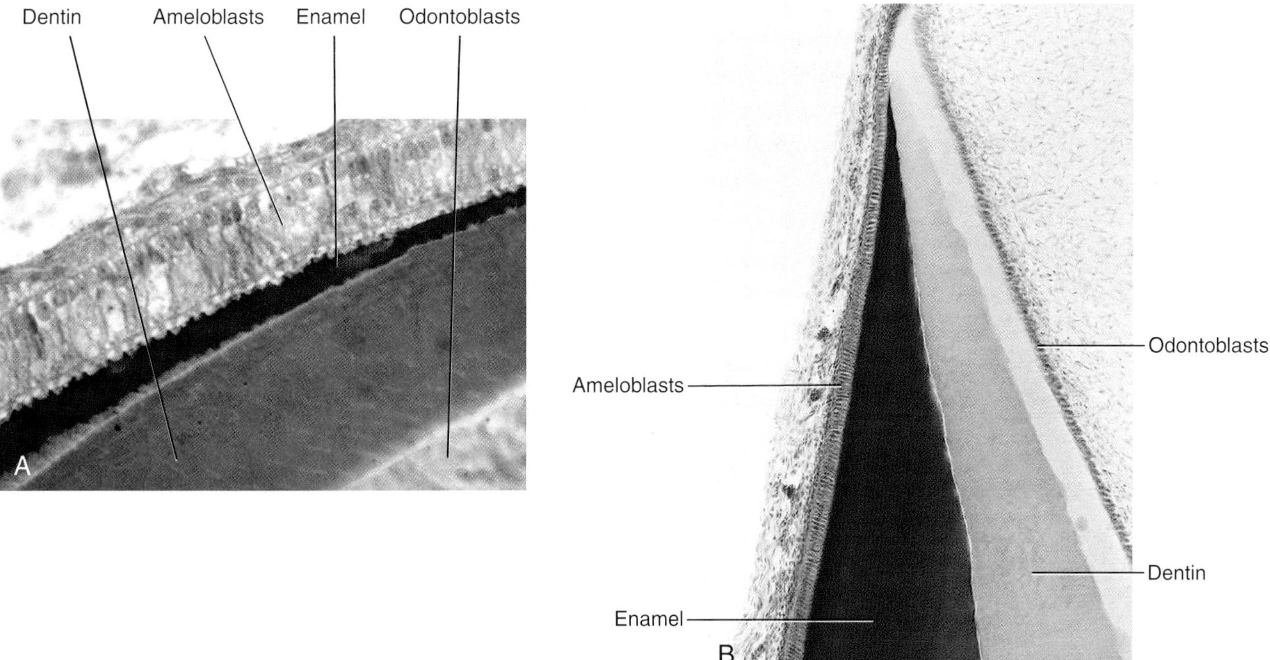

Fig. 6.15 Photomicrographs of enamel formation from ameloblasts and dentin formation from odontoblasts. The *dental core* of the stratum intermedium and stellate reticulum both cover the ameloblasts. (**A,** From CD-ROM from Nanci A. *Ten Cate's Oral Histology*. 6th ed. St. Louis: Elsevier; 2003. **B,** From Bernhard Gottlieb Collection, courtesy of James McIntosh, PhD, Assistant Professor Emeritus, Department of Biomedical Sciences, Baylor College of Dentistry, Dallas.)

traumatic birth, systemic infections, nutritional deficiencies, or dental fluorosis.

Any tooth in which amelogenesis is active during the metabolic interference may be affected and changes in either local regions or the entire tooth or even an entire dentition may occur. A type of enamel dysplasia, **enamel hypoplasia** (hahy-puh-**pley**-zhuh), results from a reduction in the *quantity* of enamel matrix due to factors that interfere with enamel matrix formation. As a result, the teeth appear with pitting and grooves in the enamel surface or in the development of horizontal lines across the enamel of the crown.

Enamel hypoplasia is often seen as one component of many different syndromes. In this scenario, enamel hypoplasia can be noted in the presence of the tooth abnormalities of Hutchinson incisors and mulberry molars, which are both caused by the teratogen of syphilis (see Fig. 3.17 and **Chapters 16 and 17**). From the labial view, Hutchinson incisors have a crown with a screwdriver shape that is wide cervically and narrow incisally with a notched incisal edge. Mulberry molars have enamel tubercles or extra extensions from the cusps on the occlusal surface.

Enamel dysplasia may also involve **enamel hypocalcification** (hahy-puh-kal-sey-fih-**kay**-shuhn). This disturbance results in reduction in the *quality* of the enamel maturation due to factors that interfere with enamel mineralization and maturation. The teeth appear more opaque, yellower, or even browner within because of an intrinsic staining of enamel. A single affected area or white "sparkle spot" is considered a *Turner spot* and if the entire permanent crown is affected, it is considered a *Turner tooth.*

Enamel hypoplasia and enamel hypocalcification may occur together and affect entire dentitions, which is a common finding in **dental fluorosis** (floo-**roh**-sis) or mottled enamel (see Fig. 12.5). This hypomineralization occurs due to an excess systemic fluoride level such as from naturally fluoridated water systems. The severity of the condition is dependent on the dose, duration, and age of the individual during the exposure; it may occur due to oxidative stress to the ameloblasts from the excess fluoride.

A certain type of enamel dysplasia, **amelogenesis imperfecta** (im-per-**fek**-tuh), has a hereditary etiology and can affect all teeth of both dentitions (Fig. 6.16). With this disturbance, the teeth have very thin enamel that chips off or have no enamel at all. Therefore the crowns are yellow because they are mostly composed of softer dentin that undergoes extreme attrition, the mechanical loss of tooth material resulting from mastication. Full-coverage crowns are needed for esthetic appearance as well as to prevent further attrition.

In addition, **dentin dysplasia**, which is the faulty development of dentin, can result from an interference with the metabolic processes of the odontoblasts during dentinogenesis. This condition is rarer than enamel dysplasia but can also be due to local or systemic factors (similar to enamel dysplasia) and can involve either dentin hypoplasia or hypocalcification or both disturbances at the same time.

One type of dentin dysplasia is **dentinogenesis imperfecta**, which has a hereditary basis (Fig. 6.17). This disturbance results in blue-gray or brown teeth with a rainbow-like opalescent sheen. The enamel appears as usual but chips off because of a lack of support by the abnormal underlying dentin, leaving only crowns of dentin; the dentin also has an irregular maturation quality (having increased amounts of interglobular dentin) (see Fig. 13.4). The result is severe attrition because the dentin is less mineralized overall; full-coverage crowns are needed for esthetic appearance as well as to prevent further attrition. Several types of the condition are recognized; most are Type II, whereas Type I is associated with systemic syndrome of osteogenesis imperfecta.

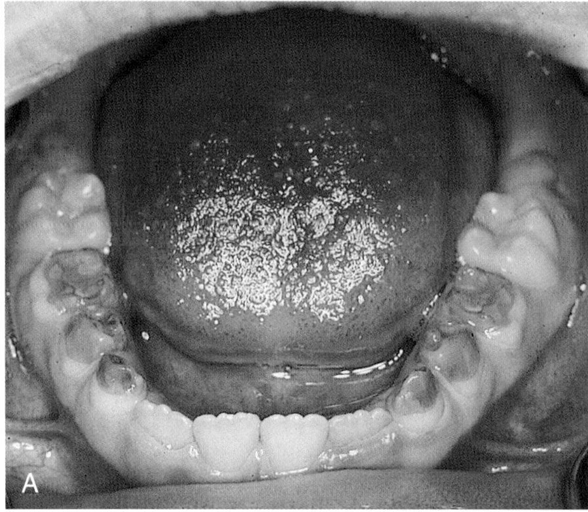

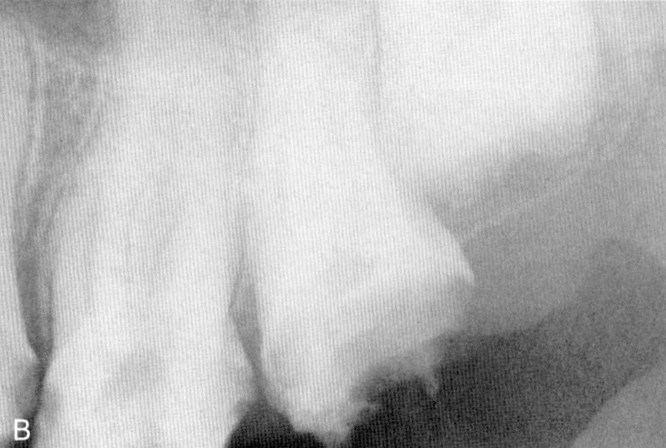

Fig. 6.16 Amelogenesis Imperfecta in the Permanent Dentition. A hereditary type of enamel dysplasia where the teeth have either no enamel or very thin enamel that chips off, leaving the yellow crowns of dentin, which undergo extreme attrition. **A,** Clinical view. **B,** Radiograph. (Courtesy of Margaret J. Fehrenbach, RDH, MS.)

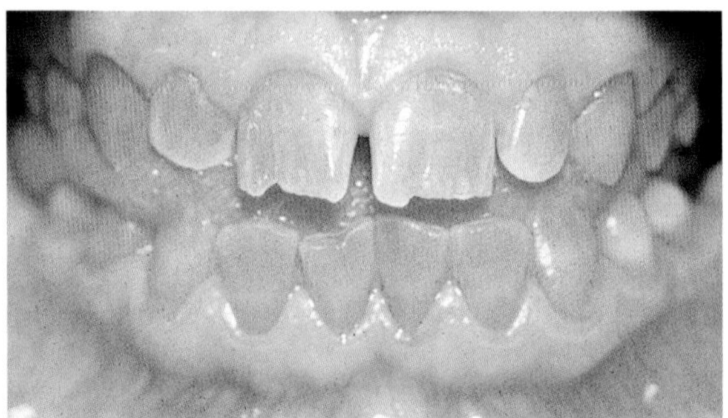

Fig. 6.17 Dentinogenesis Imperfecta in the Permanent Dentition. A hereditary type of dentin dysplasia that results in blue-gray teeth with an opalescent sheen, chipped enamel, and crowns of dentin with severe attrition. (Courtesy of Margaret J. Fehrenbach, RDH, MS.)

ROOT DEVELOPMENT

It is clear that during early tooth development, reciprocal and sequential interactions between the epithelium and mesenchyme eventually lead to the formation of root dentin, cementum, and periodontal tissue, similar to the interactions discussed in the formation of the face, neck, and even the crown of the tooth.

The process of root development takes place long after the crown is completely formed and the tooth is starting to erupt into the oral cavity (see Fig. 6.22 noting root development over time). Most find it unbelievable that the tooth is formed starting with the crown and then moving to the apex of the root (unlike rooted plant life), unless they have studied dentistry or looked closely at their dental office radiographs (see Fig. 6.27, *A*). The structure responsible for root development is the **cervical loop** (**ser**-vih-kal) (Fig. 6.18, *A*). The cervical loop is the most cervical part of the enamel organ, a bilayer rim that consists of only IEE and OEE.

To form the root region, the cervical loop begins to grow deeper into the surrounding ectomesenchyme of the dental sac, elongating and moving away from the newly completed crown to enclose more of the dental papilla, forming the **Hertwig epithelial root sheath (HERS)** (**hurt**-wig ep-uh-**thee**-lee-uhl) (see Fig. 6.18, *B-C*). The function of this sheath is to shape the root(s) by inducing dentin formation in the root so that it is continuous with coronal dentin. Thus, HERS will determine if the root will be curved or straight, short or long as well as single or multiple. This chapter first discusses root development in a single-rooted tooth and then later in a multirooted tooth.

ROOT DENTIN FORMATION

Root dentin forms when the outer cells of the dental papilla in the root area undergo induction and then differentiation and become odontoblasts (Fig. 6.19). This induction occurs similarly to the process that happens in the crown area to produce coronal dentin but under the influence of the IEE of HERS. Lacking the intermediate layers of the stellate reticulum and stratum intermedium, HERS induces odontoblastic differentiation but fails to have IEE differentiate into enamel-forming ameloblasts. This accounts for the usual absence of enamel in the roots.

After the differentiation of odontoblasts in the root area, these cells undergo dentinogenesis and begin to secrete predentin. As in the crown area, a basement membrane is located between the IEE of the sheath and the odontoblasts in the root area.

When root dentin formation is completed, this part of the basement membrane also disintegrates as does the entire HERS. After this disintegration of the root sheath, its cells may become the **epithelial rests of Malassez (ERM)** (mal-uh-**say**)**.** These groups of cells of epithelium are then located in the mature periodontal ligament but can become cystic, presenting future periodontal infections. In addition, these cells are also demonstrating an involvement in periodontal ligament repair and regeneration (see Fig. 14.26).

CEMENTUM AND PULP FORMATION

The process of **cementogenesis** (si-men-toh-**jen**-i-sis) from appositional growth of cementum in the root area also occurs when the HERS disintegrates (Fig. 6.20). This disintegration of the sheath allows the undifferentiated cells of the dental sac to contact the newly formed surface of root dentin. This contact of the dental sac cells with the

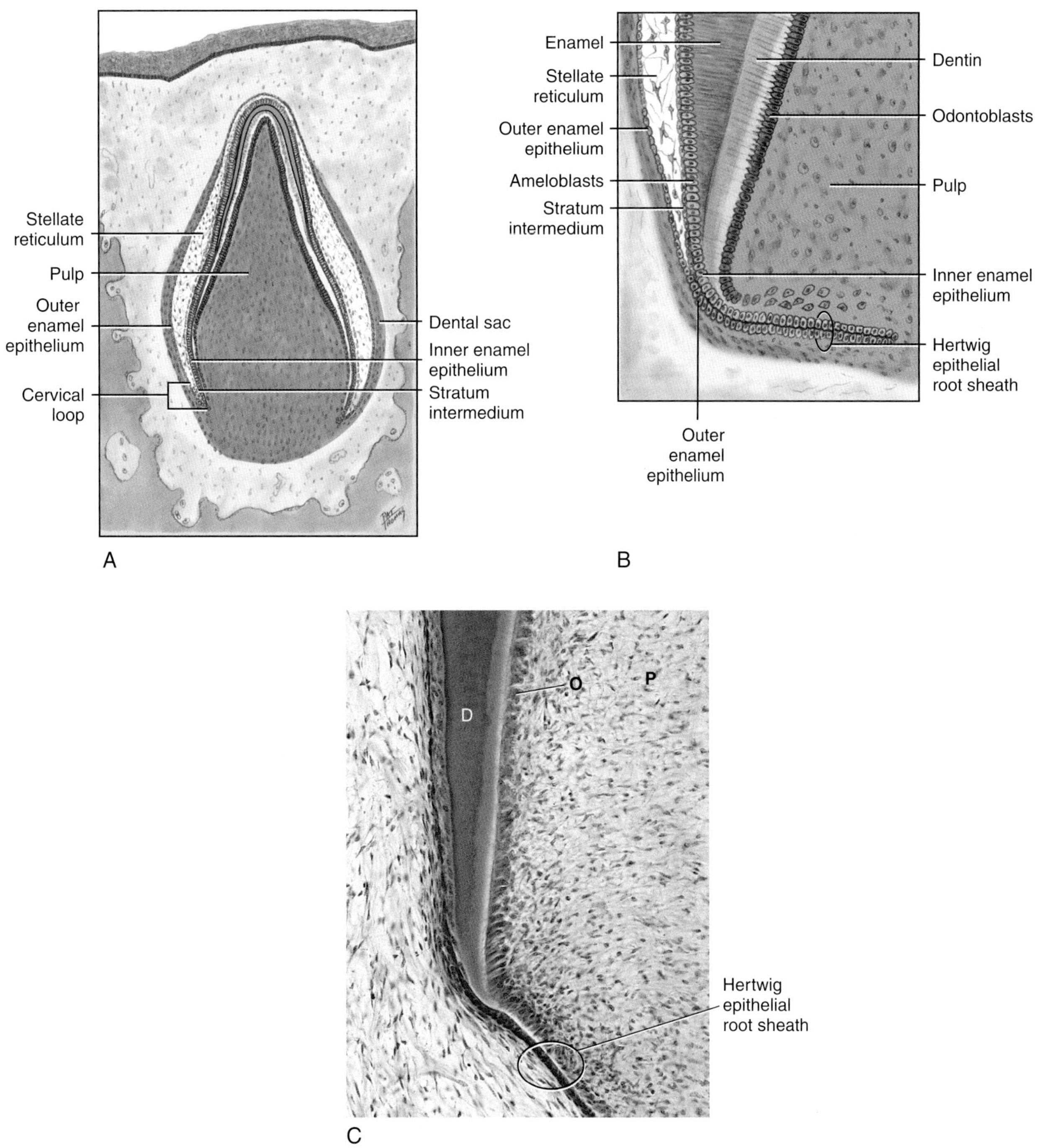

Fig. 6.18 Root Development. **A,** Cervical loop of a primary tooth, which is composed of the most cervical part of the enamel organ, with only the inner and outer enamel epithelium. **B,** Hertwig epithelial root sheath is formed from elongation of the cervical loop *(circle)*, which is responsible for the shape of the root (or roots) and the induction of root dentin. **C,** Microscopic section of the root sheath *(circle)*. Odontoblasts *(O)* are within the pulp *(P)* after forming dentin *(D)*. (From Bernhard Gottlieb Collection, courtesy of James McIntosh, PhD, Assistant Professor Emeritus, Department of Biomedical Sciences, Baylor College of Dentistry, Dallas.)

dentin surface induces these cells to become immature **cementoblasts** (si-**men**-tuh-blastz).

These cementoblasts move to cover the root dentin and undergo cementogenesis, laying down cementum matrix or **cementoid** (si-**men**-toid). Unlike ameloblasts and odontoblasts, which leave no cellular bodies in their secreted products, many cementoblasts become entrapped by the cementum they produce and become mature **cementocytes** (si-**men**-toh-sahytz) in the later stages of appositional growth. As the cementoid surrounding the cementocytes becomes mineralized or matured, it is then considered cementum (see Fig. 14.2).

As a result of the appositional growth of cementum over the dentin, the **dentinocemental junction (DCJ)** (den-tin-oh-si-**ment**-uhl) is formed where the disintegrating basement membrane between the two tissue types was located. At this time, the central cells of the dental papilla are also forming into the pulp, which later becomes surrounded by the newly formed dentin (see Fig. 13.9).

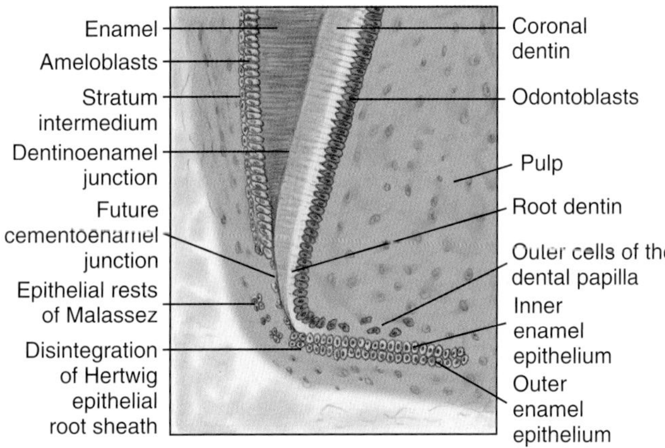

Fig. 6.19 Appositional growth of dentin in the root area resulting from the induction of the outer cells of the dental papilla to differentiate into odontoblasts. Hertwig epithelial root sheath is disintegrating to produce the epithelial rests of Malassez.

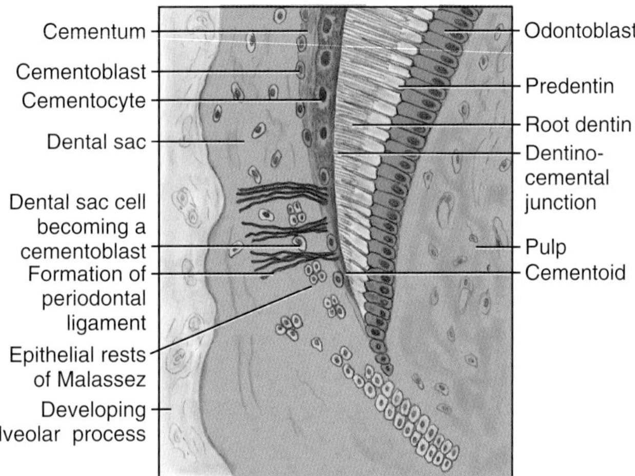

Fig. 6.20 Appositional growth of cementum in the root area after Hertwig epithelial root sheath disintegration and the induction of dental sac cells to differentiate into cementoblasts. The cementoblasts produce cementoid, entrapping the cells to become cementocytes. Nearby both the alveolar process and periodontal ligament are also beginning to develop further.

Clinical Considerations with Cementum Formation Disturbances

Excess cementum formation can occur with **concrescence** (kon-**kres**-uhns) (see Box 6.1, *Q*). This rare occurrence is the union of the root structure of two or more teeth through the cementum only, mostly occurring with permanent maxillary molars (see **Chapter 17**). The teeth involved were originally separate but now are joined because of the excessive cementum deposition on one or more teeth after eruption. Traumatic injury or crowding of the teeth during the apposition and maturation stage of tooth development may be the cause. This may present complications during extraction and endodontic therapy and thus preoperative radiographs are important in the detection of this disturbance.

MULTIROOTED TOOTH DEVELOPMENT

Like anterior teeth, multirooted premolars and molars originate as a single root on the base of the crown. This part of posterior teeth is considered the *root trunk*. The cervical cross section of the root trunk initially follows the form of the crown (see Fig. 15.8, *B*). However, the root of a posterior tooth later divides from the root trunk into the correct number of root branches for its tooth type (see Fig. 17.7).

To produce multiple roots, there is differential growth of HERS that causes the root trunk of each multirooted tooth to divide into two or three roots (Fig. 6.21). During the formation of the enamel organ on a multirooted tooth, elongation of its cervical loop occurs, which allows the development of long tongue-like horizontal extensions or flaps within it. Two or three such extensions can be present on multirooted teeth, depending on the similar number of roots of the mature tooth.

The usually single cervical opening of the coronal enamel organ is then divided into two or three openings by the horizontal extensions. On the pulpal surfaces of these openings, dentin formation starts after the induction of the odontoblasts and disintegration of HERS and the associated basement membrane. Cementoblasts are induced to form cementum on the newly formed dentin only at the periphery of each opening. Root development then proceeds in the same way as described for a single-rooted tooth.

Clinical Considerations with Root Formation Disturbances

In some cases, misplaced ameloblasts can migrate to the surface of root by the localized failure of the HERS to separate from the dentin, which causes the enamel to be abnormally ectopically formed over the cemental root surface, which produces an **enamel pearl** (see Box 6.1, *R-S*). It appears as a small spherical enamel projection on the root surface in close proximity to the cementoenamel junction (CEJ) or in the furcations on molars where the roots divide. It may have a tiny dentin and pulp core and appear radiopaque (or light) on radiographs.

Enamel pearls in this location near the CEJ can contribute to the retention of dental biofilm that can, in turn, lead to a risk of periodontal lesions since it interferes with homecare. An enamel pearl may also be confused with a calculus deposit upon exploration of the root surface but cannot be removed by scaling alone. In many cases, the enamel pearl needs to be removed by a dental bur.

If amelogenesis is not turned off after the enamel of the crown has been laid down, the enamel organ may continue to produce enamel over the root dentin. This additional enamel often takes the shape of *enamel projections/spurs* that project into the furcation of multirooted teeth. These projections may increase the risk of periodontal lesions in the affected furcations. Successful treatment of periodontal pockets caused by this anomaly requires again grinding away the enamel projection with a dental bur. By restoring the normal contour of the tooth and exposing the underlying dentin, it is more likely that new attachment procedures will succeed in eliminating the lesion.

Another disturbance that can occur during root development is **dilaceration** (dih-las-uh-**rey**-shuhn), resulting in either distorted root(s) or severe associated crown angulation in a formed tooth (see **Chapter 16** and Fig. 17.36). Dilaceration is caused by a distortion of HERS due to an injury or pressure; it can occur in any tooth or group of teeth during tooth development. It may cause complications during extraction and endodontic therapy and underlines the importance of preoperative radiographic examination; sometimes the bend is pronounced enough to prevent eruption of the tooth. This is in contrast to the disturbance of *flexion,* which is a deviation or bend restricted just to the root; usually the bend is less than 90° to the crown.

As to contributing to alteration of the HERS and dilaceration, possibly the following may occur: As a tooth is erupting or experiences delayed eruption, there are other relative dentoskeletal alterations occurring, such as the mesial drift of the dentition and transverse growth of the maxilla or mandible. Thus during the physiologic and growth-related alteration of the alveolar process and basal bone, parts of developing tooth could be found within one or more of the plasticity zones.

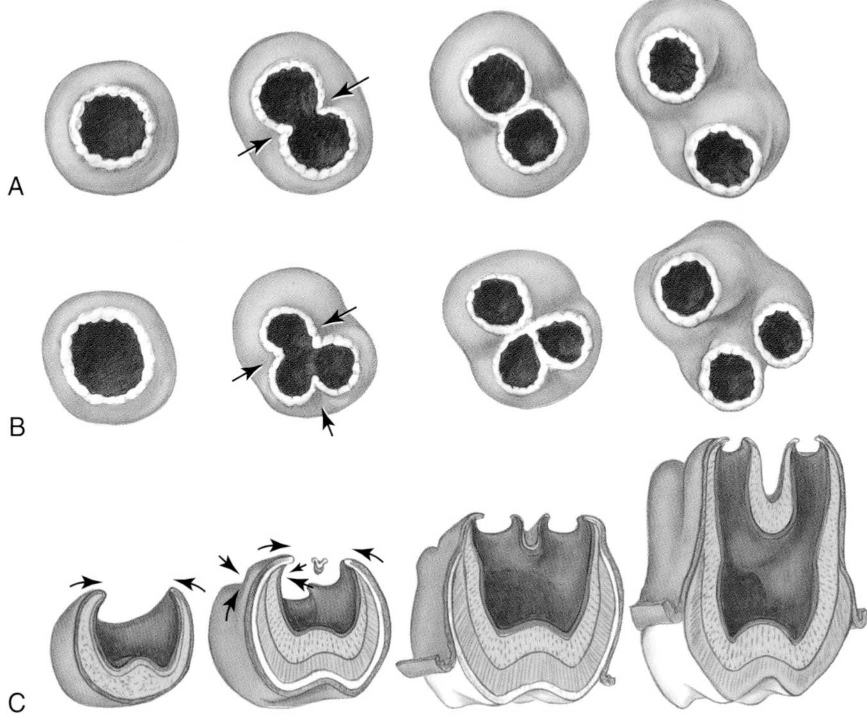

Fig. 6.21 Apical view of multirooted tooth development from horizontal extensions *(arrows)* of the cervical loop for **(A)** a two-rooted tooth and **(B)** a three-rooted tooth. The detailed cross-section shows the division that produces three roots **(C)** on a permanent maxillary molar.

Teeth may also have **accessory roots** (or supernumerary roots). These extra roots may be due to trauma, pressure, or metabolic disease that affects HERS. Any tooth may be affected, but it occurs more commonly with the permanent third molars and is rare with incisors. These accessory roots can present complications in extraction and endodontic therapy; thus preoperative radiographic examination is again necessary to rule out this disturbance.

Developmental root anatomy variants may involve linguogingival (or palatogingival) grooves as well as proximal root (or radicular) grooves. Linguogingival grooves, found primarily on permanent maxillary incisors are associated with increased dental biofilm accumulation, clinical attachment level loss, and bone loss. Proximal root grooves on permanent incisors and maxillary premolars also predispose to dental biofilm accumulation, loss of clinical attachment level, and bone loss.

PERIODONTAL LIGAMENT AND ALVEOLAR PROCESS DEVELOPMENT

As the crown and root develop, the surrounding supporting tissue types of the tooth also develop from the dental sac (see Fig. 6.20). The ectomesenchyme from the dental sac begins to form the periodontal ligament (PDL) adjacent to the newly formed cementum. The correct formation and degeneration of the HERS are also critical for PDL development. The PDL formation starts with the migration of dental sac cells in contact with the HERS in between the newly formed root and the developing alveolar process. This event coincides with the beginning of HERS disintegration. During migration, a number of cytoplasmic processes project from the leading edges of the NCC-derived dental sac cells and begin secreting collagen fibers.

These collagen fibers of the PDL are initially disorganized, but as development progresses, they thicken and become arranged in a structured manner (see Fig. 14.27). The proper secretion and distribution of these collagen fibers contribute to the correct orientation and attachment of the PDL, which is critical for its ability to connect the root and alveolar process together, stabilizing and preparing the tooth for mastication. The ends of these fibers insert into the outer layers of the cementum and the surrounding alveolar process to support the tooth and are now considered *Sharpey fibers*. The ectomesenchyme of the dental sac also begins to mineralize to form the tooth sockets, which are now considered the *alveoli* of each alveolar process surrounding the PDL (see Fig. 14.14).

The role of HERS in root development, especially as it relates to the initiation of cementogenesis, has become a focus of research. It is now generally accepted that there is a transient period of secretion of proteins, including bone sialoprotein, osteopontin, and amelin, by the cells of HERS. Also growth and differentiation factors may play roles in the development of the attachment apparatus of PDL with reduced enamel epithelium. Interestingly, pluripotent cells from HERS have been shown to differentiate into osteoblasts, cementoblasts, or PDL fibroblasts.

PRIMARY TOOTH ERUPTION AND SHEDDING

Eruption of the primary dentition takes place in chronologic order as does the permanent dentition (Fig. 6.22). This process involves **active eruption**, which is the actual vertical movement of the tooth. This is not the same as **passive eruption**, which occurs with aging, when the gingival tissue recedes, uncovering the clinical root and increasing instead the size of the clinical crown, but no actual tooth movement takes place. In a fully erupted tooth without the influence of aging, the gingival margin becomes located on the enamel 0.5 to 2.0 mm coronal to the CEJ. The timelines for active eruption and root completion using approximate ages are useful for the clinician (for primary dentition with shedding, see Table 18.1 and Fig. 20.5 for sequence; for permanent dentition, see Table 15.2, **Appendix D**, and Fig. 20.6 for sequence).

How active eruption occurs is understood but *why* can only be theorized. No one can certify what forces "push" teeth through the oral soft tissue or can identify the timing mechanism that coincides with these eruptions; each theory for eruption presents a challenge in its conception of its answer to the why. The processes of root growth, existence of a temporary ligament, vascular pressure, contractile collagen, and hormonal signals to genetic targets all have been used to explain eruption.

Active eruption of a primary tooth has many stages in the movement of the tooth. After enamel appositional growth ceases in the crown of each primary or permanent tooth, the ameloblasts place an acellular dental cuticle on the newly formed outer enamel surface. In addition, the layers of the enamel organ become compressed, forming the **reduced enamel epithelium (REE)** (Figs. 6.23 and 6.24). The REE appears as a few layers of flattened cells overlying the enamel surface. When this formation of the REE occurs for a primary tooth, it can then begin to erupt into the oral cavity.

The external cells of the REE are mostly from the stratum intermedium cells but may also include cellular remnants of the stellate reticulum and OEE. Thus these undifferentiated epithelial cells will divide and multiply and eventually give rise to the junctional epithelium of the tooth.

To allow for the eruption process, the REE first has to fuse with the oral epithelium lining the oral cavity (Fig. 6.25). Second, enzymes from the REE then disintegrate the central part of the fused tissue,

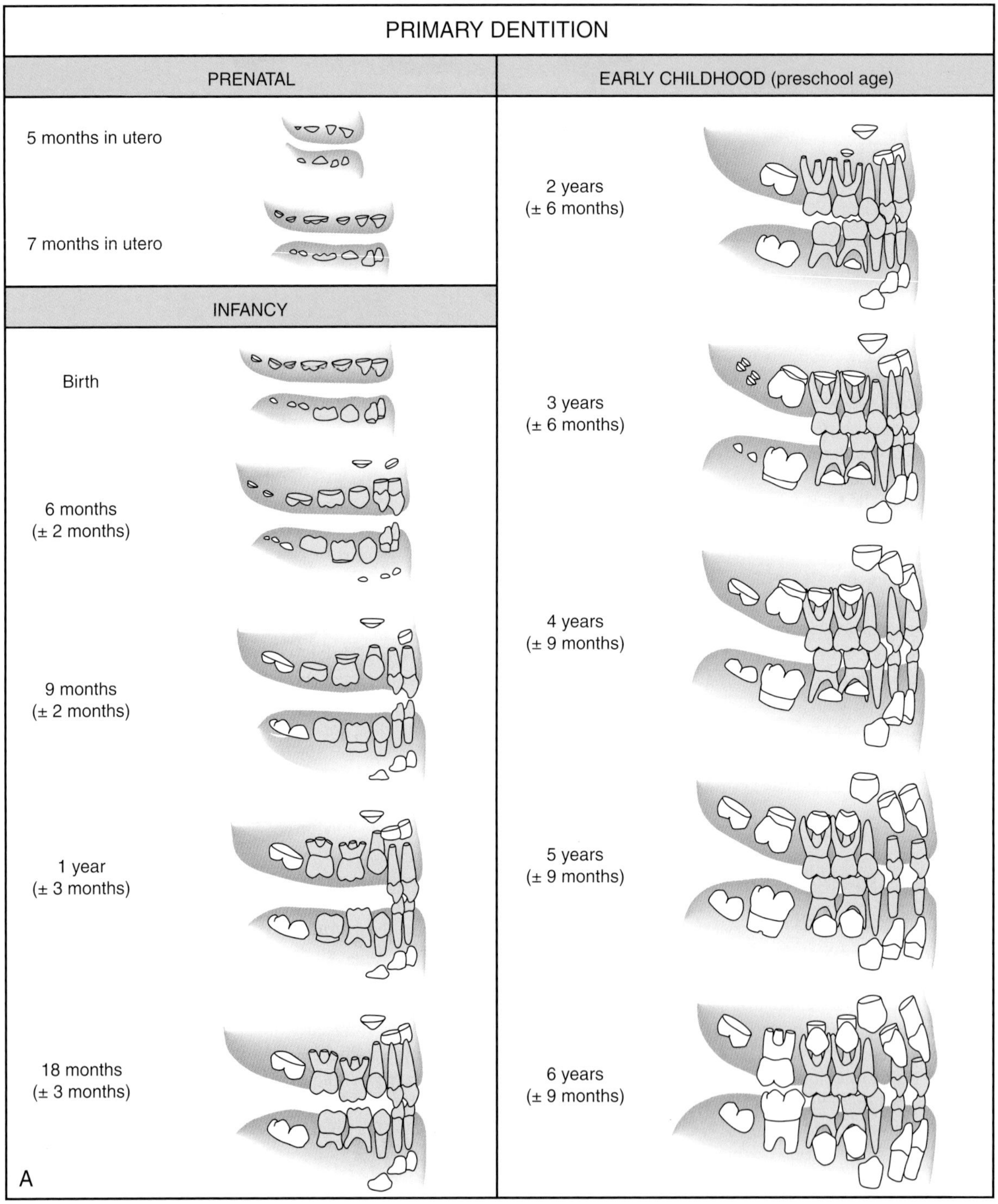

Fig. 6.22 Chronologic order of the eruption of **(A)** the primary (blue) dentition and **(B)** the permanent (white) dentition (continued on next page).

Continued

PERMANENT DENTITION

MIXED DENTITION Late childhood (school age)	PERMANENT DENTITION Adolescence and adulthood
7 years (± 9 months)	11 years (± 9 months)
8 years (± 9 months)	12 years (± 6 months)
9 years (± 9 months)	15 years (± 6 months)
10 years (± 9 months)	21 years
B	35 years

Fig. 6.22 cont'd Chronologic order of the eruption of (A) the primary (blue) dentition and (B) the permanent (white) dentition. (Modified from Schour I, Massler M. The development of the human dentition. *J Am Dent Assoc.* 1941;28:1153-1160.)

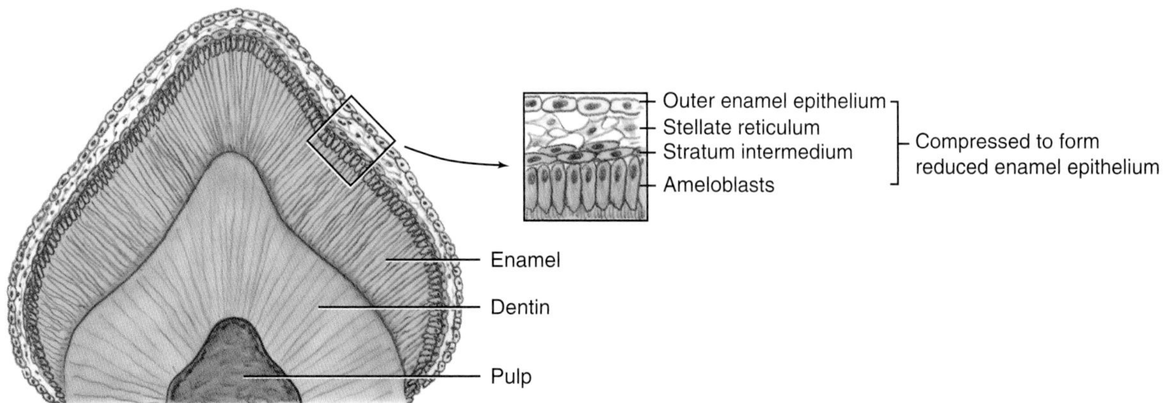

Fig. 6.23 Reduced enamel epithelium produced after the completion of enamel appositional growth when the enamel organ undergoes compression of its many layers on the enamel surface.

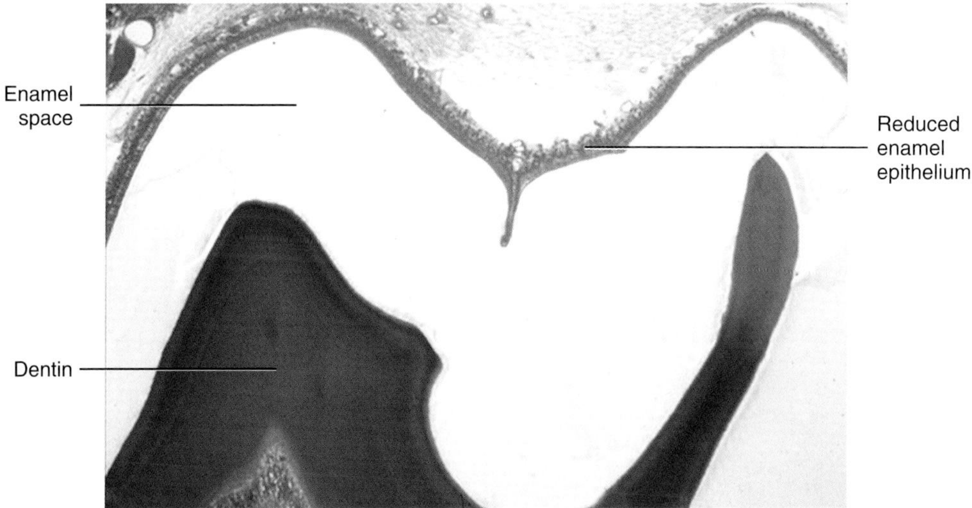

Fig. 6.24 Photomicrograph of reduced enamel epithelium after the completion of enamel appositional growth when the enamel organ undergoes compression of its many layers on the enamel surface (noted as enamel space). (From Nanci A. *Ten Cate's Oral Histology*. 9th ed. St. Louis: Elsevier; 2018.)

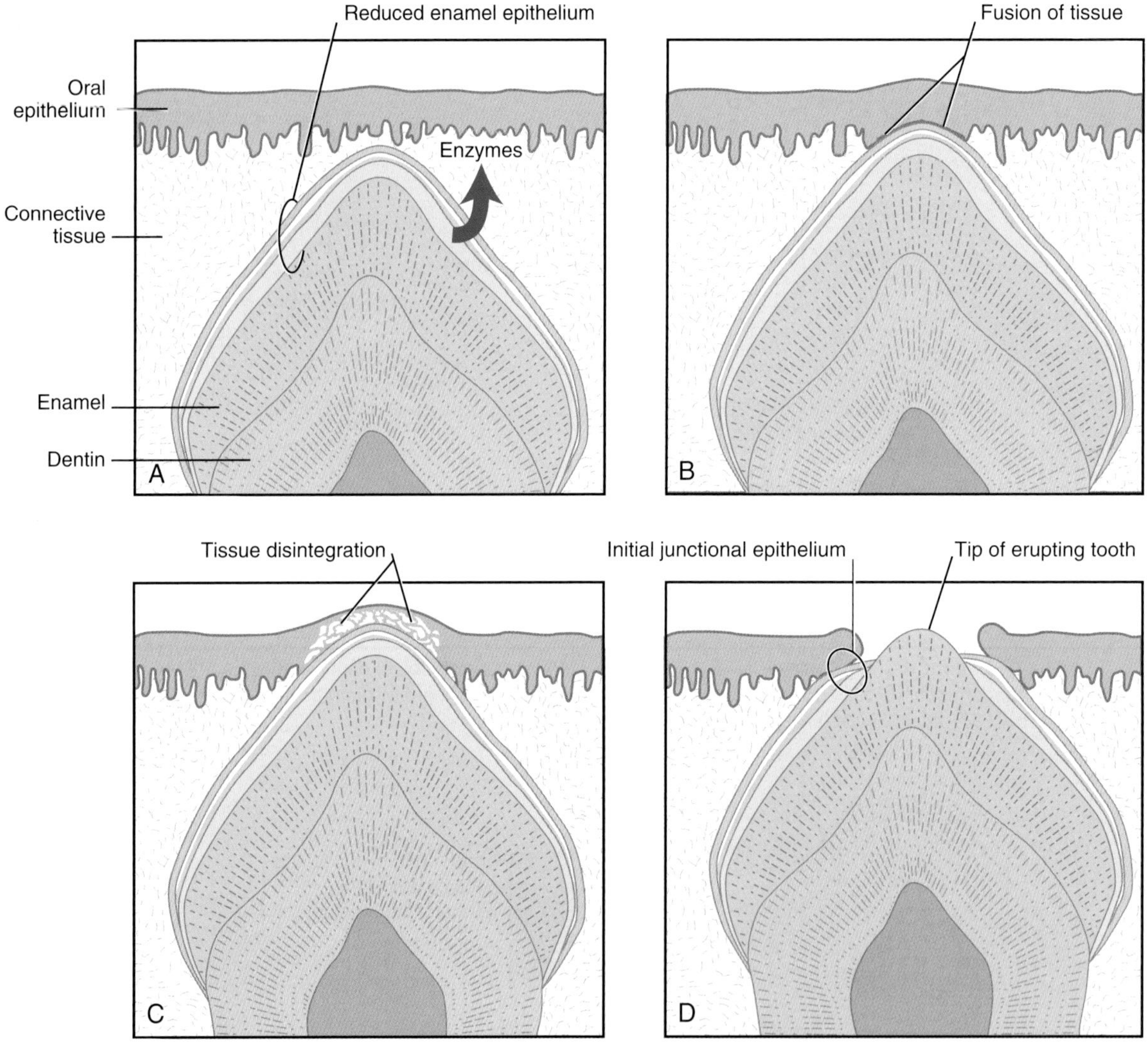

Fig. 6.25 Process of Tooth Eruption. A, Oral cavity before the eruption process begins with reduced enamel epithelium *(circle)* covering the newly formed enamel; enzymes from the reduced enamel epithelium are present for tissue disintegration *(arrow)*. **B,** Fusion of the reduced enamel epithelium with the oral epithelium. **C,** Disintegration of the central fused tissue, leaving an epithelial-lined eruption tunnel for tooth movement. **D,** Coronal fused epithelial tissue peels back from the crown during eruption, leaving the initial junctional epithelium *(circle)*.

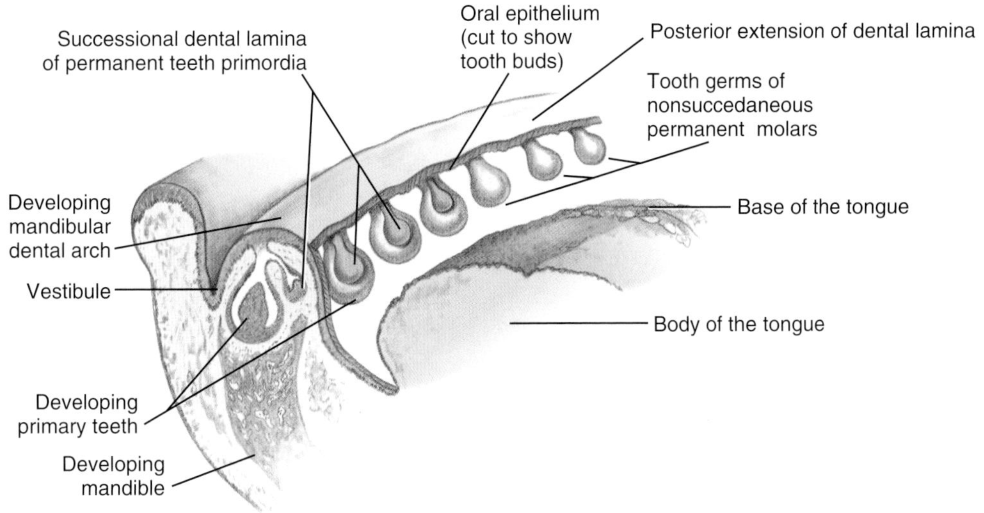

Fig. 6.26 Development of the succedaneous permanent teeth in a lingual position to the primary teeth on a section of a fetal mandible.

leaving a protective epithelial-lined eruption tunnel for the tooth to erupt through the surrounding oral epithelium into the oral cavity. This tissue disintegration causes the usually present inflammatory response known as "teething," which may be accompanied by tenderness and edema of the local tissue. Instituting thorough homecare can reduce the amount of inflammation and thus most of the discomfort associated with these oral changes in infants as their first teeth erupt as well as in young adults when the third molars erupt.

As a primary tooth actively erupts, the coronal part of the fused epithelial tissue peels off the crown, leaving the cervical part still attached to the neck of the tooth like a banana being peeled. This fused tissue that remains near the CEJ after the tooth erupts then serves as the initial junctional epithelium of the tooth, creating a seal between the tissue and the tooth surface. This tissue is later replaced by a definitive junctional epithelium as the root becomes completely formed (see Fig. 10.1).

The primary tooth is then shed as the succedaneous permanent tooth develops lingual to it. The process involving shedding of the primary tooth consists of differentiation of multinucleated osteoclasts from fused macrophages of the surrounding area, which absorb the alveolar process between the two teeth from their *ruffled borders* (see Fig. 8.15). The dental sac surrounding a succedaneous permanent tooth retains its connection with the lamina propria of the oral mucosa by means of a strand of fibrous cord containing remnants of the dental lamina within the **gubernacular canal (GC)** (goo-ber-**nak**-yuh-lahr). As a succedaneous permanent tooth erupts, its GC is widened rapidly by local osteoclastic activity removing the surrounding alveolar bone, delineating the eruptive pathway for the tooth.

In addition, **odontoclasts** (oh-**don**-tuh-klastz) are formed from undifferentiated mesenchyme. These cells cause mostly primary tooth root resorption with the removal of dentin and cementum. Special fibroblasts, now considered **fibroclasts** (**fahy**-bruh-klastz), destroy any remaining connecting collagen fibers holding the primary tooth within its surrounding PDL.

The PDL develops only after root formation has been initiated; when established, the PDL must be remodeled to accommodate continued eruptive tooth movement. The remodeling of PDL fiber bundles is achieved by the both fibroblasts and fibroclasts, which simultaneously create and break down the collagen fibrils as required across the entire extent of the ligament.

The process of shedding the primary tooth is intermittent ("tight/loose") because at the same time that osteoclasts differentiate to resorb bone and odontoclasts differentiate to resorb dental tissue, the always ready odontoblasts and cementoblasts work to replace the resorbed parts of the root as well as the fibroblasts to repair the PDL. Thus, a loose primary tooth may become tightened just when the supervising adult takes a child to the dental office to have it checked (perhaps because the child playing with it is driving the supervising adults crazy). When the primary tooth is finally shed, the mythologic **tooth fairy** (and helpers) goes into action with rates of return now approaching very high levels.

PERMANENT TOOTH ERUPTION

The succedaneous permanent tooth usually erupts into the oral cavity in a position lingual to the roots of the shedding primary tooth, just as it develops that way (Figs. 6.26, 6.27, and 6.28). The only exception to this is the permanent maxillary incisors, which move to a more facially placed position as they erupt into the oral cavity.

The process of eruption for a succedaneous permanent tooth is the same as for the primary tooth after the widening of the GC discussed earlier, the REE fuses with the oral epithelium and then degenerates, leaving an epithelial-lined eruption tunnel. The process of the nonsuccedaneous eruption of the permanent teeth is similar also, but no primary tooth is shed to allow for the process as with the succedaneous permanent teeth. Both succedaneous and nonsuccedaneous permanent teeth usually erupt in chronologic order (see Fig. 6.22). Studies show that the absence of GC as noted by cone-beam computed tomography (CBCT) may indicate a disturbed eruption pattern of the tooth and may increase the risk of complications related to impaction resulting in a tooth that is more likely to remain unerupted.

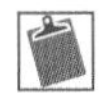 CLINICAL CONSIDERATIONS WITH ERUPTION PROCESS

A permanent tooth often starts to erupt before the primary tooth is fully shed, which may create challenges with spacing. Interceptive orthodontic therapy can prevent some of these situations. Thus, it is important for children with prolonged retention of any primary teeth to seek early dental consultation. Root fragments from primary molars may also be left from the eruption process and can create periodontal

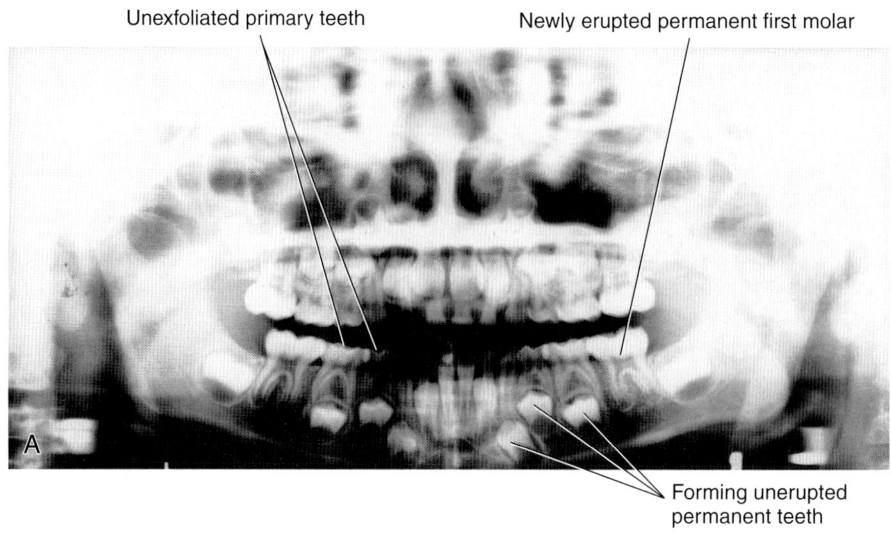

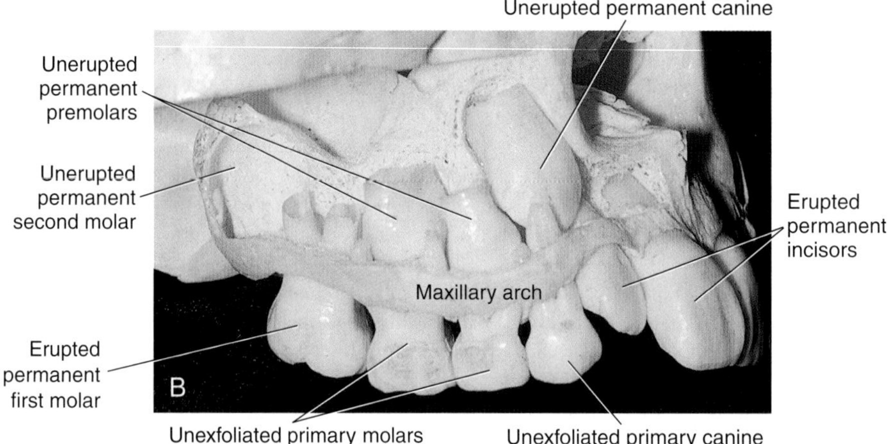

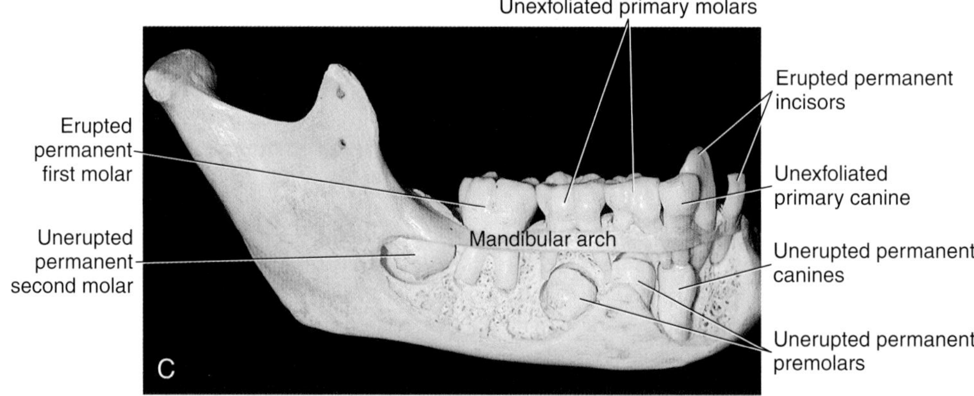

Fig. 6.27 Mixed dentition with primary teeth being shed and the permanent dentition erupting within the jaws of each arch. **A,** Panoramic radiograph. **B** and **C,** Maxilla and mandible with a section of facial cortical plate removed. (Courtesy of Margaret J. Fehrenbach, RDH, MS.)

complications for the permanent dentition. Panoramic radiographs of the mixed dentition are important in order to monitor tooth development (see Fig. 6.27, *A*).

A residue may form on newly erupted teeth of both dentitions that may leave the teeth extrinsically stained. This green-gray residue, **Nasmyth membrane** (**nas**-mith), consists of the fused tissue of the REE and oral epithelium as well as the dental cuticle placed by the ameloblasts on the newly formed outer enamel surface (Fig. 6.29). Nasmyth membrane then easily picks up coloring from food debris but can be removed by selective polishing; the child's supervising adults may need reassurance as to its background.

In addition, because the crown forms before the root, prevention of traumatic injury to the permanent teeth before they are fully anchored into the jaws is very important. Mouthguards, which consist of individually formed plastic coverings for the teeth, are recommended for children active in all types of sports. Any injury to dentition of children

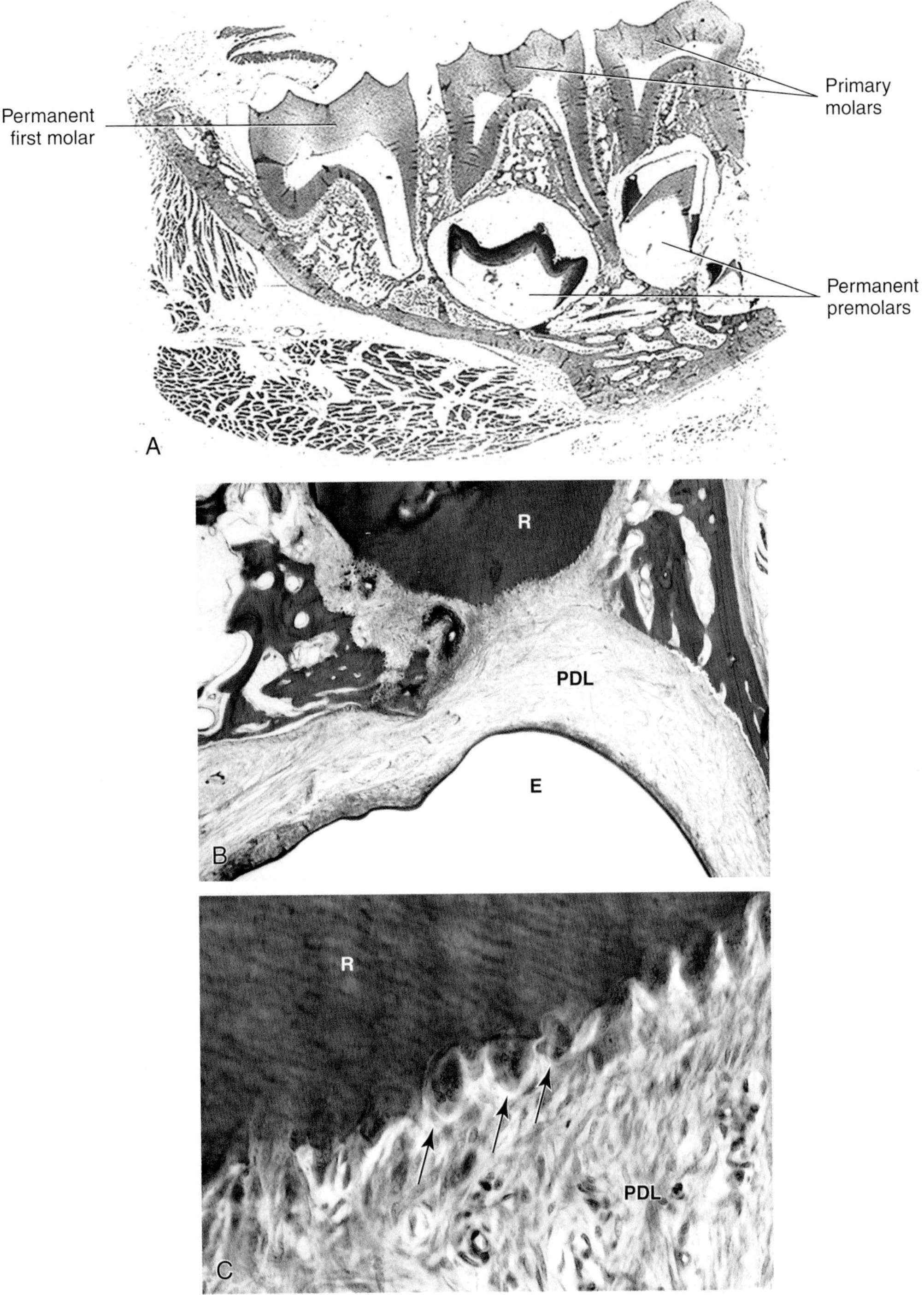

Fig. 6.28 Eruption Process. **A,** Photomicrograph of mandibular sagittal section showing a mixed dentition of posterior teeth, primary and permanent. The primary molars are undergoing root resorption due to the nearby succedaneous permanent premolars and also present is the nearby formation of the roots of the nonsuccedaneous permanent first molar that needs to erupt into the oral cavity. **B** and **C,** Close-up microscopic sections of process, the primary tooth resorption of root *(R)*, periodontal ligament *(PDL)* with its odontoclasts *(arrows)*, and enamel *(E, now as a space due to processing)* of permanent tooth undergoing eruption. (**A,** From Nanci A. *Ten Cate's Oral Histology*. 9th ed. St. Louis: Elsevier; 2018; **B** and **C,** From Bernhard Gottlieb Collection, courtesy of James McIntosh, PhD, Assistant Professor Emeritus, Department of Biomedical Sciences, Baylor College of Dentistry, Dallas.)

(such as avulsion) must be promptly cared for to prevent injury to the forming teeth and its supporting tissue types.

An odontogenic cyst that forms from the REE after the crown has completely formed and matured is considered a **dentigerous cyst** (den-**tij**-er-uhs) (or follicular cyst) (Fig. 6.30). This initially asymptomatic cyst forms around the crown of a nonerupted impacted or developing tooth, most commonly associated with the permanent third molars. When this cyst becomes larger within the bone of the jaws, it may cause displaced teeth, jaw fracture, and pain; it must be completely removed surgically because it may otherwise become neoplastic.

If a dentigerous cyst appears on a partially erupted tooth, it is considered an *eruption cyst* and appears as fluctuant blue vesicle-like gingival lesion (Fig. 6.31). Unlike the other types of dentigerous cysts, the eruption cyst disintegrates with eruption of the tooth and no further treatment is needed. Because it appears to enlarge as the tooth erupts, the child's supervising adults may need reassurance as to its background.

As discussed earlier, the disintegration of the dental lamina after eruption results in the formation of discrete clusters of epithelial cells that usually degenerate, but some may persist and form **epithelial pearls.** These clusters of cells may form small cysts or eruption cysts as noted over the developing tooth and delay eruption, may give rise to an odontoma (discussed next), or may be activated to form supernumerary teeth (discussed earlier).

The ability to form supernumerary teeth suggests that these structures of the epithelial pearls have been exposed to all necessary signals and retain memory. Thus the epithelial pearls may hold the key to tooth regeneration. Epithelial pearls could also serve as a potential source of dental stem cells for new strategies in tooth bioengineering and regeneration.

An **odontoma** (oh-don-**toh**-mah) is a benign neoplasm of odontogenic origin (i.e., linked to tooth development) that can come from the presence of epithelial pearls. Odontomas are inherited or are due to a mutagene or interference, possibly postnatal, with the genetic control of tooth development. An odontoma should be surgically removed before it can interfere with eruption of teeth in the area.

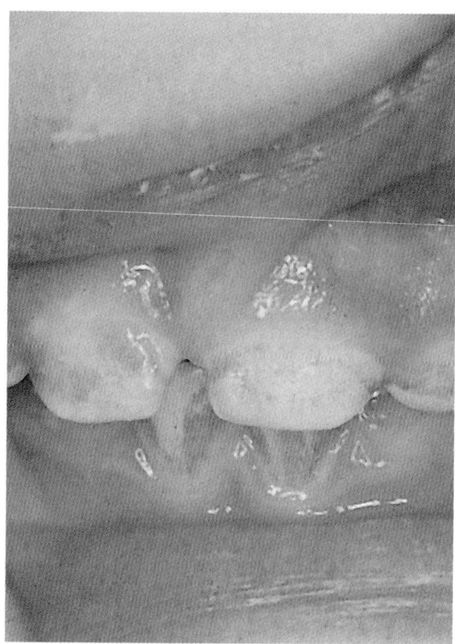

Fig. 6.29 Extrinsic Staining with Nasmyth Membrane After Eruption of the Teeth. Entire crowns of the primary dentition may be affected as well as those of the permanent dentition. (Courtesy of Margaret J. Fehrenbach, RDH, MS.)

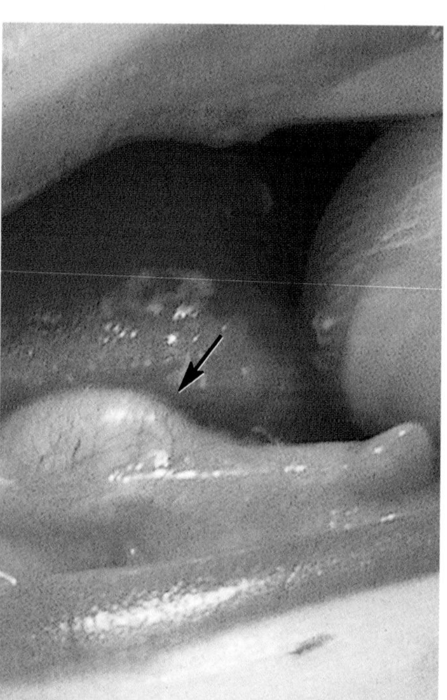

Fig. 6.31 Eruption Cyst in a Child. This less serious type of dentigerous cyst *(arrow)* has formed over the crown of an erupting primary mandibular incisor. (Courtesy of Margaret J. Fehrenbach, RDH, MS.)

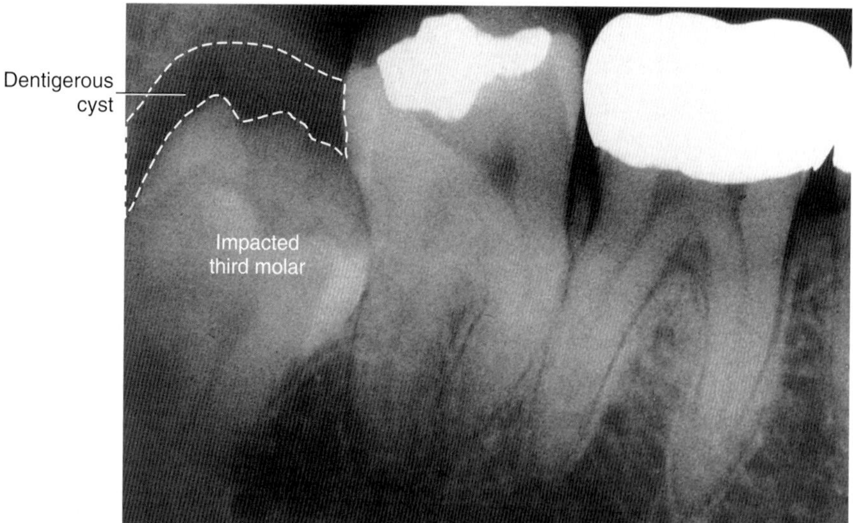

Fig. 6.30 Radiograph of a dentigerous cyst *(dashed lines)* that is formed around the crown of an unerupted permanent mandibular third molar as a result of impaction. (Courtesy of Margaret J. Fehrenbach, RDH, MS.)

7

Cells

Additional resources and practice exercises are provided on the companion Evolve website for this book: http://evolve.elsevier.com/Fehrenbach/illustrated.

LEARNING OBJECTIVES

1. Define and pronounce the key terms in this chapter.
2. Discuss cell properties and components, including the cell membrane, cytoplasm, organelles, and inclusions.
3. Identify the components of the cell on a diagram.
4. Outline the cell cycle, describing the phases of mitosis that are involved.
5. Describe the extracellular materials surrounding the cell and its intercellular junctions.
6. Integrate the study of cell anatomy into the further study of dental histology.

CELL PROPERTIES

As an introduction to **Unit 3**, the microscopic organization of the body is discussed in this chapter. **Histology** (hi-**stol**-uh-jee) is the study of the microscopic structure and function of cells and the associated tissue. Another term for histology is *microanatomy* because the dimensions of the anatomic structures studied are on a microscopic scale; see **Appendix B** for information on the units of measurement used. A dental professional must have a clear understanding of the basic structural unit of the body, the cell and its components as well as understanding the larger concepts involved in the histology of tissue, such as those found in the oral cavity. This chapter gives an overview of the cell and its various components and then **Chapter 8** presents a review of basic tissue types in the body. A discussion of the histology of each of the tissue types within the oral cavity follows in later chapters of **Unit 3** along with clinical considerations related to histology.

The smallest living unit of organization in the body is the **cell** because each cell is capable of performing any necessary functions without the aid of other cells (Figs. 7.1 and 7.2, Table 7.1). Each cell has a cell membrane, cytoplasm, organelles, and inclusions. Thus, every cell is a world unto itself like a small gated community or walled city surrounded by a boundary, having "factories" and other "industries" that make it almost self-sufficient.

Cells also interact with one another similar to how a city interacts with other cities. Cells with similar characteristics of form and function are grouped together to form a **tissue,** which is analogous to how states or provinces are then formed from cities having a common goal (see Table 7.1). Thus, a tissue is a collection of similarly specialized cells, which are most often surrounded by extracellular materials. Various tissue types are then bonded together to form an **organ,** a somewhat independent body part that performs a specific function or functions, similar to countries formed from like-minded states or provinces. Organs can further function together globally as a **system.**

Cells in a tissue undergo cell division to reproduce and replace the dead tissue cells. As a result of the division process, two daughter cells that are identical to each other and to the original parent cell are formed. This process consists of different phases, which are discussed later in this chapter in regard to the different components of the cell.

However, cells also interact with the extracellular environment in many ways. Cells can perform **exocytosis** (ek-soh-sahy-**toh**-sis), which is an active transport of material from a vesicle within the cell out into the extracellular environment. Exocytosis occurs when there is fusion of a vesicle membrane with the cell membrane and subsequent expulsion of the contained material.

The uptake of materials from the extracellular environment into the cell is **endocytosis** (en-doh-sahy-**toh**-sis). Endocytosis can take place as an invagination of the cell membrane. Endocytosis can also take the form of **phagocytosis** (fag-uh-sahy-**toh**-sis), which is the engulfing and then digesting of solid waste and foreign material by the cell through enzymatic breakdown of the material (discussed later in this chapter).

CELL ANATOMY

The **cell membrane** (or plasma membrane) surrounds the cell (see Figs. 7.1 and 7.2). Despite its fragile microscopic structure, it is a tough and resourceful "gatekeeper" for the cell's interior. The usual cell membrane is an intricate bilayer, consisting mostly of phospholipids and proteins. The phospholipids serve mostly as a diffusion regulator. The proteins of the cell membrane serve as structural reinforcements as well as receptors for specific hormones, neurotransmitters, and immunoglobulins (or antibodies). The cell membrane is associated with many of the mechanisms of intercellular junctions and other functions of the cell.

The **cytoplasm** (**sahy**-tuh-plaz-uhm) includes the semifluid part contained within the cell membrane boundary as well as the skeletal system of support or cytoskeleton (discussed later in this chapter). The cytoplasm contains not only a number of structures but also cavities or **vacuoles** (**vak**-yoo-ohlz).

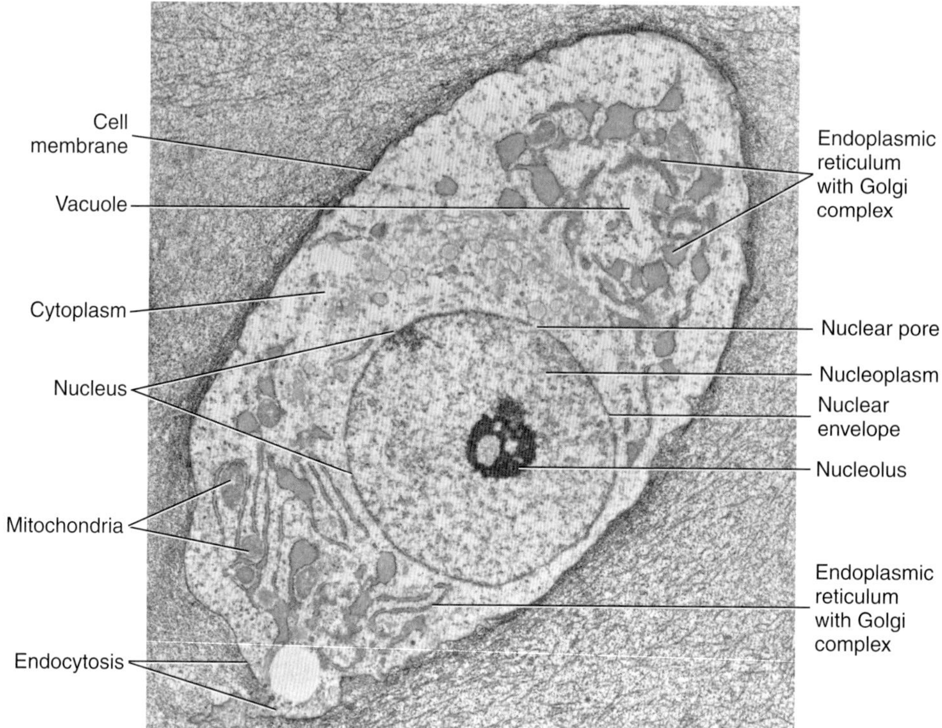

Fig. 7.1 Electron Micrograph of the Cell and its Most Visible Contents: Cell Membrane and Nucleus.

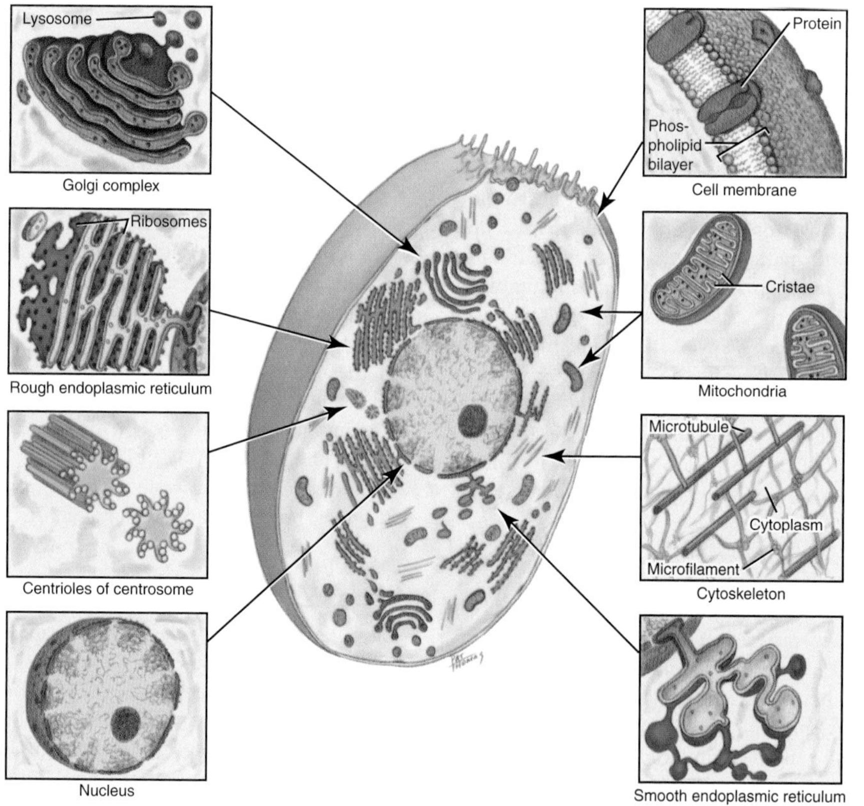

Fig. 7.2 The Cell with its Organelles and Cell Membrane Examined.

ORGANELLES

The **organelles** (awr-guh-**nels**) are metabolically active specialized structures within the cell (see Figs. 7.1 and 7.2). The organelles allow each cell to function according to its genetic code. Organelles also subdivide the cell into compartments. The major organelles of the cell include the nucleus, mitochondria, ribosomes, endoplasmic reticulum, Golgi complex, lysosomes, and the cytoskeleton.

Nucleus

The **nucleus** (**noo**-klee-uhs) (plural, **nuclei** [**noo**-klee-ahy]) is the largest, densest, and most conspicuous organelle in the cell when it is

TABLE 7.1 Body Components

Body Components	Description : Examples
Cell	Smallest living unit of organization: epithelial cell, neuron, myofiber, chondrocyte, osteocyte, fibroblast, erythrocyte, macrophage, sperm
Tissue	Collection of similarly specialized cells: epithelium, nervous tissue, muscle, cartilage, bone, connective tissue, blood
Organ	Independent body part formed from tissue: skin, brain, heart, liver
System	Organs functioning together: central nervous system, respiratory system, immune system, cardiovascular system

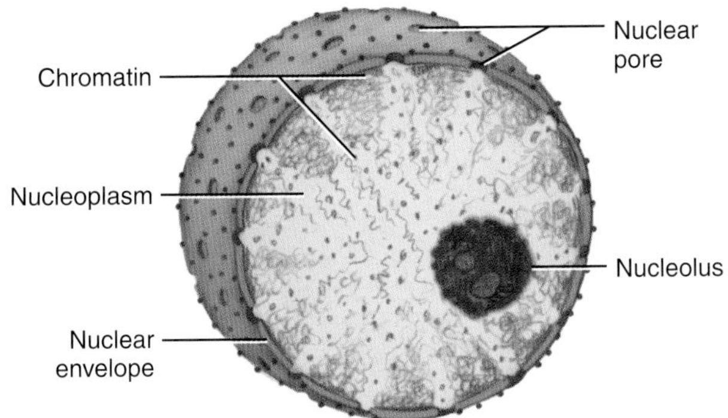

Fig. 7.3 Nucleus and its Various Components, Chromatin, Nucleoplasm, Nuclear Envelope, Nuclear Pore, and Nucleolus.

examined microscopically (Fig. 7.3; see Figs. 7.1 and 7.2). A nucleus is found in all cells of the body except mature red blood cells and most cells have a single nucleus. However, some cells are multinucleated, such as osteoclasts or skeletal muscles (see Figs. 8.15 and 8.18).

The main nucleic acid in the nucleoplasm is deoxyribonucleic acid (DNA), in the form of **chromatin** (**kroh**-muh-tin), which looks like diffuse stippling when the cell is viewed at lower power microscopically. In an actively dividing cell, the chromatin condenses into visible and discrete rodlike **chromosomes** (**kroh**-muh-sohms) (see Table 7.2). Each chromosome has a **centromere** (**sen**-truh-meer), a clear constricted area near the middle. Chromosomes then become two filamentous or threadlike **chromatids** (**kroh**-muh-tids) as daughter chromosomes joined by a centromere during cell division. After cell division, major segments of the chromosomes again become uncoiled and dispersed among the other components of the nucleoplasm as before.

The nucleus is the cell's "data bank" because it stores the genetic code. From its sequence of nucleotides in the chromatin, the DNA and ribonucleic acid (RNA) contain instructions for everything the cell is and will become. Thus, they control all functions the cell performs. The nucleus is also the "command center" of the cell, controlling the other organelles in the cell; it is influenced by what occurs inside the cell as well as outside the cell. Only certain genes are "turned on" to participate in the production of specific proteins at any particular time.

The chemical messages that result in genes switching on or off in the nucleus come from the cytoplasm, where in turn, they are generated as a result of interaction between the surface membrane and the environment. Although genes contain the total range of the cell's possibilities, the cellular environment dictates which of these possibilities for differentiation, growth, development, and specialization will be expressed.

As would be expected, the nucleus is constantly active. Before cell division, new DNA must first be synthesized with every single gene replicated. These genes, linked into chromosomes, are then separated into duplicate sets during cell division. In the nucleus, three very important types of RNA are produced, the messenger RNA (mRNA) molecules, which are complementary copies of distinct segments of DNA, and transfer RNA (tRNA) molecules, which are capable of specifically binding to and transporting amino acid units for protein synthesis as well as ribosomal RNA (rRNA) molecules, which will be discussed later.

In addition to all the activity associated with cell division, the genes on the DNA selectively direct the synthesis of thousands of enzymes and other integral and cytoplasmic proteins as well as any secretory products. This process involves transcription of information from various parts of the DNA molecules into new strands of mRNA, which carry the encoded instructions into the cytoplasm for processing through the process of translation, which involves tRNA, rRNA, and amino acids.

The fluid part within the nucleus is the **nucleoplasm** (**noo**-klee-uh-plaz-uhm), which contains important molecules used in the construction of ribosomes, nucleic acids, and other nuclear materials. The nucleus is surrounded by the **nuclear envelope** (**noo**-klee-er), a membrane similar to the cell membrane, except that it is double layered. The nuclear envelope is associated with many other organelles of the cell. The nuclear envelope may be pierced by **nuclear pores,** which act as avenues of communication between the inner nucleoplasm and the outer cytoplasm. The number and distribution of these nuclear pores vary with the cell type, with the level of cell activity, and with states of differentiation level of the same cell type.

Contained in the nucleus is the **nucleolus** (noo-**klee**-uh-luhs), a prominent and rounded nuclear organelle that is centrally placed in the nucleoplasm when the cell is examined microscopically (see Fig. 7.3). The nucleolus mostly produces rRNA and the nucleotides of the two other types of RNA. Without a nucleolus, no protein synthetic activity would occur within the cell; the nucleolus acts similarly to a "city hall" in managing the activity within the cell. The roles of the nucleolus and ribosomes with rRNA in protein synthesis are discussed later.

Mitochondria

The **mitochondria** (mahy-tuh-**kon**-dree-uh) are the most numerous organelles in the cell. They are associated with energy conversion and thus are the "power stations" for the cell (see Figs. 7.1 and 7.2). They are a major source of adenosine triphosphate (ATP) and thus are the site of many metabolic reactions. Microscopically mitochondria resemble small bags with a larger bag fitted inside because each bag is folded back on itself. These inner folds exist to increase the surface area for more dense packing of the particular proteins and enzyme molecules involved in aerobic cellular respiration. Internal to the folds, mitochondrial DNA, calcium and magnesium granules, enzymes, electrolytes, and water are present in a matrix. A matrix is a surrounding medium to a structure as discussed in **Chapter 6**.

Most of a cell's energy comes from mitochondria, produced by two of the pathways of aerobic cellular respiration. These involve both the Krebs cycle (or citric acid cycle) with its multienzyme system as well as the hydrogen pathway, which uses the electron transport chain of enzymes. Besides supplying energy, mitochondria help with the balance of the concentration of water, calcium, and other ions in the cytoplasm. Cells with high levels of mitochondria are also known for high levels of activity, such as with "young" fibroblasts in healthy oral mucosa; the reverse is noted with the cellular changes encountered with inflammatory periodontal disease having lower levels of mitochondria in the "older" fibroblasts (see **Chapter 8**). This may also explain the possible interrelationship between two prominent inflammatory diseases, periodontal disease and cardiovascular disease (CVD).

TABLE 7.2 **Cell Cycle**

Cell Cycle Phases	Microscopic Structures	
Interphase: G1, S, G2 Phases Cells between divisions engage in growth, metabolism, organelle replacement, and substance production, including chromatin and centrosome replication.	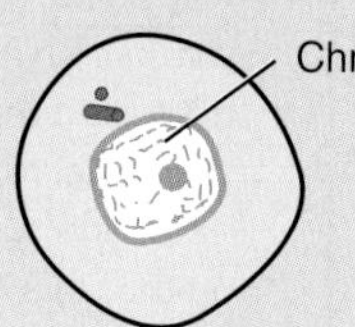	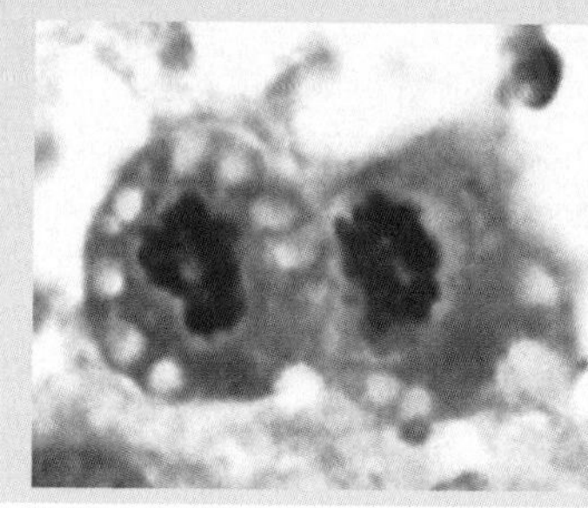
Mitosis Phases ***Prophase*** Chromatin condenses into chromosomes in cell. Replicated centrioles migrate to opposite poles. Nuclear membrane and nucleolus disintegrate.	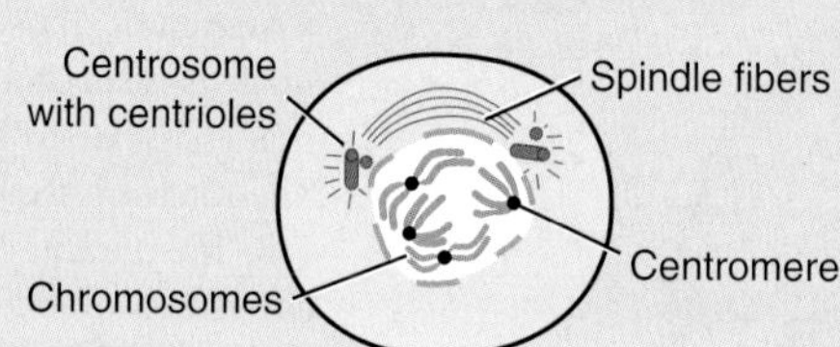	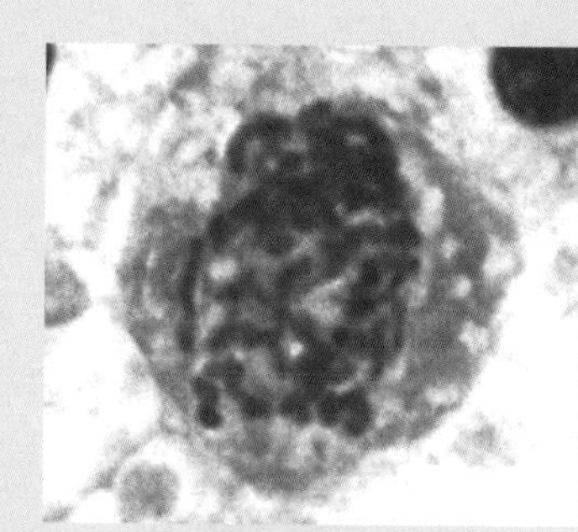
Metaphase Chromosomes move so that their centromeres are aligned in equatorial plane. Mitotic spindle forms.	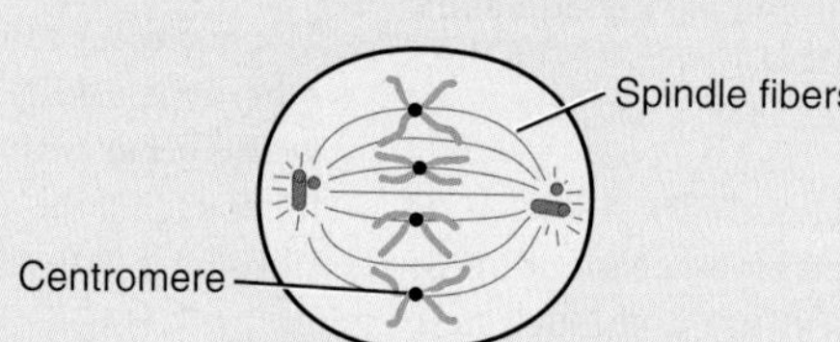	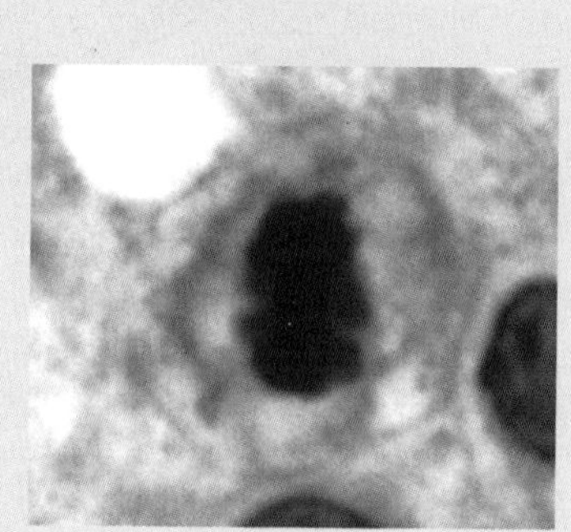
Anaphase Centromeres split and each chromosome separates into two chromatids. Chromatids migrate to opposite poles by mitotic spindle.	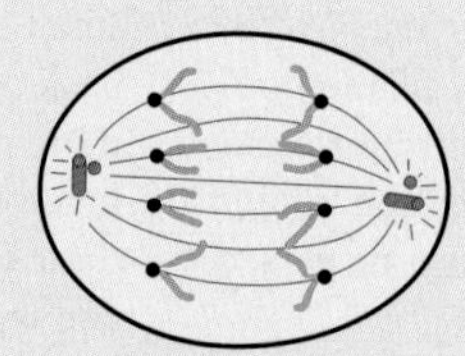	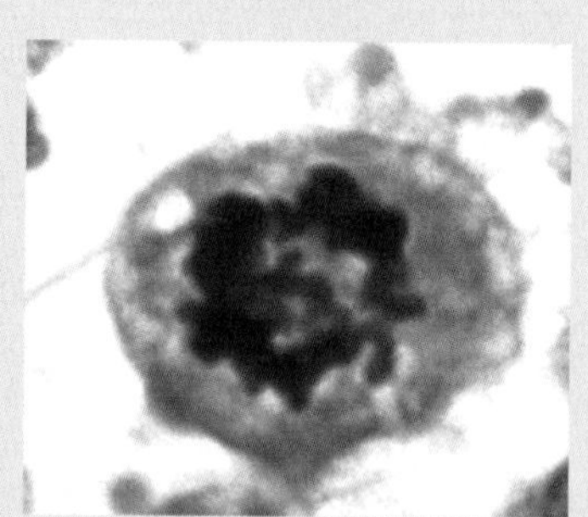
Telophase Division into two daughter cells occurs. Nuclear membrane reappears.	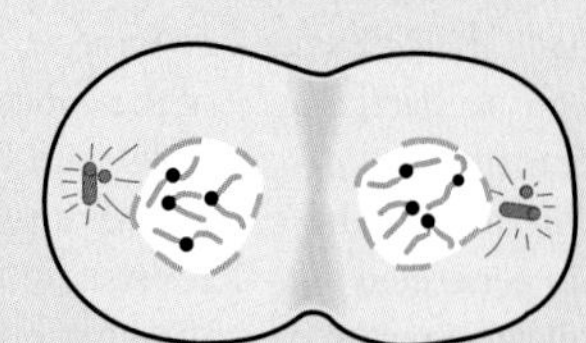	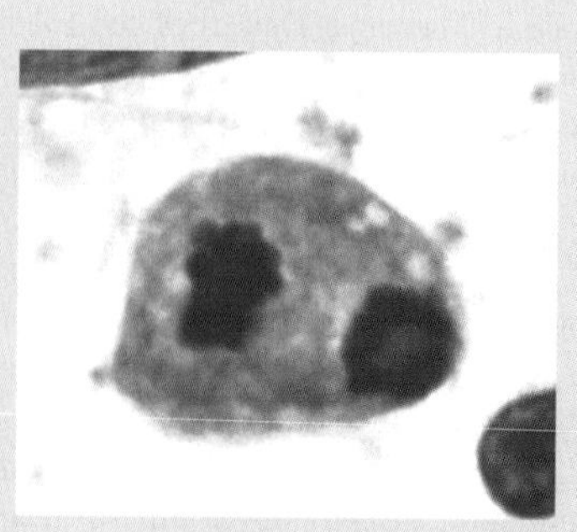

Electron micrographs from Stevens A, Lowe J. *Human Histology*. 5th ed. St. Louis: Elsevier; 2010.

Ribosomes

The **ribosomes** (**rahy**-buh-sohms) are the tiny sphere-shaped organelles in the cell (see Fig. 7.2). The ribosomes are produced in the nucleolus from rRNA and protein molecules and are assembled in the cytoplasm. They function as mobile "protein factories" for the cell; their location changes based on the type of protein being made for the cell. They can be within mitochondria, free in the cytoplasm, or bound to membranes, either to the outer nuclear membrane or onto the surface of the rough endoplasmic reticulum (discussed next).

Ribosomes can also be found singly or in clusters within the cell. As many as 30 separate ribosomes may be attached sequentially to a single molecule of mRNA, with each ribosome making its own protein copy as it works its way along the length of the mRNA transcript. Within these ribosomes, free amino acids are being joined together according to the particular order specified by the mRNA transcript corresponding to the sequence of the required protein chain.

Endoplasmic Reticulum

The **endoplasmic reticulum (ER)** (**en**-duh-**plaz**-mik) is so referred to because it is more concentrated in the cell's inner or endoplasmic region as compared to the peripheral or ectoplasmic region (see Figs. 7.1 and 7.2). The ER consists of parallel membrane-bound channels. All the membranes of the ER interconnect, forming a system of channels and folds microscopically, and are continuous with the nuclear envelope like a "highway" system for the cell.

The ER can be classified as either smooth or rough, which is determined by the absence or presence of ribosomes, giving each a differing outer microscopic texture structure as well as differing in function. The smooth ER (SER), which is free of ribosomes, appears microscopically smooth in surface texture. The rough ER (RER) as discussed earlier is dotted with ribosomes on its outer surface, which makes it appear microscopically rough.

The outer layer of the nuclear envelope connects with all the ER in the cell, both smooth and rough. The ER's primary functions are modification, storage, segregation, and finally transport of proteins that the cell manufactures on the ribosomes for use in other sections of the cell or even outside the cell.

Golgi Complex

Once the ER has modified a new protein, it is then transferred to the **Golgi complex** (**gawl**-jee) (or Golgi apparatus) for subsequent segregation, packaging, and transport of protein compounds just like a "distribution center" for the cell (see Figs. 7.1 and 7.2). The Golgi complex is the second largest organelle after the nucleus and is composed of stacks of 3 to 20 flattened smooth-membrane vesicular sacs arranged parallel to one another.

Vesicles of protein molecules from the RER fuse with the Golgi complex, transferring protein molecules to be further modified, concentrated, and packaged by the Golgi complex. After this modification and packaging, the Golgi complex wraps up large numbers of these molecules into a single membranous vesicle and then sends it on its way to the cell's surface to be released by the process of exocytosis. These protein molecules, which include hormones, enzymes, and other secretory products, are released into the extracellular space or into capillaries as these vesicles fuse with the cell membrane. These products that are put together in the Golgi complex can include such substances as mucus secretory product for the salivary glands or insulin for the pancreas.

The modifications by the Golgi complex to the protein molecules include adding carbohydrates, thus forming glycoproteins as it does in the production of mucus. The Golgi complex also may remove part of a polypeptide chain as it does in the case of insulin. The Golgi complex not only prepares proteins for export by exocytosis but also produces a separate organelle, lysosome (discussed next).

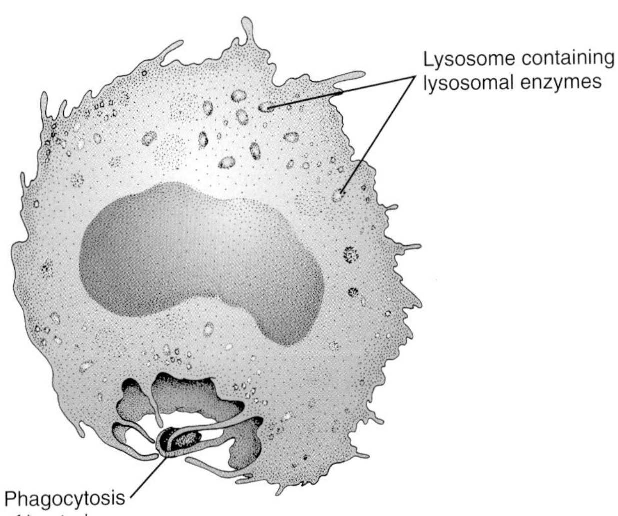

Fig. 7.4 Phagocytosis, which is the engulfing and digesting of solid waste and foreign material (such as with the bacterium shown here) by a white blood cell (monocyte) through enzymatic breakdown of the matter from its enclosed lysosomes. (From Fehrenbach MJ. Inflammation and repair. In: Ibsen OAC, Phelan JA, eds. *Oral Pathology for Dental Hygienists*. 7th ed. St. Louis: Elsevier; 2018.)

Lysosomes

The **lysosomes** (**lahy**-suh-sohmz) are organelles produced by the Golgi complex and function in both intracellular and extracellular digestion by the cell (see Fig. 7.2). This digestive function is due to their ability to lyse or digest various waste and foreign materials in or around the cell, which occurs during phagocytosis like a "sewer system" for the cell (Fig. 7.4). Lysosomes break down many kinds of molecules using the powerful hydrolytic and digestive enzymes contained within them (see Fig. 8.15). The main hydrolytic enzyme in lysosomes is hyaluronidase. Lysosomes are membrane-bound vesicles that develop as a bud that pinches off the end of one of the Golgi complex's flattened sacs. The enzymes of the lysosomes originally are produced on the RER and then are transported for packaging in the Golgi complex, where the lysosomes originate.

As the substances are broken down into sufficiently small and simple products, the usable material diffuses out of the lysosome into the cell's cytoplasm to be incorporated into new molecules being synthesized, a type of cellular "recycling." Indigestible material remains in the lysosome and becomes a residual body. It either migrates to the cell surface to be released by exocytosis or remains as a remnant in the lysosome and becomes an inclusion (discussed later in this chapter). Although all cells, except red blood cells, are capable of some digestive activity, other cells such as certain white blood cells (e.g., neutrophils) have differentiated to specialize in digestive processes, especially during phagocytosis (see Fig. 8.17). Phagocytosis is very active at the junction between healthy gingival tissue and the tooth surface (see **Chapter 10**).

Centrosome

The **centrosome** (**sen**-truh-sohm) is a dense and somewhat oval-shaped organelle that contains a pair of cylindrical structures, the **centrioles** (**sen**-tree-ohlz) (see Fig. 7.2). The centrosome is always located near the nucleus, which is important because it plays a significant role in forming the mitotic spindle apparatus during cell division. There are two centrioles within the centrosome and each is composed of triplets of microtubules arranged in a cartwheel pattern. Without this self-replicating centriole-centrosome unit, a cell from the body cannot reproduce (discussed later in this chapter).

Cytoskeleton

The interior of the cell is neither liquid nor gel in nature but somewhat between the two types of substances. Within the cell there is a three-dimensional system of support using cellular scaffolding, the **cytoskeleton (CSK)** (sahy-tuh-**skel**-i-tn) (see Fig. 7.2). The components of the CSK include microfilaments, intermediate filaments, and microtubules as a shifting lattice arrangement of structural and contractile components distributed throughout the cell cytoplasm. This design lends basic stability to the cell as a whole, functioning like reinforced girders. It also acts to compartmentalize the cytoplasm, creating preferred "freeways" for the movement of molecules formed by cellular processes.

Both **microfilaments** (mahy-kruh-**fil**-uh-muhnts) and **microtubules** (mahy-kroh-**too**-byoolz) consist of specialized proteins. Microfilaments are delicate threadlike microscopic structures. Microtubules are slender hollow tubular microscopic structures that may appear individually, doubly, or as triplets. Microtubules assist microfilaments in the maintenance of overall cell shape and in the transport of intracellular materials. Additionally, microtubules form the internal framework of cilia and flagella, centrioles, and the mitotic spindle for cell division (discussed later in this chapter).

Certain cells exhibit projections that help move substances along the surface of the cell or are for moving the entire cell in the extracellular environment. If the projections on the cell are shorter and more numerous, they are **cilia** (**sil**-ee-uh); if the projections are fewer and longer, they are **flagella** (fluh-**jel**-uh).

Both the projections of cilia and flagella are useful in human reproduction. An ovum is propelled within the fallopian tube by cilia, and sperm are propelled by their own flagella (see Fig. 3.1). Structurally, there is no major difference between cilia and flagella except for their relative lengths. Both consist of pairs of multiple microtubules that form a ring around two single microtubules. Cilia are also noted in the respiratory mucosa lining the nasal cavity and paranasal sinuses as they move the mucous coating of these tissue types along the surface (see Fig. 11.20).

The **intermediate filaments** (**fil**-uh-muhnts) are of various types of thicker threadlike microscopic structures within the cell. One type of intermediate filaments, the **tonofilaments** (tohn-oh-**fil**-uh-muhnts), have a major role in intercellular junctions (discussed later in this chapter). Another type of intermediate filaments is one that forms keratin, which is found in a calloused type of epithelium located in the oral cavity on the attached gingiva as well as the dorsal surface of the tongue (see Fig. 9.4).

INCLUSIONS

The cell also contains **inclusions** (in-**kloo**-zhuhns), which are metabolically inert substances that are also considered transient over time in the cell (see Fig. 7.2). These include masses of organic chemicals and often are recognizable microscopically. These inclusions are released from storage by the cell and used as demand dictates. Lipids and glycogen can be decomposed for energy from inclusions in the cell. Melanin is stored as inclusions in certain cells of the skin and oral mucosa being responsible for the pigmentation of these tissue types (see Figs. 9.23 and 9.24). Inclusions also include residual bodies, which are spent lysosomes and their digested material.

CELL DIVISION

Cell division or **mitosis** (mahy-**toh**-sis) is a complex process involving many of the organelles of the cell (Table 7.2). Mitosis functions during tissue growth or regeneration and its activity is dependent on the length of the individual cell's lifespan. Before cell division, the DNA is replicated during **interphase** (**in**-ter-feyz) as part of the cell cycle, which is the cell's "living" time. Interphase has three phases: Gap 1or *G1* (or initial resting phase that has cell growth and functioning); synthesis or *S* (or cell DNA synthesis by duplication); and Gap 2 or *G2* (or second resting phase that resumes cell growth and functioning).

Following interphase, mitosis occurs with the cell's nuclear material dividing so that the resulting production is of two daughter cells that are identical to the parent cell as well as to each other (see **Chapter 3**). Then, at the same time, the other cytoplasmic components of the cell also are divided. The cell division that takes place during mitosis consists of four phases: **prophase** (**proh**-feyz), **metaphase** (**met**-uh-feyz), **anaphase** (**an**-uh-feyz), and **telophase** (**tel**-uh-feyz); cell division is followed again by interphase continuing the overall cell cycle (see again Table 7.2).

EXTRACELLULAR MATERIALS

The cells in each tissue type are surrounded by extracellular materials, which include both tissue fluid and intercellular substance. **Tissue fluid** (or interstitial fluid) provides a medium or matrix for dissolving, mixing, and transporting substances and for carrying out chemical reactions. Similar to blood plasma in its content of ions and diffusible substances, tissue fluid contains a small amount of plasma proteins.

Tissue fluid enters the tissue to surround the cells by diffusing through the capillary walls as a filtrate from the plasma of the blood. Tissue fluid then drains back into the blood as lymph through osmosis, via the lymphatics (see **Chapter 8**). The amount of tissue fluid varies from tissue to tissue, with smaller variations occurring over time within any one tissue. An excess amount can accumulate when an injured tissue undergoes an inflammatory response, leading to edema with its tissue enlargement (see Fig. 10.8).

Intercellular substance (in-ter-**sel**-yuh-ler) (or ground substance) is a shapeless, colorless, and transparent material in which the cells of a tissue are imbedded; it also fills the spaces between the cells in a tissue. The intercellular substance serves as a barrier to the penetration of foreign materials into the tissue as well as a medium for the exchange of gases and metabolic substances. The surrounding cells produce the intercellular substance and one of its most common elements is hyaluronic acid.

INTERCELLULAR JUNCTIONS

Certain cells in varying tissue are joined by the mechanism of **intercellular junctions.** These are mechanical attachments formed between cells and also between cells and adjacent noncellular surfaces. With the formation of these intercellular junctions, the cell membranes of different cells come close together but do not completely attach. Higher-power magnification is needed to visualize these attachments, which appear as dense bodies. All intercellular junctions involve some type of intricate attachment device. The attachment device includes an attachment plaque that is located within the cell as well as adjacent tonofilaments.

An intercellular junction between cells is formed by a **desmosome** (**dez**-moh-sohm), such as that present in the superficial layers of the skin or oral mucosa (Fig. 7.5). The desmosome appears to be disc-shaped and as such can be likened to a "spot weld" within the structure of a tissue. The desmosomal junctions are also released during tissue turnover and then become reattached in new locations as the cells migrate, such as during repair after an injury to the skin or oral mucosa (see Fig. 8.3).

Desmosomes can create an artifact when cells in the stratified squamous epithelium are fixed for prolonged microscopic study. The regularly plump cells in the prickle cell layer appear prickly or spiky at their outer edges as they still maintain their junctional stronghold from the desmosomes. The individual dehydrated cells have shrunk from the drying fixation chemicals as a result of cytoplasm loss (see Fig. 9.8).

Another type of intercellular junction is formed by a **hemidesmosome** (hem-eye-**dez**-moh-sohm), which involves an attachment of a cell to an adjacent noncellular surface (Fig. 7.6). This type of attachment

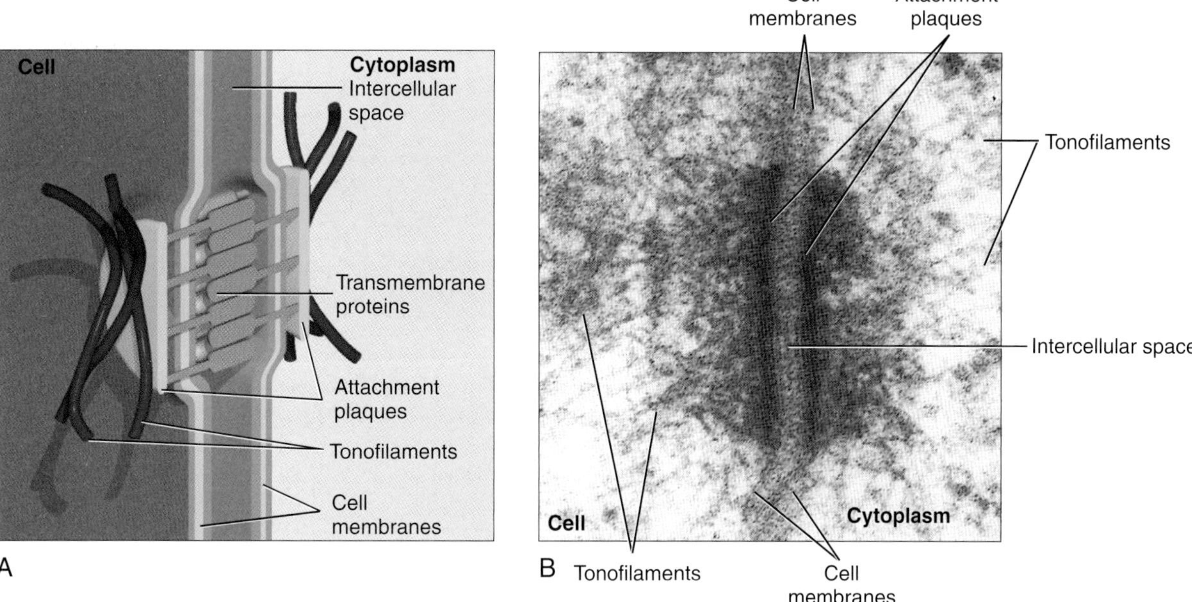

Fig. 7.5 Intercellular Junction Between Cells via a Desmosome. **(A)** Diagram. **(B)** Electron micrograph. The cell adhesion between cell membranes is mediated by transmembrane proteins. This type occurs within the epidermis of the skin (shown here) as well as within the epithelium of the oral mucosa. Note the attachment plaque, which is an attachment device involving tonofilaments. (From Lowe JS, Anderson PG. *Stevens and Lowe's Human Histology.* 5th ed. St. Louis: Elsevier; 2020.)

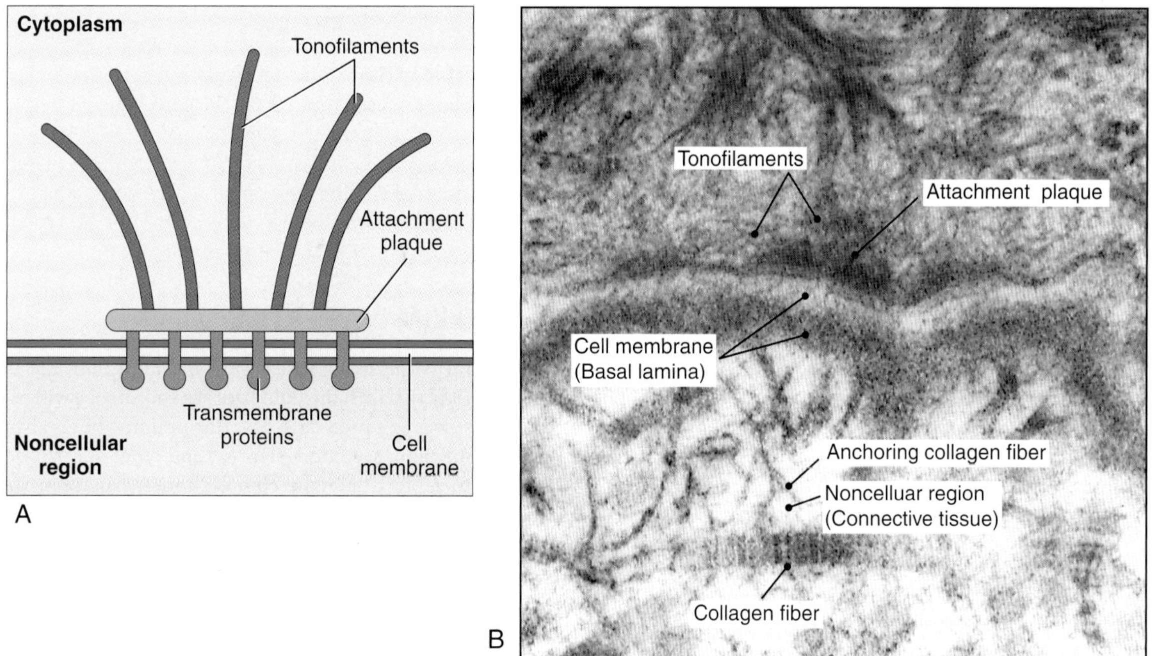

Fig. 7.6 Intercellular Junction Between a Cell with its Cytoplasm and Noncellular Surface via a Hemidesmosome. **(A)** Diagram. **(B)** Electron micrograph. The attachment of cells is to an adjacent noncellular surface is by the adhesion of the noncellular surface mediated by transmembrane protein. This type occurs at the basement membrane between epithelium and connective tissue within the dermis of the skin or lamina propria of oral mucosa (as shown here) as well as at the attachment of gingival tissue to the tooth surface. Note the smaller attachment plaques of the hemidesmosomal junction with tonofilaments on the cellular side. (From Lowe JS, Anderson PG. *Stevens and Lowe's Human Histology.* 5th ed. St. Louis: Elsevier; 2020.)

is used for attaching the epithelium to connective tissue, such as with the basement membrane in the skin and oral mucosa (see Fig. 8.4). The attachment device of a hemidesmosome represents half of a desmosome because it involves a smaller attachment plaque and has tonofilaments from only the cellular side. Therefore it appears as a thinner disc because the noncellular surface cannot produce the other half of the attachment mechanism. Hemidesmosomes are also involved as a mechanism allowing gingival tissue to be secured to the tooth surface by the epithelial attachment (see Figs. 10.6 and 10.7), which is similar to the attachment between the nails and adjoining nail beds.

8

Basic Tissue

Additional resources and practice exercises are provided on the companion Evolve website for this book: http://evolve.elsevier.com/Fehrenbach/illustrated.

LEARNING OBJECTIVES

1. Define and pronounce the key terms in this chapter.
2. Discuss basic tissue properties.
3. Describe epithelium properties, including its histology, classification, regeneration, turnover, and repair.
4. Describe basement membrane properties, including its histology.
5. Integrate the study of the histology of both epithelium and the basement membrane into the further study of dental histology.
6. Discuss connective tissue properties, including its histology, classification, turnover, regeneration, and repair.
7. Describe specialized connective tissue properties.
8. Describe cartilage properties, histology, development, repair, and aging.
9. Describe bone properties, histology, development, remodeling, repair, and aging.
10. Describe blood properties, plasma, and blood components.
11. Integrate the study of the basic histology of connective tissue into understanding the clinical considerations of the orofacial region.
12. Describe muscle properties, classifications, and histology.
13. Describe nerve tissue properties and histology as well as the nervous system divisions.
14. Identify the components of each basic tissue on a diagram.
15. Integrate the study of the histology of both muscle and nerve tissue into the further study of dental histology.

BASIC TISSUE PROPERTIES

Dental professionals must have a clear understanding of the histology of the basic tissue types before studying the distinct tissue types present in the oral cavity and associated regions of the face and neck. This information will help dental professionals fully understand the processes involving tissue renewal and repair and the process of aging during clinical care to promote orofacial health as well as the underlying pathologic processes that can occur.

As was discussed in **Chapter 7**, the smallest living unit of organization in the body is the cell because each cell is capable of performing any necessary functions without the aid of other cells (see Figs. 7.1 and 7.2). It was also noted that a group of cells with similar characteristics of form and function together form a tissue (see Table 7.1). A tissue is a collection of similarly specialized cells that will then form into organs.

Tissue types are categorized according to four basic histologic types. These basic histologic tissue types include epithelial, connective, muscle, and nerve tissue (Table 8.1). In addition, these basic tissue types have subcategories that serve specialized functions. It is during prenatal development that embryonic cell layers differentiate into the various basic embryologic tissue types, including ectoderm, mesoderm, and endoderm, that will later form in some manner into these basic histologic tissue types of the body (see Table 3.4).

Most tissue of the body undergoes **regeneration** (ri-jen-uh-**rey**-shuhn) as the individual cells die and are removed from the tissue and new ones take their place. Regeneration is the natural renewal of a tissue and thus an organ; it is produced by growth and differentiation of new cells and intercellular substances. Regeneration occurs through growth from the same type of tissue that has been destroyed or from its precursor. Regeneration is a continuous physiologic process that occurs with most tissue types and in most organs; it even occurs with injury and disease. However, tooth enamel is an example of a tissue type that sadly does not undergo regeneration.

The **turnover time** is the time it takes for the newly divided cells to be completely replaced throughout the tissue. The turnover time differs for each of the basic tissue types in the orofacial region as well as for specific regions of the oral cavity. A more complete understanding of turnover time may be the future basis for how the aging process as well as disease processes in the body are delayed or prevented, including those occurring in the oral cavity (see **Chapter 9**).

EPITHELIUM PROPERTIES

Epithelium is the tissue that covers and lines both the external and internal body surfaces, including vessels and small cavities. Epithelium not only serves as a protective covering or lining but is also involved in tissue absorption, secretion, sensory, and other specialized functions. It serves to protect the more complex inner structures from physical, chemical, and pathogenic attack as well as dehydration and heat loss by its formation as an epithelial barrier.

Depending on individual classification, epithelial tissue can be derived from any of the three embryonic cell layers based on the location when developing. Importantly for dental professionals, both the epithelium of the skin and that of the oral mucosa are of similar ectodermal origin. In comparison, those lining the respiratory and digestive tract are of endodermal origin, and those lining the urinary tract are derived from mesoderm.

EPITHELIUM HISTOLOGY

In general, epithelium consists of closely grouped polyhedral cells surrounded by very little or no intercellular substance or tissue fluid (Fig. 8.1). Epithelium is avascular, having no blood supply of its own. Cellular nutrition consisting of oxygen and metabolites is obtained by diffusion from the adjoining connective tissue, which is usually highly vascularized, sharing its source of nutrition.

TABLE 8.1 **Basic Tissue Classification**

Tissue	Types : Examples
Epithelium	Simple: Squamous, cuboidal, columnar, pseudostratified
	Stratified: Squamous (keratinized, nonkeratinized), cuboidal, columnar, transitional
Connective tissue	Solid soft: Connective tissue proper, specialized (adipose, fibrous, elastic, reticular)
	Solid firm: Cartilage
	Solid rigid: Bone
	Fluid: Blood, lymph
Muscle	Involuntary: Smooth, cardiac
	Voluntary: Skeletal
Nerve	Afferent: Sensory
	Efferent: Motor

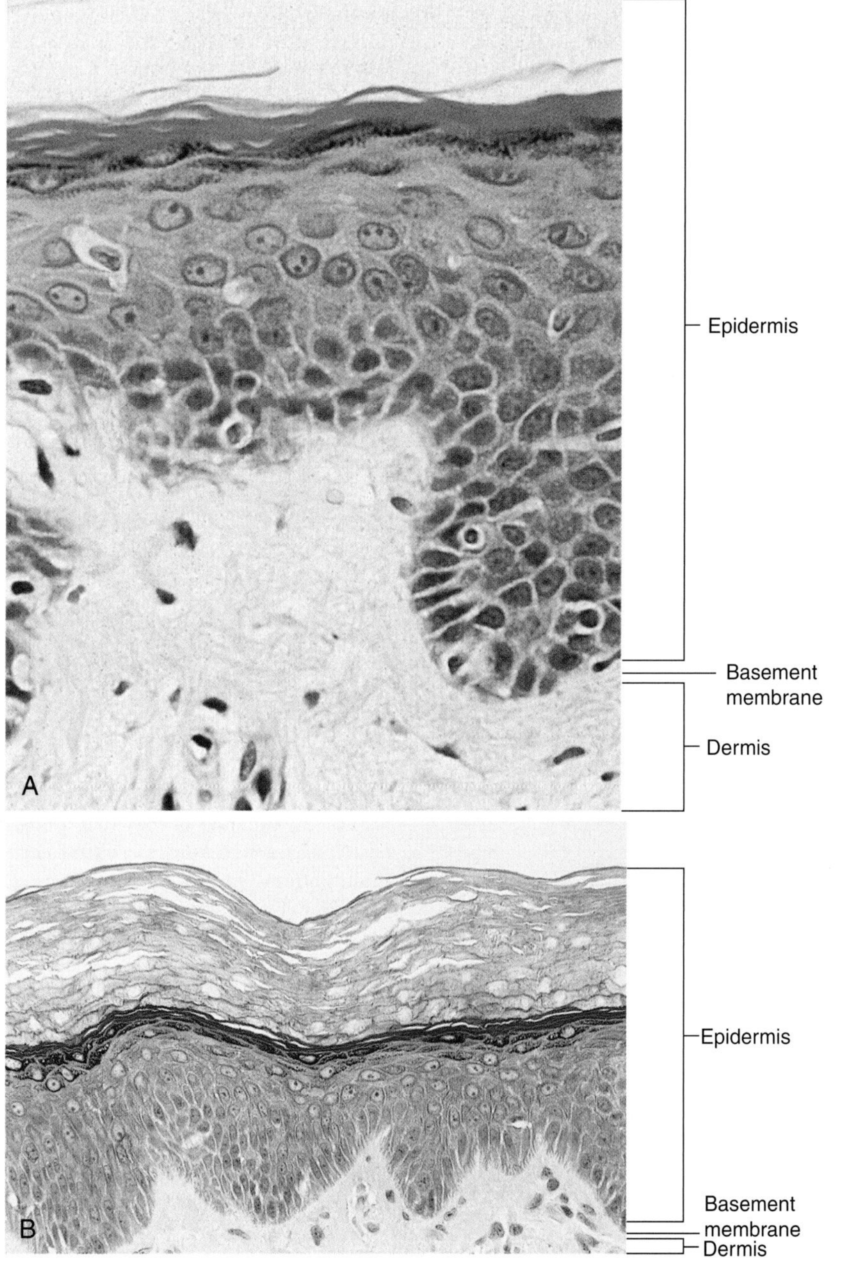

Fig. 8.1 Microscopic Sections of the Skin. The epidermis and dermis (**A** and **B**) of the skin, which is epithelium and connective tissue, respectively. A basement membrane is located between these two tissue types. (**A,** From Stevens A, Lowe J. *Human Histology.* 5th ed. St. Louis: Elsevier; 2020. **B,** From Bernhard Gottlieb Collection, courtesy of James McIntosh, PhD, Assistant Professor Emeritus, Department of Biomedical Sciences, Baylor College of Dentistry, Dallas.)

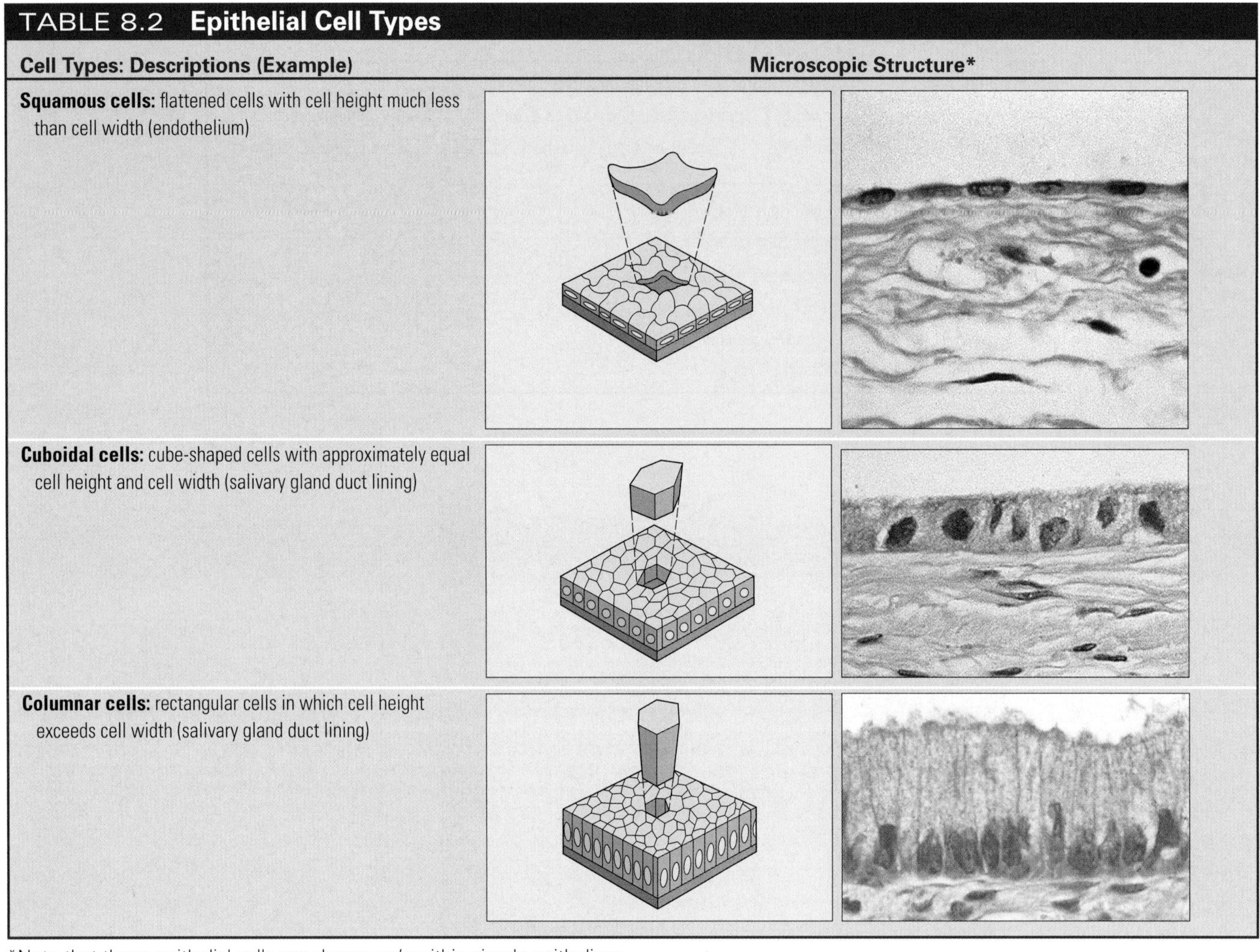

TABLE 8.2 **Epithelial Cell Types**

Cell Types: Descriptions (Example)	Microscopic Structure*
Squamous cells: flattened cells with cell height much less than cell width (endothelium)	
Cuboidal cells: cube-shaped cells with approximately equal cell height and cell width (salivary gland duct lining)	
Columnar cells: rectangular cells in which cell height exceeds cell width (salivary gland duct lining)	

*Note that these epithelial cells are shown *only* within simple epithelium.
Images from Stevens A, Lowe J. *Human Histology*. 5th ed. St. Louis: Elsevier; 2020.

This tissue is capable of rapid cellular turnover. In fact, epithelium is highly regenerative because its deeper germinal cells are capable of reproduction by mitosis (see Table 7.2). Epithelial cells usually undergo cellular differentiation as they move from the deeper germinal layers to the surface of the tissue to be shed or lost. An exception to the process of cellular maturation is the junctional epithelium of the gingival sulcular region that is attached to the tooth surface.

Epithelial cells are usually tightly joined to each another by intercellular junctions provided for by the desmosomes except in the more superficial layers (see Fig. 7.5). The epithelial cells are also tightly joined in some cases to adjacent noncellular surfaces by hemidesmosomes as is the case with its relationship to the basement membrane (see Fig. 7.6) as well as the junctional epithelium of the gingival sulcular region that is attached to the tooth surface (see Figs. 10.6 and 10.7).

A basement membrane is located between most epithelium and deeper connective tissue, such as with both the skin and oral mucosa. Components of basement membrane are produced by both the overlying epithelium as well as the adjoining connective tissue (discussed later in this chapter).

EPITHELIUM CLASSIFICATION

Epithelium can be classified into two main categories based on the arrangement into layers of cells, simple and stratified (see Table 8.1). **Simple epithelium** consists of a single layer of epithelial cells. The further classification of the tissue involves different types of epithelial cells according to cellular structure; they can be classified as either simple squamous, simple cuboidal, or simple columnar (Table 8.2).

Simple squamous epithelium consists of flattened platelike epithelial cells or **squames** (**skwaymz**), lining blood and lymphatic vessels, heart, and serous cavities as well as interfaces in the lungs and kidneys. **Endothelium** (en-doh-**thee**-lee-uhm) refers to the simple squamous epithelium lining of these vessels and serous cavities.

Simple cuboidal epithelium consists of cube-shaped cells that line the ducts of various glands, such as certain ducts of the salivary glands (see Fig. 1.6). Simple columnar epithelium consists of rectangular cells, such as in the lining of other salivary gland ducts as well as the inner enamel epithelium of a maturing tooth germ, whose cells become enamel-forming ameloblasts (see Figs. 6.9 to 6.12).

Epithelium can also be considered **pseudostratified columnar epithelium** (soo-doh-**strat**-uh-fahyd), which is named as such since it falsely appears as multiple cell layers when viewed with lower-power magnification due to the cells' nuclei appearing at different levels (Fig. 8.2). However, in reality as viewed with higher-power magnification, only cells of different heights are noted. Thus this is a type of simple epithelium because all the cells line up to contact the inner surface of the basement membrane even if not all the cells reach the outer surface of the tissue. Pseudostratified columnar epithelium lines the upper respiratory tract, including the

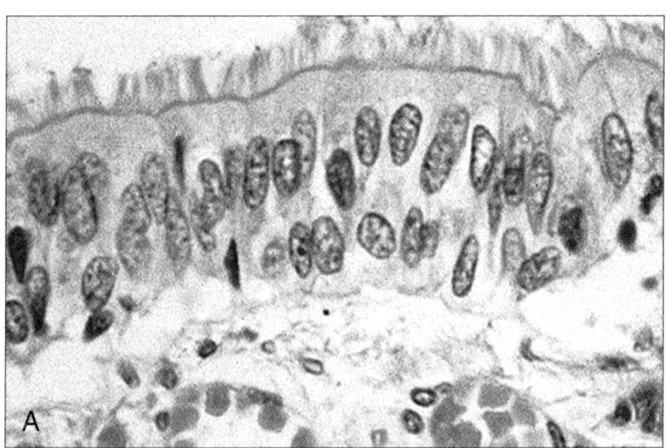

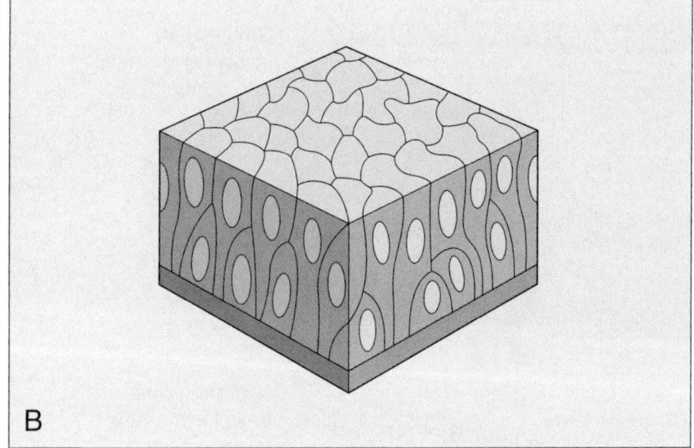

Fig. 8.2 Pseudostratified Columnar Epithelium. **A,** Photomicrograph. **B,** Diagram. This type of epithelium can line the respiratory system. The tissue falsely appears as multiple cell layers when viewed under lower-power magnification because the cells' nuclei appear at different levels. However, in reality, cells of different heights are present. And because all have a direct relationship with the basement membrane, it is considered simple epithelium. (From Stevens A, Lowe J. *Human Histology*. 5th ed, St. Louis: Elsevier; 2020.)

nasal cavity and paranasal sinuses (see Fig. 11.20). This type of epithelium may have cilia or be nonciliated at the tissue surface (see **Chapter** 7).

In contrast to simple epithelium, **stratified epithelium** (**strat**-uh-fahyd) consists of two or more layers of cells, with only the deepest layer lining up to contact the basement membrane (see Table 8.1). It is important to note that only the cellular shape of the surface layer is used to determine the classification of stratified epithelium. Thus stratified epithelium can consist of cuboidal, columnar, or squamous epithelial cells, or a combination of cell types as seen in a transitional epithelium.

Most epithelium in the body consists of **stratified squamous epithelium** (**skwey**-muhs), which includes the superficial layer of both the skin and oral mucosa (see Figs. 8.1 and 8.7 and **Chapter 9**). Only the most superficial layers of this tissue are flat cells or squames; the deeper cells vary from the deeper cuboidal to the more superficial polyhedral. Interdigitation of the outer epithelium with the deeper connective tissue occurs with the epithelial tissue forming **rete ridges** (**ree**-tee) (or rete pegs); however, there is always a basement membrane located between these two tissue types.

Stratified squamous epithelium can be nonkeratinized or keratinized. Nonkeratinized tissue can be found in certain regions of the oral mucosa as well as keratinized tissue. The keratin found within the keratinized tissue is a tough, fibrous, opaque, and waterproof protein that is impervious to pathogenic invasion and resistant to friction (see **Chapter 9**). Keratin is produced during the maturation of the keratinocyte epithelial cells as they migrate from near the basement membrane to the surface of the keratinized tissue (see Fig. 9.4).

Another example of keratinized stratified squamous epithelium is **epidermis** (ep-i-**dur**-mis), which is the superficial layer of the skin (see Figs. 8.1 and 8.7). The epidermis overlies a basement membrane and the adjoining deeper layers of connective tissue (dermis and hypodermis, respectively, which is discussed later). The skin has varying degrees of keratinization depending on the region of the body. Areas such as the palms of the hands and bottom of the feet have thicker layers of keratin, which form calluses. However, the keratin is less densely packed in both the skin and oral cavity as compared with the densely packed hard keratin of the nails and hair.

EPITHELIUM REGENERATION, TURNOVER, AND REPAIR

Turnover of both the epithelium in skin and oral mucosa occurs as a result of the cell division during the regeneration process. Cellular turnover of epithelium occurs as the newly formed deepest cells migrate superficially from their formation near the basement membrane. Thus, the turnover time is the time needed for a cell to divide during mitosis and pass through the entire thickness of tissue. In order to migrate, the cells release and then regain their desmosomal connections at the intercellular junctions in the more superficial location.

The turnover time is faster for all types of epithelium as compared to connective tissue. This faster turnover time is a result of the higher level of mitosis in those deepest dividing cells near the basement membrane. Thus, the older, superficial epithelial cells are being shed or lost at the same rate as the deeper germinal cells are dividing into more cells during turnover time.

These overall faster turnover times vary only slightly but sometimes importantly for the different types of epithelium. In general, the epithelium of the oral mucosa has a faster turnover time than the epidermis of the skin (see Table 9.6). More specifically within the oral cavity, the epithelium of the buccal mucosa that lines the cheek tissue has a faster turnover time of 14 days than the epithelium that covers the skin, which is 20 to 30 days, depending whether one is a younger or older adult. This difference becomes apparent when dental professionals sadly note a traumatic superficial injury to the facial skin lasting for weeks from a tight overlying rubber dam and at the same time, happily observe the quicker healing after the patient accidentally bites down on the superficial surface of the inner cheeks when taking dental radiographs.

The differences of turnover time are especially noted during repair or healing of the tissue after injury. Immediately after an injury to either the skin or oral mucosa, a clot from blood-related products forms in the area and the inflammatory response is triggered by the white blood cells from the blood supply as they migrate into the tissue (Fig. 8.3). If the source of injury is removed, tissue repair can begin within the next few days. The epithelial cells at the periphery of the injury lose their desmosomal intercellular junctions and then are able to migrate to form a new epithelial surface layer beneath the clot.

Thus, a clot is very important in repair of the epithelium and must be retained in the first days of repair because it acts as a guide to form a new surface. A clot stays moist in the oral cavity but dries out on the skin, which is considered a *scab* when on the skin. Later, after the epithelial surface is repaired, the clot is then broken down by enzymes because it is no longer needed for healing. Repair of the epithelium is a process that is also tied to repair in the deeper connective tissue (discussed later in this chapter).

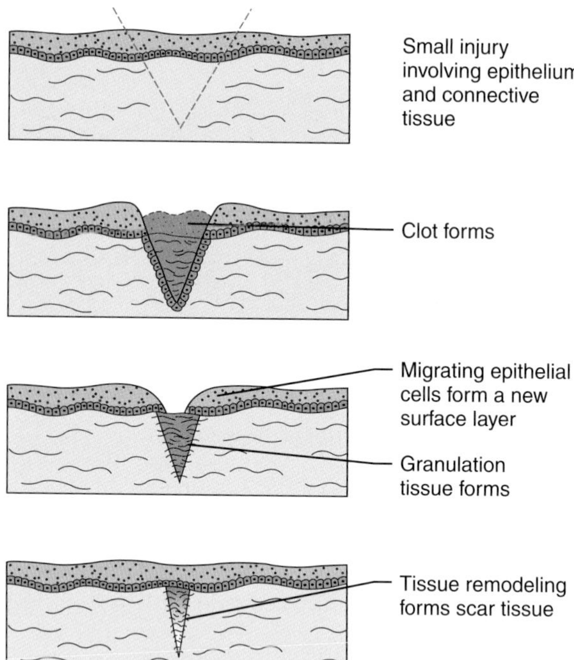

Fig. 8.3 Repair Process of the Skin or Oral Mucosa After an Injury. Note the initial formation of the clot and migrating epithelial cells from the surrounding intact tissue and formation of granulation tissue in the later days of repair. Later, the tissue will remodel and form scar tissue. (From Fehrenbach MJ. Inflammation and repair. In: Ibsen OAC, Phelan JA, eds. *Oral Pathology for Dental Hygienists.* 7th ed. St. Louis: Elsevier; 2018.)

BASEMENT MEMBRANE PROPERTIES

As discussed earlier, the **basement membrane** is a thin acellular structure always located between any form of epithelium and the underlying connective tissue as noted in both the skin and oral mucosa (Fig. 8.4, see Figs. 7.6 and 8.7). This type of structure is even present between the components of the tooth germ during tooth development (see Fig. 6.7).

BASEMENT MEMBRANE HISTOLOGY

The details of the basement membrane are not seen when it is viewed by scanning or lower-power magnification; only its location can be indicated. A higher-power magnification, such as that afforded by an electron microscope, is needed to visualize the intricacies of the basement membrane. The basement membrane consists of two layers, basal lamina and reticular lamina. The terms *basement membrane* and *basal lamina* are sometimes used interchangeably but the basal lamina is, in fact, only a part of the basement membrane. The use of "basal lamina" refers to electron microscopy, whereas the use of "basement membrane" refers to lower-power light microscopy.

The superficial layer of the basement membrane is the **basal lamina** (**bey**-suhl), which is produced by the epithelium and is about 40 to 50 nm thick. Microscopically the basal lamina consists of two sublayers: the **lamina lucida** (**loo**-si-duh) is a clear layer that is closer to the epithelium and the **lamina densa** (**den**-suh) is a dense layer that is closer to the connective tissue. The deeper layer of the basement membrane is usually the **reticular lamina** (reh-**tik**-yuh-ler); the exception is lung alveoli and kidney with fusion of basal laminae. The reticular lamina consists of collagen fibers and reticular fibers produced and secreted by the underlying connective tissue (discussed later).

Attachment mechanisms are also part of the basement membrane. These involve hemidesmosomes with the attachment plaque as well as tonofilaments from the epithelium and the **anchoring collagen fibers** (**kol**-uh-juhn) from the connective tissue (see Fig. 7.6). The tonofilaments from the epithelium loop through the attachment plaque, whereas the collagen fibers of the reticular lamina loop into the lamina densa of the basal lamina, forming a flexible attachment between the two tissue types.

It is important to note that the interface between the epithelium and connective tissue of both the skin and oral mucosa where the basement membrane is located is not two-dimensional as noted in microscopic cross sections of the tissue with its epithelial rete ridges and connective tissue papillae (discussed next). Instead in reality, the interface consists of three-dimensional interdigitation of the two tissue types. This complex arrangement increases the amount of surface area for the interface, thus increasing the mechanical strength of the interface as well as the nutrition potential for the avascular epithelium from the vascularized connective tissue.

CONNECTIVE TISSUE PROPERTIES

All of the **connective tissue** of the body when taken together represents by weight, the most abundant type of basic tissue in the body, even if it is epithelium that is mostly noted when clinically examining the body. Connective tissue is derived from the somites during prenatal development (see Fig. 3.13). The functions of connective tissue are as varied as its types; connective tissue is involved in support, attachment, packing, insulation, storage, transport, repair, and defense.

CONNECTIVE TISSUE HISTOLOGY

Compared with epithelium, connective tissue is usually composed of fewer cells spaced farther apart and containing larger amounts of matrix between the cells (except for adipose connective tissue) (see Fig. 8.1). Within connective tissue, the matrix is composed of intercellular substance and fibers.

Most connective tissue is renewable because its cells are capable of mitosis and because most of its cells can even produce their own matrix of intercellular substance and fibers. In most cases, connective tissue is vascularized (except cartilage), each having its own blood supply.

Differing cells are found within the various types of connective tissue. The most common cell in all types of connective tissue is the **fibroblast** (**fahy**-bruh-blast) (Fig. 8.5). Fibroblasts synthesize certain types of protein fibers and intercellular substances needed to sustain the connective tissue. They are flat and elongated spindle-shaped cells with cytoplasmic processes at each end. Subpopulations of fibroblasts may be possible within connective tissue. Fibroblasts are considered fixed cells in connective tissue because they do not leave the tissue to enter the blood as compared to cells with mobility, such as white blood cells.

Young fibroblasts that are actively engaged in the production of fibers and intercellular substance appear to have large amounts of cytoplasm, mitochondria, and rough endoplasmic reticulum. Fibroblasts can show aging and inactivity, along with a reduction in cytoplasm, mitochondria, and rough endoplasmic reticulum, which is evident in the later stages of chronic advanced periodontal disease (see **Chapter 10**). If adequately stimulated during repair, however, fibroblasts may revert to a more active state.

Other cells found in connective tissue include migrated white blood cells from the blood supply, such as monocytes (within tissue as macrophages), basophils, mast cells, lymphocytes (including associated plasma cells), and neutrophils (discussed later in this chapter). Certain other transient cell types are found in specific classifications of connective tissue and are discussed later in this chapter.

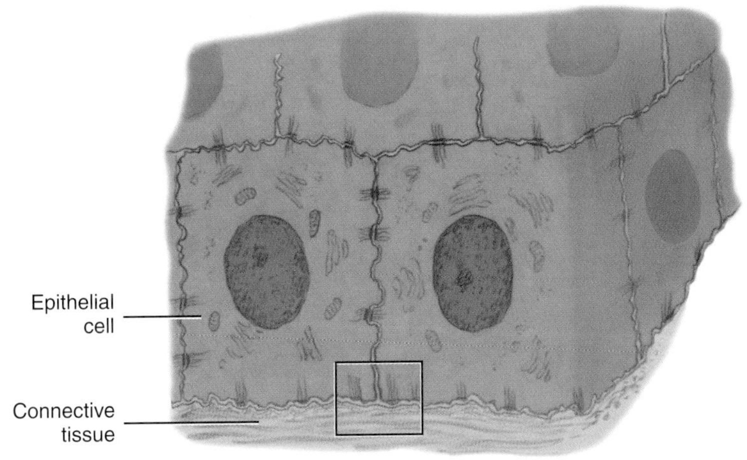

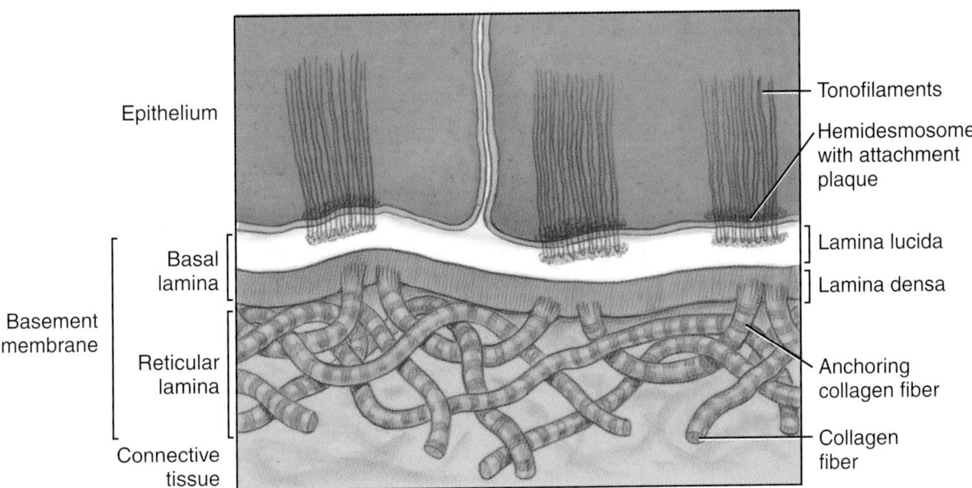

Fig. 8.4 Basement Membrane with its Basal Lamina and Reticular Lamina. Close-up view shows the attachment devices from an epithelial cell by way of hemidesmosomes and tonofilaments with attachment plaques connecting to the connective tissue by way of anchoring collagen fibers.

Differing types of protein fibers are found in various types of connective tissue. The main connective tissue fiber type found in the body is the **collagen fibers** (Fig. 8.6). Tissue containing a large amount of collagen fibers is considered a **collagenous connective tissue** (**kuh**-laj-uh-nuhs), but most connective tissue (except blood) contain some collagen fibers. Collagen fibers are composed of the protein collagen, including distinct types that have been shown by immunologic study to have great tensile strength. All collagen fibers are composed of smaller subunits or **fibrils** (**fahy**-bruhlz), which are composed of even smaller subunits or **microfibrils** (mahy-kroh-**fahy**-bruhlz), similar to a strong intact rope that is composed of smaller entwined strands of roping material.

Over 29 types of collagen have been identified and described; however, over 90% of the collagen in the body or in fetal tissue is composed of only Types I to IV collagen (Table 8.3). The most common type of collagen protein is Type I collagen, which is found in the teeth, lamina propria of the oral mucosa, dermis of the skin, bone, tendons, and virtually all other types of connective tissue. Cells responsible for the synthesis of Type I collagen include fibroblasts and osteoblasts, which produce fibers and intercellular substance as well as bone, respectively, and odontoblasts, which produce dentin (see Fig. 6.11).

The **elastic fibers** (e-**las**-tik) are another type of fiber, composed of microfilaments embedded in the protein elastin, which results in a very elastic type of tissue. Thus this tissue has the ability to stretch and then to return to its original shape after contraction or extension. Certain regions in the oral cavity, such as the soft palate, contain elastic fibers in the connective tissue of lamina propria to allow this type of tissue movement (see Fig. 9.10).

The **reticular fibers** can be found in relationship to an evolving embryonic tissue and thus are found more rarely in the adult body. Reticular fibers are composed of the protein reticulin and are very fine hairlike fibers that branch, forming a network in the tissue that contains them. However, reticular connective tissue still predominates in the lymph nodes and spleen in an adult.

CONNECTIVE TISSUE CLASSIFICATION

One method of classifying connective tissue is according to texture, which can be soft, firm, rigid, or fluid in nature (see Table 8.1). Soft connective tissue includes the tissue found in the deeper layers of both the skin and oral mucosa, such as a connective tissue proper. The firm connective tissue consists of different types of cartilage. The rigid hard form of connective tissue consists of bone. The fluid connective tissue consists of blood with all its components and lymph.

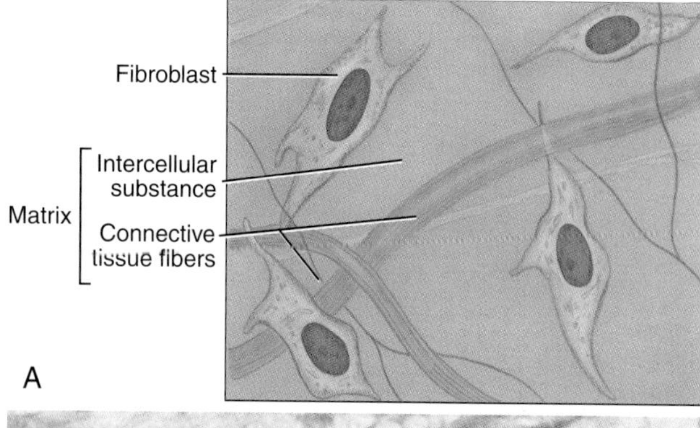

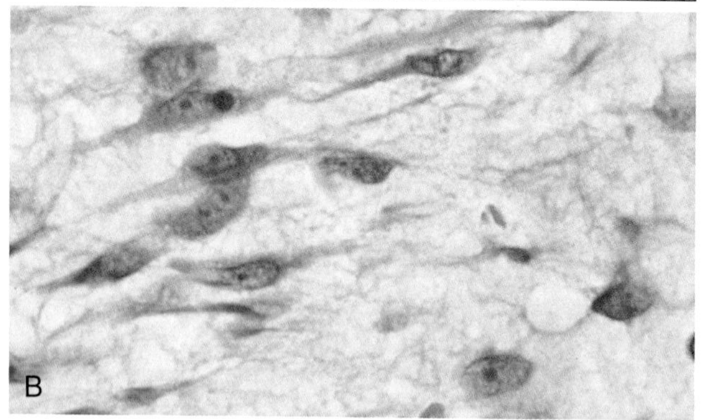

Fig. 8.5 Fibroblasts. A, Diagram. **B,** Photomicrograph. The fibroblasts are within loose connective tissue, showing their spindle or fusiform shape. The cell forms the fibers of the connective tissue as well as the intercellular substance between the tissue components. (**B,** From Stevens A, Lowe J. *Human Histology*. 5th ed. St. Louis: Elsevier; 2020.)

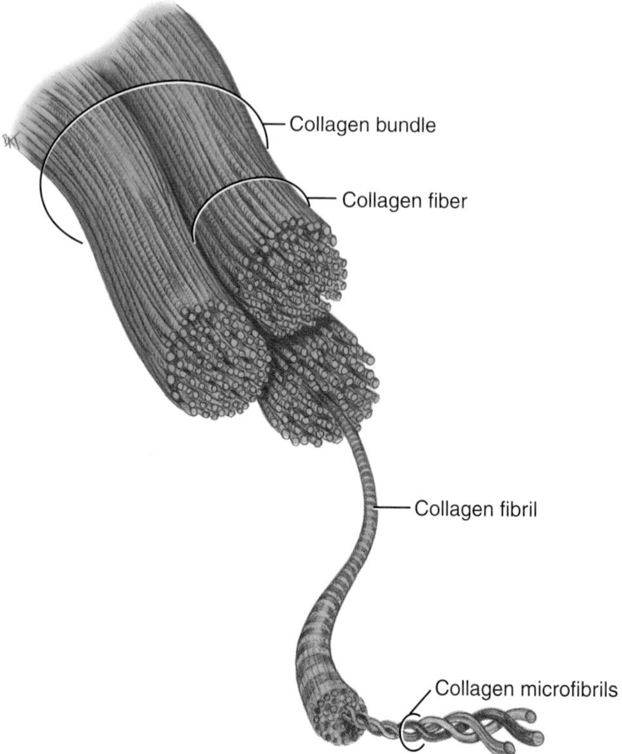

Fig. 8.6 Collagen bundle that is composed of fibers with smaller subunits, the fibrils and microfibrils.

TABLE 8.3 Collagen Types

Main Types of Collagen	Features with Locations
Type I	Most common type in dermis of skin, skeletal bone, tendons; virtually all connective tissue of the body as well as lamina propria of oral mucosa, dentin, pulp, periodontium, jaws
Type II	In hyaline and elastic cartilage
Type III	In granulation tissue, produced quickly by young fibroblasts before tougher Type I synthesized, thus commonly found alongside Type I; main component of reticular fibers but also found in artery walls, skin, intestines, uterus
Type IV	In basal laminae of basement membrane, eye lens, filtration system of capillaries, kidney's nephron glomeruli

CONNECTIVE TISSUE PROPER

Soft connective tissue can be classified as loose, dense, or specialized. Both loose and dense types of connective tissue are found together in two adjoining layers as the **connective tissue proper**. The connective tissue proper is found deep to the epithelium and basement membrane, in the deeper layers of both the skin and oral mucosa.

The connective tissue proper in the skin is the **dermis** (**dur**-mis) and is found deep to the epidermis (discussed earlier; Fig. 8.7, see Fig. 8.1). Even deeper to the dermis is the **hypodermis** (hahy-puh-**dur**-mis), a subcutaneous tissue that is composed of loose connective tissue and adipose connective tissue, which is a specialized connective tissue as well as glandular tissue, large blood vessels, and nerves. Cartilage, bone, and muscle can be present deep to the hypodermis of the skin, depending on the region of the body. In oral mucosa, the deep connective tissue proper is considered the lamina propria, and the even deeper connective tissue sometimes present is the submucosa, similar to the hypodermis in the skin (see Figs. 9.1 and 9.6).

Loose Connective Tissue

The superficial layer of both the dermis of the skin and lamina propria of the oral mucosa is composed of **loose connective tissue** (see Fig. 8.7). In both the dermis and lamina propria of oral mucosa, this layer of loose connective tissue is also considered the **papillary layer** (**pap**-uh-ler-ee). The papillary layer forms **connective tissue papillae,** which is interdigitated with the epithelial rete ridges discussed earlier. This papillary layer has no overly prominent connective tissue element; all of the components of the papillary layer are present in equal amounts. Thus equal amounts of cells, intercellular substance, fibers, and tissue fluid are in an irregular and loose arrangement. This loose layer of the connective tissue proper serves as protective padding for the deeper structures of the body.

Dense Connective Tissue

Deep to the loose connective tissue is **dense connective tissue,** such as that found in the deepest layers of both the dermis and lamina propria (see Fig. 8.7). Similar to the loose connective tissue, all of the same components of connective tissue are still present. However, in contrast to the loose connective tissue, dense connective tissue is tightly packed with a regular arrangement, and it also consists mostly of protein fibers, which give this tissue its strength.

The dense connective tissue in both the dermis and lamina propria is also considered the **dense layer** (or reticular layer). Therefore the dense layer is deep to the papillary layer in the connective tissue proper. In contrast, tendons, aponeuroses, and ligaments are a type of dense connective tissue that has a regular arrangement of strong parallel collagen fibers with few fibroblasts or cells.

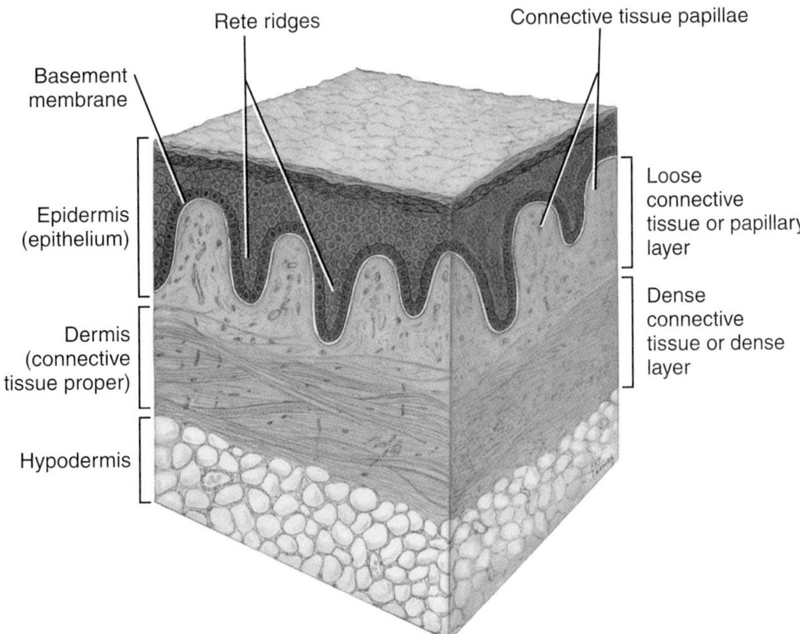

Fig. 8.7 Skin with its Epidermis and Dermis Layers. The hypodermis is present deep to the dermis. Note the interdigitating rete ridges of the epidermis with the connective tissue papillae of the dermis.

Connective Tissue Proper Turnover, Regeneration, and Repair

Turnover of both the connective tissue proper in skin or oral mucosa occurs as a result of the production of fibers and intercellular substance by the fibroblasts during regeneration (see Fig. 8.5). Other types of cells can also undergo mitosis and create additional cells, such as certain white blood cells and endothelial cells. The overall turnover time for a connective tissue proper is slower than its adjoining epithelium; it also demonstrates individual variance from region to region.

When injured, the connective tissue proper in both the skin and oral mucosa goes through stages of repair that are related to the events in the more superficial epithelium (see Fig. 8.3). After a clot forms and an inflammatory response is triggered with white blood cells, fibroblasts migrate to produce an immature connective tissue deep to the clot and newly forming epithelial surface.

This immature connective tissue is considered **granulation tissue** (gran-yuh-**ley**-shuhn) and has few fibers and an increased amount of blood vessels. Granulation tissue can clinically appear as a redder soft tissue that bleeds easily after injury or surgery, such as in the oral cavity after a tooth extraction. In addition, this tissue may become abundant, interfering with the repair process. Surgical removal of excess granulation tissue may be necessary to allow for optimum repair; this sometimes occurs after chronic advanced periodontal disease.

Later, during the repair process, this temporary granulation tissue is replaced by paler and firmer scar tissue in the area. It is paler because scar tissue contains an increased amount of fibers and fewer blood vessels. The amount of scar tissue varies, depending on the type and size of the injury, amount of granulation tissue, and movement of tissue after injury. Interestingly, the skin shows more scar tissue production both clinically and microscopically after repair than does the oral mucosa. This difference may be based on differing developmental origins of the tissue producing differing types of fibroblasts and thus different types of fibers.

The repair process can also be affected by hormones such as noted with systemic glucocorticoids (e.g., cortisone) that hinder repair by depressing the inflammatory reaction or by inhibiting the growth of fibroblasts, the production of collagen, and the formation of endothelial cells. Systemic stress, thyroidectomy, testosterone, adrenocorticotropic hormone, and large doses of estrogen suppress the formation of granulation tissue and impair healing. Progesterone increases and accelerates the vascularization of granulation tissue and appears to increase the susceptibility of the gingival tissue to mechanical injury by causing dilation of the marginal vessels.

Clinical Considerations with Aging Process in Skin

At birth, the skin has not developed a sufficient protective layer or facilitated the synthesis of immune cells. It often looks to be transparent and therefore is sensitive to damage, so it must be protected by extra clothing and kept away from environmental stress. At puberty, glandular and hair development as well as the immune system begins to function at an increased rate, giving extra protection to the skin against the coming adult world. During this time, the skin is in a very active metabolic state but still vulnerable to sensitization by allergens.

By age 20, however, the skin begins to deteriorate and by the age of 50 is in a rapid state of degradation due to the aging process. Collagen fibers begin to fall apart; elastic fibers stiffen and thicken, wrinkling the skin. Oil glands in skin cease production, and melanin production decreases, leading to more pallid color and gray hairs. Keratin cells cease production and already produced keratin becomes thin and stiff.

Most importantly to dental professionals, the skin with aging begins to heal poorly after injury (see earlier discussion) with fibroblasts now having less replication activity (considered replicative senescence). The skin also becomes susceptible to disease states that include inflammation (such as with dermatitis), infection (such as with herpes zoster), and cancer (such as with basal cell carcinoma and melanoma). Solar damage will accelerate the aging process in skin as does increased environmental toxicity (such as with chronic alcohol and tobacco use) (see Fig. 1.8 for solar damage of the lips). The aging of the oral mucosa will be further discussed in **Chapters 9 and 10.**

SPECIALIZED CONNECTIVE TISSUE PROPERTIES

Specialized connective tissue includes adipose, elastic, or reticular. **Adipose connective tissue** (**ad**-uh-pohs) is a fatty tissue that is found beneath the skin, around organs and various joints, and in regions of the oral cavity. Unlike most connective tissue, this type of connective tissue has cells packed tightly together with little or no matrix. After fibroblasts, the predominant type of cell found in this tissue is the adipocyte, which stores fat intracellularly.

Elastic connective tissue has a large number of elastic fibers in its matrix, which combine strength with elasticity, such as in the tissue of the vocal cords. **Reticular connective tissue** is a delicate network of interwoven reticular fibers forming a supportive framework for blood vessels and internal organs.

CARTILAGE PROPERTIES

The firm but flexible nonmineralized connective tissue in the body is **cartilage** (Fig. 8.8). Cartilage forms most of the temporary skeleton of the embryo and then serves as structural support for certain soft tissue after birth. Additionally, cartilage serves as a model or template in which certain bones of the body subsequently develop. Cartilage is also present at articular surfaces of most freely movable joints, such as the temporomandibular joint (see Fig. 19.3).

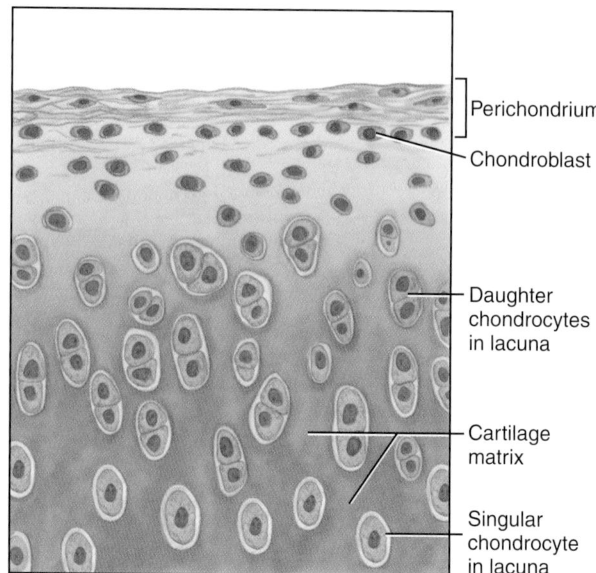

Fig. 8.8 Cartilage, including its cells, the chondroblasts and chondrocytes, as well as the outer layer of perichondrium, which is a formative connective tissue sheath.

Cartilage Histology

Cartilage is composed of cells and matrix. Its matrix or surrounding medium is composed of fibers, mostly collagen, and intercellular substance. Thus this matrix is similar to soft connective tissue in composition, except that the matrix of cartilage is firmer. The connective tissue surrounding most cartilage (except at joints) is the **perichondrium** (per-i-**kon**-dree-uhm), a fibrous connective tissue sheath containing blood vessels. Since cartilage itself is avascular (having no blood vessels), it receives its nutrition from this associated surrounding tissue.

Two types of cells found in cartilage are the immature **chondroblasts** (**kon**-droh-blastz), which lie internal to the perichondrium and produce cartilage matrix and the **chondrocytes** (**kon**-droh-sahytz), which are mature chondroblasts that maintain the cartilage matrix (see Fig. 8.8). After the production of cartilage matrix, the chondrocyte becomes surrounded and enclosed by the matrix. Only a small space surrounds the chondrocyte within the cartilage matrix, the **lacuna** (luh-**kyoo**-nuh) (plural, **lacunae** [luh-**kyoo**-nee]).

There are three types of cartilage, hyaline, elastic, and fibrocartilage, with each having slightly different histologic features. Histologists believe that this distinction between types of cartilage is not to be overly stressed and that most cartilage contains a combination of the different types.

Hyaline cartilage (**hahy**-uh-lin) is the most common type found in the body and contains only collagen fibers as part of its matrix. The associated collagen fibers of hyaline cartilage are much finer in substance than those within dense connective tissue, thus it is the weakest type. Hyaline cartilage can be found in the embryonic skeleton and in subsequent growth centers, such as within the mandibular condyle (see Fig. 19.4). All cartilage starts as hyaline cartilage and is then modified into the other two types of cartilage according to need.

Elastic cartilage is similar to hyaline, except that it has numerous elastic fibers in its matrix, in addition to its numerous collagen fibers. Elastic cartilage is found in the external ear, auditory tube, epiglottis, and parts of the larynx that need its elastic nature.

Fibrocartilage (fahy-broh-**kahr**-ti-lij) is never found alone and merges gradually with its neighboring hyaline cartilage, such as in the outer part of the of the bones of the temporomandibular joint (see Fig. 19.3). Unlike elastic cartilage, fibrocartilage is not merely a modification of hyaline. Rather, it is a transitional type of cartilage between hyaline cartilage and dense connective tissue of tendons and ligaments. The cells of the tissue are enclosed in capsules of matrix, giving it great tensile strength. Unlike both elastic and hyaline cartilage, fibrocartilage has no true layer of perichondrium overlying it.

Cartilage Development

Cartilage can develop or grow in size in two different ways, interstitial growth and appositional growth as does other tissue such as bone (see **Chapter 3**). Interstitial growth is growth from deep within the tissue by the mitosis of each chondrocyte, thus producing larger numbers of daughter cells within a single lacuna (each of which secretes more matrix) and expanding the tissue (see Fig. 8.8). This interstitial growth is important in the development of bone that uses cartilage as a model for its own formation during endochondral ossification (discussed next).

Appositional growth is layered growth on the outside of the tissue from an outer layer of chondroblasts within the perichondrium. This layer of chondroblasts is always present on the external surface of cartilage to allow appositional growth of cartilage after an injury or remodeling.

Cartilage Repair and Aging

Unlike rigid bone that is discussed next, cartilage has some flexibility resulting from its fibers in the matrix; however, it has no inorganic or mineralized materials. Cartilage, unlike most connective tissue, is also avascular. Much like epithelium, this tissue depends on its surrounding connective tissue for its cellular nutrition, such as oxygen and metabolites. Because it has no vascularity of its own, cartilage takes longer to repair than vascularized bone. Cartilage also has no nerve supply within its tissue. Thus cartilage even when subjected to trauma or surgery does not produce overly painful symptoms.

During repair, avascular cartilage is dependent on neighboring connective tissue from the perichondrium for nutrition to transform it slowly into cartilage. With this transformation, the newly formed cartilage slowly proliferates and fills in the defect by appositional growth. In contrast, fractured mature cartilage is often united by dense connective

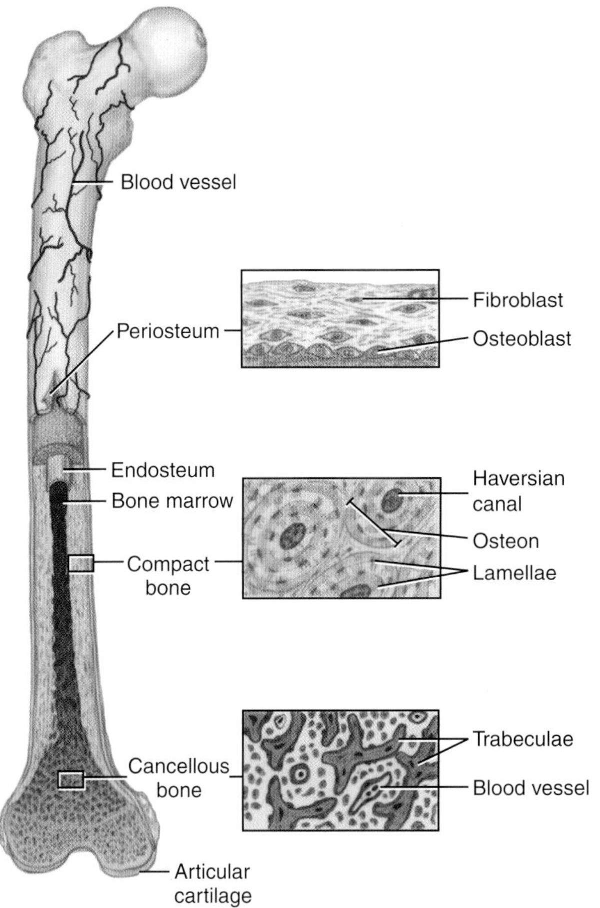

Fig. 8.9 Anatomy of bone showing close-up views of its periosteum, compact bone, and cancellous bone. Note also the endosteum and bone marrow of the bone.

tissue and if vascularization is initiated, then healing cartilage may eventually be replaced by bone.

As cartilage ages, it becomes less cellular with its chondrocytes dying. It may start to contain firm fibers splayed out in parallel groups or it may even form areas of scattered mineralization. These tend to coalesce over time with the tissue becoming hard and brittle and losing flexibility. Furthermore, in regard to the temporomandibular joint, cartilage may form abnormally within an aging joint disc that is usually only composed of dense fibrous connective tissue, which may cause difficulties with movement (see **Chapter 19**).

BONE PROPERTIES

The hard and rigid form of connective tissue that constitutes most of the mature skeleton is the **bone** (Fig. 8.9). Thus, bone serves as protective and structural support for soft tissue and as an attachment mechanism. It also aids in movement, manufactures blood cells through its red bone marrow, is an energy bank through its yellow marrow, and is a storehouse for calcium and other minerals. Bone also surrounds the root(s) of a tooth, creating the alveolus as the alveolar bone proper (see Fig. 14.14).

Because bone is vascularized with its own blood supply, it repairs quickly compared with avascular cartilage. Even though bone is rigid, it is important to remember that it does not consist of an inanimate inner rod being moved by the skeletal muscles. Instead, it is a living and functioning tissue in the body. Bone has also undergone the most developmental differentiation of all the connective tissue.

When bone is examined grossly, the outer part of bone is covered by **periosteum** (per-ee-**os**-tee-uhm) (see Fig. 8.9). Periosteum is a double-layered dense connective tissue sheath. The outer layer contains blood vessels and nerves. The inner layer contains a single layer of cells that give rise to bone-forming cells, the osteoblasts.

Deep to the periosteum is a dense layer of **compact bone** (**kuhm**-pakt). Deep to the compact bone is a spongy bone or **cancellous bone** (kan-**suh**-luhs). Both compact bone and cancellous bone have the same cellular components, but each has a different arrangement of those components (discussed next).

It is important to understand that the differences between these two types of bone include the relative amount of solid bone and also the size and number of soft tissue spaces in each; however, no sharp boundary exists between these two types of bone within an individual bone. Each bone type is located where it best serves the needs for either strength or lightness of weight. Compact bone is strong because it has fewer soft tissue spaces, but it is heavy. In contrast, cancellous bone is light because it is formed by pieces of solid bone that join to form a lattice; it is not as strong because it has more soft tissue spaces.

Lining the medullary cavity of bone on the inside of the layers of compact bone and cancellous bone is the **endosteum** (en-**dos**-tee-uhm) (see Fig. 8.9). The endosteum has the same composition as the periosteum but is thinner. On the innermost part of bone in the medullary cavity is the **bone marrow** (**mar**-oh). This gelatinous substance is where the stem cells of the blood are located, lymphocytes are created, and B cells mature (discussed later). These stem cells can continue to produce most of the components of the blood.

Bone Histology

Bone consists of cells and a partially mineralized matrix that is 60% inorganic or mineralized material (Fig. 8.10). It is this inorganic substance in a crystalline formation of mostly **calcium hydroxyapatite** (**kal**-see-uhm hahy-drok-see-**ap**-uh-tahyt), having the chemical formula $Ca_{10}(PO_4)_6(OH)_2$ that gives bone its hardness. This same type of inorganic crystal is found in differing percentages in the hard dental tissue, such as enamel, dentin, and cementum (see Table 6.2 for comparison of dental hard tissue types). Smaller amounts of other minerals (such as magnesium, potassium, calcium carbonate, and fluoride) are also present. This inorganic material has matrix packed between its bone cells. The matrix is composed of organic collagen fibers and intercellular substance.

Bone matrix is initially formed as **osteoid** (**os**-tee-oid), which later undergoes mineralization. The osteoid is produced by **osteoblasts** (**os**-tee-uh-blastz), which are cuboidal cells that arise from fibroblasts. Osteoblasts are also involved in the later mineralization of osteoid to form bone. Always present in the periosteum is a layer of osteoblasts at the external surface of the compact bone; it allows remodeling of bone and repair of injured bone.

Within fully mineralized bone are **osteocytes** (**os**-tee-uh-sahytz), which are entrapped mature osteoblasts. Similar to the chondrocyte, the cell body of the osteocyte is surrounded by bone, except for the space immediately around it, the lacuna. The cytoplasmic processes of the osteocyte radiate outward in all directions in the bone and are located in tubular canals of matrix or **canaliculi** (kan-l-**ik**-yuh-lahy). These canals provide for interaction between the osteocytes. However, unlike chondrocytes, osteoblasts never undergo mitosis during tissue formation and thus only one osteocyte is ever found in a lacuna.

Bone matrix in compact bone is formed into closely apposed sheets or **lamellae** (luh-**mel**-ee). Within and between the lamellae are embedded osteocytes with their cytoplasmic processes in the canals. This highly organized arrangement of concentric lamellae in compact bone is the **Haversian system** (huh-**vur**-zuhn).

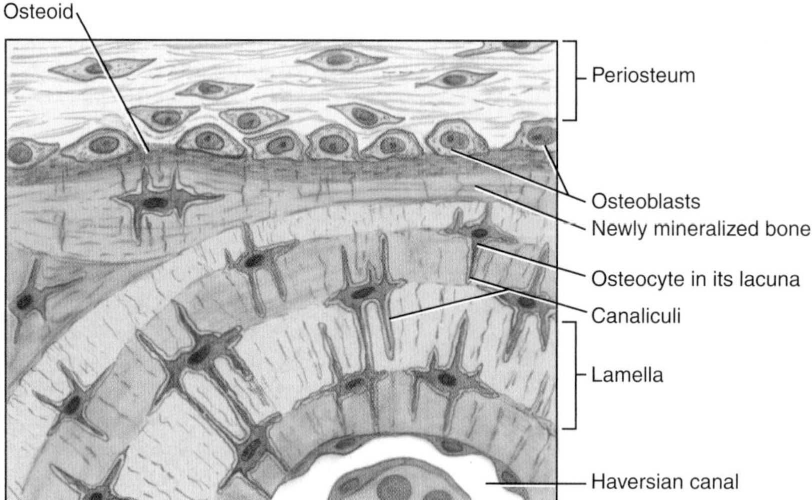

Fig. 8.10 Histology of Compact Bone. Note the cells of bone, osteoblasts, and osteocytes as well as the periosteum, the outer formative sheath of connective tissue. The initial bone matrix or osteoid will mineralize later into primary bone first and then secondary bone.

In the Haversian system, these lamellae form concentric layers of matrix into cylindrical units of bone or **osteons** (**os**-tee-onz) (Fig. 8.11). The osteon is the unit of structure in compact bone and consists of 5 to 20 parallel lamellae. This arrangement in the osteon is like the growth rings in a cross section of a tree trunk. However, unlike tree rings that form at a rate of around one per year, an entire Haversian system is produced all at the same time, no matter the number of concentric lamellae that may be involved.

The **Haversian canal** (or central canal) is a central vascular canal within each osteon surrounded by the lamellae. It contains longitudinally running blood vessels, nerves, with a small amount of connective tissue, which is overall lined by endosteum. The Haversian canals communicate not only with each other but also with the osteocytic processes in the canaliculi, providing cellular nutrition for the surrounding bone. This organized system of bone is noted within the structure of the alveolar bone proper (see Fig. 14.15).

Located on the periphery of the Haversian system in compact bone are **Volkmann canals** (**fawlk**-mahn) or similar nutrient canals that contain the same vascular and nerve components as the Haversian canals, being also lined by endosteum. Volkmann canals pass obliquely or at 90° to the Haversian canals of the osteons and communicate with them as well as with the larger blood supply external to the bone further linking the Haversian canals to one another. These more perpendicular canals are noted within the alveolus or tooth socket so that it is sometimes referred to as the *cribriform plate* because they appear grossly as perforating holes (see Fig. 14.14, *B*).

In contrast to the highly organized compact bone, cancellous bone has its bone matrix formed into **trabeculae** (truh-**bek**-yuh-lee) or joined matrix pieces forming a lattice (see Fig. 8.9). Lamellae of the matrix of cancellous bone are not arranged into concentric layers around a central blood vessel as with the compact bone, but their concentric rings are instead formed into cone-shaped spicules. Osteocytes in lacunae with their cytoplasmic processes are located between the lamellae of the trabeculae. Surrounding the trabeculae are soft tissue spaces that consist of vascular canals with blood vessels, nerves, and varying amounts of connective tissue. These spaces also serve as a nutritional source for the lattice structure of bone.

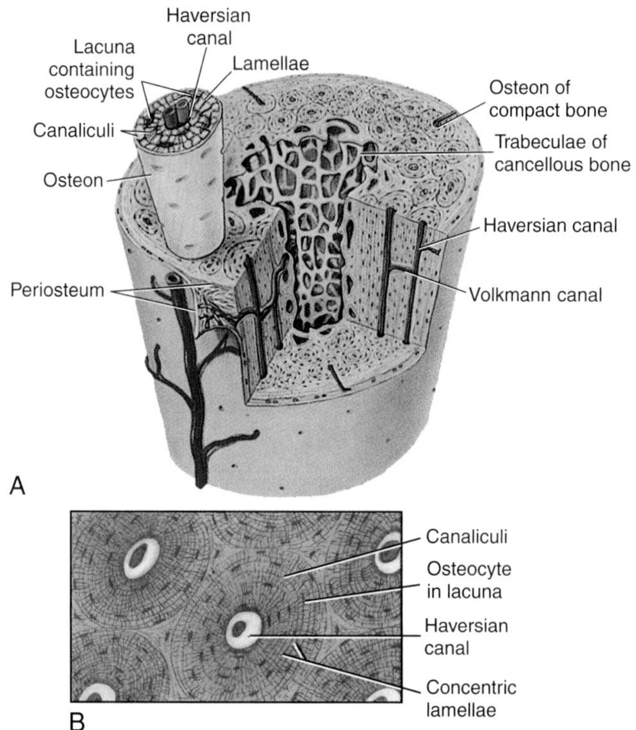

Fig. 8.11 Haversian System in Compact Bone. A, Lamellae creating osteons. Note the Volkmann canal and its communication with larger blood vessels external to the bone. **B,** Close-up view highlighting osteons with the central Haversian canals, osteocytes, and canaliculi. (**A,** From Applegate EJ. *The Anatomy and Physiology Learning System.* 4th ed. St. Louis: Elsevier; 2011.)

Bone Development

Bone development is considered **ossification** (os-uh-fi-**key**-shun) and has two methods for development: intramembranous and endochondral ossification. The bone produced by both these developmental methods is microscopically the same; only the process of formation is different. **Intramembranous ossification** (in-trah-**mem**-bruh-nuhs) is formation of osteoid between two dense connective tissue sheets, which then eventually replaces the outer

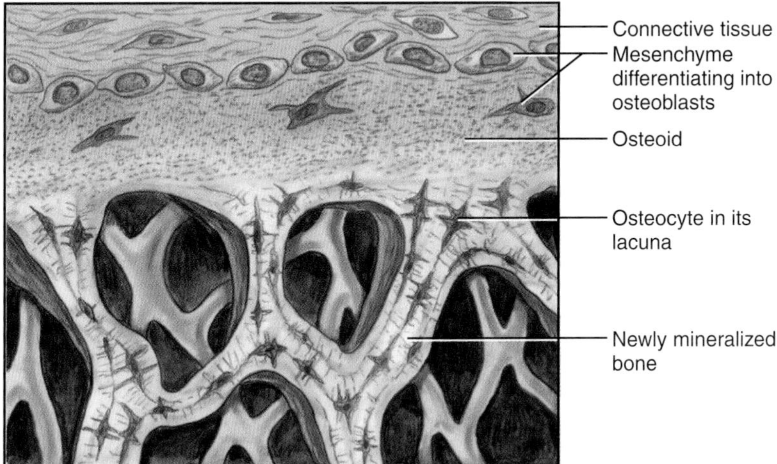

Fig. 8.12 Intramembranous ossification, which is the formation of osteoid within two dense connective tissue sheets that will eventually replace the initially formed connective tissue. During intramembranous ossification, mesenchyme differentiates into osteoblasts to form osteoid, which later matures into bone.

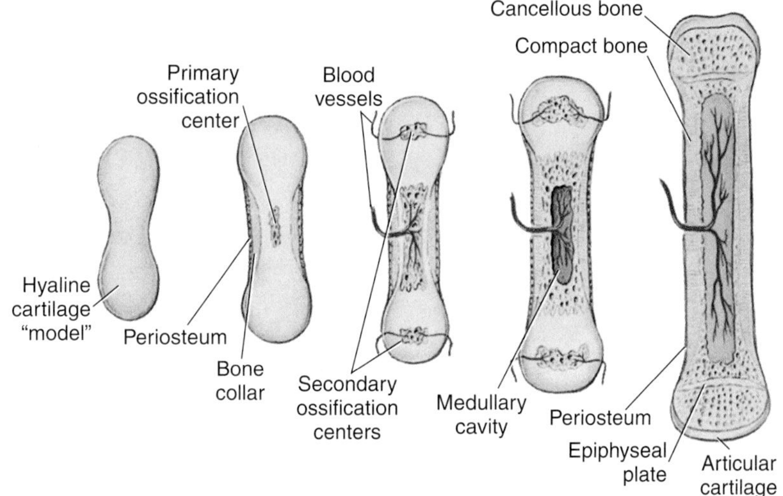

Fig. 8.13 Endochondral ossification over time, which is the formation of the osteoid within a cartilage model that subsequently becomes mineralized and dies. Osteoblasts penetrate the disintegrating cartilage and form a primary ossification center that continues forming osteoid toward the ends of the bone during prenatal development. Later after birth, secondary ossification centers form, which allows further growth of bones. (From Applegate EJ. *The Anatomy and Physiology Learning System*. 4th ed. St. Louis; Elsevier; 2011.)

connective tissue (Fig. 8.12). During intramembranous ossification, mesenchymal cells differentiate into osteoblasts to form the osteoid.

Intramembranous ossification uses a method of appositional growth similar to that of cartilage with layers of osteoid being produced. The osteoid later becomes mineralized to form bone. Certain bones in the body (such as the flat bones and clavicle) can form this way, enlarging over time as the appositional growth of bone occurs. The maxilla and the majority of the mandible are formed by intramembranous ossification (see Fig. 6.6 and **Chapter 14**).

Endochondral ossification (en-doh-**kon**-druhl) is the formation of the osteoid within a hyaline cartilage model that subsequently becomes mineralized and dies (Fig. 8.13). Osteoblasts penetrate the disintegrating cartilage and form primary ossification centers that continue forming osteoid toward the ends of the bone during prenatal development. Thus bone matrix eventually replaces the earlier cartilage model. This type of ossification first uses the method of interstitial growth of the initial cartilage tissue to form the model, or pattern, of the future bone's shape. Later, appositional growth of osteoid, with layers laid down on the outer perimeter, occurs to complete the final bone mass within the model.

Most long bones of the body are formed this way because it allows bone to grow in length from deep within the tissue. Later after birth, secondary ossification centers, which allow further growth of the bones until puberty end, are also formed. In particular, the head of the mandibular condyle is formed by endochondral ossification that has a multidirectional growth capacity (see **Chapter 14** and Fig. 19.4).

Regardless of its method of development, bone also goes through similar specific stages of development (Fig. 8.14). The first bone to be produced by either method of ossification is an immature bone, the **primary bone** (or woven bone). Within primary bone, the lamellae are indistinct because of the irregular arrangement of the collagen fibers and lamellae, whether located within the Haversian system or trabeculae.

Primary bone is a temporary tissue that is replaced by the more mature **secondary bone**. In contrast to primary bone, secondary bone

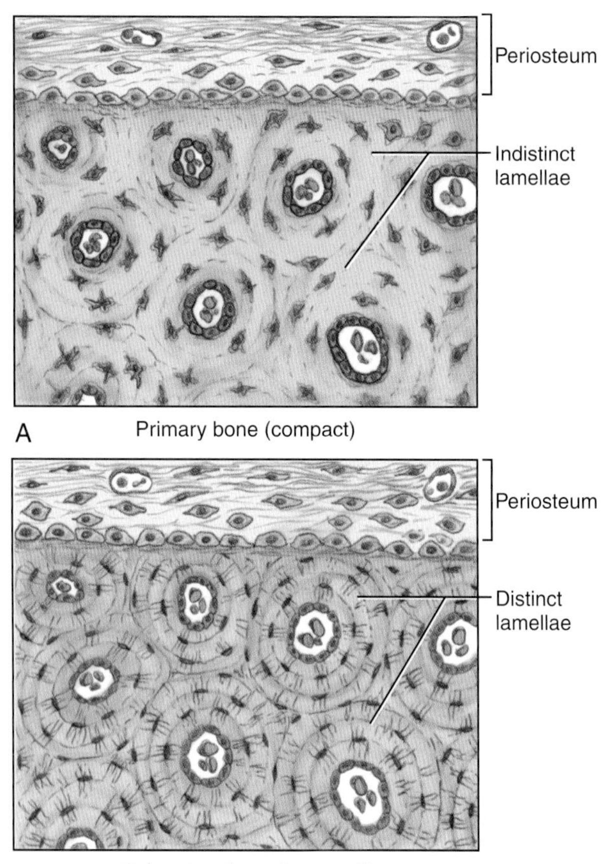

Fig. 8.14 Stages of bone development, in this case that of compact bone, from primary bone **(A)** to secondary bone **(B)**. These two stages occur during both methods of ossification as well as during the repair of bone.

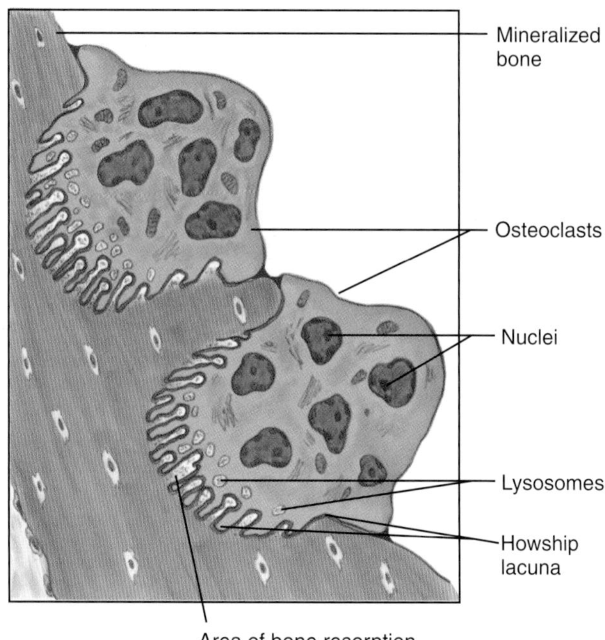

Fig. 8.15 Osteoclasts within Howship lacunae resorbing bone from their ruffled borders. Note the multiple nuclei within their cytoplasm, which contain lysosomes that break down the bone when discharged into the surrounding tissue.

has a well-organized arrangement of collagen fibers and distinct lamellae. Depending on the specific needs of the bone in any given area, secondary bone can be compact or cancellous.

Bone Remodeling, Repair, and Aging

It is important to keep in mind that a bone's overall structure is not static and, therefore, never remains the same. Throughout life, bone in the body is constantly being remodeled or regenerated despite its solid appearance. Bone undergoes removal in certain areas and new bone formation in other areas with the two processes balancing each other within a healthy body so function of the bone can be maintained. Appositional growth with layered formation of bone along its periphery is accomplished by the osteoblasts, which later become entrapped as osteocytes (see Fig. 8.10).

After bone fracture and during the repair of bone, bone also goes through the stages of bone formation, no matter how the bone initially developed. In the area to be repaired, bone forms initially as primary bone, which matures into secondary bone to complete the repair (see Fig. 8.14). The repair of bone depends on adequate blood supply, the presence of periosteum with active osteoblasts, and adequate mineral and vitamin levels.

Resorption of bone involves the removal of bone (Fig. 8.15). The cell that causes resorption of bone is the **osteoclast** (**os**-tee-uh-klast). The osteoclast is a large multinucleated cell located on the surface of secondary bone in a large shallow pit created by this resorption, a **Howship lacuna** (**how**-ship). The osteoclast is formed from the fusion of numbers of macrophage blood cells (discussed later in this chapter). Each osteoclast contains a large number of lysosomes in its cytoplasm and these are discharged into the surrounding tissue. The enzymes of the lysosomes then break down the bone when the osteoclast attaches by way of its ruffled border.

Localized resorption (ri-**sawrp**-shuhn) occurs in a specific area of a bone as a result of infection, altered mechanical stress, or pressure on the bone so that it adapts by removing bone tissue. In contrast, **generalized resorption** occurs over the entire skeleton in varying amounts because of endocrine activity to increase blood levels of calcium and phosphate needed by the body.

Microscopically a cross section of bone demonstrates layers related to its development that look like growth rings in a tree, similar to those noted in cementum (see Figs. 14.10 and 14.13). The **arrest lines** or resting lines appear as smooth lines between the layers of bone because of osteoblasts having rested, formed bone, and then rested again after appositional growth. Thus arrest lines show the incremental or layered nature of appositional growth. In contrast, **reversal lines** appear as scalloped lines between the layers of bone. Reversal lines represent areas where bone resorption has first taken place, followed quickly by appositional growth of new bone. As a person grows from fetal life through childhood, puberty, and finishes growth as a young adult, the bones of the skeleton change in size and shape; these changes can be noted on radiographs. The "bone age" of a child is the average age at which children reach this stage of bone maturation and a child's current height and bone age can be used to predict adult height. With aging, the generalized loss of bone mass or density is increased.

Clinical Considerations with Bone Tissue

Resorption of bone can occur in an uncontrolled manner during active advanced periodontal disease (considered periodontitis), which is in contrast to that occurring in a controlled manner with orthodontic therapy (see **Chapters 14 and 20,** respectively). At the same time as resorption, regeneration of bone occurs even in the presence of injury and disease. Excess generalized bone resorption as well as excess bone

TABLE 8.4 Blood Components

Type	Microscopic Structure	Histologic Features	Function
Red blood cell (or erythrocyte)		Biconcave disc without nucleus	Binds and transports oxygen and carbon dioxide
Platelets (or thrombocytes)		Discs without nucleus; cell fragments derived from special line of blood cell	Clotting mechanism
White blood cell (or leukocyte)	See Table 8.5	Rounded cells with nucleus, many variations possible (see Table 8.5)	Inflammatory response and immune response

appositional growth can occur in certain systemic bone disorders when the two processes are no longer balanced, such as with Paget disease.

Bone mass or density can increasingly be lost in women after menopause with the bones losing calcium and other minerals. This can become accelerated with the systemic bone disease of osteoporosis, especially for mature women. The spinal column also becomes curved, compressed, and shorter; bone spurs may also form on the vertebrae that have become thinner with mineral and fluid loss. Now bones become more brittle and may break more easily, especially those involved with the hip. This tissue degeneration can also affect the bones involved with the temporomandibular joint.

BLOOD PROPERTIES

The **blood** is a fluid connective tissue that serves as a transport medium for cellular nutrients, such as respiratory gases like oxygen and carbon dioxide as well as metabolites for the entire body. Blood is carried in endothelium-lined blood vessels and its medium consists of plasma with blood components (Table 8.4).

Plasma

The **plasma** (**plaz**-muh) is the fluid substance in the blood vessels that carries the plasma proteins, blood cells, and metabolites. It is more consistent in composition than tissue fluid and lymph, yet it contains most of the same materials with the addition of red blood cells (see **Chapter 7**). Serum, another fluid product, is distinguished from the plasma from which it is derived due to the removal of clotting proteins. If a sample of blood is treated with an agent to prevent clotting and is spun in a centrifuge, the plasma fraction is the least dense and will float as the top layer.

Blood Components

Blood cells and associated derivatives are also considered the *formed elements* of the blood. Most blood cells develop from a common stem cell in the bone marrow (Fig. 8.16). The formed elements of the blood include the numerous red blood cells. Not only are these cells present in the blood and its associated vessels but certain related components are also present in surrounding connective tissue.

Thus the most common cell in the blood is the **red blood cell (RBC)** or **erythrocyte** (ih-**rith**-ruh-sahyt) (see Table 8.4). An RBC is a biconcave disc that contains hemoglobin, which binds and then transports the oxygen and carbon dioxide. It has no nucleus and does not undergo mitosis because it is directly formed from the bone marrow's stem cells. There are 5 to 6 million per cubic milliliter of blood and are more common than other blood cells. In centrifuged blood, the RBCs settle to the bottom because they are also denser than the rest; this fraction is the *hematocrit*.

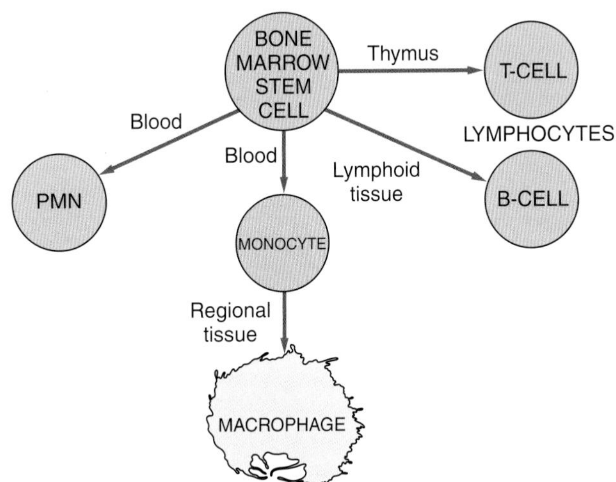

Fig. 8.16 Flowchart demonstrating that most blood cells develop from a common stem cell type in the bone marrow. B-cell lymphocytes stay and mature in the bone marrow, and T-cell lymphocytes travel to mature in other glands or tissue in the body, such as the thymus. Later, both types of lymphocytes will engage in immune responses throughout the body. Note also the polymorphonuclear leukocyte (*PMN;* or neutrophil) and monocyte (or macrophage). (From Fehrenbach MJ. Immunity and immunologic oral lesions. In: Ibsen OAC, Phelan JA, eds. *Oral Pathology for Dental Hygienists.* 7th ed. St. Louis: Elsevier; 2018.)

The blood also contains **platelets** (**pleyt**-litz) or **thrombocytes** (**throm**-buh-sahyts), which are smaller than RBCs, disc-shaped, and also have no nucleus. However, these formed elements are not considered true blood cells but instead fragments of bone marrow cells (or megakaryocytes) and platelets are also found in much lesser numbers than RBCs at 250,000 to 400,000 per cubic milliliter. Platelets function in the clotting mechanism.

In even smaller numbers in the blood is the **white blood cell (WBC)** or **leukocyte** (**loo**-kuh-sahyt) (see Tables 8.4 and 8.5). Like RBCs, WBCs form from bone marrow stem cells. The WBCs later mature in the bone marrow or in various lymphatic organs. They are involved in the defense mechanisms of the body, including the inflammatory and immune responses. Therefore WBCs are also usually found in both epithelium and connective tissue after they migrate from the blood by moving through openings between the cell junctions of the endothelial lining of the vessel to participate in defense mechanisms.

TABLE 8.5 Blood Cells and Related Tissue Cells

Cells	Microscopic Structure	Features	Functions
Polymorphonuclear leukocyte (or neutrophil)		Multilobed nucleus with granules	Inflammatory response: Phagocytosis
Lymphocyte		Eccentric round nucleus without granules: B, T, and natural killer cells	B and T cell immune response: Humoral and cell-mediated. Natural killer cells: defense against tumor- and virally infected cells.
Plasma cell		Round cartwheel nucleus derived from B-cell lymphocytes	Humoral immune response: Produces immunoglobulins (or antibodies)
Monocyte (in blood)/macrophage (in tissue)		Bean-shaped nucleus with poorly staining granules	Inflammatory and immune response: Phagocytosis as well as process and present immunogens (or antigens)
Eosinophil		Bilobed nucleus with granules	Hypersensitivity response
Basophil		Irregularly shaped bilobed/trilobed nucleus with granules	Hypersensitivity response
Mast cell (in tissue)		Irregularly shaped bilobed nucleus with granules	Hypersensitivity response

The WBCs differ from RBCs because they possess a nucleus, have more cytoplasm, and have the power of active amoeboid movement in order to migrate from the blood to the tissue; thus, unlike RBCs, WBCs perform their functions not only in the blood but also in other tissue. They are also even less numerous than platelets at only 5000 to 10,000 per cubic milliliter. There are five main types based on their microscopic structure, the neutrophils, lymphocytes, monocytes, eosinophils, and basophils. The fraction of centrifuged blood that settles on the surface of the hematocrit consists of the WBCs along with platelets, forming the intermediately placed buffy coat with the plasma fraction superior to it.

The most common WBC in the blood is the **neutrophil** (**noo**-truh-fil) or **polymorphonuclear (PMN) leukocyte** (pol-ee-mawr-fuh-**noo**-klee-er) (Fig. 8.17). These are the first cells to appear at an injury site when the inflammatory response is triggered; thus large numbers of the PMNs can be present in the suppuration or pus, which in certain cases forms locally at the injury site. The PMNs constitute 54% to 62% of the total blood WBC count. They have a short lifespan, contain lysosomal enzymes, are active in phagocytosis, and respond to chemotactic factors (see **Chapter 7**).

The second most common WBC in the blood is the **lymphocyte (lim-**fuh-sahyt**)**, which makes up 25% to 33% of the count. There are three functional types of lymphocytes, the **B cell, T cell,** and **natural killer (NK) cell**. The B cells mature in the bone marrow and gut-associated lymphoid tissue such as lymph nodes (see Fig. 11.16), whereas the T cells mature in the thymus gland (see Fig. 8.16). The NK cells also mature in the bone marrow; they are large cells that are involved in the first line of defense against tumor- or virally infected cells by killing them and thus are not considered part of the immune response.

Cytokines are produced by both B and T cells and are one of the major chemical mediators of the immune response (see the discussion in **Chapter 14** related to periodontal disease). Thus, both of these types of lymphocytes are involved in the immune response (see Table 8.5). In the past, the immune response was broken into two strict divisions, the humoral immune response with B cells and cell-mediated immune response with T cells. However, the distinction between the two divisions is now considered less important because they are so strongly related.

One important difference between the two divisions remains, the B-cell lymphocytes divide during the immune response to form

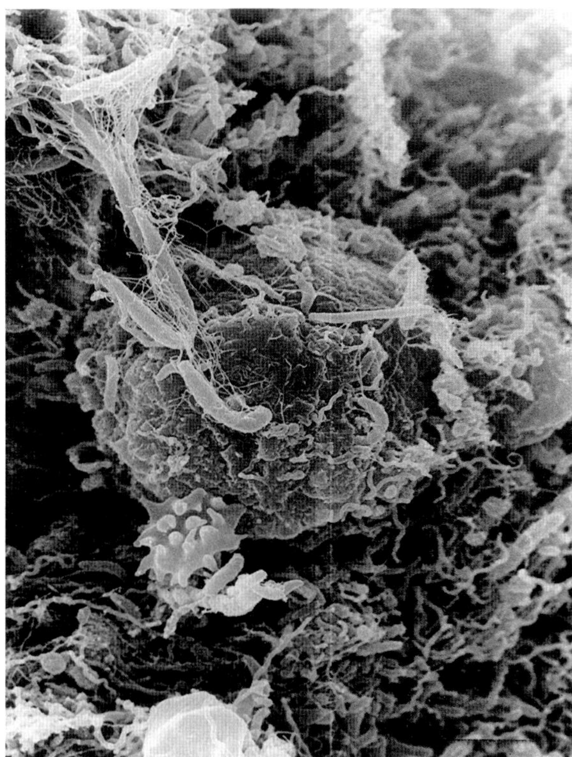

Fig. 8.17 Electron micrograph of a polymorphonuclear leukocyte (*PMN;* or neutrophil), which is the most common white blood cell. (Courtesy of Jan Cope, RDH, MS.)

plasma cells. Once mature, plasma cells produce an **immunoglobulin (Ig)** (im-yuh-noh-**glob**-yuh-lin), which is also considered an **antibody** (**an**-ti-bod-ee) and one of the blood proteins. There are five distinct classes of immunoglobulins: IgA (including serum or secretory types), IgD, IgE, IgG, and IgM (Table 8.6). Each plasma cell produces only one specific class of immunoglobulin in response to a specific **immunogen** (ih-**myoo**-nuh-juhn) or **antigen** (**an**-ti-juhn). Immunogens are mostly proteins that are seen by the body as foreign and are capable of triggering an immune response.

Although immunoglobulin structure overall is very similar, a small region at the tip of the protein (hypervariable region) is extremely variable, allowing generation of an infinite number with slightly different tip structures or antigen-binding sites to exist. An immunoglobulin, along with its specific immunogen (at epitope variable region), often forms an immune complex in an effort to render the immunogen unable to cause disease. Immunoglobulins can be extracted from the blood of recovering patients and used for passive immunization against certain infectious diseases.

However, the most common WBC in the connective tissue proper is the **macrophage** (**mak**-ruh-feyj), which is considered a **monocyte** (**mon**-uh-sahyt) before it migrates from the blood into the tissue. They have a longer lifespan than PMNs but constitute only 2% to 10% of the WBC count. After migration, macrophages arrive at the site of injury later and in fewer numbers than PMNs when the inflammatory response is triggered. Macrophages contain lysosomal enzymes, are involved in phagocytosis (as are PMNs), are actively mobile, and have the ability to respond to chemotactic factors and cytokines (see Fig. 7.4). Macrophages also assist in the immune response to facilitate immunoglobulin production. In certain disease states, numbers of macrophages may fuse together, forming giant cells with multiple nuclei. In bone connective tissue, these are then considered osteoclasts that will resorb bone (discussed earlier).

TABLE 8.6 Known Immunoglobulins (or Antibodies) from Plasma Cells

Immunoglobulin	Features : Functions
IgA	Has two subgroups: serous in blood; secretory in saliva, tears, and breast milk; both aid in defense against pathogens in body fluids
IgD	Functions in activation of B-cell lymphocytes as antigen receptor; has been shown to activate basophils and mast cells to produce antimicrobial factors
IgE	Involved in hypersensitivity response; binds to mast cells and basophils and releases bioactive substances such as histamine
IgG	Has four subgroups; major immunoglobulin in blood serum and can pass placental barrier to form first passive immunity for newborn
IgM	Involved in early immune responses against pathogens because of involvement with IgD in activation of B-cell lymphocytes before sufficient immunoglobulin production

The **eosinophil** (ee-uh-**sin**-uh-fil) is usually only 6% of the WBC count, but its percentage is increased during a hypersensitivity response (or allergy) and in parasitic diseases because its primary function is the phagocytosis of immune complexes.

The **basophil** (**bey**-suh-fil) is usually found to be less than 1% of the WBC count and is also involved in the hypersensitivity response releasing bioactive products. Other WBCs located in the connective tissue include the **mast cell,** which is similar in structure to the basophil. Mast cells are involved in a type of primitive hypersensitivity response that also releases bioactive products but are not involved with immunoglobulins such as IgE. However, even though both cells are derived from the bone marrow, they may originate from different stem cells within the bone marrow. Mast cells have been implicated in the progression of periodontal disease due to their bioactive products as well as many confounding systemic diseases.

Clinical Considerations with Blood-Related Products

Dental professionals must understand certain laboratory procedures that patients may have undergone when viewing the medical record. These procedures include a complete blood count (CBC), which is an evaluation of both RBC and WBC types to detect infections, anemia, or leukemia. A platelet count can also be performed to determine the number of platelets if bleeding problems are a consideration due to past medical history; a coagulation (bleeding) test can also be performed to test platelet function. These procedures may also be recommended to the dental patient if there is clinical evidence or history of bleeding difficulties, especially before periodontal surgery, tooth extraction, or dental implant placement as well as if they have an unusual level of periodontal disease, such as an aggressive periodontitis with its uncontrolled loss of periodontal support. Also these tests can be done if there is failure to form a clot after any dental surgical procedures.

There is now an increase in the use during dental surgery of **platelet-rich plasma (PRP),** which is an autologous conditioned plasma that is a concentrate of PRP protein derived from whole blood centrifuged to remove RBCs. This is used to support both soft and hard tissue healing (i.e., osteoid, blood vessels, and even collagen), a process already well known postsurgically in medicine. This increased healing level occurs because the PRP contains vast amount of growth factors

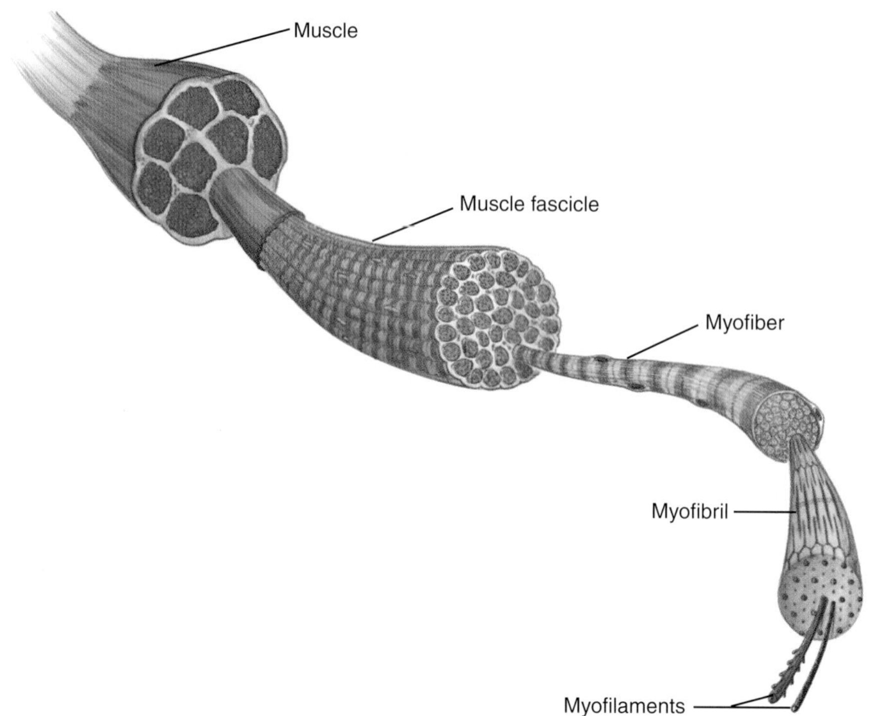

Fig. 8.18 Skeletal muscle with its striations and which is composed of smaller muscle bundles, fascicles, myofibers, myofibrils, and myofilaments.

as well as having other various healing mechanisms along with the high concentration of platelets. The PRP is used to coat dental implants and is also placed within the soft tissue flaps created following periodontal surgery to promote repair of bony defects as well as with graft placement.

Another use of blood-related products within a dental setting is with the use of postexposure prophylaxis of dental healthcare personnel (DHCP) by a passive injection of hepatitis B immunoglobulin (HBIG). It is given if there is evidence that the person is without seroconversion after the usually required vaccination for the infection. It is made from human plasma containing immunoglobulins made in response to the type B form of hepatitis.

MUSCLE PROPERTIES

The **muscle** in the body is part of the muscular system and similar to connective tissue; most muscles are derived from somites (see Fig. 3.13). Each muscle shortens under neural control, causing soft tissue and bony structures of the body to move. The three types of muscle are classified according to structure, function, and innervation, skeletal, smooth, and cardiac (see Table 8.1).

MUSCLE CLASSIFICATION

Each type of muscle has its own type of action, which is the movement accomplished when the muscle cells contract. Smooth muscle and cardiac muscle are considered involuntary muscles because they are under autonomic nervous system control (discussed next). Smooth muscles are located in organs, glands, and the linings of blood vessels. Cardiac muscle is in the wall of the heart (myocardium).

Skeletal muscles are considered voluntary muscles because they are under voluntary control, involving the somatic nervous system (Fig. 8.18). All the major muscles of the body's appendages and trunk are skeletal muscles. Thus skeletal muscles are usually attached to bones of the skeleton. Skeletal muscles also include the muscles of the facial expression, tongue, pharynx, and upper esophagus as well as the muscles of mastication that assist the temporomandibular joint in the actions involved in mastication (see Fig. 19.8).

SKELETAL MUSCLE HISTOLOGY

Skeletal muscles are also considered *striated muscles* because the muscle cells appear striped microscopically. Each muscle is composed of numerous muscle bundles or **fascicles** (**fas**-i-kuhlz) like the bundles of fibers that go together to create a rope, which then are composed of numerous muscle cells or **myofibers** (mahy-uh-**fahy**-berz). Each myofiber extends the entire length of the muscle and is composed of smaller subunits of **myofibrils** (**mahy**-uh-fahy-bruhlz) surrounded by the other organelles of the cell. Each myofibril is composed of even smaller subunits of **myofilaments** (mahy-uh-**fil**-uh-muhntz).

NERVE TISSUE PROPERTIES

Nerve tissue forms the nervous system in the body, being derived from the neuroectoderm within the embryo (see Fig. 3.10). Nerves function to carry messages or impulses based on electrical potentials. Nerve tissue in the body causes muscles to contract, resulting in facial expressions and joint movements, such as those associated with mastication and speech. The tissue stimulates glands to secrete hormones and regulates many other systems of the body, such as the cardiovascular system. It also allows for the perception of sensations, such as pain, touch, taste, and smell.

NERVE TISSUE HISTOLOGY

A **neuron** (**noor**-on) is the functional cellular component of the nervous system and is composed of three parts, one neural cell body with two different types of neural cytoplasmic processes (Fig. 8.19). The

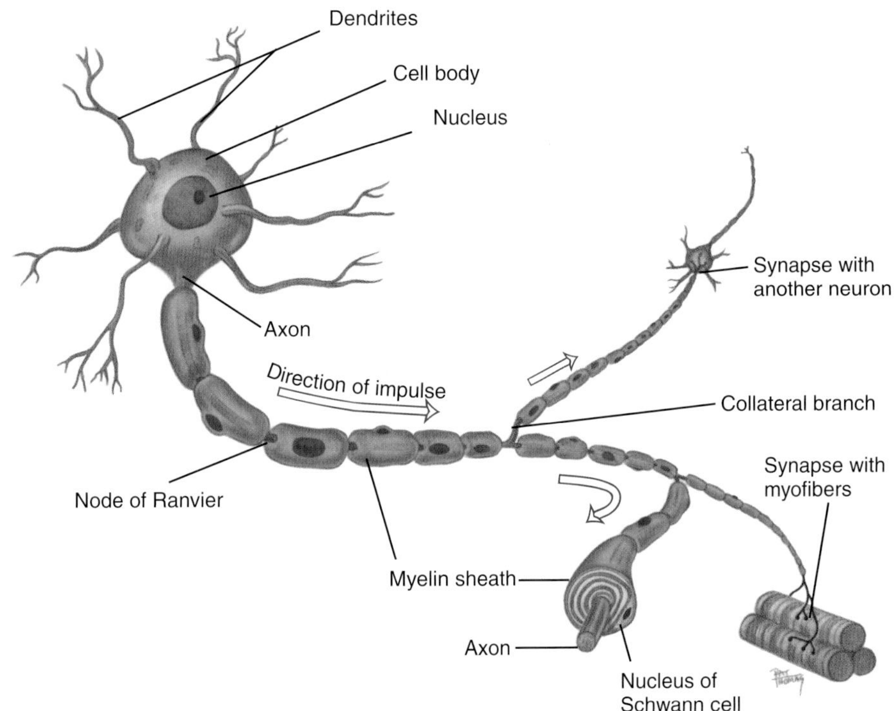

Fig. 8.19 Neuron with its dendrites, cell body, and axon, showing a synaptic relationship with the muscle as well as with another neuron.

neural cell body is not involved in the process of impulse transmission but provides the metabolic support for the entire neuron.

One type of process associated with the cell body is an **axon** (**ak**-son), a long, thin, singular, cable-like process that conducts impulses away from the cell body. An axon is encased in its own cell membrane, having nerve excitability and conduction due to changes that develop in the nerve membrane. Certain axons can also be additionally covered by a **myelin sheath** (**mahy**-uh-lin).

The myelin sheath consists of tightly wrapped layers of phospholipid-rich membrane surrounding the Schwann cell cytoplasm; there is very little cytoplasm sandwiched between them. It is only in the outermost layer of the myelin sheath where the Schwann cell and its nucleus are located. Along a myelinated axon are the nodes of Ranvier, which form gaps between the adjacent Schwann cells. The insulating properties of the myelin sheath and its gaps allow the axon to conduct impulses more quickly. The other type of process associated with the cell body is the **dendrite** (**den**-drahyt), a threadlike process that usually contains multiple branches, which functions to receive and conduct impulses toward the cell body.

A **nerve** is a bundle of neural processes outside the central nervous system (CNS) and in the peripheral nervous system (PNS). A **synapse** (**sin**-aps) is the junction between two neurons or between a neuron and an effector organ (such as a muscle or gland) where neural impulses are transmitted by chemical means (neurotransmitter substance). To function, most tissue or organs have innervation, through supply of nerves. A nerve allows information to be carried to and from the brain, which is the central information center. An aggregation of neuron cell bodies outside the CNS is a **ganglion** (**gang**-glee-uhn) (plural, **ganglia** [**gang**-glee-uh]).

Within the innermost part of the nerve or core region are the fasciculi of the **core bundles**. Core bundles are exposed later to local anesthetic agents in more diluted or lower concentrations because the bundles are located farther away with more anatomic barriers. Core fibers tend to innervate the anterior mandible, including the chin and lips. Lips, chin, and anterior dentition as well as supporting structures anesthetize later and with more difficulty. A lack of labial and mental soft tissue signs and symptoms of anesthesia after an inferior alveolar nerve block indicates core bundles are not yet adequately anesthetized. In contrast, **mantle bundles,** which are the fasciculi located near the outer surface of a nerve, tend to innervate the molar region; molar regions anesthetize earlier and more easily.

The two functional types of nerves are afferent and efferent nerves. An **afferent nerve** (**af**-er-uhnt) or *sensory nerve* carries information or relays impulses from the periphery of the body to the brain (or spinal cord). Thus an afferent nerve carries sensory information (such as taste, pain, or proprioception) to the brain. Proprioception is information concerning the movement and position of the body. This sensory information is sent on to the brain to be analyzed, acted upon, associated with other information, and stored as memory.

An **efferent nerve** (**ef**-er-uhnt) or *motor nerve* carries information away from the brain to the periphery of the body. Thus an efferent nerve carries information to the muscles or glands in order to activate them, often in response to information received by the afferent nerve pathway. One motor neuron with its branching fibers may control hundreds of muscle fibers. Autonomic nerves are (by definition) always efferent.

Within the pulp, the nerves include sensory types. In addition, the afferent axons of these sensory pulp nerves are also located in the dentinal tubules that make up the dentin. Thus when the either dentin or pulp is injured or restored, the sensation of pain is perceived by the brain.

NERVOUS SYSTEM

The nervous system has two main divisions, the CNS and the PNS (Table 8.7). These two systems are not separate but rely on each other and thus constantly interact. The CNS consists of the brain and spinal cord. The PNS consists of the spinal and cranial nerves and includes both the somatic nervous system and the autonomic nervous system

TABLE 8.7 Nervous System Divisions

Divisions	Components
Central nervous system	Brain and spinal cord
Peripheral nervous system	Spinal and cranial nerves of somatic nervous system and autonomic nervous system (includes sympathetic and parasympathetic systems)

(ANS). The spinal nerves extend from the spinal cord to the periphery of the body. The cranial nerves are initially attached to the brain, which then pass through openings in the skull. Certain cranial nerves are associated with the oral cavity, especially the fifth cranial nerve or trigeminal nerve. The somatic nervous system operates with conscious control of the individual to move the skeletal muscles.

The ANS is a part of the PNS and operates without conscious control as the caretaker of the body. Autonomic nerves are efferent processes and they are always in two-neuron circuits. The first neuron carries autonomic impulses to a ganglion, where they are transmitted to the body of the second neuron. The ANS itself has two divisions, a sympathetic system and parasympathetic system (see Table 8.7). Most tissue or organ systems are supplied by both divisions of the ANS.

The sympathetic nervous system is involved in fight-or-flight responses, such as in the inhibition of salivary gland secretion (known as hyposalivation). Such a response by the sympathetic system leads to a dry mouth (known as xerostomia) (see Fig. 11.9). Sympathetic neurons arise in the spinal cord and synapse in ganglia arranged in a chain extending almost the entire length of the vertebral column on both sides. Therefore all the sympathetic neurons in the head have already synapsed in a ganglion. Sympathetic fibers reach the cranial tissue that they supply by traveling with the arteries.

The parasympathetic nervous system is involved in rest-or-digest responses, such as the stimulation of salivary gland secretion. Such a response leads to salivary flow to aid in digestion. Parasympathetic fibers associated with glands of the head and neck region are carried in various cranial nerves and their ganglia are located in the head. Therefore, parasympathetic neurons in this region may be either preganglionic neurons (before synapsing in the ganglion) or postganglionic neurons (after synapsing in the ganglion).

9

Oral Mucosa

Additional resources and practice exercises are provided on the companion Evolve website for this book: http://evolve.elsevier.com/Fehrenbach/illustrated.

LEARNING OBJECTIVES

1. Define and pronounce the key terms in this chapter.
2. List and describe the types of oral mucosa, characterizing each type of epithelium associated with the oral cavity.
3. Discuss the clinical considerations for oral mucosa pathology, integrating it into patient care.
4. Identify the components of each type of oral mucosa on a diagram.
5. List and discuss the clinical correlations associated with the regional differences in the oral mucosa, integrating it into patient care.
6. Discuss tongue and lingual papillae properties as well as oral mucosa pigmentation and the clinical considerations for each.
7. Discuss the turnover times for regions of the oral cavity and associated clinical correlations as well as repair and aging considerations, integrating it into patient care.

ORAL MUCOSA PROPERTIES

Dental professionals must have a clear understanding of the basic histology of the oral mucosa, its regional differences, and any related clinical considerations. Only then will they be able to further understand the clinical considerations involved with the process of aging as well as injury to the oral mucosa. This injury to the oral mucosa can include that which occurs with trauma, inflammation, infection, and cancer as discussed later in this chapter. With this information, they then can promote the health of the oral mucosa.

Oral mucosa almost continuously lines the oral cavity. Microscopically the oral mucosa is composed of stratified squamous epithelium overlying a connective tissue proper or lamina propria, with possibly a deeper submucosa (Fig. 9.1). In the skin, these two similar tissue types are considered the *epidermis* and *dermis*, respectively (see **Chapter 8**).

Even though the entire oral cavity has an epithelial covering with connective tissue making up the bulk of lamina propria, regional differences are noted throughout in the oral mucosa. For example, the oral mucosa is perforated in various regions by the ducts of salivary glands (see Fig. 11.6). Other areas have thinner or thicker epithelium and some areas of the lamina propria contain specialized fibers. This chapter also discusses these regional differences; however, the gingival sulcular region is discussed in more detail in **Chapter 10.**

As always, a basement membrane lies between the epithelium and connective tissue of the oral mucosa (see Figs. 7.6 and 8.4). It serves not as a separation between the two tissue types but as a continuous structure linking the two. Studies are focusing on trying to understand the interactions between these two tissue types and the basement membrane may hold these answers.

Three main types of oral mucosa are found in the oral cavity, the lining, masticatory, and specialized mucosa (Table 9.1). This classification of oral mucosa is based on the general histologic features of the tissue. As noted before, the specific histologic features of each oral region are discussed later in this chapter. Overall, the clinical appearance of the tissue reflects the underlying histology, both in health and disease. Thus the oral cavity has correctly been described as a mirror that reflects the health of the individual. Changes indicative of disease are seen as alterations in the oral mucosa lining the mouth, which can reveal systemic conditions such as diabetes or vitamin deficiency or the local effects of chronic tobacco or alcohol use.

LINING MUCOSA

The **lining mucosa** is a type of oral mucosa noted for its softer surface texture, moist surface, and ability to stretch and be compressed, acting as a cushion for the underlying structures. Lining mucosa includes that of the buccal mucosa, labial mucosa, alveolar mucosa as well as the oral mucosa lining the ventral surface of the tongue, floor of the mouth, and soft palate.

Microscopically the lining mucosa is a type that is associated with nonkeratinized stratified squamous epithelium (Fig. 9.2). In contrast to masticatory mucosa, which is discussed next, the interface between the epithelium and the lamina propria is generally smoother with fewer and less-pronounced rete ridges and connective tissue papillae. In addition to these factors, the presence of elastic fibers in the lamina propria also provides the tissue with a movable base.

A submucosa deep to the lamina propria is usually present in lining mucosa, overlying muscle and allowing compression of the superficial tissue. These general histologic features allow this type of mucosa to serve in regions of the oral cavity where a movable base is needed, such as during speech, mastication, and swallowing. Thus surgical incisions in this tissue frequently require sutures for closure due to tissue movement. Local anesthetic injections into lining mucosa are also easier to accomplish than in masticatory mucosa with less discomfort and easy dispersion of the agent, but infections also spread rapidly. And dental medications have less difficulty being absorbed since this type is the most permeable to liquid.

MASTICATORY MUCOSA

The **masticatory mucosa** (mass-ti-**keyt**-tor-ee) is a type of oral mucosa noted for its rubbery surface texture and resiliency. Masticatory mucosa includes that of the hard palate, attached gingiva, and dorsal surface of the tongue. Microscopically the masticatory mucosa is associated with orthokeratinized stratified squamous epithelium

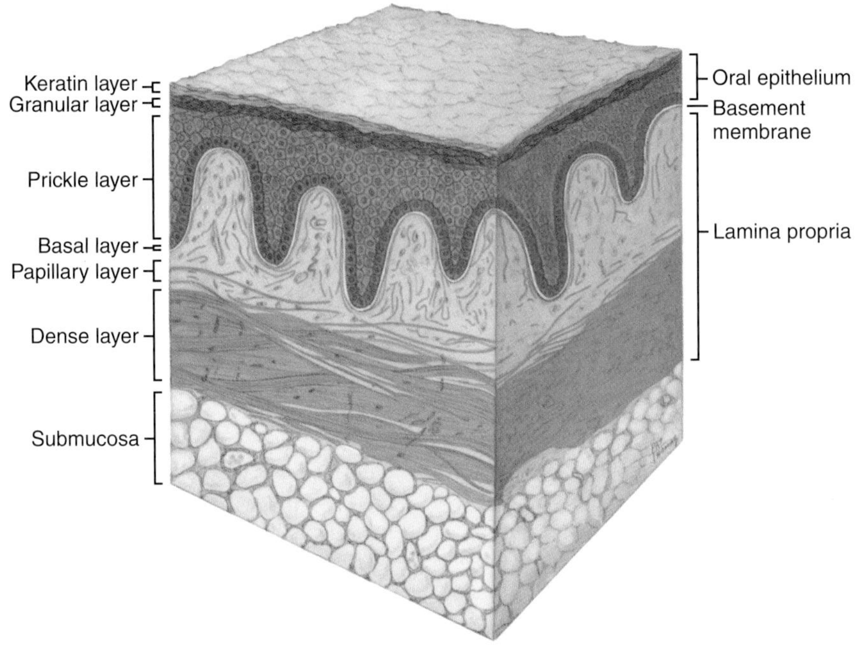

Fig. 9.1 General histologic features of a masticatory oral mucosa composed of keratinized stratified squamous epithelium overlying lamina propria with a deeper submucosa present.

TABLE 9.1 Oral Mucosa Types

Types	Regions	General Clinical Appearance	General Histologic Features
Lining mucosa	Buccal mucosa, labial mucosa, alveolar mucosa, ventral surface of the tongue, floor of the mouth, and soft palate	Softer surface texture, moist surface, ability to stretch and be compressed, acting as a cushion	Nonkeratinized epithelium with smooth interface, few rete ridges and connective tissue papillae, with elastic fibers in lamina propria and submucosa
Masticatory mucosa	Attached gingiva, hard palate, and dorsal surface of the tongue	Rubbery surface texture and resiliency, serving as firm base	Keratinized epithelium and interdigitated interface with many rete ridges and connective tissue papillae with thin layer of submucosa or none
Specialized mucosa	Dorsal and lateral surface of the tongue	Associated with lingual papillae	Discrete structures of epithelium and lamina propria; many with taste buds (see Table 9.5)

as well as parakeratinized stratified squamous epithelium, which will both be discussed later in this chapter (Figs. 9.3, 9.4, and 9.5). Unlike lining mucosa discussed earlier, the interface between the epithelium and lamina propria in masticatory mucosa is highly interdigitated with numerous and more-pronounced rete ridges and connective tissue papillae, giving it a firm base. In addition, the deeper submucosa is an extremely thin layer or is absent. When masticatory mucosa overlies bone, with or without submucosa, it increases the firmness of the tissue.

These general histologic features allow masticatory mucosa to function in the regions that need a firm base, such as during mastication and speech. Therefore sutures are rarely needed for this tissue after surgery because it has less tissue movement. However, local anesthetic injections are more difficult and cause greater discomfort in masticatory mucosa than those in lining mucosa due to its firmness as well as when any swelling from an infectious source occurs in the tissue due to the inherent pressure. And dental medications have more difficulty being absorbed because this type is least permeable to liquid.

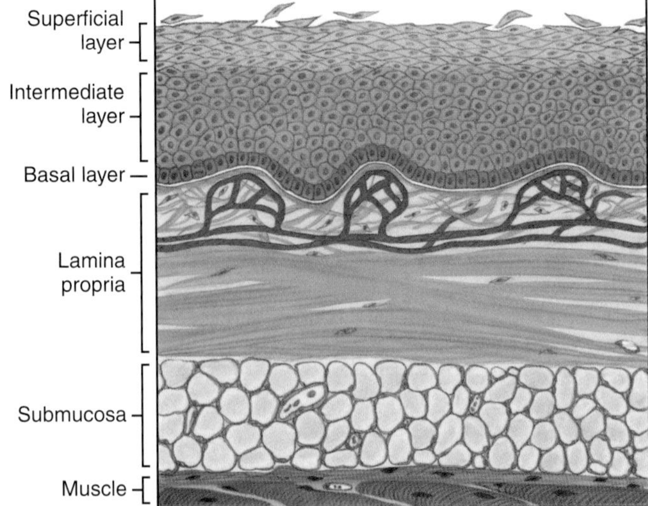

Fig. 9.2 General histologic features of a lining mucosa composed of nonkeratinized stratified squamous epithelium (with its three layers) overlying lamina propria. A deeper submucosa is usually present overlying muscle.

SPECIALIZED MUCOSA

The **specialized mucosa** is a type of oral mucosa found on both the dorsal and lateral surface of the tongue in the form of the lingual

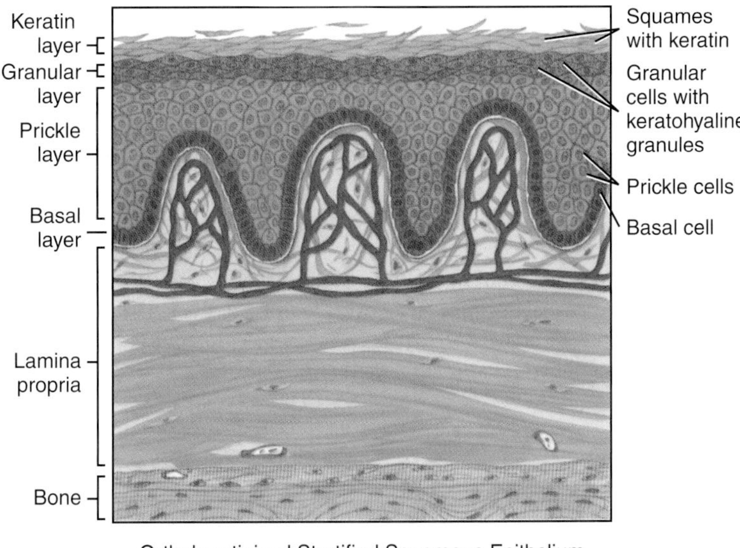

Fig. 9.3 General histologic features of masticatory mucosa composed of orthokeratinized stratified squamous epithelium (with its four layers) overlying lamina propria. A deeper thin submucosa may or may not be present and may overlay bone (as shown here). Note that the cells in the keratin layer have lost their nuclei and are filled with keratin. However, the artifact of the spiky look of the prickle layer has not been shown.

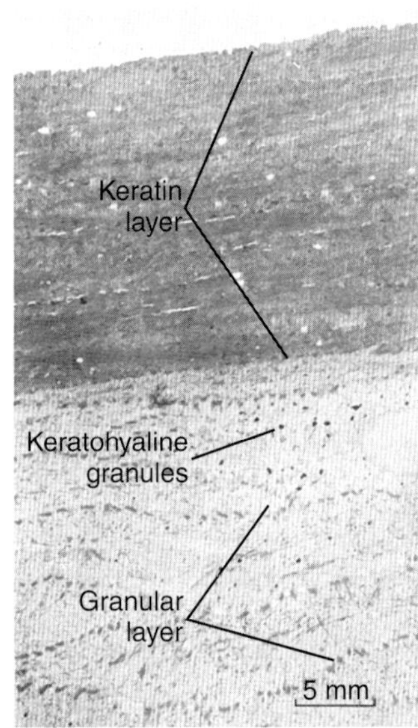

Fig. 9.4 Electron micrograph of keratinized epithelium showing both the granular and keratin layers. Small keratohyaline granules are visible in the granular layer; the cells of the keratin layer are flattened and contain keratin. However, it is hard to discern at this lower-power magnification whether this tissue is orthokeratinized or parakeratinized based on the presence of nuclei of the keratin layer. (From Nanci A. *Ten Cate's Oral Histology*. 9th ed. St. Louis: Elsevier; 2018.)

papillae (see Figs. 2.14 and 2.15). Microscopically the lingual papillae are discrete structures composed of keratinized epithelium and lamina propria (discussed later in this chapter).

EPITHELIUM OF ORAL MUCOSA

Three types of stratified squamous epithelium are found within the oral cavity, the nonkeratinized, orthokeratinized, and parakeratinized (Table 9.2). Although all three types of epithelium are similar in many ways, they are also different, primarily in the surface layers of the epithelium as will be discussed in this chapter.

Nonkeratinized epithelium is associated with lining mucosa. Orthokeratinized and parakeratinized epithelium are both associated with masticatory mucosa as well as specialized mucosa. All types of epithelium usually act as an environmental barrier to pathogenic invasion and mechanical irritation as well as offering protection against dryness. These protective features are accentuated in the types of epithelium that contain **keratin** (**ker**-uh-tin). Histologists use the term **keratinocytes** (ker-**raht**-uh-sahytz) for the epithelial cells in oral mucosa that can produce keratin either at the usual levels if it is a keratinized tissue or at higher levels when the tissue becomes traumatized, even in previously nonkeratinized tissue (Table 9.3).

The **nonkeratinocytes** (nohn-ker-**raht**-tn-uh-sahytz), those cells that do not produce keratin in epithelium, are present in much smaller numbers in oral mucosa (see Table 9.3). These cells include melanocytes (discussed later in this chapter) along with their associated production of melanin pigmentation. Also present in epithelium of oral mucosa are Granstein and Langerhans cells, both of which arise from the bone marrow and help the tissue's immune responses as well as Merkel cells, which are involved in tactile sensory information. White blood cells are also present, with the polymorphonuclear leukocyte being the most commonly occurring one in all forms of healthy oral mucosa (see Fig. 8.17).

Using recent ultrastructural studies, the superficial surface layer of most types of epithelium in oral mucosa has now been shown to contain cellular ridge-like folds, **microplicae (MPL)** (mahy-kroh-**plih**-kee). These microridges are known to be typical of the surfaces of the body covered with protective mucus or in the case of the oral cavity, saliva. However, MPL may merely represent the remnants of intercellular interdigitations or a modified expression of microvillous-like extensions. However, it is speculated that grooves they produce may function to hold a layer of lubricating and cushioning mucin designed to protect the underlying cell from abrasive abuse, similar to that of mucus or saliva. The cell surface itself is of potentially great significance as it harbors many biomarkers for refined prognosis and targets for oral mucosal diseases and cancer therapy.

Nonkeratinized Stratified Squamous Epithelium

The **nonkeratinized stratified squamous epithelium** (nohn-**ker**-uh-tn-izd **strat**-uh-fahyd **skwey**-muhs) is located in the superficial layers of lining mucosa, such as in the labial mucosa, buccal mucosa, and alveolar mucosa, as well as in the oral mucosa lining the ventral surface of the tongue, the floor of the mouth, and the soft palate (see Fig. 9.2). Lining mucosa has similar epithelial histologic features, even though it has its own regional differences. Nonkeratinized epithelium is the most common form of epithelium in the oral cavity.

Each area of lining mucosa has at least three layers within the epithelium. A **basal layer** or *stratum basale* is the deepest of the three layers. The basal layer is a single layer of cuboidal epithelial cells overlying the basement membrane, which in turn is situated superior to the lamina propria. The basal layer produces the basal lamina of the basement membrane.

The basal layer is also considered germinative because mitosis of the epithelial cells occurs within this layer; however, this cell division is seen only under higher-power magnification of the tissue (see Table 7.2). Future ultrastructural studies may show the existence of an epithelial stem cell in the basal layer that produces other stem and daughter cells, similar to the situation for blood cells in the bone marrow.

The layer of epithelium superficial to the basal layer in nonkeratinized epithelium is the **intermediate layer** or *stratum intermedium.* The intermediate layer is composed of larger stacked polyhedral-shaped cells. These cells appear larger and plumper than the basal layer cells because they have larger amounts cytoplasm. However, as they migrate superficially, the cells of the intermediate layer have lost the ability to undergo mitosis. The intermediate layer makes up the bulk of nonkeratinized stratified squamous epithelium.

At the most superficial level in nonkeratinized epithelium is the **superficial layer** or *stratum superficiale.* It is hard to discern the exact division between the superficial layer and the deeper intermediate layers in lining mucosa when viewing microscopic sections. The superficial layer shows even larger, similarly stacked polyhedral epithelial cells but with the outer cells flattening into squames. The squames in these layers show shedding or loss as they age and die during the turnover of the tissue. In summary, maturation within this nonkeratinized tissue is at a lesser level than keratinized tissue, noting only the increase in the size of cells as they migrate superficially, unlike the more complex changes that occur in the most superficial layers of keratinized tissue.

Orthokeratinized Stratified Squamous Epithelium

In contrast to nonkeratinized tissue, the **orthokeratinized stratified squamous epithelium** (ohr-thoh-**ker**-uh-tn-izd) demonstrates a keratinization of the epithelial cells throughout its most superficial layers (see Figs. 9.3 and 9.4). Orthokeratinized epithelium is the least common form of epithelium found in the oral cavity. It is associated with the masticatory mucosa of the hard palate and the attached gingiva. It is also associated with the specialized mucosa of the lingual papillae on the dorsal surface of the tongue. As this tissue matures, it forms keratin within its most superficial cells as well as showing a visible and physiologic difference in the cells as they migrate superficially.

Like nonkeratinized epithelium, orthokeratinized epithelium has a single basal layer or *stratum basale* undergoing mitosis. This layer also produces the basal lamina of the adjacent basement membrane. Unlike nonkeratinized epithelium, however, orthokeratinized epithelium has more layers superficial to the basal layer, with four separate layers with somewhat distinct divisions.

Superficial to the basal layer is the **prickle layer** or *stratum spinosum.* This refers to an artifact that occurs when the regularly plump epithelial cells of this layer are fixed for prolonged microscopic study; the cells shrink as a result of cytoplasm loss from the drying fixation chemicals (see Fig. 7.5). Thus a prickly or spiky look results when the individual dehydrated cells are still joined at their outer edges by desmosomes. In live tissue, they migrate to this superior level in the tissue

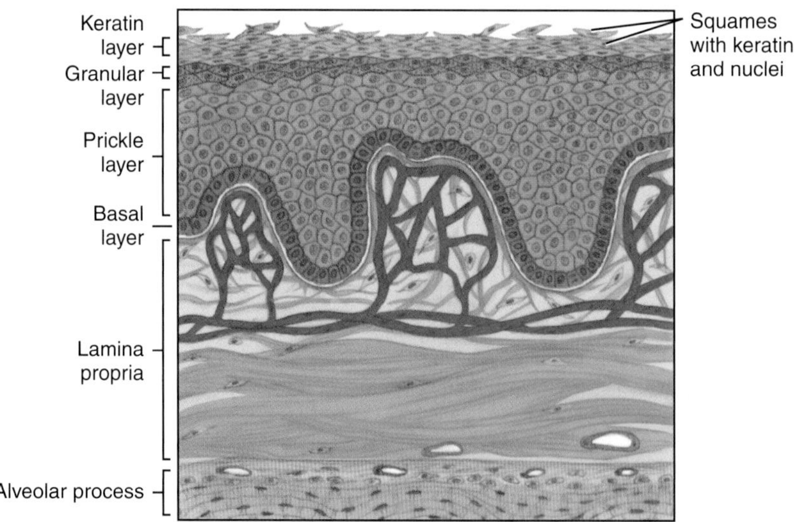

Fig. 9.5 General histologic features of masticatory mucosa, which is composed of parakeratinized stratified squamous epithelium (with its three to four layers) overlying lamina propria. Note that the cells in the keratin layer have retained their nuclei and are filled with keratin. However, the artifact of the spiky look of the prickle layer that can occur with microscopic fixation is not demonstrated. A deeper thin submucosa may or may not be present. If the submucosa is not present (as shown here), the oral mucosa and periosteum of the bone combine and are then considered a mucoperiosteum that is directly attached to the underlying bone of the alveolar process.

and also lose the ability to undergo mitosis, such as noted in the deeper basal layer. The prickle layer makes up the bulk of orthokeratinized epithelium.

Superficial to the prickle layer is the **granular layer** or *stratum granulosum.* The epithelial cells in this layer are flat and stacked in a layer three to five cells thick. In their cytoplasm, each of the cells has a nucleus with prominent **keratohyaline granules** (ker-uh-toh-**hyah**-uh-lin), which appear microscopically as dark spots. The keratohyaline granules form a chemical precursor for the keratin (keratohyalin) that is found in the more superficial layers.

The most superficial layer in orthokeratinized epithelium is the **keratin layer** or *stratum corneum,* which shows variable thickness depending on the oral cavity region. The cells in the keratin layer are flat and have no nuclei, and their cytoplasm is filled with keratin. The soft opaque waterproof keratin is formed from a complex of keratohyaline granules and intermediate filaments from the cells and it appears microscopically as a translucent dense material. The outer cells of the keratin layer or squames show increased flattening and also shedding or loss because they are no longer viable.

In addition, parts of the keratin material are also shed as a result of the turnover of the tissue. However, these squames and their cornified cell envelope make up a major part of the epithelial barrier discussed earlier and are continuously being renewed as cells mature from the deeper layers. The epithelial barrier serves as protection from physical, chemical, and pathogenic attack, as well as dehydration and heat loss that sometimes can occur in the oral cavity environment.

Parakeratinized Stratified Squamous Epithelium

The **parakeratinized stratified squamous epithelium** (pahr-uh-**ker**-uh-tn-izd) is associated with the masticatory mucosa of the attached gingiva in higher levels than the presence of orthokeratinization (see Figs. 9.4 and 9.5). Most histologists believe that parakeratinized epithelium is an immature form of orthokeratinized epithelium. The presence of this form of keratinization on the skin is considered a disease state; therefore, parakeratinization is one of the unique histologic features of the healthy oral cavity. Parakeratinized epithelium along with orthokeratinized epithelium is also associated with the specialized mucosa of the lingual papillae on the dorsal surface of the tongue.

Parakeratinized epithelium may have all the same layers of epithelium as orthokeratinized epithelium (such as the basal layer, prickle layer, granular layer, and keratin layer), although the granular layer may be indistinct or absent altogether.

The main difference between parakeratinized epithelium and orthokeratinized epithelium is in the cells of the keratin layer. In parakeratinized epithelium, the most superficial layer is still being shed and lost similar to orthokeratinized epithelium. However, these cells of the keratin layer contain not only keratin but also nuclei, unlike those of orthokeratinized epithelium. This distinction is sometimes difficult to discern under lower-power magnification in microscopic sections. Studies have shown that even though the epithelial cells have nuclei in the parakeratinized epithelium, they may be no longer viable, which is similar to the orthokeratinized epithelium. Further ultrastructural studies need to be done to see if this main difference in the cells of the keratin layers between the two types of tissue plays out in their functioning.

TABLE 9.2 Epithelium of Oral Mucosa

Types of Epithelium	Associated Oral Mucosa	General Histologic Features
Nonkeratinized epithelium	Lining mucosa	Basal, intermediate, superficial layers
Orthokeratinized epithelium	Masticatory mucosa	Basal, prickle, granular, keratin layers (cells contain only keratin and no nuclei)
Parakeratinized epithelium	Masticatory mucosa	Basal, prickle, granular, keratin layers (cells contain keratin and nuclei)

LAMINA PROPRIA OF ORAL MUCOSA

All forms of epithelium, whether associated with lining, masticatory, or specialized mucosa, have an adjoining connective tissue proper located deep to the basement membrane. In the case of oral mucosa, it is considered the **lamina propria** (**proh**-pree-uh) (see Fig. 9.1). The main fiber group in the lamina propria is Type I collagen fibers, but elastic fibers are present in certain regions of the oral cavity (see Table 8.3). The lamina propria, like all forms of connective tissue proper, has two layers, papillary and dense (Fig. 9.6).

The **papillary layer** is the more superficial layer of the lamina propria. It consists of loose connective tissue within the connective tissue papillae, along with blood vessels and nerve tissue. The tissue has an equal amount of fibers, cells, and intercellular substance. The **dense layer** is the deeper layer of the lamina propria. It consists of dense connective tissue with a large amount of fibers. Between the papillary layer and the deeper layers of the lamina propria is a **capillary plexus** (**kap**-uh-ler-ee **plek**-suhs), which provides nutrition for the all layers of the oral mucosa by way of the adjacent basement membrane, sending capillaries into the surrounding connective tissue papillae.

TABLE 9.3 Cells Types in Epithelium*

Types	Features	Functions
Epithelial cell	Rapidly renewing cell that usually undergoes pathway of differentiation with desmosomes; can be derived from all three embryonic cell layers	Forms cohesive sheet that resists physical forces and usually serves as barrier to infection
Granstein cell	Similar to Langerhans cell	Same as Langerhans cell
Langerhans cell	Dendritic bone marrow–derived cell with Langerhans granule; mostly suprabasal	Immune response with T-cell lymphocytes; antigen trapping and processing
Melanocyte	Dendritic cell of neural crest cell origin; premelanosomes and melanosomes present; forms a continuous network in basal layers	Synthesis of melanin pigmentation inclusion granules (melanosomes) with transfer to adjacent keratinocytes by injection
Merkel cell	Nondendritic neural cell noted in basal layers; characteristic electron-dense vesicles and associated nerve axon	Tactile sensory information

*White blood cells are not included in this table.

A **submucosa** (sub-myoo-**koh**-suh) may or may not be present deep to the dense layer of the lamina propria, depending on the region of the oral cavity (see Figs. 9.1 and 9.11). If present, the submucosa usually contains loose connective tissue and may also contain adipose connective tissue or salivary glands as well as overlying the bone or muscle within the oral cavity.

Lining mucosa does not have prominent connective tissue papillae that alternate with the rete ridges present in masticatory mucosa. In addition, elastic fibers are present in the papillary layer, thus allowing the lining mucosa to stretch and recoil during speech, mastication, and swallowing. In contrast to lining mucosa, masticatory mucosa has numerous and prominent connective tissue papillae, giving the oral mucosa a firm base, which is needed for speech and mastication.

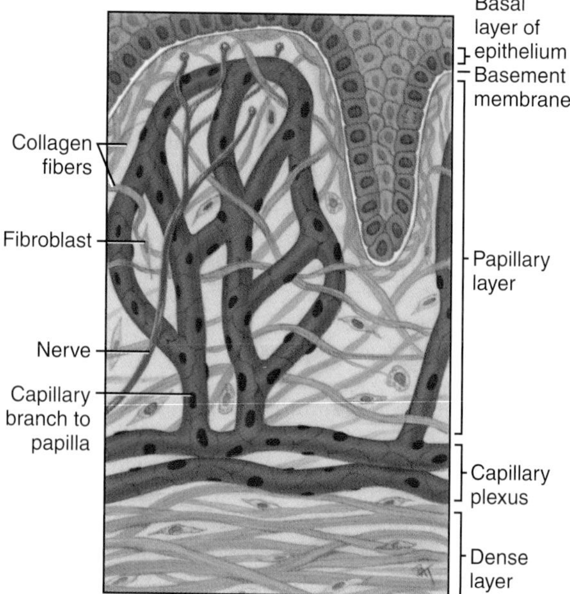

Fig. 9.6 General histologic features of the lamina propria (with its two layers) of the oral mucosa and its relationship to the adjoining basement membrane and overlying epithelium.

The most common cell in the lamina propria of all types of oral mucosa, similar to differing locations of connective tissue proper, is the fibroblast (see Fig. 8.5). Fibroblasts synthesize different types of protein fibers and intercellular substance. Histologists believe that subpopulations of the fibroblast may exist and that controlling the beneficial productive groups may be the answer to periodontal disease and age-related changes that occur in the lamina propria and other components of the periodontium. Other cells present in the lamina propria in smaller numbers are white blood cells, such as polymorphonuclear leukocytes, macrophages, lymphocytes, and mast cells (see Table 8.5).

Clinical Considerations for Oral Mucosa Pathology

Unlike keratinized epithelium, nonkeratinized epithelium usually has no superficial layers showing keratinization. Nonkeratinized epithelium may, however, readily transform into a keratinizing type in response to frictional or chemical trauma, in which case it undergoes **hyperkeratinization** (hahy-per-ker-uh-tn-ah-**zey**-shuhn).

This change to hyperkeratinization commonly occurs on the usually nonkeratinized buccal mucosa when the linea alba forms a white ridge of calloused tissue that extends horizontally at the level where the maxillary and mandibular teeth come together and occlude (see Fig. 2.3, *B*). Microscopically, an excess amount of keratin is noted from the tissue obtained from the linea alba, and the tissue has all the layers of an orthokeratinized tissue, including its granular and keratin layers.

In patients who have habits such as clenching or grinding (with bruxism) their teeth, a larger area of the buccal mucosa than just the nearby linea alba becomes hyperkeratinized (Fig. 9.7). This larger white rough raised lesion needs to be recorded so that changes may be made in the dental treatment plan regarding the patient's parafunctional habits (see **Chapter 20**). Even keratinized tissue can undergo a further level of hyperkeratinization; an increase in the amount of keratin is produced as a result of chronic trauma to the region. This occurs to attached gingiva in the form of fibrosis during the later stages of advanced periodontal disease.

Changes such as hyperkeratinization are reversible if the source of the injury is removed, but it takes time for the keratin to be shed by the tissue. Hyperkeratinized tissue is also associated with the chronic heat production on the hard palate in the form of nicotinic stomatitis from smoking or taking in hot fluids as well as with the chronic placement of spit tobacco in the oral vestibules (see Fig. 11.12). Thus, it is important

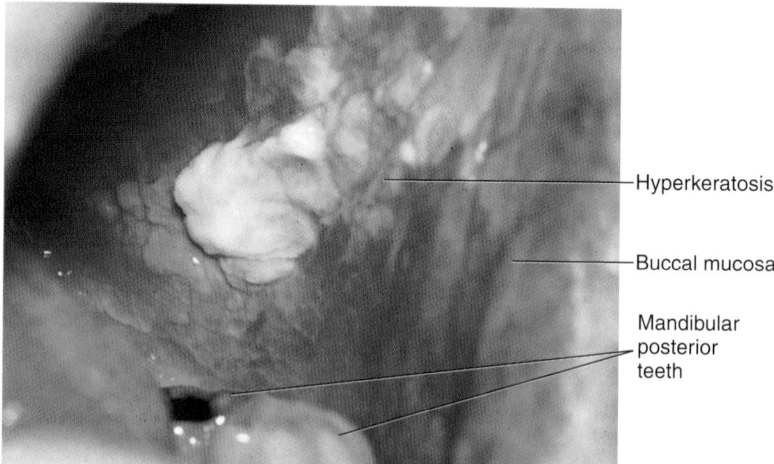

Fig. 9.7 Hyperkeratinization of the buccal mucosa shown by larger white rough and raised calloused lesion than that of the nearby linea alba. Buccal mucosa usually has nonkeratinized epithelium but this tissue has undergone chronic physical injury to the area as a result of grinding or *bruxism* of the teeth. Thus the epithelium has become keratinized in response. Other more serious lesions of the oral cavity must be ruled out when considering this lesion. (Courtesy of Margaret J. Fehrenbach, RDH, MS.)

to rule out malignant changes, and a baseline biopsy and microscopic study of any whitened tissue may be indicated. This is especially true if the patient is within a high-risk cancer category, such as those with a history of chronic tobacco or alcohol use or those who are human papillomavirus (HPV) positive.

ORAL MUCOSA REGIONAL DIFFERENCES

Specific histologic features are noted in the different regions of the oral cavity (Table 9.4). These specific histologic features are the basis for the differences observed clinically when these regions are examined. One way to integrate these two interrelated concepts is to review the clinical appearance of the different regions of oral mucosa when armed with the new knowledge of the specific underlying histologic features.

Thus, the novice dental professional must first look closely at the clinical photographs of the different regions of the oral cavity as well as in the descriptions of their clinical appearances presented in **Chapter 2** and compare these with the histologic features discussed in this chapter. Next, practice finding these regional differences in the oral cavity using a mirror and this textbook for review in order to improve skills of examination. Later, locate them on peers and then on patients in a clinical setting during an intraoral examination.

LABIAL MUCOSA AND BUCCAL MUCOSA

Clinical Appearance

The labial mucosa and buccal mucosa line the inner lips and cheeks (see Figs. 2.2 and 2.3). Both of these regions appear clinically as an opaque pinkish color, shiny, moist, compressible tissue that stretches easily. Areas of melanin pigmentation may be noted (discussed later in this chapter). A variable number of Fordyce spots (or granules) are scattered throughout the tissue. These are a variant usually present in the oral cavity, which are visible as small yellowish bumps on the surface of the oral mucosa. They correspond to deposits of sebum from misplaced sebaceous glands in the submucosa. The oral mucosa of the inner lips and cheeks is classified as a lining mucosa.

Histologic Features

The nonkeratinized stratified squamous epithelium of the labial mucosa and buccal mucosa is extremely thick and overlies and obscures a lamina propria with an extensive vascular supply, giving the overall mucosa an opaque and pinkish clinical appearance (Fig. 9.8 and see Fig. 11.8). The lamina propria has irregular and blunt connective tissue papillae but contains elastic fibers in addition to its collagen fibers, giving the tissue the ability to stretch and return to its original shape.

TABLE 9.4 Regional Differences in Oral Mucosa

Region and Clinical Appearance	Epithelium	Lamina Propria	Submucosa
Lining Mucosa			
Labial mucosa and buccal mucosa: Opaque pink, shiny, moist with possible areas of melanin pigmentation and Fordyce spots	Thick nonkeratinized	Irregular and blunt connective tissue papillae, some elastic fibers, extensive vascular supply	Present with adipose connective tissue and minor salivary glands with firm attachment to muscle
Alveolar mucosa: Reddish-pink, shiny, moist, extremely mobile	Thin nonkeratinized	Connective tissue papillae sometimes absent, many elastic fibers, with extensive vascular supply	Present with minor salivary glands and many elastic fibers with loose attachment to muscle or bone
Ventral surface of the tongue and floor of the mouth: Reddish pink, moist and shiny, compressible with vascular blue areas; mobility varies	Extremely thin nonkeratinized	Extensive vascular supply **Ventral surface of the tongue:** Numerous connective tissue papillae, some elastic fibers, minor salivary glands **Floor of the mouth:** Broad connective tissue papillae	Present **Ventral surface of the tongue:** Extremely thin and firmly attached to muscle **Floor of the mouth:** Adipose connective tissue with submandibular and sublingual salivary glands, loosely attached to bone or muscles
Soft palate: Deep pink with yellow hue and moist surface; compressible and extremely elastic	Thin nonkeratinized	Thick lamina propria with numerous connective tissue papillae and distinct elastic layer	Extremely thin with adipose connective tissue and minor salivary glands with a firm attachment to underlying muscle
Masticatory Mucosa			
Hard palate: Pink, immobile and firm medial zone along with palatal rugae and median palatine raphe; cushioned lateral zones	Thick orthokeratinized; medial zone considered part of the mucoperiosteum to the underlying bone	Medial zone considered part of the mucoperiosteum to underlying bone, along with the features of palatal rugae and median palatine raphe	Present only in lateral zones with anterior part having adipose connective tissue and posterior part having minor salivary glands; absent in medial zone along with palatal rugae and median palatine raphe
Attached gingiva: Opaque pink, dull and firm, immobile with areas of melanin pigmentation possible and varying amounts of stippling	Thick keratinized (mostly parakeratinized, some orthokeratinized); part of mucoperiosteum to underlying bone	Tall narrow connective tissue papillae, extensive vascular supply; part of mucoperiosteum to underlying bone	Not present

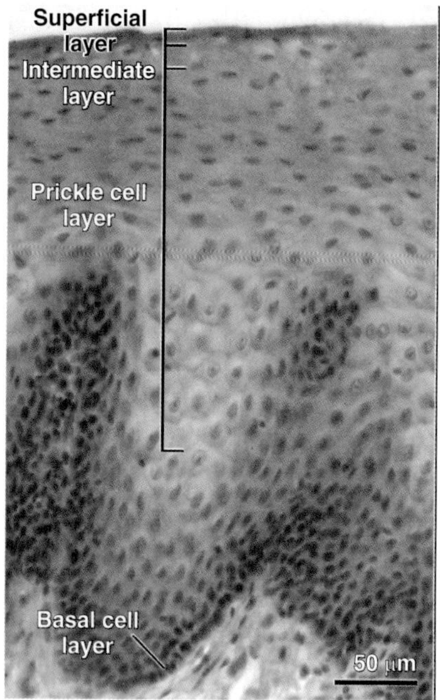

Fig. 9.8 Photomicrograph of the buccal mucosa with extremely thick nonkeratinized stratified squamous epithelium and its four layers overlying a deeper extensively vascular lamina propria. However, the deeper submucosa usually overlying muscle is not shown. Note the prickly or spiky look to the cells of the prickle cell layer due to microscopic fixation causing the individual dehydrated cells to shrink; the desmosomes create this artifact due to the maintenance of their junctional stronghold. (From Nanci A. *Ten Cate's Oral Histology*. 9th ed. St. Louis: Elsevier; 2018.)

The lamina propria overlies a submucosa that contains adipose connective tissue and minor salivary glands, giving the tissue its compressibility and moisture, respectively. The submucosa is firmly attached to the underlying muscle in the region of the labial and buccal mucosa, thus preventing any of the nearby tissue from interfering during mastication or speech because the oral mucosa and muscle function as one unit.

ALVEOLAR MUCOSA

Clinical Appearance

The alveolar mucosa is a reddish tissue with blue vascular areas (see Figs. 2.2, 2.9, and 2.10). This shiny moist region is extremely mobile and lines the vestibules of the oral cavity. The alveolar mucosa is classified as a lining mucosa.

Histologic Features

The epithelium of the alveolar mucosa is extremely thin nonkeratinized stratified squamous epithelium that overlies but does not obscure an extensive vascular supply in the lamina propria, making the alveolar mucosa redder than the pinkish labial mucosa or buccal mucosa (see Figs. 9.12 and 9.13). Connective tissue papillae are sometimes absent and numerous elastic fibers are present in the lamina propria, thus allowing mobility of the tissue. Where the alveolar mucosa meets the attached gingiva is the anatomic feature of the mucogingival junction (discussed in more detail with the attached gingiva).

The submucosa associated with the alveolar mucosa has minor salivary glands and again there are numerous elastic fibers present in a loose connective tissue, thus giving the tissue its moisture and additional mobility, respectively. The submucosa is loosely attached to the underlying muscle or bone, increasing the ability of the tissue to move because the alveolar mucosa is located between the moving lips and the stationary attached gingiva. Local anesthetic injections placed in the height or depth of vestibule within the alveolar mucosa (such as with the posterior superior alveolar nerve block or incisive nerve block) have less discomfort levels noted than those involving the bones of the palate or the bony jaws.

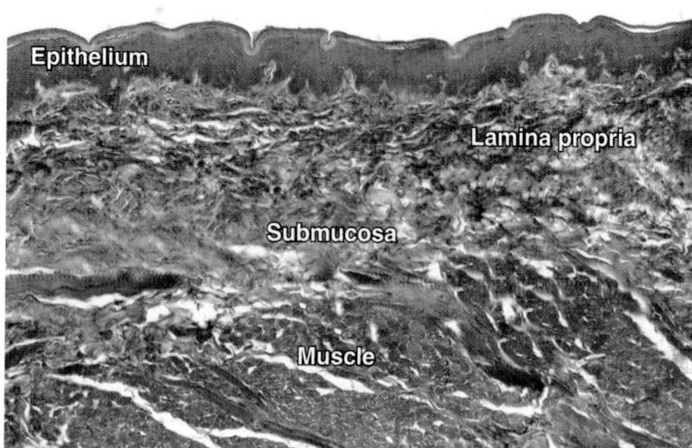

Fig. 9.9 Photomicrograph of the ventral surface of the tongue that demonstrates the extremely thin nonkeratinized stratified squamous epithelium overlying (but not obscuring) a lamina propria with an extensive vascular supply and numerous connective tissue papillae. The deeper submucosa is also extremely thin but firmly attached to the underlying tongue muscle. (From Nanci A. *Ten Cate's Oral Histology*. 9th ed. St. Louis: Elsevier; 2018.)

VENTRAL SURFACE OF THE TONGUE AND FLOOR OF THE MOUTH

Clinical Appearance

Both the ventral surface of the tongue and floor of the mouth appear as a reddish-pink tissue with vascular blue areas of veins (see Figs. 2.16 and 2.17). The tissue is also moist, shiny, and compressible. Although the floor of the mouth has some mobility, the ventral surface of the tongue is firmly attached, yet it allows some stretching along with the tongue muscles. Both the ventral surface of the tongue and the floor of the mouth are classified as a lining mucosa.

Histologic Features

Both the ventral surface of the tongue and the floor of the mouth have an extremely thin nonkeratinized stratified squamous epithelium overlying but not obscuring a lamina propria with an extensive vascular supply, thus making both regions redder and the veins (such as the deep lingual veins) more apparent (Fig. 9.9).

The connective tissue papillae of the lamina propria of the ventral surface of the tongue are numerous. Some elastic fibers and a few minor salivary glands provide the ability to stretch and supply moisture. The submucosa associated with the ventral surface of the tongue is extremely thin and firmly attached to the underlying tongue muscle. This arrangement allows the oral mucosa and muscles to function as one unit, thus reducing mobility during mastication and speech.

The connective tissue papillae of the lamina propria are also broad in the floor of the mouth. The submucosa deep to the lamina propria consists of loose connective tissue with adipose connective tissue and includes the submandibular salivary gland and sublingual salivary gland, giving the tissue its compressibility and moisture, respectively. The submucosa associated with the floor of the mouth is loosely attached to the underlying bone and muscles, thus giving the tissue

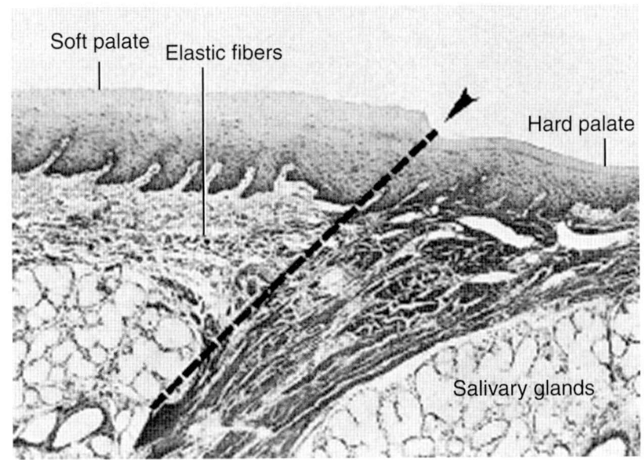

Fig. 9.10 Photomicrograph of the junction of the soft palate and hard palate *(arrow with dotted line)*, which is also a junction between a lining mucosa and a masticatory mucosa as well as a junction between non-keratinized epithelium and keratinized epithelium. (From Nanci A. *Ten Cate's Oral Histology*. 9th ed. St. Louis: Elsevier; 2018.)

its mobility when the attached tongue moves during mastication and speech.

SOFT PALATE

Clinical Appearance

The posterior part of the palate, the soft palate, is deep pink with a yellowish hue and a moist surface (see Figs. 2.11 and 2.12). The tissue is compressible and extremely elastic to allow speech and swallowing. The soft palate is classified as a lining mucosa.

Histologic Features

The soft palate has a thin nonkeratinized stratified squamous epithelium overlying a thick lamina propria (Fig. 9.10). The lamina propria has numerous connective tissue papillae and a distinct elastic connective tissue layer for increased mobility with its elastic fibers.

The submucosa associated with the oral mucosa of the soft palate is extremely thin and has a firm attachment to the underlying muscle to allow the mechanisms of speech and swallowing. Again, this arrangement allows the oral mucosa and muscles to function as one unit. The submucosa contains adipose connective tissue, which gives the tissue its yellow hue and compressibility, and minor salivary glands, which give the tissue its moisture.

HARD PALATE

Clinical Appearance

The anterior part of the palate, the hard palate, appears as a whiter pink tissue that is immobile and firm (see Figs. 2.11 and 2.12). However, a cushioned feeling is noted when the hard palate is palpated in the posterior lateral zones and a firmer feeling in the adjacent medial zone. The palatine rugae and the median palatine raphe are also firm to the touch. Palatine rugae are permanent and unique to each person and can be used to establish identity through discrimination, like fingerprints. The mucogingival junction is absent between the tissue of the hard palate and the lingual surfaces of attached gingiva of the maxillary teeth; instead the two types of tissue blend into each other. The hard palate is classified as a masticatory mucosa.

Histologic Features

The hard palate has a thick layer of orthokeratinized stratified squamous epithelium overlying a thick lamina propria (Fig. 9.11). This palatal epithelium is continuous with the nearby lingual surfaces of the attached gingiva of the maxillary teeth. Because the palate is devoid of freely movable alveolar mucosa, there is no mucogingival junction present between the two types of tissue. In addition, only the lateral zones of the hard palate have a submucosa overlying the bones of the palate, giving the tissue here a cushioned feeling when palpated (see Figs. 9.1 and 9.11, *A*).

The submucosa in the anterior part of the lateral zone (from the canines to the premolars) contains adipose connective tissue. The submucosa in the posterior part of the lateral zone of the hard palate (around the molars) contains minor salivary glands. However, the submucosa in these areas of the hard palate is thinner than that associated with lining mucosa, which becomes apparent when injections of local anesthetic are placed in the lateral zones of the hard palate (such as with the anterior middle superior alveolar nerve block or the greater palatine nerve block) because they can produce more discomfort; these levels can be modified with pressure anesthesia methods.

Submucosa is absent in the medial zone of the hard palate; thus the tissue has a firmer feeling when palpated (see Fig. 9.11, *B*). This firm feeling is enhanced because the oral mucosa is directly attached to the periosteum of the underlying bones of the palate by way of the lamina propria. Thus the overlying oral mucosa when combined with the periosteum of the bones of the palate in this situation is considered a mucoperiosteum (see Fig. 9.4). A **mucoperiosteum** (myoo-koh-per-ee-**os**-tee-uhm) is a structure consisting of a mucous membrane combined with the periosteum of the adjacent bone. Here, the mucoperiosteum attaches directly to the underlying bones of the palate without the usual intervening submucosa, providing a firm inelastic attachment. The oral mucosa and periosteum are so intimately united as to nearly form one single membrane.

Because there is no submucosa present, local anesthetic injections placed in the medial zone of the hard palate (such as with the nasopalatine nerve block) can be discomforting unless pressure anesthesia methods are also used. Both surface landmarks on the hard palate, the palatine rugae and the median palatine raphe, have histologic features similar to those of the medial zone of the hard palate.

ATTACHED GINGIVA

Clinical Appearance

Healthy attached gingiva is opaque pink and areas of melanin pigmentation may be present (discussed later in this chapter) (see Figs. 2.9 and 2.10). When dried, the tissue is dull, firm, and immobile. **Stippling** is observed clinically as small pinpoint depressions, which give the surface of the attached gingiva an orange-peel appearance; this is analogous to the button tufting on upholstery as will be demonstrated with the discussion of its histologic features. The amount of stippling varies even within healthy oral cavities. The attached gingiva that covers the alveolar process of each of the dental arches is classified as a masticatory mucosa.

Also noted is the mucogingival junction, which is a sharply defined scalloped junction between the pinker attached gingiva and the redder alveolar mucosa. Thus there are three areas where this anatomic landmark of the mucogingival junction can be noted in the oral cavity, on the facial of the maxillary arch and on both the facial and lingual of the mandibular arch; however, this latter landmark is not present on the palate of the maxillary arch. The clinical importance of the mucogingival junction is in measuring the width of attached gingiva by demarcating its apical border; the amount of attached gingiva determines the

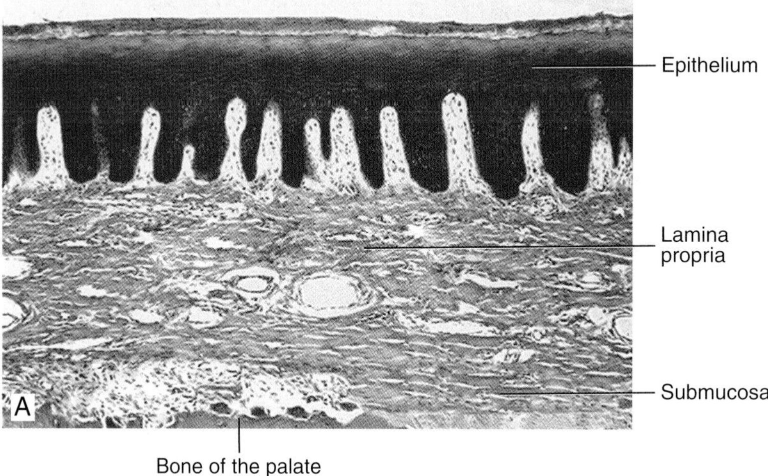

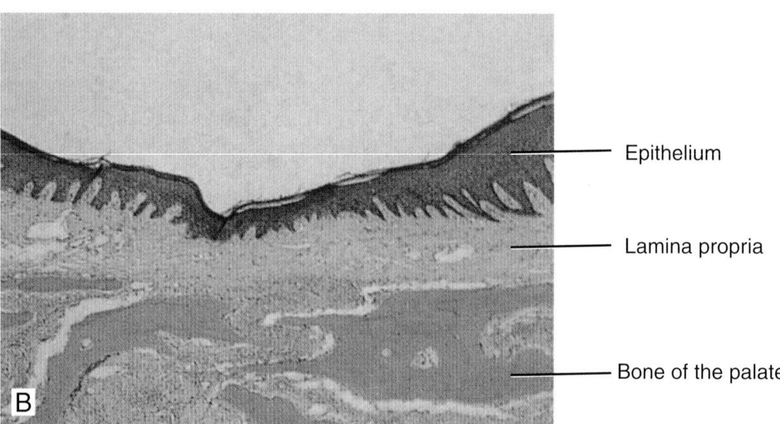

Fig. 9.11 Photomicrographs of the Hard Palate with Orthokeratinized Epithelium Overlying Lamina Propria. A, The cushioned lateral zone of the hard palate that has a deeper thin submucosa overlying bones of the palate, which can contain either adipose tissue (anterior part) or salivary glands (posterior part). **B,** The firmer medial zone of the hard palate that has no submucosa present, so the oral mucosa combines with the periosteum of the underlying bones of the palate to form a mucoperiosteum. (**A,** From Nanci A. *Ten Cate's Oral Histology*. 8th ed. St. Louis: Elsevier; 2013. **B,** From Berkowitz B, Moxham B. *Oral Anatomy, Histology, and Embryology*. 5th ed. St. Louis: Elsevier; 2018.)

support level that the tooth has by way of both the periodontal ligament and alveolar process. The attached gingiva as well as other types of gingival tissue such as those that line the gingival sulcus and attach deep to the tooth surface are discussed further in **Chapter 10.**

Histologic Features

The attached gingiva has a thick layer of mostly parakeratinized stratified squamous epithelium that obscures the extensive vascular supply in the lamina propria, making the tissue appear opaque and pinkish (Fig. 9.12). Again the cells of the keratin layer that have nuclei along with keratin may be difficult to see under lower-power magnification in microscopic sections. However, minor amounts of orthokeratinized stratified squamous epithelium without nuclei may still be present in the keratin layer (see Fig. 9.12).

The lamina propria of the attached gingiva also has tall and narrow connective tissue papillae; its clinically noted stippling is due to a strong attachment or pull of the epithelium toward the lamina propria in these areas (see Fig. 9.12). No submucosa is present, which is similar to the medial zone of the hard palate and palatal landmarks. The lamina propria is directly attached to the underlying alveolar process of the jaws, making the attached gingiva firm and immobile. Thus the overlying oral mucosa when combined with the periosteum of the alveolar process in this situation is considered a mucoperiosteum (see Figs. 9.5 and 9.12). A mucoperiosteum is a structure consisting of a mucous membrane combined with the periosteum of bone. Here the mucoperiosteum attaches directly to the underlying alveolar process of the jaws without the usual intervening submucosa, providing a firm inelastic attachment. The oral mucosa and periosteum are so intimately united as to nearly form one single membrane.

Microscopically the mucogingival junction can be seen as a dividing zone between the keratinized attached gingiva and the nonkeratinized alveolar mucosa and thus is between a masticatory mucosa and a lining mucosa (Figs. 9.13 and 9.14). It is also a junction between a tissue with a thick epithelial layer in the pinkish attached gingiva and a tissue with a thin epithelial layer in the redder alveolar mucosa, even though both tissue types have a similar extensive vascular supply in the lamina propria.

TONGUE AND LINGUAL PAPILLAE PROPERTIES

Microscopically the tongue is a mass of striated muscle in its core, covered by oral mucosa (Fig. 9.15). In the mobile anterior part of the

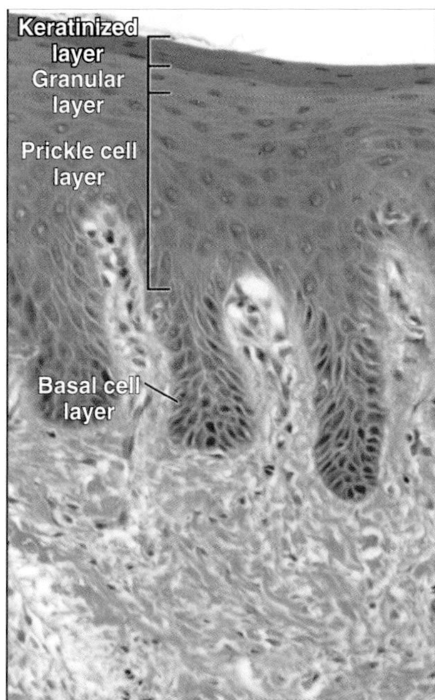

Fig. 9.12 Photomicrograph of the attached gingiva with mostly parakeratinized epithelium and its four layers overlying a deeper extensively vascular lamina propria. Note that the cells in the keratin layer have retained their nuclei and are filled with keratin, although it is hard to see at this lower-power magnification. Stippling on surface is due to a strong attachment or pull of the epithelium toward the lamina propria in these areas. The oral mucosa when combined with the periosteum of the underlying alveolar process forms a mucoperiosteum where there is no intervening submucosa present. However, the deeper alveolar process with its periosteum is not shown. (From Nanci A. *Ten Cate's Oral Histology*. 9th ed. St. Louis: Elsevier; 2018.)

tongue, the striated muscle bundles are tightly packed with relatively little intervening adipose connective tissue in the core. In the bulkier and less-mobile posterior part of the tongue, the adipose connective tissue is more abundant in the core. Collections of minor salivary glands are numerous in the submucosa and muscular core of the posterior part of the tongue, particularly close to the junction between the posterior and anterior parts.

The V-shaped line, the sulcus terminalis, divides the dorsal surface of the tongue into the anterior two-thirds or body of the tongue and the posterior one-third, which is the base of the tongue (see Fig. 2.14). The dorsal surface of the tongue has both a masticatory mucosa and specialized mucosa present. A masticatory mucosa of orthokeratinized stratified squamous epithelium covers most of the surface of the muscle associated with the tongue.

The specialized mucosa found on the dorsal surface is associated with the lingual papillae, which are small discrete structures or appendages of keratinized epithelium with both orthokeratinized and parakeratinized epithelium present overlying a lamina propria (see Figs. 2.14 and 2.15). Lingual papillae are also found on the lateral surface of the tongue. There are four types of lingual papillae, filiform, fungiform, foliate, and circumvallate (Table 9.5). The development of the lingual papillae and the tongue is discussed in **Chapter 5**.

Three types of lingual papillae are associated with taste buds, the fungiform, foliate, and circumvallate. A **taste bud** is a barrel-shaped organ of taste derived from the epithelium (Fig. 9.16). Each taste bud is composed of 30 to 80 spindle-shaped cells that extend from the basement membrane of the oral mucosa to the epithelial surface of the lingual papilla. The turnover time of the taste bud cells is a fairly rapid process of about 10 days.

The two types of taste bud cells are the supporting cells and the taste cells. However, the difference between the two is hard to discern under lower-power magnification of most microscopic sections and indifferent immature forms are also noted. The *supporting cells* maintain the taste bud and are usually located on the outer part of the taste bud. The *taste cells* are usually located in the central part of the taste bud and produce taste sensations (see Figs. 9.15 and 9.16).

To produce a taste sensation, dissolved molecules of food in the oral cavity contact the taste receptors of the taste cells at the **taste pore,** which is an opening in the most superficial part of the taste bud (Fig. 9.17). Taste cells are also associated with sensory neuron processes among the cells in the inferior part of the taste bud. These sensory neuron processes receive messages of taste sensation through the taste receptors. The message generated is then sent to the central nervous system by the connecting nerves where it is identified as a certain type of taste.

Evidence suggests that the four fundamental taste sensations, sweet, sour, salty, and bitter, are different because of four slightly differentiated taste cells. However, the tastes experienced are the result of the blending of the four fundamental taste sensations and the addition of other sensations by the tongue as well as the interplay of the sense smell with that of taste. In the past, the tongue was thought to have a specific mapping of taste sensations, but studies have proved this assumption false. Other taste sensations through current studies have now branched out to include umami (or savory) and fatty acid tastes.

FILIFORM LINGUAL PAPILLAE

Clinical Appearance

The filiform lingual papillae are the most common lingual papillae located on the body of the dorsal surface of the tongue (see Fig. 2.14). They are shaped like fine-pointed cones of 2 to 3 mm with the tips naturally turned toward the pharynx, giving the dorsal surface of the tongue its velvety texture. Filiform are sensitive to changes in the body and thus are associated with certain clinical considerations (discussed later in this chapter).

Histologic Features

A filiform is a pointed structure with a thick layer of orthokeratinized or parakeratinized epithelium overlying a core of lamina propria (Fig. 9.18). An increased amount of keratin is also at the surface of each filiform, forming a flocked "Christmas tree" arrangement and whiter color noted for this lingual papilla. No taste buds are present in the epithelium. The filiform may have a rudimentary mechanical function as a result of their rougher surface texture, which is related to the increased amount of surface keratinization present and thus may aid in guiding food back to the pharynx for swallowing.

FUNGIFORM LINGUAL PAPILLAE

Clinical Appearance

The fungiform lingual papillae are found in lesser numbers than are the filiform on the body of the dorsal surface of the tongue (see Fig. 2.14). They appear as smaller reddish dots, which on closer inspection are slightly raised and mushroom-shaped with a 1 mm diameter. Fungiform are not found near the sulcus terminalis.

Histologic Features

A fungiform is a small mushroom-shaped structure with a thin layer of orthokeratinized or parakeratinized epithelium overlying a highly

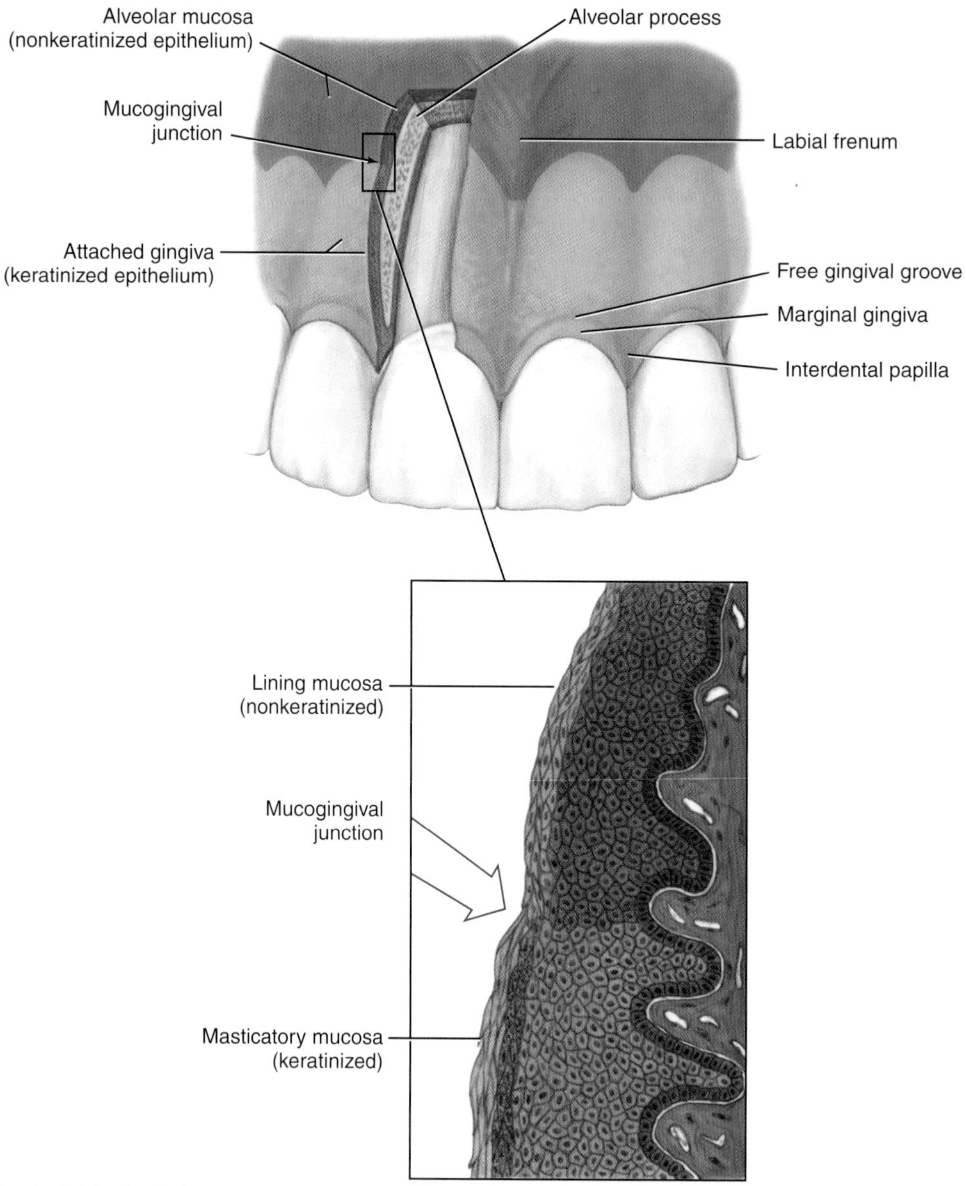

Fig. 9.13 Histologic features of the mucogingival junction *(arrow),* which is a junction between the alveolar mucosa and attached gingiva as well as between a lining mucosa (also nonkeratinized) and masticatory mucosa (also keratinized).

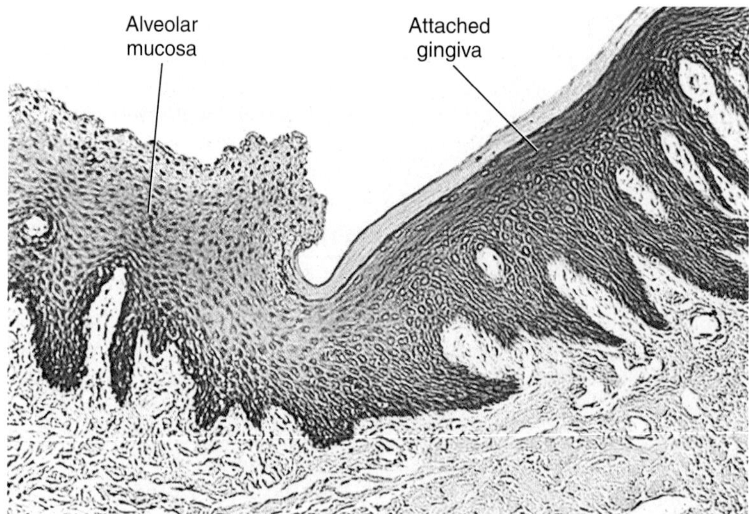

Fig. 9.14 Photomicrograph of the mucogingival junction, which is a junction between the nonkeratinized alveolar mucosa and the keratinized attached gingiva as well as between a lining mucosa and a masticatory mucosa. (From CD-ROM from Nanci A. *Ten Cate's Oral Histology.* 6th ed. St. Louis: Elsevier; 2002.)

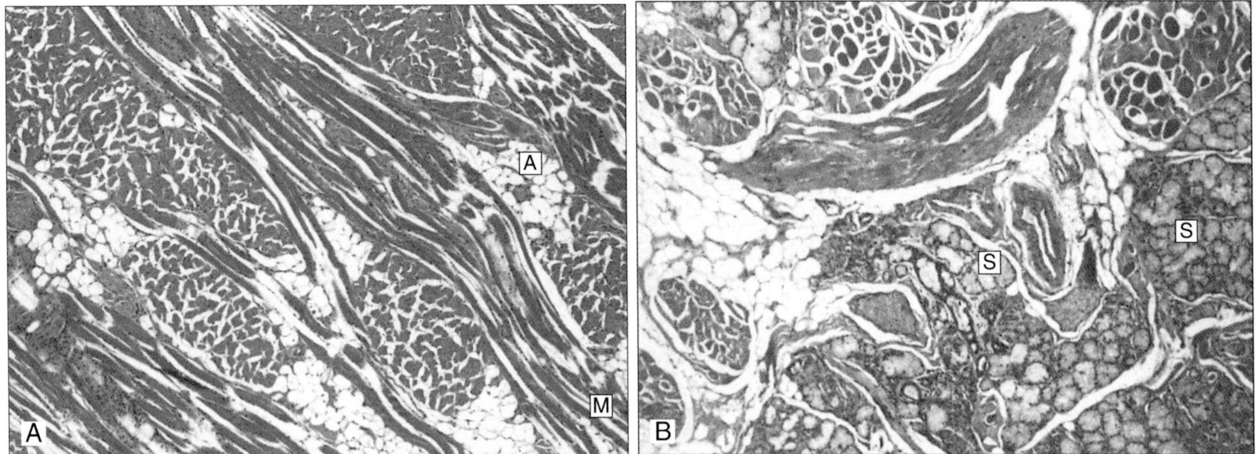

Fig. 9.15 Photomicrographs of the Muscular Core of the Tongue. A, In the mobile anterior tongue, the striated muscle bundles *(M)* are tightly packed with relatively little intervening adipose connective tissue *(A)*, unlike the less mobile posterior. **B,** Collections of salivary glands *(S)* are numerous in the submucosa and muscular core of the posterior tongue. (From Stevens A, Lowe J. *Human Histology*. 5th ed. St. Louis: Elsevier; 2020.)

TABLE 9.5 Comparison of Lingual Papillae

Comparisons	Filiform	Fungiform	Foliate	Circumvallate
Clinical appearance	Most common on body; fine-pointed cones giving tongue velvety texture	Lesser numbers on body; mushroom-shaped small red dots	About 4 to 11 vertical ridges on lateral surface of posterior tongue	About 7 to 15 large raised mushroom-shaped structures anterior to sulcus terminalis
Histologic features	Pointed structure with thick layer of keratinized epithelium, overlying core of lamina propria; no taste buds	Mushroom-shaped structure with thin layer of keratinized epithelium overlying core of lamina propria with taste buds in most superficial part	Leaf-shaped structure of keratinized epithelium overlying core of lamina propria with taste buds in superficial lateral part	Mushroom-shaped structure with similar histology to fungiform but also sunken deep to tongue surface, taste buds in papilla base, and surrounded by trough with von Ebner minor salivary glands in submucosa
Function	May be mechanical	Taste	Taste	Taste

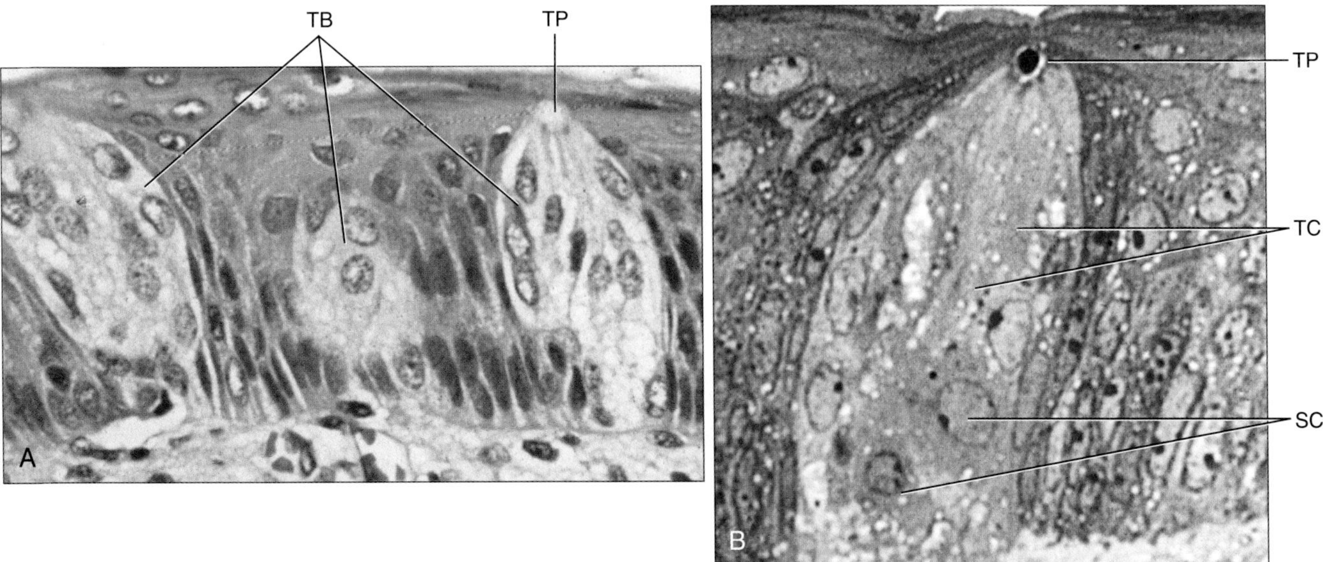

Fig. 9.16 A and **B,** Microscopic sections of taste buds *(TB)* with supporting cells *(SC)* and taste cells *(TC)*; immature forms are also present. However, it is hard to discern the associated nerves and differences between the two cell types at this lower-power magnification. Note taste pores *(TP)* at most superficial parts. (From Stevens A, Lowe J. *Human Histology*. 5th ed. St. Louis: Elsevier; 2020.)

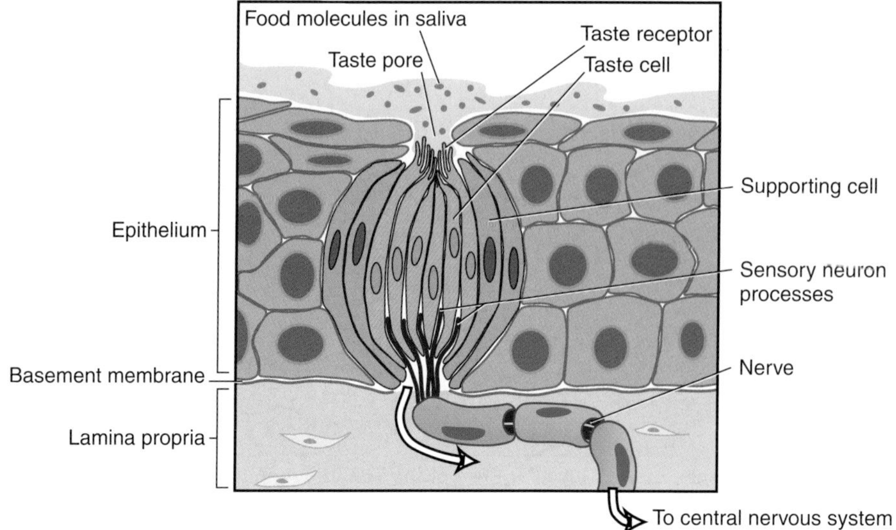

Fig. 9.17 Events Involved in Taste Sensation with a Taste Bud. Dissolved food contacts the taste receptors of the taste cells at the taste pore. Taste cells are also associated with sensory neuron processes in the inferior part of the taste bud, among the cells that receive messages of taste sensation from the taste receptors. The message produced is then sent by the nerve to the central nervous system, where it is identified as a certain type of taste.

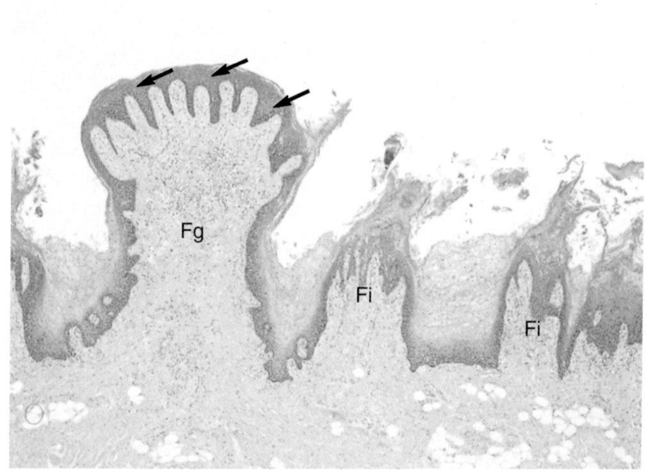

Fig. 9.18 Microscopic section of the dorsal surface of the tongue showing a fungiform lingual papilla *(Fg)* and filiform lingual papillae *(Fi)*. Note the mushroom shape of the fungiform and the tree shape of the filiform. However, the taste buds *(arrows)* at the superficial surface of fungiform are difficult to discern at this low level of magnification. (From Young B, Heath JW. *Wheater's Functional Histology*. 6th ed. Edinburgh: Elsevier; 2014.)

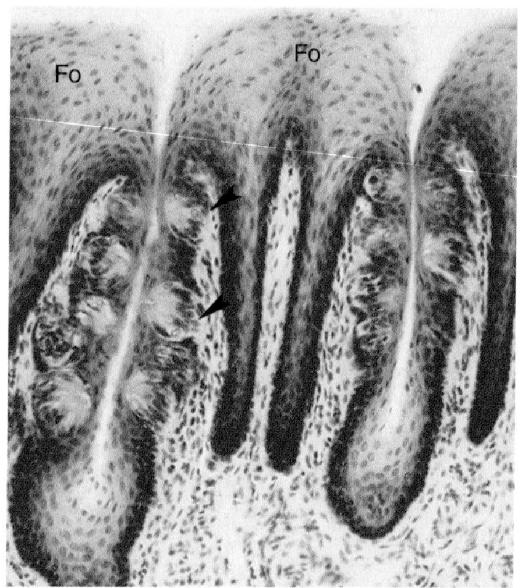

Fig. 9.19 Microscopic section of the lateral surface of the tongue with foliate lingual papillae *(Fo)*. Taste buds *(arrowheads)* are located in the epithelial layer on the lateral parts of the leaf-shaped structure. (Courtesy of B. Kablar.)

vascularized core of lamina propria, thus producing the redder clinical appearance of this lingual papilla (see Fig. 9.18). A variable number of taste buds are located in the most superficial part of the epithelial layer; however, taste buds are not located near the base of the structure. Thus the function of the fungiform is taste sensation.

FOLIATE LINGUAL PAPILLAE

Clinical Appearance

The foliate lingual papillae appear as 4 to 11 vertical ridges parallel to one another on the lateral surface of the tongue in its most posterior part (see Fig. 2.15).

Histologic Features

The foliate are leaf-shaped structures with a layer of orthokeratinized or parakeratinized epithelium overlying a core of lamina propria (Fig. 9.19). Taste buds are located in the epithelial layer on the lateral parts of the leaf-shaped structure. Thus the function of the foliate is taste sensation. Some histologists believe that the foliate are not true lingual papillae because of their rudimentary clinical appearance, developmental background, and location.

CIRCUMVALLATE LINGUAL PAPILLAE

Clinical Features

The circumvallate lingual papillae are lined up in an inverted V-shaped row on the dorsal surface of the tongue facing the pharynx, just

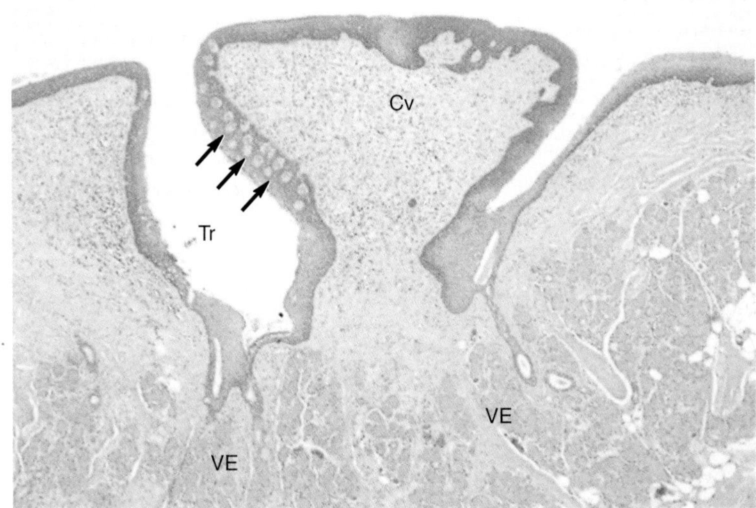

Fig. 9.20 Microscopic section of the posterior part of the dorsal surface of the tongue showing a circumvallate lingual papilla *(Cv)*, with taste buds *(arrows)* within the epithelial layer and surrounded by a circular trough *(Tr)*. Note von Ebner salivary glands *(VE)*, which flush the trough between tastes. (From Young B, Heath JW. *Wheater's Functional Histology*. 6th ed. Edinburgh: Elsevier; 2014.)

anterior to the sulcus terminalis. The circumvallate have a larger diameter than the fungiform, measuring from 3 to 5 mm. When the tongue is arched and extended, the circumvallate lingual papillae appear as 7 to 15 raised large mushroom-shaped structures, mimicking the outline of the sulcus terminalis (see Fig. 2.14, *A*). With the tongue in a more relaxed and natural position, the circumvallate are sunken as deep as the tongue surface because they are surrounded by a circular trough or trench.

Histologic Features

The circumvallate are larger mushroom-shaped structures with orthokeratinized or parakeratinized epithelium overlying a core of lamina propria (Fig. 9.20). Hundreds of taste buds are located in the epithelium surrounding the entire base of each lingual papilla, opposite the circular trough lined by the surrounding tongue surface tissue.

It is important to note that von Ebner salivary glands are also present in the submucosa deep to the lamina propria of the circumvallate. These are minor salivary glands with only serous cells present (see **Chapter 11**). With ducts that open into the trough, they flush the area near the taste pores so as to introduce new taste sensations from several sequential food molecules. Thus the function of the circumvallate is taste sensation.

 Clinical Considerations for Tongue Pathology

Two lesions associated with the dorsal surface of the tongue involve the filiform lingual papillae. Neither lesion is considered a serious condition, but both should be noted on the patient record if present. One of these tongue lesions is **geographic tongue,** which appears as red and then paler pink to white patches on the body of the tongue (Fig. 9.21). These patches change shape with time, resembling a geographic map. The lesion is found in all age groups and shows the sensitivity of the filiform lingual papillae to changes in their environment.

These red and white surface patches of geographic tongue correspond to groups of filiform undergoing changes from parakeratinized epithelium that appears redder to orthokeratinized epithelium that appears whiter. This lesion is sometimes associated with soreness or slight burning on the surface of the tongue. However, no treatment is needed for geographic tongue, although dental professionals should reassure the patient and rule out any other more serious tongue lesions.

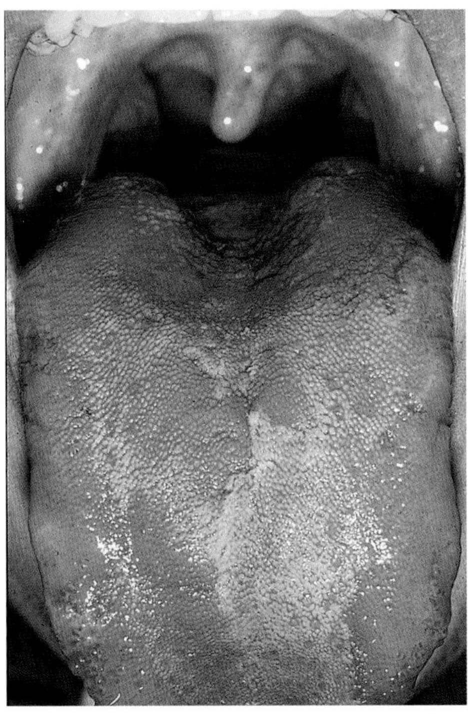

Fig. 9.21 Geographic tongue showing the sensitivity of the filiform lingual papillae. This results in redder to paler pink and whiter patches appearing and disappearing on the dorsal surface of the body of the tongue over time. (Courtesy of Margaret J. Fehrenbach, RDH, MS.)

A less common lesion noted on the dorsal tongue surface is **black hairy tongue** (Fig. 9.22). With this lesion, the usual level of shedding of epithelium of the filiform lingual papillae does not occur. As a result, a thick layer of dead cells and keratin builds up on the tongue surface,

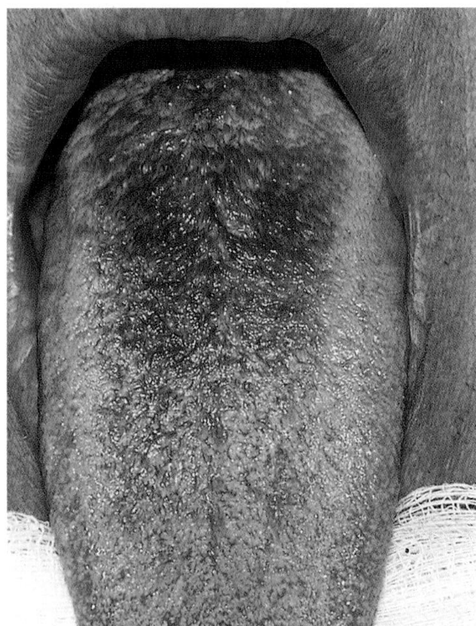

Fig. 9.22 Black hairy tongue on the dorsal surface of the tongue where the usual level of shedding of epithelium of the filiform lingual papillae is lacking. This results in the formation of a thick layer of dead cells and keratin, which becomes stained. (Courtesy of Margaret J. Fehrenbach, RDH, MS.)

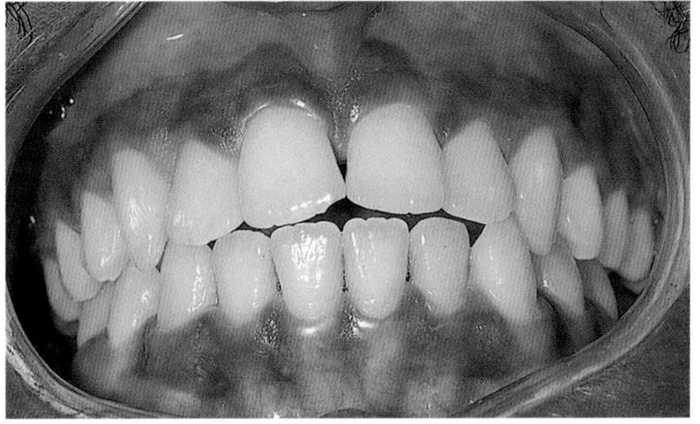

Fig. 9.23 Pigmentation of the attached gingiva associated with the permanent dentition that is most abundant at the base of the interdental gingiva. (Courtesy of Margaret J. Fehrenbach, RDH, MS.)

which becomes extrinsically stained by tobacco, medications, or chromogenic (or colored) oral bacteria. Studies show that this condition in some cases might be an effect of fungal overgrowth, possibly as a result of high doses of antibiotics or radiation therapy. Brushing the tongue is recommended in this case to promote tissue shedding and remove debris.

Generally, brushing the dorsal surface of the tongue is important for overall homecare of the oral cavity and to reduce bad breath (also known as malodor or halitosis) because microbial colonization by dental biofilm on the tongue's surface is a contributing factor.

ORAL MUCOSA PIGMENTATION

The oral mucosa can range in color from pink to reddish pink (see **Chapter 2**). The presence of melanin pigmentation within the epithelium may give rise to localized flat areas of the oral mucosa that range in color from brown to brownish black (Fig. 9.23).

Melanin is a pigment formed by **melanocytes** (muh-**lan**-uh-sahtz), which are epidermal cells derived from the neural crest cells. Melanocytes are clear cells that occupy a position in the basal layer of the stratified squamous epithelium between the dividing epithelial cells (Fig. 9.24). The melanocytes have small cytoplasmic granules as inclusions, the **melanosomes** (muh-**lan**-uh-sohms), which store the melanin pigment. They inject these granules into the neighboring newly formed epithelial cells of the basal layer.

As the tissue undergoes regeneration during its turnover time, the injected cells migrate to the surface of the oral mucosa and appear clinically as a group of localized flat pigmented areas or macules. Because melanocytes are evenly distributed throughout the oral mucosa, clinical levels of pigmentation are based on the degree of melanin-producing activity of the melanocytes, which is controlled by genetic programming. Thus this is a variation that can be present in the oral cavity; it appears most abundant in the attached gingiva at the base of the interdental gingiva with both dentitions (see Fig. 9.23).

 Clinical Considerations with Oral Mucosa Pigmentation

The pathology involved in a nevus (known as a mole) is different from that of a variation of melanin pigmentation levels within a tissue. The nevus is a benign tumor of melanin; in further contrast is the melanoma, which is a cancer involving melanin. Both lesions can appear in the oral cavity usually as one distinct small flat macule or raised papule. The melanoma may or may not appear at the site of an existing nevus.

The pigmentation of both the oral mucosa and skin may increase with certain endocrine diseases. Additionally, if dramatic localized pigment changes are recently noted in the oral cavity, biopsy and microscopic study are recommended to rule out any malignancies. Many oral pathologists also recommend the removal of any nevus within the oral cavity to reduce the risk of carcinomatous change.

ORAL MUCOSA TURNOVER TIME, REPAIR, AND AGING

Overall, the turnover time for the oral mucosa is faster than that for the skin as the tissue undergoes the regeneration process (see **Chapter 8**). Regional differences in the turnover times, however, do exist within the oral cavity (Table 9.6). The gingival epithelium in the gingival sulcular region that attaches deep to the tooth surface, the junctional epithelium, has the fastest turnover time of all the oral tissue at 4 to 6 days (see **Chapter 10**). One of the lowest turnover times is for the hard palate at 24 days. The turnover times of all other oral mucosa regions fall between these two end points—between 4 and 24 days. Regional differences in the pattern of epithelial maturation or keratinization appear to be associated with different turnover times; nonkeratinized buccal mucosa turns over faster than keratinized attached gingiva, around 1.5 times faster; thus, lining mucosa turns over faster than masticatory mucosa.

In general, the epithelium of any region of oral mucosa has a faster turnover time than cells of the lamina propria, although the turnover time of its matrix, both fibers and intercellular substance, is quite rapid in response. As stated before, all regions of the oral cavity have a faster turnover time than the skin, which has a turnover time of 20 to 30 days, depending on being a younger or older adult. Such differences noted in turnover times for oral mucosa regions can have important implications for healing and rate of recovery time from injury such as periodontal disease or tooth extraction. Skin regions also have varying levels of turnover times; for example, the face is faster than the legs.

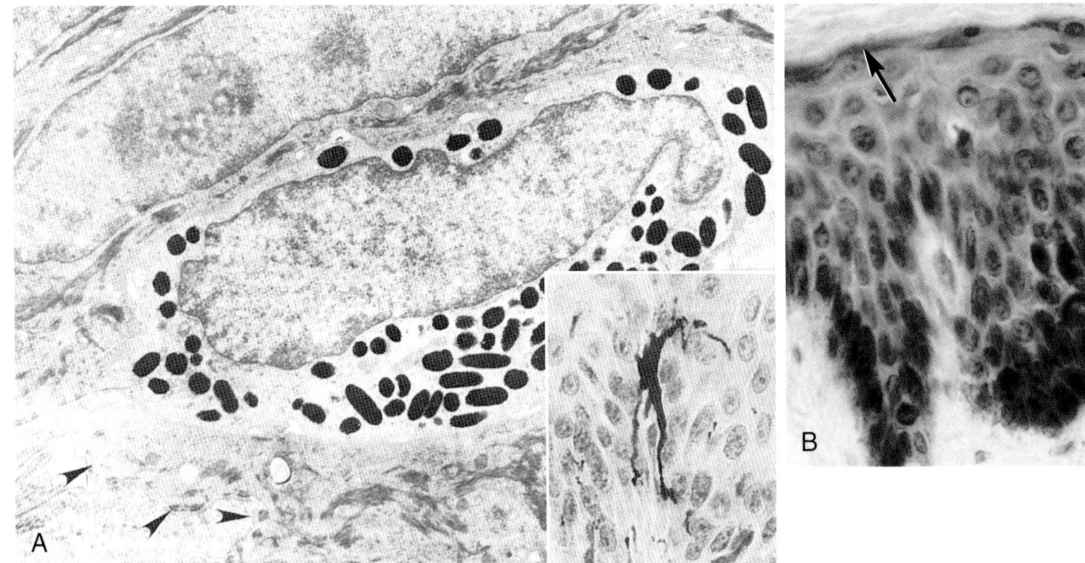

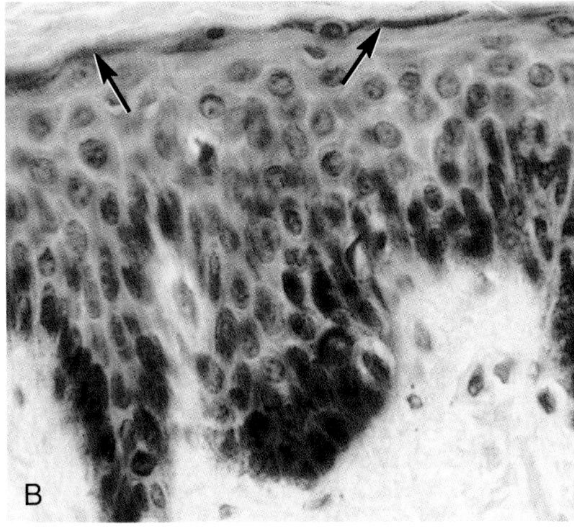

Fig. 9.24 Pigmentation Process. **A,** Electron micrograph of a melanocyte in the basal layer of pigmented oral epithelium where the dense melanosomes are abundant near the basement membrane *(arrowheads)*. *Inset:* Photomicrograph showing a melanocyte, which appears dark because it has been stained to reveal the presence of melanin. **B,** Photomicrograph of the attached gingiva, showing the pigmentation process within the oral mucosa. Note the granular layer *(arrows)* and the deposits of melanin, particularly in the basal layer. (**A** and inset, From Nanci A. *Ten Cate's Oral Histology*. 9th ed. St. Louis: Elsevier; 2018. **B,** Courtesy of TS Leeson, Professor Emeritus, Cell Biology and Anatomy, Medicine and Oral Health, University of Alberta, Edmonton.)

TABLE 9.6 Oral Tissue Mean Turnover Time*

Oral Tissue	Mean Turnover Time
Hard palate	24 days
Floor of the mouth	20 days
Buccal and labial mucosa	14 days
Attached gingiva	10 days
Taste buds	10 days
Junctional epithelium (attached to tooth)	4 to 6 days

*Note that for comparison, the turnover time for the skin is 20 days in young adults and lengthens by 10 days to 30 days for older adults From Maeda, K: New method of measurement of epidermal turnover in humans. *Cosmetics*. 2017;4(4):47.

The repair process of the oral mucosa is similar to that of the skin, except that it involves a moist clot and not a dried scab like the skin (see Fig. 8.3). After an injury to the oral mucosa, the clot from blood products forms in the area, and the inflammatory response is triggered with its white blood cells. In the next days as tissue repair begins, the epithelial cells at the periphery of the injury will lose their desmosomal junctions and migrate to form a new epithelial surface layer beneath the clot. Thus, the clot is highly important in repair of the epithelium and must be retained in the first days of repair because it acts as a guide to form a new surface. Instructions must be given to patients before tooth extractions outlining behaviors to avoid in order not to disturb the clot, thus preventing a condition referred to as *dry socket,* a postextraction infection. Later, after the epithelial surface is repaired, the clot breaks down through enzymatic activity because it is no longer needed.

At the same time, fibroblasts migrate to produce an immature connective tissue in the injured lamina propria deep to the clot and newly forming epithelial surface (see Fig. 8.5). This immature connective tissue is now considered granulation tissue and has fewer fibers and an increased number of blood vessels. Granulation tissue appears as a soft bright red tissue that bleeds easily.

This temporary granulation tissue is later replaced by firmer and paler scar tissue in the affected area. Replacement tissue is characterized by an increased amount of fibers and fewer blood vessels. The amount of scar tissue varies depending on the type and size of the wound, amount of granulation tissue, and movement of tissue after injury. The oral mucosa shows less scar tissue, either clinically or microscopically after repair than does the skin, because fewer fibers are located in this area than in the skin when it undergoes a similar injury. Studies show that the minimal scar tissue formation in oral mucosa after repair is similar to fetal tissue repair.

The formation of a lesser amount of scar tissue in the oral mucosa is useful both esthetically and functionally when oral or periodontal surgery is performed. Histologists believe it may be linked to the differing embryologic origins of the fibroblasts from the two tissue types; skin fibroblasts are derived from the mesoderm, and oral mucosa fibroblasts are derived from neural crest cells. Recent studies have found distinct differences in the aging profiles of cells using both oral mucosa and patient-matched skin fibroblasts isolated from these tissue types; thus, increased replicative potential of oral mucosa fibroblasts may confer upon them preferential wound-healing capacities.

After the source of injury is removed, the repair of the oral mucosa usually follows a time frame similar to its turnover time. Studies show that epithelial cells possess receptors for growth factors and respond also to chemical mediators of the inflammatory process. Future studies may show a way to speed repair and even prevent aging in the oral mucosa.

The process of aging of the oral mucosa mirrors some of the changes observed in the skin and lips (Fig. 9.25). Unlike skin and lips, the deeper oral mucosa is protected from changes due to solar damage (see Fig. 1.8). However, similar to skin, it is important to remember that it is sometimes difficult to distinguish changes caused by the aging

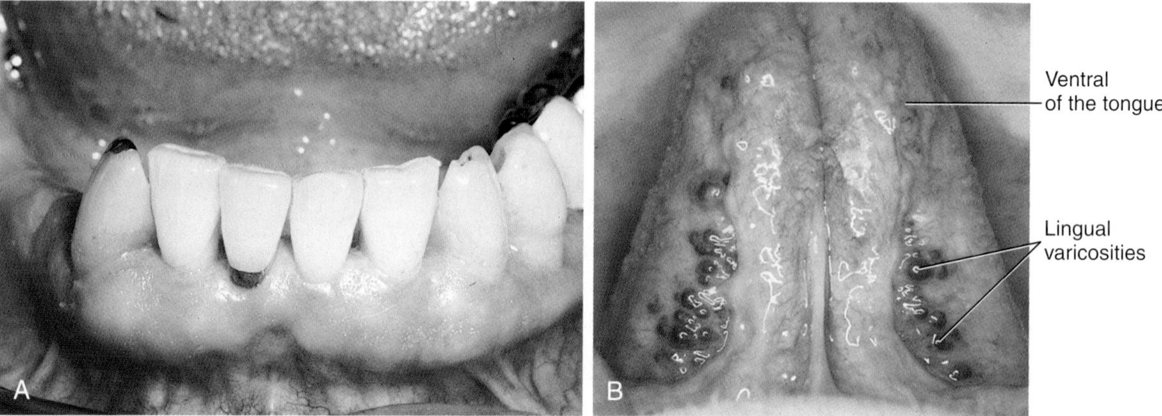

Fig. 9.25 Various Changes Resulting From the Aging Process in the Oral Cavity. **A,** Loss of stippling of the attached gingiva. **B,** Lingual varicosities on the ventral surface of the tongue. (Courtesy of Margaret J. Fehrenbach, RDH, MS.)

process in the oral mucosa from those changes caused by chronic disease (discussed next). In addition, there is emphasis on biologic aging and not chronologic aging.

Aging of the oral mucosa is seen clinically as a reduction of stippling on the attached gingiva, an increase of Fordyce spots in the labial and buccal mucosa, and an enlargement of the lingual veins to form lingual varicosities on the ventral surface of the tongue. The number of lingual papillae and associated taste buds, especially the foliate lingual papillae, is also reduced and may be related to changes noted in taste perception as a person ages over time. Many of the changes in the oral cavity may be due to changes in the salivary glands that result in less production of saliva (or hyposalivation); these changes make the oral mucosa drier (or xerostomia) and thus less protective. However, these changes in saliva are not directly due to the aging process but usually due to medications taken by mature individuals or concurrent disease processes (see Fig. 11.9).

Microscopically the thickness and number of rete ridges in the epithelium diminish as the oral mucosa ages, showing the overall sagging and lack of firmness of the tissue. The interconnecting pattern of MPL is reduced with age as noted in studies. In addition, the degree of keratinization of the masticatory mucosa declines, especially in the attached gingiva. Cell division at the basal layer of the epithelium does not slow down, but studies show that the turnover times do slow down for all regions of the oral cavity.

Microscopic changes also occur in the composition of the matrix of the lamina propria and in a less-defined division between the papillary and dense layers in mature oral mucosa. Collagen fibers appear thickened and are arranged into dense bundles resembling those found in tendons or ligaments. Elastic fibers, if present in the lamina propria, appear changed, even though more of them are present. This change in elastic fibers may explain the loss of resiliency found in aged oral mucosa. The fibroblasts decrease in quantity, appear smaller, and are less active in mature oral mucosa. The entire lamina propria has a slower collagen turnover time. Overall, with the aging process, the ability of the oral mucosa to repair itself is reduced and the length of the repair time is increased, just as turnover time is increased.

With increasing aging of the patient base, dental professionals must consider the associated effects of aging on the oral mucosa during dental treatment—one being longer times for healing. Age-associated changes (such as loss of stippling and lingual varicosities) should be distinguished from conditions resulting from oral or systemic disease.

In the future, many changes associated with the aging process may be delayed or prevented. With present knowledge, cases of gingival recession might be prevented by appropriate toothbrushing techniques, placement of a protective mouthguard against occlusal forces, or institution of crown-lengthening procedures. Other changes, such as a drier mouth (or xerostomia with hyposalivation) and loss of resiliency, should be considered and complications prevented when treatment is performed on mature patients.

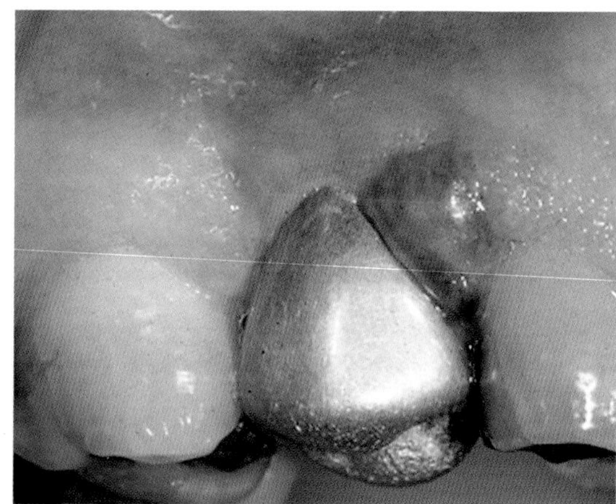

Fig. 9.26 Postoperative excessive granulation tissue, in this case after endodontic therapy, that may interfere with the repair process and need to be surgically removed. (From Gutmann JL, Dumsha TC, Lovdahl PE. *Problem Solving in Endodontics*. 5th ed. St. Louis: Elsevier; 2011.)

Recent tissue engineering of oral mucosa combines cells and materials to produce a three-dimensional reconstruction of the tissue type so as to simulate its anatomic structure and function. This shows promise for clinical use, such as the replacement of soft tissue defects in the oral cavity occurring with gingival recession and tissue trauma occurring with oral cancer. This also impacts the approaches to biocompatibility evaluation of dental materials and oral homecare products as well as therapies associated with implant-soft tissue interfaces. Newer approaches used today for replacing injured oral mucosa are the use of autologous grafts and cultured epithelial sheets.

Clinical Considerations with Oral Mucosa Pathology

Granulation tissue may become abundant and may actually interfere with the repair process in oral mucosa. Surgical removal of excess granulation tissue may be necessary to allow for optimal repair, such as after a tooth extraction or certain periodontal surgical techniques with advanced chronic periodontal or pulpal disease (Fig. 9.26).

Dental professionals must also consider the faster turnover time and faster repair times for oral regions as compared to the skin when diagnosing lesions of the oral mucosa. Should the lesion be traumatic, complete healing takes up to approximately 2 weeks, depending on the region involved and if the source of the injury is first removed. Possible sources of injury to the oral mucosa may be physical, chemical, or infectious; assumptions should never be made about the source of any lesion of the oral mucosa. Biopsy followed with microscopic study is the only way to effectively diagnose any lesion.

A delay of approximately 2 weeks to allow a lesion to undergo healing before obtaining a referral or instigating a more serious clinical treatment plan does not adversely affect a patient's health. However, a longer delay (e.g., until the next maintenance visit) before the lesion is checked is not in the best interest of a patient. This is because malignant changes involved with cancer in a worst-case scenario do not heal but grow in size and may metastasize. The larger lesion that has metastasized gives the patient a poorer prognosis if the lesion is later determined to be malignant after microscopic study.

Turnover times also have implications during the treatment of cancer by surgical, chemical, and radiologic means because these methods can injure the oral mucosa while they are used to halt or reduce the cancerous growth. Healing that is required also varies according to the original turnover times of the tissue, even if it takes longer due to the trauma of therapy. Thus, the buccal mucosa heals faster than the hard palate when subjected to cancer therapy methods.

As was stated before, it is important to remember that it is sometimes difficult to distinguish changes caused by the aging process in the oral mucosa from those changes caused by chronic disease. Exposure of the dental tissue from gingival recession of attached gingiva in the aged population is argued to be more a sign of disease than of age (see Fig. 10.10). Also thought to be a sign of disease in the aged is creasing and then cracking at the labial commissures, which may be related to a loss of vertical dimension of the dentition and jaws (see Fig. 14.22 and **Chapter 20**).

10

Gingival and Dentogingival Junctional Tissue

Additional resources and practice exercises are provided on the companion Evolve website for this book: http://evolve.elsevier.com/Fehrenbach/illustrated.

LEARNING OBJECTIVES

1. Define and pronounce the key terms in this chapter.
2. List and describe the properties of each type of gingival tissue.
3. Describe the histologic features of each type of gingival tissue and the clinical considerations for gingival tissue esthetics, integrating it into patient care.
4. Identify the components of each type of gingival tissue on a diagram.
5. Describe dentogingival junctional properties, histology, and development.
6. Identify the structure of the dentogingival junctional tissue on a diagram.
7. Discuss the clinical considerations for gingival tissue pathology, integrating it into patient care.
8. Discuss turnover of the dentogingival junctional tissue and its clinical implications.

GINGIVAL TISSUE PROPERTIES

Gingival tissue in the oral cavity is the most important tissue of the orofacial region for dental professionals to know and understand and the most challenging as well. All of the periodontal therapy initiated and homecare instruction given are for the purpose of creating a healthy environment for the gingival tissue. Even with restorative treatment of the teeth, the impact on the gingival tissue must be considered to ensure the restoration's longevity. When healthy, it presents an effective barrier to the barrage of insults to deeper periodontal tissue.

When the gingival tissue is not healthy, it can provide a gateway for periodontal disease to advance into the deeper tissue of the periodontium, leading to a poorer prognosis for long-term retention of the teeth. Thus, the dental professional must have a clear understanding of the histology of the healthy gingival tissue. This helps in understanding the pathologic changes that occur during the disease states involving the gingival tissue. It is important to keep in mind that the clinical appearance of the tissue reflects the underlying histology, both in health and disease.

GINGIVAL TISSUE ANATOMY

Gingival tissue surrounds the maxillary and mandibular teeth in each alveolus and also covers each alveolar process (Fig. 10.1; see Figs. 2.9 and 2.10). When examining the gingival tissue in a clinical setting, different types are present in the oral cavity. The gingival tissue that tightly adheres to the alveolar process that surrounds the roots of the teeth is the attached gingiva. The gingival tissue between adjacent teeth adjoining the attached gingiva is the interdental gingiva, forming the individual extensions of the interdental papillae. The interdental papillae fill in the area between the teeth apical to their contact areas to prevent food impaction (see **Chapter 15**). The interdental papillae assume a conical shape for the anterior teeth and a blunted shape buccolingually for the posterior teeth.

Apical to the contact area, the interdental gingiva assumes a nonvisible concave shape between the facial and lingual gingival surfaces forming the gingival **col** (**kohl**) (Fig. 10.2). The col varies in depth and width, depending on the expanse of the contacting tooth surfaces. It is usually present in the broad interdental gingiva of the posterior teeth and is visible clinically only when teeth are extracted. In comparison, it is usually not present with the interproximal tissue associated with anterior teeth because this latter tissue is narrower. In the absence of contact between adjacent teeth, the attached gingiva extends uninterrupted from the facial to the lingual aspect.

The attached gingiva is considered a masticatory mucosa (see **Chapter 9**). Healthy attached gingiva is pink in color with some areas of melanin pigmentation possible (see Figs. 2.9 and 9.23). When dried it is dull firm immobile tissue, with varying amounts of stippling.

The width of the attached gingiva is measured by the distance between the mucogingival junction that remains stationary after the permanent dentition eruption and the projection on the external surface of the apex of the gingival sulcus (see Fig. 2.9 and discussion in **Chapter 9**). The width of the attached gingiva on the facial aspect varies according to its location and is an important clinical parameter of periodontal health. The attached gingiva has the greatest usually in width for the incisor region at 3.5 to 4.5 mm for the maxillary arch and 3.3 to 3.9 mm for the mandibular arch; in contrast, the narrowest is for the maxillary posterior quadrants at 1.9 mm and 1.8 mm for mandibular first premolars.

The palatal surface of the attached gingiva in the maxillary arch blends with the equally firm and resilient oral mucosa of the hard palate. On the lingual aspect of the mandibular arch, the attached gingiva terminates at the junction of the lingual alveolar mucosa, which is continuous with the oral mucosa lining the floor of the mouth.

At the gingival margin of each tooth is the marginal gingiva (or free gingiva), which is continuous with the attached gingiva. The gingival tissue that faces the tooth, the dentogingival junctional tissue, which is not easily examined within the oral cavity is discussed later. Both the attached gingiva and the marginal gingiva are more easily examined within the oral cavity, whether the gingival tissue is healthy or not.

The marginal gingiva varies in width from 0.5 to 2.0 mm from the free gingival crest to the attached gingiva (see Fig. 2.10). The marginal gingiva follows the scalloped pattern established by the contour of the cementoenamel junction (CEJ) of the teeth. When dried, the

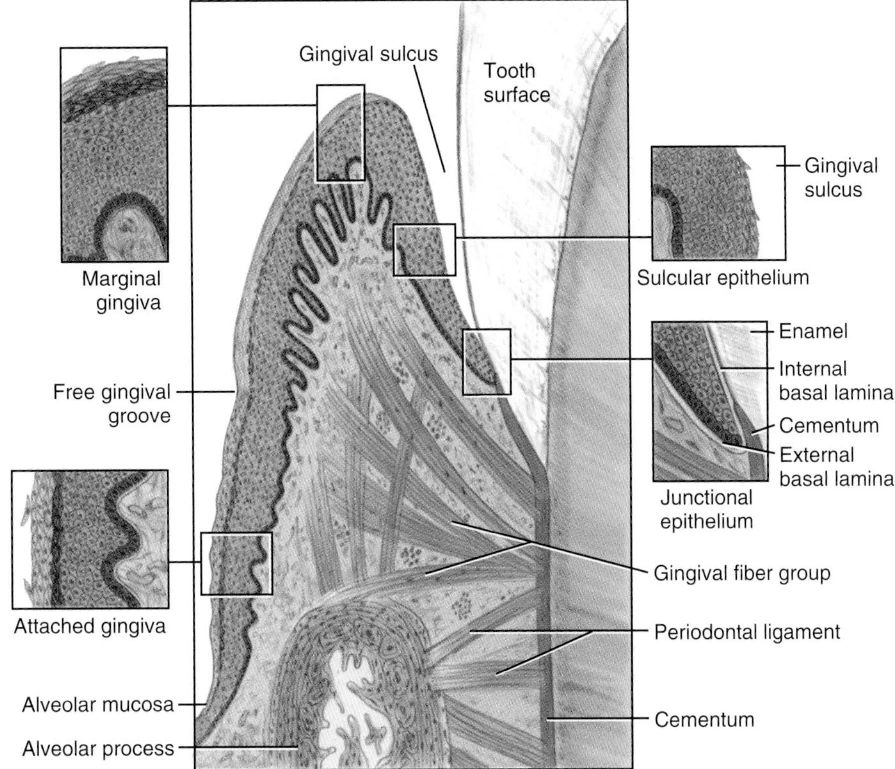

Fig. 10.1 Gingival and dentogingival junctional tissue highlighting the histology of the marginal gingiva, attached gingiva, sulcular epithelium, and junctional epithelium.

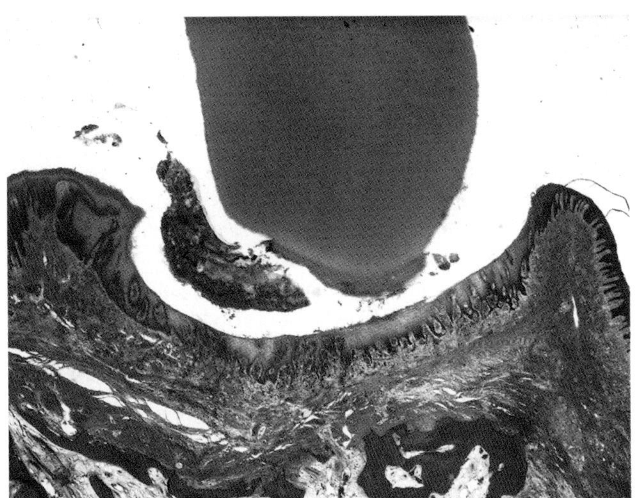

Fig. 10.2 Faciolingual microscopic section showing the col between the facial and lingual interdental papillae inferior to the cervix of the tooth. The col is covered with nonkeratinized stratified squamous epithelium with the surrounding marginal gingiva demonstrating keratinization. (From Newman MG, Takei HH, Klokkevold PR, Carranza F. *Newman and Carranza's Clinical Periodontology*. 13th ed. Philadelphia: Elsevier; 2019.)

marginal tissue is similar in clinical appearance to the attached gingiva, including pinkness, dullness, and firmness. This similarity between marginal gingiva and attached gingiva is because the marginal gingiva is also considered a masticatory mucosa. However, the marginal gingiva lacks the presence of stippling and the tissue is mobile or free from the underlying tooth surface, which can be demonstrated with a periodontal probe or blowing air into the gingival sulcus. In addition, the marginal gingiva is more translucent than the attached gingiva, so much so that the darker subgingival calculus and even the dark margins of poorly executed prosthetic crowns can show through if present.

GINGIVAL TISSUE HISTOLOGY

The attached gingiva and the marginal gingiva share similar histology because both are considered masticatory mucosa; however, each has histologic features specific to the tissue (Fig. 10.3, *A*). The attached gingiva has an overlying thick layer of mostly parakeratinized stratified squamous epithelium, which obscures its extensive vascular supply in the underlying lamina propria, making the tissue appear pinkish instead of the vascularized reddish or bluish (see Fig. 9.12). The lamina propria also has tall narrow connective tissue papillae alternating with the rete ridges, giving the tissue its varying amounts of stippling. Thus the interface between the epithelium and lamina propria is highly interdigitated. The lamina propria is directly attached to the underlying bony jaws, making the attached gingiva firm and immobile. The lamina propria thus serves as a mucoperiosteum along with the periosteum of the alveolar process.

In contrast, the marginal gingiva has an overlying surface layer of only orthokeratinized stratified squamous epithelium. The associated underlying lamina propria also has tall narrow papillae, but this lamina propria is continuous with the lamina propria of the gingival tissue that faces the tooth. And unlike the attached gingiva, the marginal gingiva is not attached to the underlying bony alveolar process, making this tissue firm but mobile. Further the epithelium covering the col consists of the marginal gingiva of the adjacent teeth, except that in this small area it is nonkeratinized. The lack of keratinization of the col tissue may be important in the formation of periodontal disease along with its thinness and apically inclined form (see later discussion).

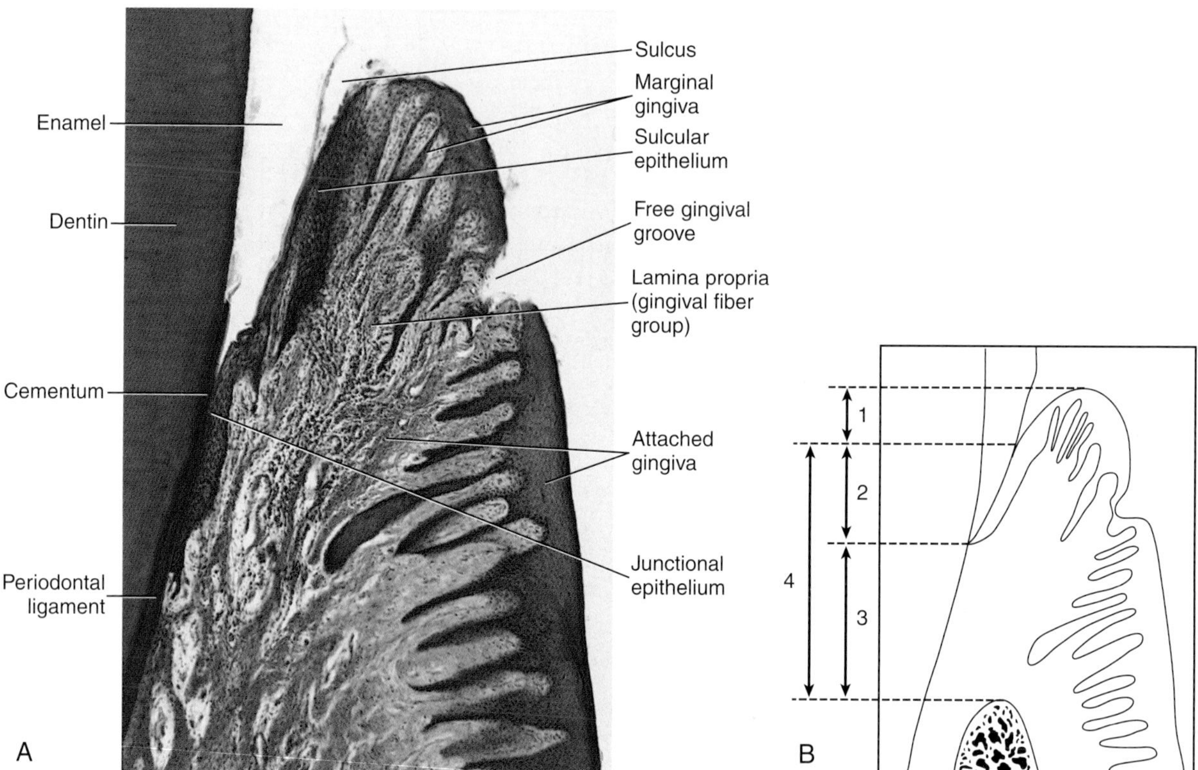

Fig. 10.3 A, Photomicrograph of both the gingival and dentogingival junctional tissue demonstrating the epithelium and lamina propria of these two types of tissue, which is continuous with the periodontal ligament that is adjacent to the hard tissue of the tooth that includes the enamel (space), dentin, and cementum. Decalcification of the specimen has removed the tooth enamel, leaving an enamel space. **B,** Diagram showing *(1)* histologic sulcus depth (0.69 mm), *(2)* length of the epithelial attachment of the junctional epithelium (0.97 mm), *(3)* lamina propria attachment length (1.07 mm), *(4)* biologic width (2.4 mm from *2+3*). (**A,** From Bernhard Gottlieb Collection, courtesy of James McIntosh, PhD, Assistant Professor Emeritus, Department of Biomedical Sciences, Baylor College of Dentistry, Dallas.)

It is important to note that the gingival fiber group is located in the lamina propria of the marginal gingiva (see Fig. 14.32). Some histologists consider the gingival fiber group part of the periodontal ligament, but this fiber group supports only the gingival tissue and not the tooth in relationship to the jaws as does the other periodontal ligament fiber groups. The lamina propria of the marginal gingiva is also continuous with the adjacent connective tissue, which includes the lamina propria of the attached gingiva as well as the periodontal ligament.

Clinical Considerations for Gingival Tissue

The **biologic width** or *supracrestal tissue attachment* describes the combined heights of the suprabony soft tissue, which is attached to the part of the tooth coronal to the crest of the alveolar bone (see Fig. 10.3, *B*). Thus the biologic width is comprised of the healthy supracrestal lamina propria and the epithelial attachment of the junctional epithelium to the root surface (and crown if not fully erupted). Based on studies, the biologic width is commonly stated to be 2.04 mm, which represents the sum of the epithelial attachment of the junctional epithelium and lamina propria measurements.

The primary significance of biologic width to the clinician is its importance relative to the position of restorative margins and its impact on postsurgical tissue position. If a restorative margin is placed too inferior to the tissue so that it violates the needed biologic width, two possible outcomes may occur. First, there may be bone resorption that recreates space for the biologic width to attach it its usual way. However, thankfully, the most common response to a biologic width violation instead is gingival inflammation around the tooth, still a significant problem on anterior restorations.

Evaluation of biologic width can be made during probing of the area noting chronic progressive gingival inflammation, possibly along with gingival hyperplasia as well as clinical attachment loss around the restoration. Bone sounding under local anesthesia and radiographic interpretation (only of interproximal violations) can also be used.

The importance of biologic width to periodontal surgery relates to its reformation following surgical intervention. Research shows it will reform through coronal migration of the gingiva to recreate not just the biologic width, but also a sulcus with the usual depth. This means if the surgery does not consider the dimensions of biologic width when replacing the gingiva relative to the underlying bone, the gingival position will not be stable, but instead will migrate in a coronal direction. Thus biologic width also has a strong influence on when and where restorative margins should be placed postsurgically.

Generally, facial gingiva is thicker in the maxilla than in the mandible. Maxillary canines and mandibular first premolars have the thinnest gingiva at 0.7 to 0.9 mm. This is a consideration when trying to determine a **gingival biotype** (**bahy**-uh-tahyp), which is also known as the *periodontal phenotype*. The gingival biotype is the thickness of the gingiva within the faciolingual dimension. According to studies, individuals with a gingival biotype that includes thin scalloped gingiva demonstrated a greater prevalence of recession, which was then correlated with a thinner underlying bone.

These differences in gingival and osseous architecture have a significant impact on the outcome of treatments for periodontal therapy, root coverage procedures, and implant placement. Therefore, clinicians recommend that the gingival biotype should be evaluated at the start of the periodontal treatment plan for the most successful as well as esthetic results. Recently, cone-beam computed tomography (CBCT) is being used as advanced diagnostic aid in measuring thickness of hard as well as soft tissue in the oral cavity.

Since gingival contours form a silhouette around the cervical section of a tooth, this fact should be acknowledged when considering overall esthetics of smile design (see Fig. 2.9). The cervical peak of the individual gingival contour is referred to as the **gingival apex of the contour**. The apex of maxillary central incisors and canines is distal to a line drawn through the midline or long axis of the tooth. The apex of a maxillary lateral incisor is equal to the midline or long axis of the tooth. The apex of a lateral incisor is also 1 mm short of the central incisor and canine's apex heights. The canine and central incisor apices are equal in height.

The gingival contour is also related to its position in regard to the lip line with continued consideration of smile design. The optimal smile line clinical appearance should reveal the least amount of maxillary facial gingival tissue as possible under the lip line. The lateral incisor may touch the lip line or be 1 to 2 mm coronal to the lip line, revealing some maxillary facial gingival tissue.

However, cases of a "gummy smile" with an excessive display of maxillary facial gingival tissue are not ideal, such as when the maxillary central incisors and canines barely touch the lip line or border of the upper lip. This can result from the abnormal eruption of the teeth; the teeth are covered by excessive tissue and appear short even though they may actually be the proper overall length. The muscles that control the movement of the upper lip could instead be hyperactive, causing the lip to rise up higher than usual so that more tissue is exposed when smiling. In addition, the excessive bulging protrusion of the maxilla may also be involved.

In most cases, orthodontic therapy along with orofacial myofunctional therapy (OMT) as well as both orthognathic surgical intervention and esthetic periodontal surgery can alter the clinical appearance of the gingival contours for a more esthetic smile (see **Chapter 20** for more discussion).

DENTOGINGIVAL JUNCTIONAL TISSUE PROPERTIES

The **dentogingival junction** (den-toh-jin-**juh**-vuhl) is the junction between the tooth surface and the gingival tissue (see Figs. 10.1 and 10.3, *A, B*). The sulcular epithelium and junctional epithelium together form the **dentogingival junctional tissue** (**juhngk**-shuhn-uhl). Both the sulcular epithelium and junctional epithelium are difficult to examine within healthy gingival tissue in a clinical setting due to their location in relationship to the gingival sulcus.

The **sulcular epithelium** (**suhl**-kuh-ler) **(SE)** stands away from the tooth, creating a gingival sulcus. The gingival sulcus is filled with **gingival crevicular fluid (GCF)** (krey-**vik**-yoo-ler) from the adjacent blood supply in the lamina propria. The usual GCF flow rate is quite slow, calculated at 1 to 2 microliters per tooth per hour. Thus, the amount of GCF is minimal at one time in the healthy state.

The GCF from the lamina propria seeps between the epithelial cells and then into the gingival sulcus. This fluid allows the components of the blood system to reach the tooth surface through the junctional epithelium from the blood vessels of the adjacent lamina propria. The GCF contains both the immunologic components and cells of the blood, although in lower amounts and in different proportions. It also contains sticky plasma proteins in the sulcus that serve as adhesive for its lining tissue, keeping it intact.

Thus, the GCF includes white blood cells (WBCs), especially the polymorphonuclear leukocytes (PMNs) as well as the immunoglobulins of IgG, IgM, and serum IgA produced by plasma cells, which all have a role in the specific defense mechanism against disease. Any immunologic reactions in the blood system are directly relevant to those found in the GCF and may affect the periodontal health of the tooth and associated gingival tissue. It also supplies complement factors that serve to initiate both vascular and cellular inflammatory responses that may damage the periodontium. Later, the GCF passes from the gingival sulcus into the oral cavity, where it mixes with saliva. Studying the GCF quantitative proteomics to know the protein level may serve as a biomarker for periodontal disease in the future.

A deeper extension of the SE is the **junctional epithelium (JE)**, which lines the floor of the gingival sulcus and is attached to the tooth surface. The JE surrounds the tooth like a turtleneck with a cross-section resembling a thin wedge. Importantly, the JE is attached to the tooth surface by way of an **epithelial attachment (EA)**. The attachment of the JE to the tooth surface can occur either on enamel, cementum, or dentin. The position of the EA on the tooth surface is initially on the cervical half of the anatomic crown when the tooth first becomes functional after eruption (discussed later). The JE is attached on the other side to the laminal propria of nearby gingiva as is the SE.

The slight depression of the free gingival groove on the outer surface of the gingiva corresponds to the apical border of the inner JE and not to the depth of the gingival sulcus. Instead, the probing depth of the gingival sulcus is measured by the use of a calibrated periodontal probe. The depth of the healthy gingival sulcus varies from 0.5 to 3 mm, with an average of 1.8 mm. However, the clinical probing depth of the gingival sulcus may be considerably different from the true microscopic gingival sulcus depth. In a healthy-case scenario and taking a more microscopic perspective of what occurs with probing, one can note that the instrument is gently inserted, then slides right by the SE, and is finally stopped by the EA of the JE.

Probing measurements of the gingival sulcus are also subject to variations depending on the clinician's insertion pressure, the accuracy of the readings, and the ability of the probe tip to easily penetrate tissue that is ulcerated or inflamed; digital probes are available for more consistent results between clinicians. Studies show that probing the gingival sulcus surrounding both teeth and implants does not seem to cause irreversible damage to the soft tissue because it quickly heals itself (discussed later in this chapter).

DENTOGINGIVAL JUNCTIONAL TISSUE HISTOLOGY

Microscopically the SE consists of stratified squamous epithelium similar to the deeper epithelium of the attached gingiva and adjacent outer marginal gingiva, making it a transition tissue between the gingival epithelium and JE (Figs. 10.4 and 10.5). Apically, it overlaps the coronal border of the JE, a structural design that minimizes ulceration of the epithelial lining in this region. However, the thinner SE is nonkeratinized, unlike the keratinized marginal gingiva and attached gingiva. In addition, the interface between the SE and the lamina propria that it shares with the outer gingival tissue is relatively smooth compared to the strongly interdigitated interface of the outer gingival tissue. The deeper interface between the JE and the underlying lamina propria is also relatively smooth, without rete ridges or connective tissue papillae.

When looking microscopically at the JE itself, the JE cells are loosely packed, with fewer intercellular junctions using desmosomes between cells as compared with other types of gingival tissue (Figs. 10.6 and 10.7). The number of intercellular spaces between the epithelial cells of the JE is also at a higher level than other types of gingival tissue and all are filled with tissue fluid. Overall the JE is more

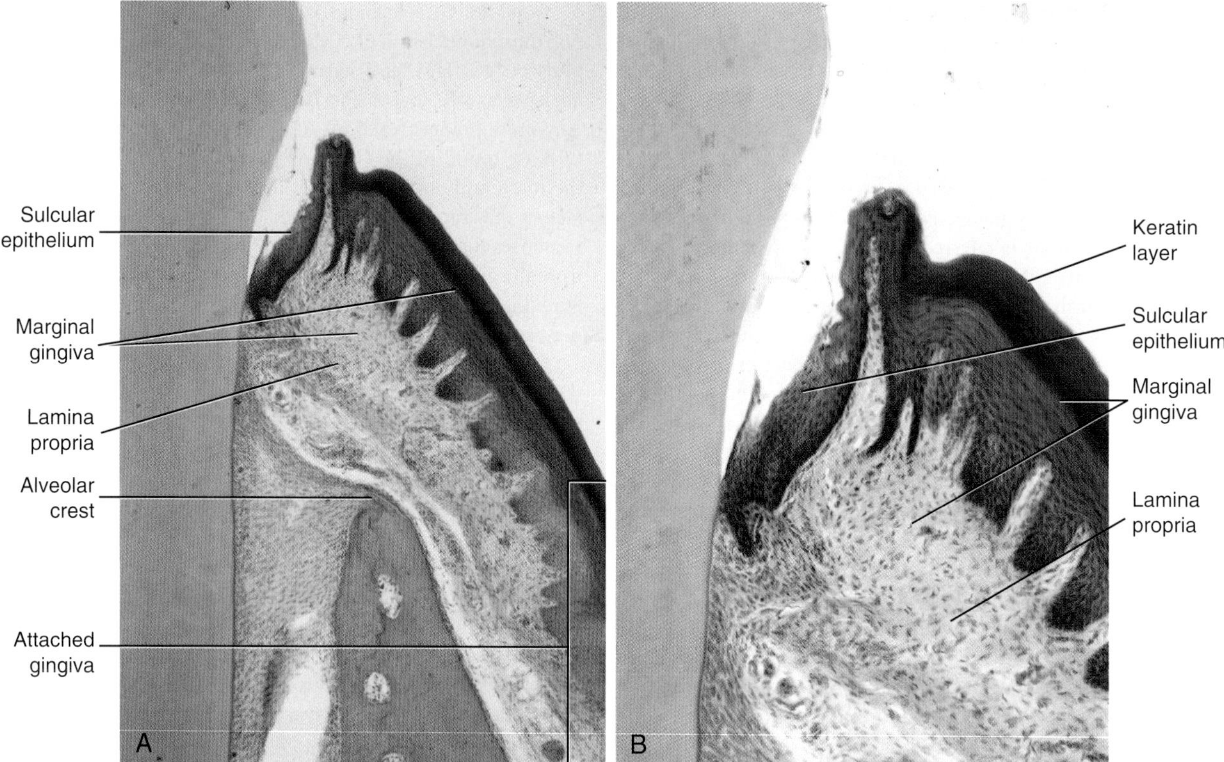

Fig. 10.4 Photomicrographs of the Sulcular Epithelium. A, Deep to the sulcular epithelium is the lamina propria of both the marginal gingiva and the attached gingiva as well as the alveolar crest of the alveolar bone proper. **B,** Close-up view showing the nonkeratinized epithelium of the inner sulcular epithelium. Note that the interface between the sulcular epithelium and the lamina propria that it shares with the marginal and attached outer gingival tissue is relatively smooth compared to the strongly interdigitated interface of the gingival tissue. (From Bernhard Gottlieb Collection, courtesy of James McIntosh, PhD, Assistant Professor Emeritus, Department of Biomedical Sciences, Baylor College of Dentistry, Dallas.)

permeable than other gingival tissue due to its lower density of desmosomal junctions and increased intercellular spaces between the cells of the JE.

This increased permeability allows for emigration of large numbers of mobile WBCs from the blood vessels in the deeper lamina propria into the JE, even in healthy tissue. This mostly involves the PMNs, with those cells actively undergoing phagocytosis (see Fig. 8.17). The PMNs also enter the GCF in the gingival sulcus in healthy mouths. In the absence of clinical signs of inflammation, approximately 30,000 PMNs migrate per minute through the JE into the oral cavity. The increased presence of these WBCs may keep the tissue healthy by protecting it from microorganisms within the dental biofilm and also associated toxins that continually form on the exposed tooth surface in the vicinity. Antigen-presenting cells that are present may be involved as well (see **Chapter 8**).

In addition, the JE is also thinner than the SE, ranging coronally from only 15 to 30 cells thick at the floor of the gingival sulcus and then tapering to a final thickness of 3 to 4 cells at its apical part. The suprabasal cells, which make up the most superficial layer of the JE, serve as part of the EA of the gingiva to the tooth surface. These more suprabasal epithelial cells of the JE provide the hemidesmosomes and an **internal basal lamina** that create the EA because this is a cell-to-noncellular type of intercellular junction (see Fig. 7.6 and Figs. 10.6 and 10.7). Furthermore, because the structure of the EA is similar to that of the junction between the epithelium and subadjacent connective tissue, such as that of the oral mucosa with its epithelium and lamina propria, this internal basal lamina also consists of a lamina lucida and lamina densa.

The internal basal lamina of the EA is also continuous with the **external basal lamina** between the JE and the lamina propria at the apical extent of the JE. The EA is very strong in a healthy state, acting as a type of protective seal between the soft gingival tissue and the hard tooth surface. Thus the JE has two basal laminas, one that faces the tooth (internal) and one that faces the lamina propria of the nearby gingiva (external).

The deepest layer of the JE or basal layer undergoes constant and rapid cell division or mitosis; this proliferative cell layer is in contact with the lamina propria of the nearby gingiva by way of the external basal lamina. This process allows a constant coronal migration of the cells as they die and are shed into the floor of the gingival sulcus at the coronal end of the JE. However, the few layers present in the JE, from its basal layer to the suprabasal layer, do not show any change in cellular structure related to maturation, unlike other types of gingival tissue. Therefore, JE does not mature like keratinized tissue, such as the marginal gingiva or attached gingiva, which fills its matured superficial cells with keratin. Nor does JE have cells like nonkeratinized tissue of the sulcular gingiva and throughout the rest of the oral cavity that enlarge and migrate superficially. Thus the JE cells do not mature and form into either a granular layer or intermediate layer.

However, without a keratinizing superficial layer at the free surface of the JE, there is no physical barrier to microbial attack as with other oral keratinized tissue, such as the attached gingiva. Other structural and functional characteristics of the JE must compensate for the absence of this barrier. The JE fulfills this difficult task with its special structural framework and the collaboration of its epithelial and nonepithelial cells

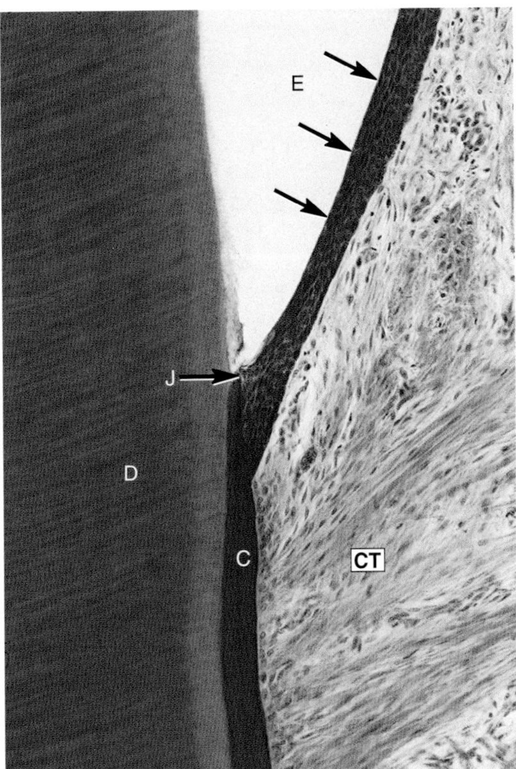

Fig. 10.5 Photomicrograph of the initial junctional epithelium before eruption *(arrows)* overlying the enamel *(E,* enamel space). Decalcification of the specimen has removed the tooth enamel, leaving an enamel space. Note the cementoenamel junction *(J),* the cementum *(C),* and dentin *(D).* Deep to the junctional epithelium is the underlying interconnecting connective tissue *(CT)* of the both lamina propria and adjacent periodontal ligament. (From Bernhard Gottlieb Collection, courtesy of James McIntosh, PhD, Assistant Professor Emeritus, Department of Biomedical Sciences, Baylor College of Dentistry, Dallas.)

that provide very potent antimicrobial mechanisms, such as the WBCs. However, these defense mechanisms do not preclude the development of extensive inflammatory lesions in the gingival tissue, and occasionally, the inflammatory lesion may eventually progress to the loss of the connective tissue attachment of the periodontal ligament to the tooth as well as the alveolar process (discussed later).

The JE cells have many organelles in their cytoplasm, such as rough endoplasmic reticulum, Golgi complex, and mitochondria, indicating a high metabolic activity. However, even with that heightened state, the JE cells remain immature or undifferentiated until they die and are shed or lost in the gingival sulcus. The key to this state of striking cellular immaturity of the JE may be found in future ultrastructural studies of the adjoining lamina propria; this lamina propria appears to be functionally different from the connective tissue underlying the other types of oral epithelium that do mature. Lysosomes are also found in large numbers in JE epithelial cells; enzymes contained within these lysosomes participate in the destruction of microorganisms contained in dental biofilm.

Clinical Considerations for Gingival Tissue Pathology

Periodontal disease is an inflammatory disease that affects the soft and hard structures that support the teeth. In its early stage, it is considered gingivitis, and in its later stages, periodontitis (discussed later in this chapter). With active periodontal disease, both the marginal gingiva and attached gingiva can become enlarged, especially the interdental papillae (Fig. 10.8). This spongy enlargement results from edema occurring in the lamina propria of the tissue caused by the inflammatory response; the marginal gingiva can become rolled. This is due to tissue fluid from the capillary plexus of the lamina propria flowing out to flush the area of its injurious agents with edema (see Fig. 9.6).

The gingival tissue can also become redder with active periodontal disease because of hyperemia or increased blood flow, which also occurs in the capillaries of the lamina propria. Later, the color can change to magenta as the inflammation becomes chronic and the blood undergoes

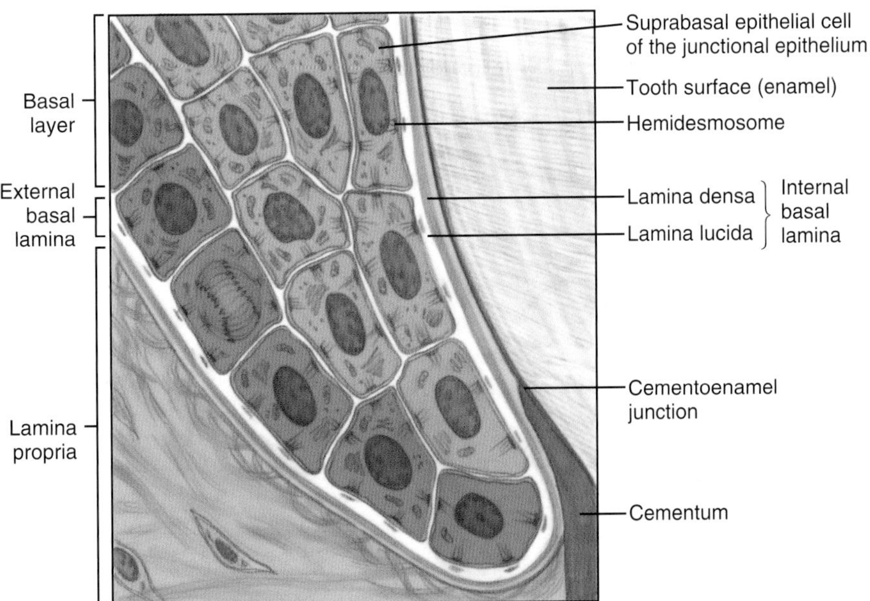

Fig. 10.6 Epithelial attachment of the junctional epithelium with its intricate attachment mechanisms to the tooth surface. Note that the interface between the junctional epithelium and the lamina propria is relatively smooth when healthy.

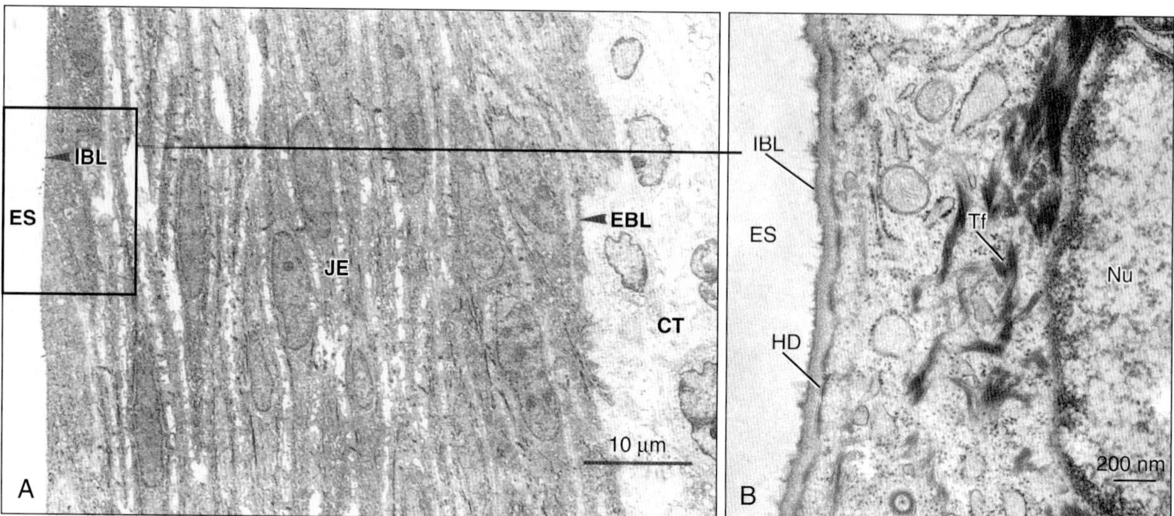

Fig. 10.7 Electron Micrographs of Junctional Epithelium and its Epithelial Attachment. Decalcification of the specimen has removed the tooth enamel, leaving an enamel space. **A,** Attachment of the junctional epithelium *(JE)* to the enamel surface (*ES,* enamel space) at the internal basal lamina *(IBL)* and to the connective tissue *(CT)* of the lamina propria by the external basal lamina *(EBL).* Note its wide intercellular spaces and the lack of cellular differentiation of the layers of epithelium that would denote maturation. **B,** Higher magnification *(close-up view of boxed area in* ***A****)* of the structure of the attachment of a single junctional epithelium cell (*Nu,* nucleus) to the enamel surface by the internal basal lamina and hemidesmosomes *(HD)* and tonofilaments *(Tf).* (**A**, From Schroeder HE, Listgarten MA. *Fine Structure of the Developing Attachment of Human Teeth.* Basel: S. Karger; 1977; **B,** From Nanci A. *Ten Cate's Oral Histology.* 9th ed. St. Louis: Elsevier; 2018.)

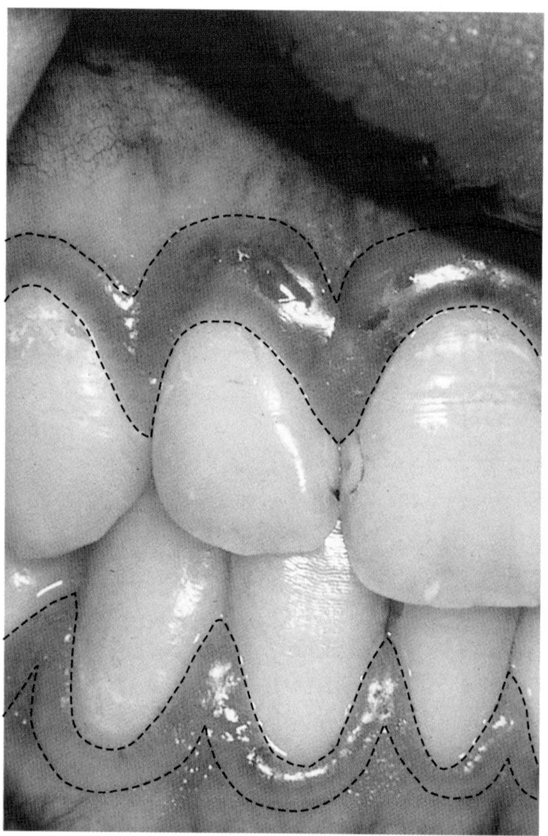

Fig. 10.8 Edema of both the marginal gingiva with its rolled margin and the attached gingiva with its tissue enlargement *(dashed lines)* as a result of acute inflammation with the active periodontal disease of gingivitis. (Courtesy of Margaret J. Fehrenbach, RDH, MS.)

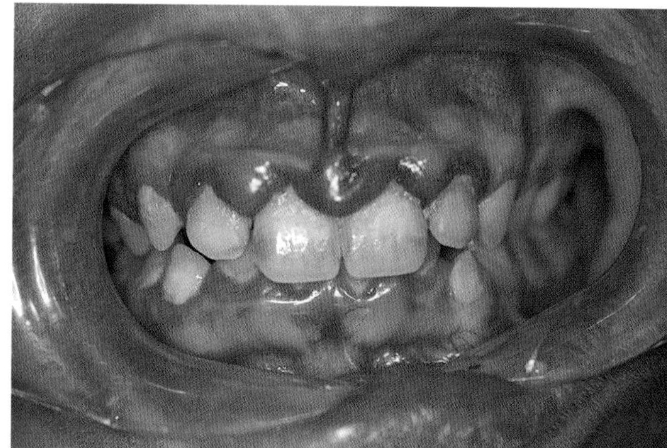

Fig. 10.9 Gingival hyperplasia caused by the intake of certain drugs and associated poor homecare. (Courtesy of Margaret J. Fehrenbach, RDH, MS.)

stasis. The stippling may also be lost because the inflammatory edema reduces the strong interdigitation between the epithelium and lamina propria. The location of the free gingival crest can also change with periodontal disease, such as when the gingival tissue becomes inflamed; the gingival margin can become more coronal with inflammation.

With increased homecare and other methods of dental biofilm control, the edema from inflammation can lessen and both the marginal and attached gingiva can shrink down to their previous levels. These are all signs of gingivitis, the inflammation of the gingiva, which can be either acute or chronic and may also overlie the deeper destruction of the periodontium (see more discussion of gingivitis in this chapter).

Another type of gingival enlargement, gingival hyperplasia, can affect both the epithelium and lamina propria, causing a permanent fibrous enlargement with the gingival margin becoming more coronal (Fig. 10.9). **Gingival hyperplasia** (hahy-per-**pley**-zhuh) is an

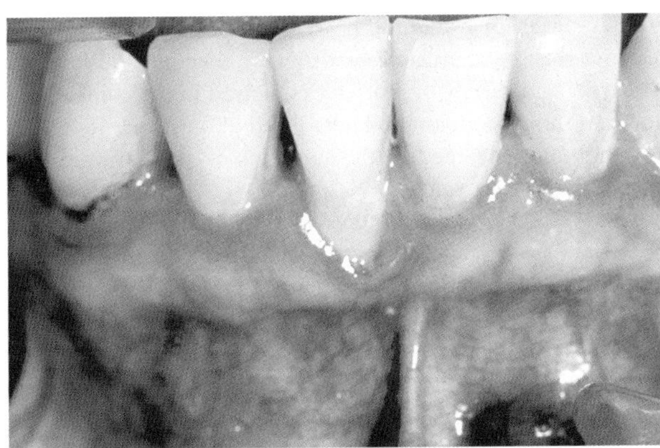

Fig. 10.10 Gingival recession of a permanent mandibular anterior tooth, which may be due to an adjacent tight frenal attachment. (Courtesy of Margaret J. Fehrenbach, RDH, MS.)

overgrowth of mostly the interproximal gingiva and can result from the intake of drugs for seizure control (such as phenytoin sodium), certain antibiotics, and specific heart medications. These drugs may either increase the populations or production outputs of certain fibroblast populations. The amount of gingival overgrowth through drug-influenced gingival hyperplasia is related to the drug dosage as well as the amount of inflammation present that is induced by dental biofilm levels.

The gingival overgrowth of gingival hyperplasia can interfere with proper homecare, increasing dental biofilm amounts, and thus may need to be periodically removed by surgery due to recurrence. Although gingivectomy was considered appropriate in the past, most cases of gingival enlargement are now treated by a flap approach that includes resection of hyperplastic tissue. The surgeon can then access alveolar process defects for management, ensure an adequate postsurgical band of keratinized gingiva and minimize the risk of postsurgical bleeding. Hyperplasia of the dentogingival junctional tissue is also a hallmark of chronic advanced periodontal disease within the tissue (discussed later).

In contrast, **gingival recession** (ri-**sesh**-uhn) results in the gingival margin becoming more apical (Fig. 10.10). This change in the gingival margin can result from periodontal disease, tooth position, abrasion by incorrect toothbrushing methods, abfraction from occlusal stresses (such as parafunctional habits), thin scalloped gingival biotype, and aging process, as well as tight frenal attachments. The width of the attached gingiva may also decrease with periodontal disease, reducing the underlying support for the tooth and should be noted in the patient's chart as well as any other changes present in the gingival tissue.

One type of graft, the free gingival graft (FGG), uses a thickness of both keratinized epithelium and lamina propria harvested from the hard palate and grafted to the root to form a new band of keratinized attached gingiva. This procedure is usually slightly less successful but the graft tends to be lighter colored and studies show that the epithelium does not survive the procedure, which means that the donor site requires extra time to heal and allow migration of the surrounding epithelium to cover the site.

In contrast, a subepithelial connective tissue graft (SECTG) consists of only lamina propria that is taken from the surrounding keratinized attached gingiva and then grafted directly to the root. Epithelial cells from the surrounding tissue migrate to cover the graft and heal the area. This procedure is highly successful; the new keratinized attached gingiva blends with the surrounding tissue and healing of the donor site is rapid. Thus the induction to form keratin in the gingival tissue's superficial layers may come from the deeper lamina propria and does not involve only the epithelium.

These two types of grafting discussed are considered passive mucogingival repair procedures. In contrast, active tissue engineering for mucogingival repair now looks very promising for the future as it produces three-dimensional models of the oral mucosa that may be soon applied to actual patient care.

DENTOGINGIVAL JUNCTIONAL TISSUE DEVELOPMENT

Before the eruption of the tooth and after enamel maturation, the ameloblasts secrete a basal lamina on the tooth surface that serves as a part of the primary EA. As the tooth actively erupts, the coronal part of the fused tissue consisting of the reduced enamel epithelium (REE) and surrounding oral epithelium peels back off the crown (see Fig. 6.25, *D*). The ameloblasts also develop hemidesmosomes for the primary EA and become firmly attached to the enamel surface (see Fig. 10.5). However, the cervical part of the fused tissue remains attached to the neck of the tooth by the primary EA. This fused tissue, which remains near the CEJ after the tooth erupts, serves as the initial JE of the tooth, creating the first tissue attached to the tooth surface. This tissue is later replaced by a definitive JE as the root is formed (see Figs. 10.6 and 10.7).

The definitive JE is formed from all the cell types present in the REE as a result of mitosis of the cells. This proliferating tissue now can provide both the basal lamina and hemidesmosomes for the secondary EA to the tooth surface. After eruption of the tooth, 3 or 4 years may pass before the initial tissue becomes the definitive JE, a multilayer nonkeratinizing squamous epithelium. Although initially controversial, studies now show that the ameloblasts undergo cellular changes that make them indistinguishable from the other newly formed JE cells, with the transformed ameloblasts eventually replaced by these new cells.

DENTOGINGIVAL JUNCTIONAL TISSUE TURNOVER

In both the SE and epithelium of the marginal gingiva, the turnover process insuring the regeneration of the tissue occurs in a manner similar to that of the epithelium of the attached gingiva; the basal cells migrate superficially after mitosis, undergo maturation, and take the place of the superficial cells, which are shed in the oral cavity as they die.

In the JE, even though it does not undergo cellular maturation, its basal cells still migrate superficially upon dividing and continuously replace the dying suprabasal cells that are desquamated into the gingival sulcus at a fast pace. The migratory route of the cells as turnover takes place in the JE is in a coronal direction, parallel to the tooth surface. Such cells continuously dissolve and reestablish their attachments by hemidesmosomes on the tooth surface. Most interestingly, the JE has the fastest turnover time in the entire oral cavity, which is approximately 4 to 6 days (see Table 9.6).

Clinical Considerations for Dentogingival Junctional Tissue Pathology: Gingivitis

When these damaging agents can enter the JE, the gingival tissue undergoes the initial signs of active periodontal disease with the presence of **gingivitis** (jin-juh-**vahy**-tis). This occurs due to the increased permeability of the JE that allows emigration of the PMN type of WBC and also allows microorganisms from the dental biofilm and associated toxins from the exposed tooth surface to enter this tissue from the deeper lamina propria. The signs of gingivitis include acute or even chronic inflammation with the formation of edema (as was discussed earlier) as well as an increased number of WBCs and epithelial ulceration with tissue thinning (see Fig. 10.8).

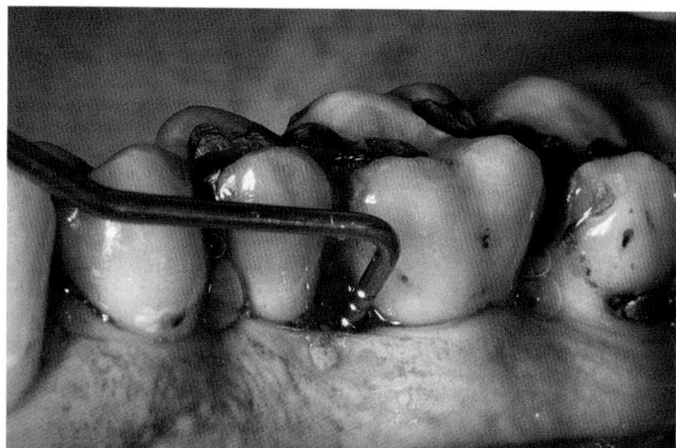

Fig. 10.11 Bleeding on probing of a periodontal pocket due to increased blood vessels in the deeper lamina propria, which are now closer to the surface because of ulceration of the junctional epithelium caused by periodontal inflammation. (Courtesy of Margaret J. Fehrenbach, RDH, MS.)

The process of gingivitis begins with the recognition of the invasion by microorganisms from the dental biofilm by the gingival epithelial cells. Embedded in the cell membrane of the gingival epithelial cells (and many others including the skin and gastrointestinal tract) are toll-like receptors (TLRs). These are transmembrane proteins that extend through the gingival epithelial cell membrane, having both internal and external parts; they recognize the presence of the bacterial endotoxins and then mobilize the inflammatory response.

The ulceration of the JE allows even more damaging agents to enter the deepest parts of periodontium, thus progressing the disease toward the bony jaw. The interface between the dentogingival junctional tissue and the lamina propria that is smooth in healthy tissue, with inflammation shows the formation of rete ridges and connective tissue papillae. The lamina propria also shows breakdown of the collagen fibers as the disease advances.

Bleeding on probing (BoP), even with a gentle touch, begins to occur even when other early signs of gingivitis are not present (Fig. 10.11). This is due to the periodontal probe damaging the increased blood vessels in the capillary plexus of the lamina propria, which are now closer to the surface because of the ulceration of the JE. Bleeding can also occur during patient homecare. The presence of bleeding is one of the first clinical signs of active periodontal disease in uncomplicated cases and should be recorded per individual tooth and tooth surface in the patient's chart. However, in patients who use nicotine products, the gingival tissue rarely bleeds because of unknown factors that do not seem related to dental biofilm and calculus formation but to the incorporated nicotine that causes vasoconstriction, a narrowing of the blood vessels.

Periodontal inflammation is also accompanied by an increase in the amount of GCF in order to fight the microbial attack, either of a serous (clinically clear) or suppurative nature (clinically yellowish white), distending the already enlarged tissue even further. Thus relatively large amounts of fluid now pass through the more permeable epithelial wall. This is noted clinically only when it involves the visible suppuration or pus, resulting from the presence of cellular debris and extensive populations of PMNs.

Current clinical practice does not usually allow measurement of these increased fluid levels in the gingival sulcus. In the future, however, this measurement may be possible in a dental office setting; it is now used usually during dental research to show the level of activity of the disease. It is important to keep in mind that GCF also supplies the minerals for subgingival calculus formation as well as a moist environment needed for dental biofilm growth.

Studies have shown that the JE cells themselves may play a much more active role in the innate defense system than previously assumed by synthesizing a variety of molecules involved in the combat against microorganisms and their products. In addition, these JE cells may express molecules that mediate the migration of PMNs toward the apical part of the gingival sulcus.

Dental professionals should consider gingivitis the "line in the sand" beyond which no patient should step. Failure to intervene at this early point will result in some patients progressing to periodontitis, which is incurable and condemns one to a lifetime of complex disease management (discussed next). Basic dental care should be aimed primarily at reduction of etiologic factors to reduce or eliminate inflammation, thereby allowing the gingival tissue to heal. Over time, appropriate modalities that include homecare and professional care is important in preventing reinitiation of inflammation.

Clinical Considerations for Dentogingival Junctional Tissue Pathology: Periodontitis

When the deeper tissue of the periodontium is affected by periodontal disease, further damage can occur, and the disease can become chronic in nature; this condition is now considered to be **periodontitis** (per-ee-oh-don-**tahy**-tis) (Fig. 10.12). With the advancement of periodontal disease, the prognosis for retention of the tooth becomes risky, then guarded as the alveolar process is lost and the lamina propria and adjacent periodontal ligament become increasingly disorganized with the inherent collagen fibers breaking down (see discussion in **Chapter 14**).

As the disease progresses apically furcations become exposed, which are areas between the roots of posterior teeth and the teeth become increasingly mobile (see Fig. 17.35). Pathologic tooth migration (PTM), the overall tooth displacement that results when the balance among the factors that maintain physiologic tooth position is disturbed, may also be present due to a weakened periodontium. The occlusal forces need not be at an abnormal level if the periodontal support is already reduced by periodontal disease (see Fig. 14.34).

True apical migration of the EA also occurs with advanced periodontal disease, causing a deepened gingival sulcus, which is now considered a **periodontal pocket** lined by **pocket epithelium (PE)** instead of dentogingival junctional tissue (see Fig. 10.11). Unlike in clinically healthy situations, superior parts of the lining can sometimes be visible in periodontally involved gingival tissue if air is blown into the periodontal pocket, exposing the newly denuded roots of the tooth. The most prominent histologic characteristics of PE are the presence of ulceration and gingival hyperplasia with the formation of rete ridges and connective tissue papillae at the once smooth tissue interface. In addition, the PE has a wrinkled papillary relief, increased levels of exfoliation of epithelial cells, WBC migration, and bacterial internalization, as well as internalization-induced programmed epithelial cell death.

Periodontal probing continues to be a key element in the diagnosis of periodontal disease and its depth must be recorded in the patient's chart to monitor periodontal disease. However, a probing depth alone does not reveal the complete state of health of the area being measured. Another measurement of the extent of the periodontal support is the **clinical attachment level (CAL)**. This is the measurement of the position of the gingiva in relation to the CEJ, which is a fixed point that does not change throughout life. Two measurements are used to calculate the CAL: the probing depth and the distance from the gingival margin to the CEJ. Three scenarios are possible for the gingival margin: the CEJ may be coronal to the gingival margin due to gingival recession; the CEJ may be at the same level as the gingival margin; or the gingival margin extends significantly over the CEJ.

However, this clinical attachment level is not the same as the **clinical attachment loss**, which is considered the *true attachment loss* based

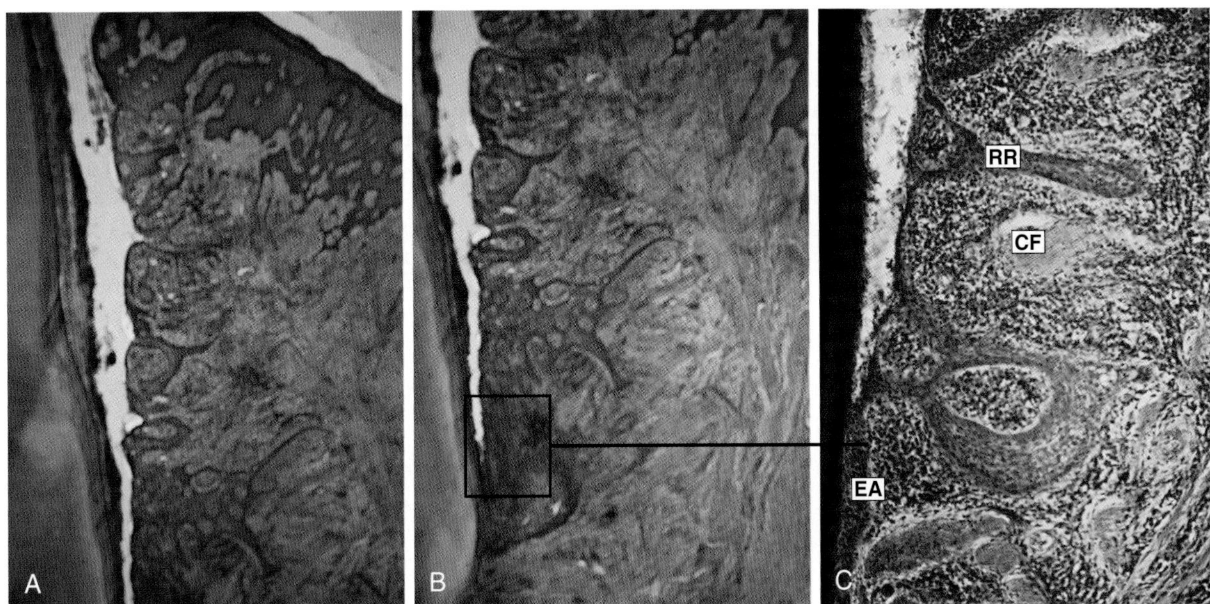

Fig. 10.12 Photomicrographs of Periodontitis as a Chronic Advanced Periodontal Disease that Progresses in an Apical Direction. A, Ulcerated junctional epithelium *(right)* that has become a lateral wall of pocket epithelium with its true apical migration of the epithelial attachment on the tooth *(left)* causing a deepened gingival sulcus or periodontal pocket. **B,** Slightly more apical view showing epithelial proliferative and atrophic changes and marked inflammatory infiltrate and destruction of collagen fibers of the pocket epithelium. **C,** Higher magnification of the newly formed pocket epithelium *(close-up view of boxed area in B)* with migrated pocket epithelium giving it a long epithelial attachment *(EA)*, increased numbers of blood vessels in the lamina propria, and formation of rete ridges *(RR)* and connective tissue papillae at the interface between the dentogingival junctional tissue and the lamina propria, as well as the breakdown of the collagen fibers *(CF)* of the lamina propria and adjacent periodontal ligament. (From Newman MG, Takei HH, Klokkevold, PR, Carranza, F. *Newman and Carranza's Clinical Periodontology*. 13th ed. Philadelphia: Elsevier; 2019.)

on histology related to CAL. If clinical attachment loss is defined as the extent of the periodontal support that has been destroyed around a tooth, then in a healthy situation the probe reading would be zero millimeters. But this situation never occurs since the tip of the periodontal probe always penetrates into the gingival tissue that is internal to the sulcus. Thus, in a patient with a healthy gingiva, the sulcus is histologically at a maximum of 0.5 mm depth, but periodontal probing will routinely yield a measurement of between 2.0 and 3.0 mm.

Periodontopathogens within a periodontal pocket are believed to play an important role in periodontitis, such as *Aggregatibacter actinomycetemcomitans (Aa)* or *Porphyromonas gingivalis (Pg)*. These pathogens have developed sophisticated methods to disturb the structural and functional integrity of the JE, including the production of gingipains or cysteine proteinases. These virulence factors may specifically degrade components of the cell-to-cell contacts of the JE, furthering the progression of disease. And an increased number of mononuclear WBCs, such as the T-cell and B-cell lymphocytes and monocytes/macrophages, together with PMNs, are also considered as factors that contribute to the focal disintegration of the JE as it forms into PE.

The placement of local antimicrobial delivery systems within the periodontal pocket to reduce localized infections may also be considered. An increasing number of studies that show positive results regarding antimicrobial photodynamic therapy (PDT) when used in both periodontics (and endodontics) against infections caused by bacteria present as biofilms. It is a therapy based on the combination of a nontoxic photosensitizer (PS) and appropriate wavelength visible light, which in the presence of oxygen is activated to produce reactive oxygen species (ROS) causing microbial death. Without intervention, a periodontal pocket can become a localized infected fascial space and may result in an abscess formation with a papule appearing on the gingival surface. Incision and drainage of the abscess may be necessary as well as systemic antibiotics if systemic signs of infection are present.

Endoscopic evaluation of the periodontal pocket is also becoming increasingly available in dental settings outside of the research facilities; it can facilitate subgingival visual examination without reliance on tactile sense and without surgical flap access. The clinician views a video monitor that displays the magnified image transmitted by a fiberoptic bundle attached to a subgingival instrument. This direct real-time visualization of the gingival sulcular region may aid the clinician in periodontal disease diagnosis and therapy. Techniques for identification and interpretation of the hard and soft tissue images, as well as the location of root fractures or deposits, defective restorations, and caries, are being developed.

Given that the turnover time of the JE is approximately 1 week (unlike most oral tissue that have slower turnover times), evaluation of periodontal therapy must occur after this time to allow initial healing of the area. Therefore, follow-up scheduling of patients should occur after this biologic temporal factor of turnover time. In addition, patients must have the information and skills necessary to enact a change in their homecare to allow optimal initial healing during this healing period. The final outcome of periodontal pocket healing depends on the sequence of events during the repair stages as discussed earlier. If the epithelium proliferates along the tooth surface before the other more supportive tissue reaches the area, the result will be a long JE. This less than stellar pattern of healing does not promote any new periodontal ligament support or alveolar process attachment associated with the tooth; thus the tooth now has a riskier prognosis.

In regard to newly placed implants, the superior tissue present originates only from epithelial cells of the oral mucosa as opposed to the JE located around natural teeth, which originates also from the REE (see earlier discussion and Fig. 14.23). Structurally, the *periimplant tissue* closely resembles a long JE and is discussed as such by many clinicians, although dissimilarities have also been reported in some studies. It is unknown if the situation of having a long JE has a risky prognosis for the implant as it does for a poorly healing periodontal case with natural teeth. However, such an adaptive potential is also observed in the regenerating JE around teeth following gingivectomy, which is performed to surgically reduce pocket depths by removal of the soft tissue pocket wall, with a completely new JE forming within 20 days.

The recent more precise staging and intuitive grading of periodontal disease guidelines by both the American Academy of Periodontology (AAP) and the European Federation of Periodontology (EFP) have started a new paradigm that includes factors for future risk analysis for the patient as well as the first-ever classifications for periimplant diseases and conditions. It is hoped that someday a patient with extensive periodontal tissue damage could have periodontal therapy performed that would allow a more coronal reattachment of the EA of the JE and also complete periodontium regeneration involving a sound periodontal ligament and alveolar process attachment. Corresponding changes would also then occur in the way periodontal therapy is performed and homecare instructions are given. Thus the practicing dental professional must keep current with changes in this area to remain current in periodontal therapy and homecare instruction.

11

Head and Neck Structures

Additional resources and practice exercises are provided on the companion Evolve website for this book: http://evolve.elsevier.com/Fehrenbach/illustrated.

LEARNING OBJECTIVES

1. Define and pronounce the key terms in this chapter.
2. Discuss gland properties.
3. Discuss salivary gland properties, including its histologic features and development as well as the clinical considerations concerning salivary gland pathology, integrating it into patient care.
4. Discuss thyroid gland properties, including its histologic features and development as well as the clinical considerations concerning thyroid gland pathology, integrating it into patient care.
5. Discuss properties of lymphatics, including the lymph nodes and intraoral tonsillar tissue, and the clinical considerations concerning lymphoid tissue pathology, integrating it into patient care.
6. Discuss the properties of the nasal cavity and paranasal sinuses as well as clinical considerations concerning each of them, integrating it into patient care.
7. Identify the components of head and neck structures on a diagram.

HEAD AND NECK STRUCTURES

Dental professionals must have a clear understanding of the histology as well as the prenatal development concerning not only the oral cavity but also the associated head and neck structures. The clinical functioning of the head and neck structures is related to their underlying histology. In addition, many pathologic lesions that are encountered in the oral cavity can be associated with changes in these associated structures of the head and neck and thus are reflected in changes in their underlying histology. The head and neck structures to be discussed in this chapter include the salivary glands, thyroid gland, lymphatics, nasal cavity, and paranasal sinuses.

GLAND PROPERTIES

A **gland** is a structure that produces a secretion necessary for body functioning. An **exocrine gland** (**ek**-suh-krin) is a gland having a duct associated with it. A **duct** is a passageway that allows the glandular secretion to be emptied directly into the location where the secretion is to be used. In contrast, an **endocrine gland** (**en**-duh-krin) is a ductless gland with its secretions conveyed directly into the blood and then carried by the blood vessels to some distant location to be used. Motor nerves associated with both types of glands help regulate the flow of the secretion. Sensory nerves are also present in each of the glands.

SALIVARY GLAND PROPERTIES

The oral fluid contains not only saliva but also other components as well, such as food debris, microorganisms and their byproducts, serum components, and desquamated oral epithelial cells. The **salivary glands** produce **saliva** (suh-**lahy**-vuh) or what is referred to as "spit." Saliva contains minerals, electrolytes, proteins, buffers, enzymes, immunoglobulins (secretory IgA), and metabolic wastes. The secretion by these glands is controlled by the autonomic nervous system (see **Chapter 8**).

Saliva lubricates and cleanses the oral mucosa, protecting it from dryness and potential carcinogens by way of its mucins and other glycoproteins. This secretory product also helps in digestion of food by enzymatic activity. Additionally, it serves as a buffer by its bicarbonate and phosphate ions as well as by salivary proteins and their byproducts, protecting the oral mucosa against acids from food products and dental biofilm and then later the stomach lining.

Saliva is also involved in antibacterial activity through its lysozyme content as well as secretory IgA (see **Chapters 7 and 8**, respectively). The glycoprotein of lactoferrin content inhibits the growth of bacteria that need iron by chelating with the element. Finally, saliva helps maintain tooth integrity because it is involved in the posteruptive maturation of enamel. It also helps continue the remineralization of the tooth surface because it is supersaturated with calcium and phosphate ions, which can be increased by having fluoride added to the saliva.

However, because it contributes to the formation of the salivary pellicle on the tooth and oral mucosa surfaces, saliva is also involved in the first step in dental biofilm formation. It also supplies the minerals for supragingival calculus formation.

Salivary glands are classified as either major or minor depending on their size, but both types have similar histologic features. Further, both the major and minor salivary glands are exocrine glands and thus have associated ducts that help convey the saliva directly into the oral cavity where it can be used. In addition, the minor glands do not have named ducts as the major glands have (discussed later in this chapter).

Salivary Gland Histology

Both major and minor salivary glands are composed of both epithelium and connective tissue (Fig. 11.1). Epithelial cells both line the ducts and produce the saliva. Connective tissue surrounds each part of the epithelia, protecting and supporting the gland. The connective tissue of the gland is divided into the **capsule** (**kap**-suhl), which surrounds the outer part of the entire gland and the septa. Each **septum** (**sep**-tuhm) (plural, **septa** [**sep**-tuh]) helps divide the inner part of the gland into the larger **lobes** and then smaller **lobules** (**lob**-yoolz). Both the capsule and septa also carry nerves and blood vessels that serve the gland.

Secretory Cells and Acini

Epithelial cells that produce the saliva are the **secretory cells** (si-**kree**-tuh-ree) (Fig. 11.2). The two types of secretory cells are classified as

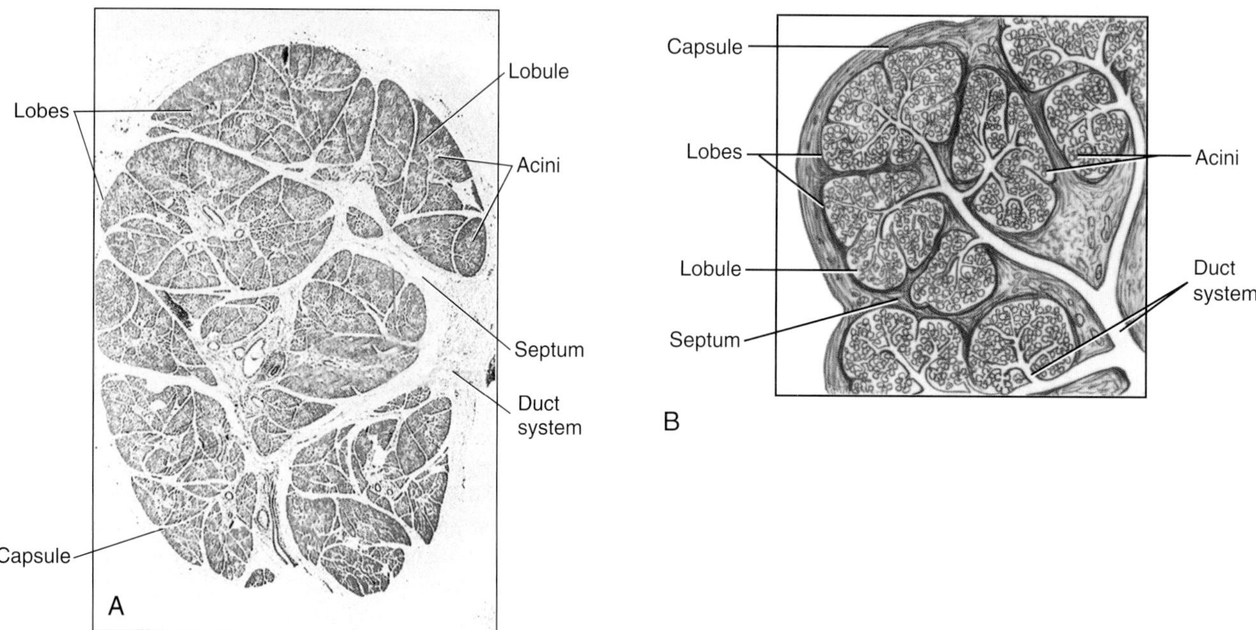

Fig. 11.1 Salivary Gland. **A,** Micrograph. **B,** Diagram. (**A,** From Nanci A. *Ten Cate's Oral Histology.* 6th ed. St. Louis: Elsevier; 2003.)

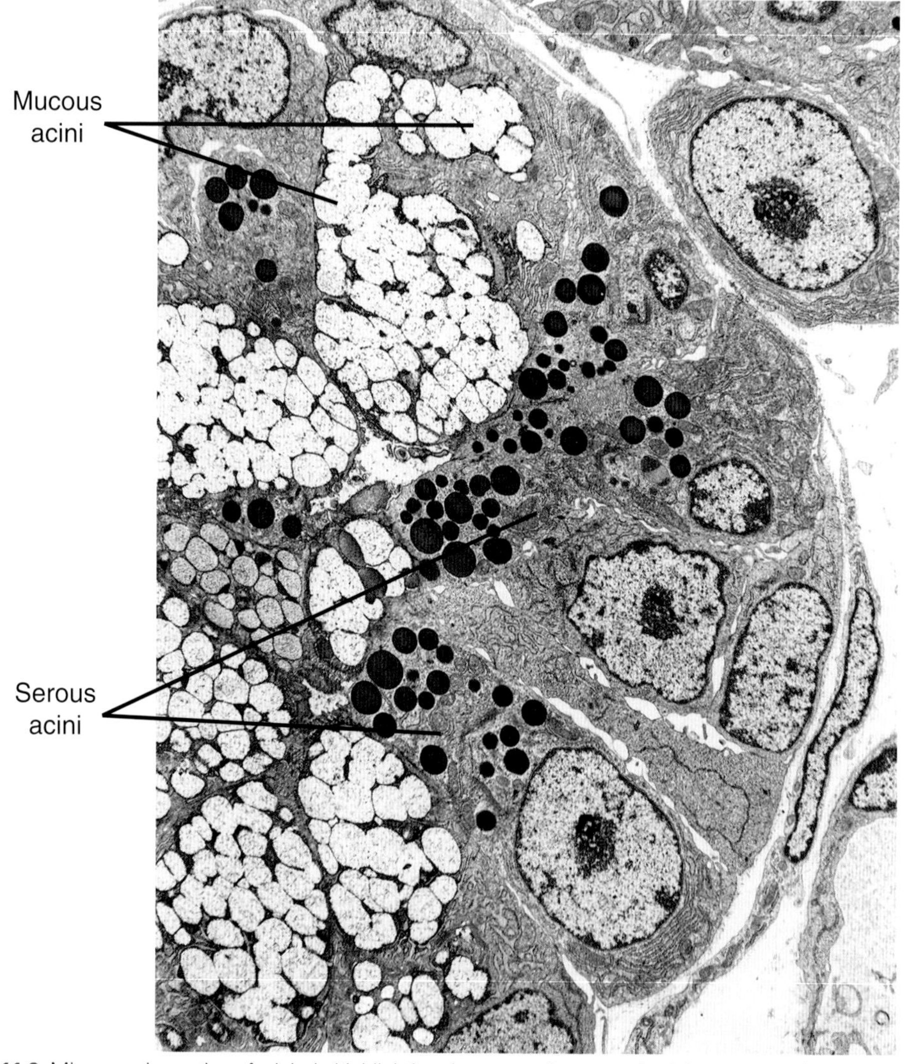

Fig. 11.2 Microscopic section of a lobule highlighting the two main types of acini: mucous acinus and serous acinus as noted in the sublingual salivary gland. See also Fig. 11.5. (From Gartner LP. *Textbook of Histology.* 4th ed. St. Louis: Elsevier; 2017.)

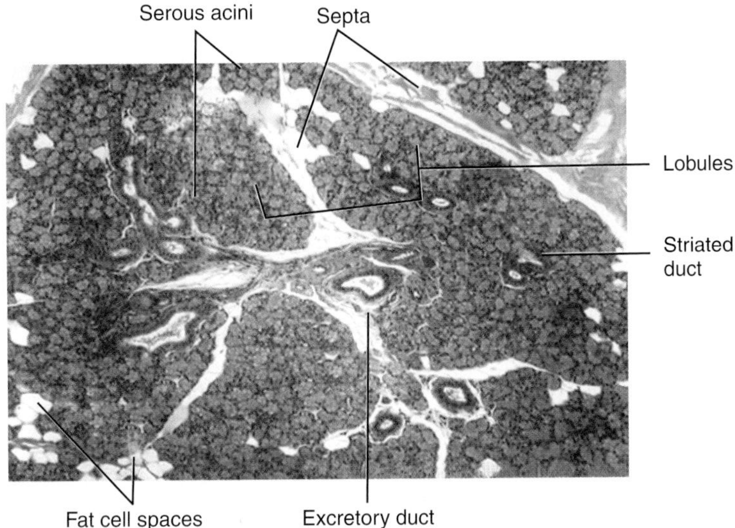

Fig. 11.3 Photomicrograph of the parotid salivary gland showing connective tissue septa dividing the serous acini into lobules to produce a mostly serous secretory product. Note also the striated and excretory ducts. (From Nanci A. *Ten Cate's Oral Histology*. 6th ed. St. Louis: Elsevier; 2003.)

either mucous or serous cells, depending on the type of secretion produced. **Mucous cells** (**myoo**-kuhs) produce a mucous secretory product with mostly mucins. Mucins in saliva lubricate and can form a surface barrier as well as aid in aggregating microorganisms. In contrast, **serous cells** (**seer**-uhs) produce a serous secretory product with proteins and glycoproteins. The serous cells also produce the enzyme amylase that catalyzes the hydrolysis of starch from food intake into sugars, which is the beginning of the chemical process of digestion.

A combination of secretory cells present in the gland can produce a mixed secretory product. However, in these mixed glands one type of cell predominates so that the product is either mostly mucous or mostly serous even if it has a range of both cell types.

Secretory cells are found in a group or **acinus** (**as**-uh-nuhs) (plural, **acini** [**as**-uh-nahy]), which resembles a cluster of grapes. Each acinus is located at the terminal part of the gland connected to the ductal system with many acini within each lobule of the gland like the stems of the grape cluster. Each acinus consists of a single layer of cuboidal epithelial cells surrounding a **lumen** (**loo**-muhn), which is a central opening where the saliva is deposited after being produced by the secretory cells.

The main two forms of acini are classified in terms of the type of epithelial cell present and the secretory product being produced. **Serous acini** are composed of serous cells producing a watery serous secretory product with rounder nuclei and narrower lumens (Fig. 11.3). In contrast, **mucous acini** are composed of mucous cells producing a viscous mucous secretory product with flatter nuclei and wider lumens. Many of these features between the two types of acini can be hard to see at lower-level microscopic power.

Some mucous acini have a **serous demilune** (**dem**-i-loon), which consists of a "bonnet" or cap of serous cells superficial to the group of mucous secretory cells and may be considered *mucoserous* or *seromucous* (Figs. 11.4 and 11.5). Small intercellular canals, not readily evident in lower-level microscopic power, permit secretions to pass from the demilunes to the lumen of the mucous acinus. In fact, recent observations suggest that demilunes are an artifact of fixation and they are serous cells that have been "squeezed" away from the lumen by fixation. However, the term demilune is still commonly used. Still important is that the mucous acini with a serous demilune contain both types of secretory cells, therefore they produce a mixed secretory product.

Both the major and minor salivary glands have differing types of acini (Table 11.1). The major glands show a range of acini types: the parotid has only serous acini, the submandibular has both including mucous acini with serous demilunes but mostly has serous acini, and the sublingual has mostly mucous acini with some having serous demilunes. Most minor salivary glands have mostly mucous acini with a few having serous demilunes as well as also having a few serous acini. However, the minor salivary glands of von Ebner are an exception, having only serous acini (discussed later). However, the types of acini are often difficult to classify at lower-power magnification of microscopic sections of the glands and some of the features noted microscopically may be artifacts.

To facilitate the flow of saliva out of each lumen into the connecting ducts, **myoepithelial cells** (mahy-oh-ep-uh-**thee**-lee-uhl) are located on the surface of some of the acini as well as on their connection to the ductal system, the intercalated ducts (Fig. 11.6). Each myoepithelial cell consists of a cell body with four to eight cytoplasmic processes radiating outward. They are specialized cells of epithelium that resemble an octopus on a rock; thus they are situated on the surface of the acini and have a contractile nature.

When the myoepithelial cells contract, the acinus and its contents are squeezed, forcing the saliva out of the lumen and into the connecting duct; more than one myoepithelial cell can sometimes be found on a single acinus. When associated with the ducts of the salivary glands in this case, the cells orient themselves lengthwise and contract to shorten or widen the ducts to keep them open. Studies show additional functions of these cells, such as signaling the secretory cells and protecting the salivary gland tissue.

Ductal System

The ductal system of salivary glands consists of hollow tubes connected initially with the acinus and then with other ducts as the ducts progressively grow larger from the inner to the outer parts of the gland (see Fig. 11.6). Each type of duct is lined by different epithelium, depending on its location in the gland (see Table 8.2). In comparison, each major salivary gland displays differences in the length or types of ducts present (see Table 11.1); minor salivary glands do not show these differences due to the shortness of their ductal system. It is important to note that the ductal system does not serve just as a pipeline for the

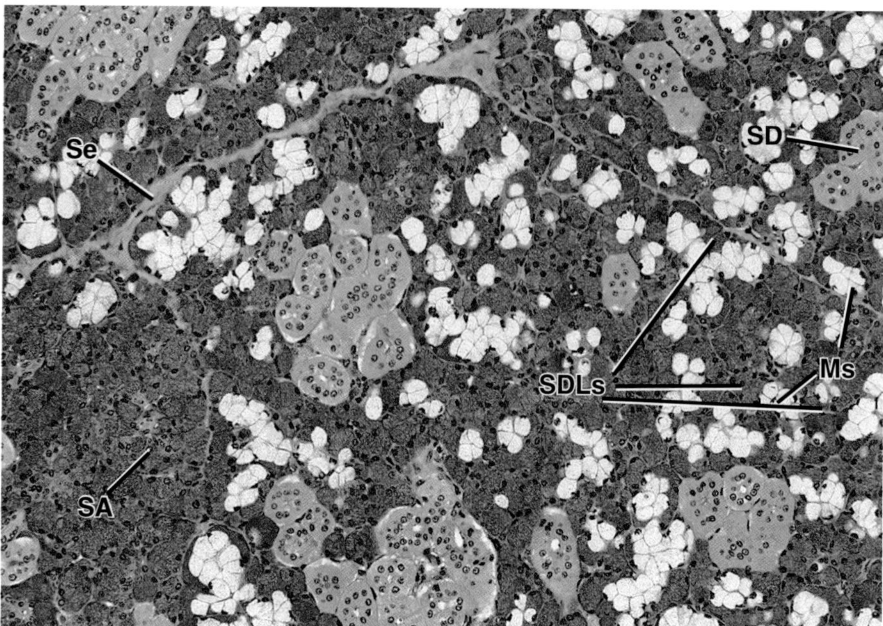

Fig. 11.4 Photomicrograph of the submandibular salivary gland highlighting a mucous acinus with its mucous cells *(Ms)* serous demilunes *(SDLs)* as well as a serous acinus *(SA)*, which indicates the gland that produces a mixed salivary that product. Note also the septum *(Se)* and striated duct *(SD)*. (Modified from Gartner LP. *Textbook of Histology*. 4th ed. St. Louis: Elsevier; 2017.)

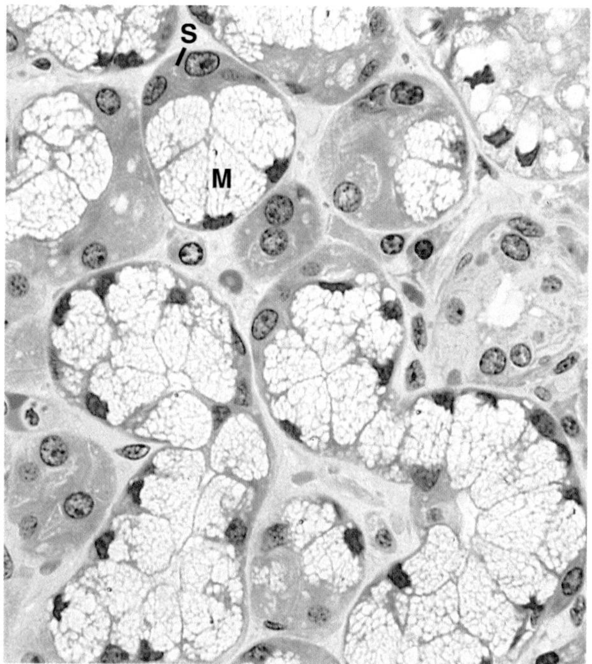

Fig. 11.5 Photomicrograph of the sublingual salivary gland highlighting a serous demilune *(S)* capping the mucous cells of a mucous acinus *(M)*, which indicates it produces a mixed secretory product because it has mostly mucous acini but also some mucous acini with serous demilunes. (From Gartner, LP. *Textbook of Histology*. 4th ed. St. Louis: Elsevier; 2017.)

passageway of saliva; many of the parts of the duct system also actively participate in the production and modification of saliva.

The duct associated with an acinus or terminal part of the gland is the **intercalated duct** (in-**tur**-kuh-ley-ted). The intercalated duct is attached to the acinus, much as a stalk is attached to a cluster of grapes. The intercalated duct consists of a hollow tube lined with a single layer of cuboidal epithelial cells. Many are found in each lobule of the gland. These ducts not only serve as a passageway for saliva, but they also contribute many macromolecular components to the saliva. These include lysozyme and lactoferrin, which are stored in the secretory granules of ductal cells.

The **striated duct** (**strahy**-ey-tid) is a part of the ductal system that is connected to the intercalated ducts in the lobules of the gland. The overall diameter of this duct is greater than that of each acinus, and its lumen is larger than those of both the acini and intercalated ducts. The striated duct consists of a hollow tube lined with a single layer of columnar epithelial cells characterized by what appear to be *basal striations*. However, these visual vertical infranuclear striations are due to the presence of numerous elongated mitochondria in narrow cytoplasmic partitions separated by highly infolded and interdigitated cell membranes. Not only does the striated duct serve as a passageway for saliva, but it also is involved in the modification of saliva. Its ductal cells actively resorb and secrete electrolytes into the saliva from the adjacent blood vessels near the visually striated regions.

The final part of the salivary gland ductal system is the **excretory duct** (**ex**-sri-tawr-ee) (or secretory duct), which is located in the septum of the gland. These ducts are larger in diameter than the striated ducts. Saliva exits by this duct into the oral cavity. The excretory duct is a hollow tube lined with a variety of epithelial cells. The cells lining the excretory duct initially consist of pseudostratified columnar epithelium, which then undergoes a transition to stratified cuboidal epithelium as the duct moves to the outer part of the gland.

On the outer part of the ductal system that empties into the oral cavity, the excretory duct lining becomes stratified squamous epithelium, blending with surrounding oral mucosa at the ductal opening. Thus the excretory duct serves as a passageway for saliva; however, it may have other functions with further research.

Major Salivary Glands

The **major salivary glands** are three large paired glands that have ducts named for them (Fig. 11.7; see Table 11.1 and Fig. 1.5). These major salivary glands are the parotid, the submandibular, and the sublingual glands.

TABLE 11.1 Comparison of Major Salivary Glands

	Parotid	Submandibular	Sublingual
Size and capsulation	Largest, capsule present	Intermediate, capsule present	Smallest, no capsule
Location	Posterior to mandibular ramus, anterior and inferior to ear	Beneath mandible	Floor of the mouth
Excretory ducts	Parotid duct (Stensen): Opens opposite maxillary second molar on buccal mucosa	Submandibular duct (Wharton): Opens near lingual frenum on floor of mouth at sublingual caruncles	Sublingual duct (Bartholin): Opens in same area as submandibular duct; may have additional ducts at submandibular folds
Striated ducts	Short	Long	Rare or absent
Intercalated ducts	Long	Short	Absent
Acini	Only serous	Mostly serous but with some mucous with serous demilunes	Mostly mucous but with some serous demilunes
Secretory product	Only serous	Mixed and but predominately serous	Mixed but predominately mucous

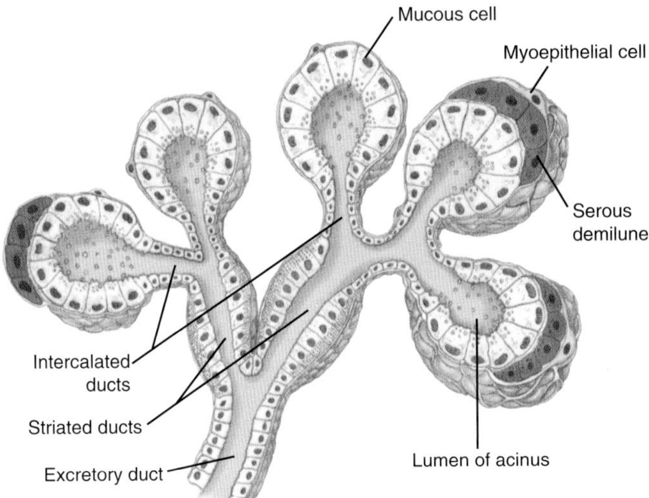

Fig. 11.6 Salivary Gland and its Ductal Epithelium. Note the serous demilunes on top of the mucous secretory cells of the mucous acini as well as the myoepithelial cells.

Although the capsulated parotid salivary gland is the largest major salivary gland, it provides only 25% of the total salivary volume. It is located in an area posterior to the mandibular ramus, anterior and inferior to the ear (see Fig. 11.7, *A*). The parotid gland has only serous acini, making the gland secrete a watery (or thin) serous secretory product as well as enzymes such as amylase (see Fig. 11.3).

The duct associated with the parotid gland is the parotid duct (or Stensen duct). This long duct emerges from the gland and then opens up into the oral cavity on the inner surface of the buccal mucosa, usually opposite the maxillary second molar at the parotid papilla (see Fig. 2.2).

The capsulated submandibular salivary gland is the second-largest major salivary gland, but it provides 60% to 65% of the total salivary volume. It lies beneath the mandible in the submandibular fossa, posterior to the sublingual salivary gland (see Fig. 11.7, *B*). However, because the submandibular gland has both serous and mucous acini with serous demilunes, the gland secretes a more viscous (or thick) mixed secretory product than the parotid, but it is mostly serous (see Fig. 11.4).

The duct associated with the submandibular gland is the submandibular duct (or Wharton duct). This long duct travels anteriorly on the floor of the mouth and opens into the oral cavity at each sublingual caruncle (see Fig. 2.17).

The sublingual salivary gland is the smallest, most diffuse, and the only major salivary gland without a capsule. It provides only 10% of the total salivary volume. It is located in the sublingual fossa, anterior to the submandibular salivary glands on the floor of the mouth (see Fig. 11.7, *C*). The sublingual gland has mostly mucous acini but with some mucous acini having serous demilunes. Thus the gland secretes a mixed secretory product, but with a predominately viscous mucous component (see Fig. 11.5).

The main duct associated with the sublingual gland is the sublingual duct (or Bartholin duct). The sublingual duct then opens into the oral cavity through the same opening as the submandibular duct, at each sublingual caruncle (see Fig. 2.17). Other smaller **duct(s) of Rivinus** (**reh**-vee-nuhs) of the sublingual gland at 8 to 20 in number also open directly along the sublingual folds.

Minor Salivary Glands

The **minor salivary glands** are much smaller than the major salivary glands but are more numerous. The minor salivary glands are also exocrine glands, but their unnamed ducts are shorter than those of any of the major salivary glands. The saliva secreted by minor salivary glands reaches the oral cavity through the short ducts that open directly onto oral mucosa surface. These glands are scattered in the tissue of the buccal, labial, and lingual mucosa, as well as the soft palate, lateral zones of the hard palate, and the floor of the mouth (Fig. 11.8).

Most minor salivary glands have mostly mucous acini, with a few having serous demilunes as well as also having a few serous acini. As a result, most minor salivary glands secrete a predominately viscous mucous secretory product with slight watery serous influence. The minor salivary glands allow a continuous slow secretory flow and thus have an important role in protecting and moistening the oral mucosa, especially at night when the major salivary glands are mostly inactive.

The exception to minor salivary glands that mostly have mucous acini is the **von Ebner salivary glands** (**von eb**-nuhr), which are associated with the larger circumvallate lingual papillae on the posterior part of the dorsal surface of the tongue (see Fig. 9.20). These glands contain only serous acini and thus secrete only a watery serous secretory product. The salivary flow from these glands "flush" the trough around the circumvallate allowing for new taste sensations when eating.

Salivary Gland Development

Between the sixth and eighth weeks of prenatal development, the three major salivary glands begin as epithelial proliferations or buds from the ectoderm lining of the primitive mouth. The rounded terminal ends of these epithelial buds grow into the underlying mesenchyme, producing the secretory cells of the glandular acini and the ductal system.

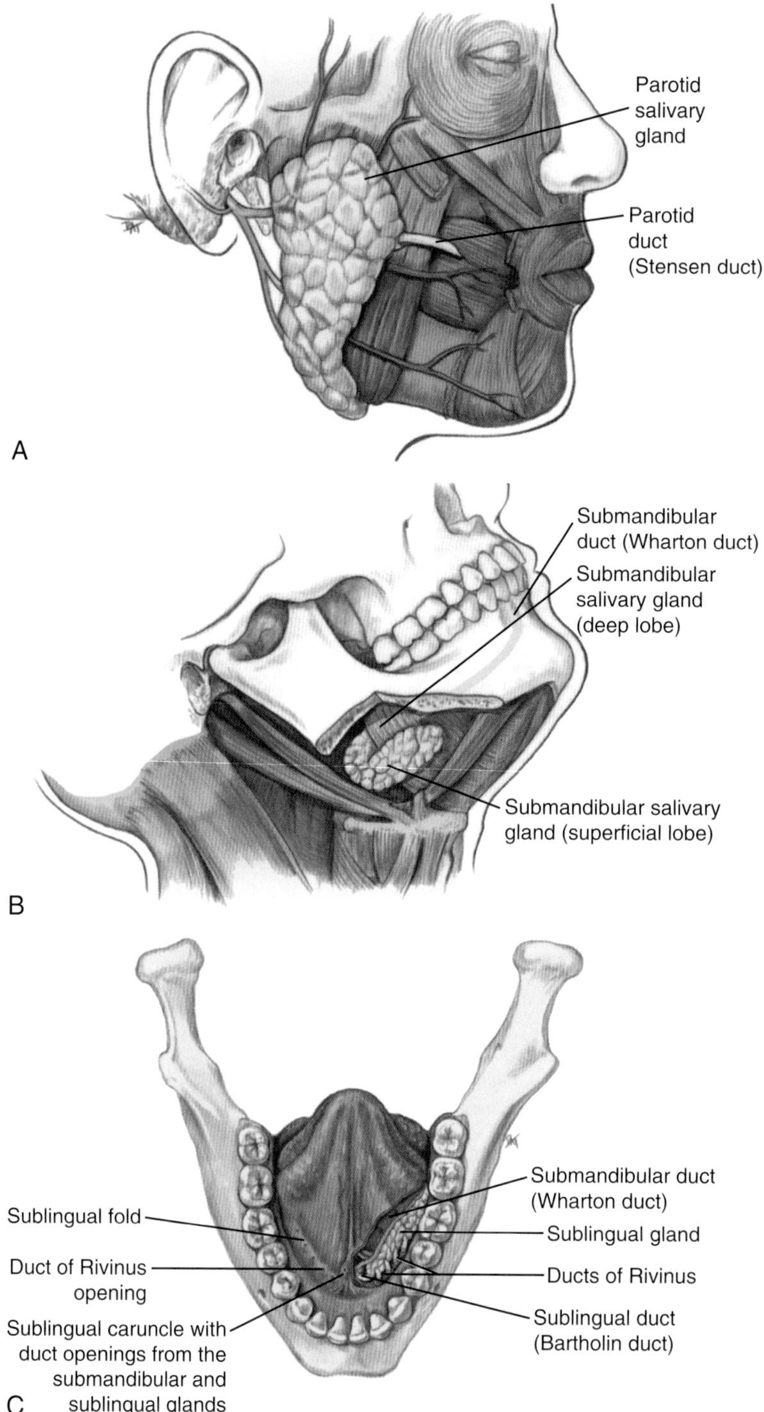

Fig. 11.7 Major Salivary Glands. **A,** Parotid. **B,** Submandibular. **C,** Sublingual with the tongue elevated and the floor of mouth sectioned. (**A** and **B,** From Fehrenbach MJ, Herring SW. *Illustrated Anatomy of the Head and Neck*. 5th ed. Philadelphia: Elsevier; 2017.)

The parts of the glands that contain supporting connective tissue, such as the outer capsule and inner septa, are produced from the mesenchyme, which is influenced by neural crest cells. It is important to note that interaction between the developing components of the epithelium, mesenchyme, nerves, and blood vessels is necessary for complete development of the salivary glands.

The parotid glands appear early in the sixth week of prenatal development and are the first major salivary glands formed. The epithelial buds of these glands are located on the inner part of the cheek, near the labial commissures of the primitive mouth. These buds grow posteriorly toward the otic placodes of the ears and branch to form solid cords with rounded terminal ends near the developing facial nerve.

Later at approximately 10 weeks of prenatal development, these cords are canalized and form ducts with the largest becoming the parotid duct for the parotid gland. The rounded terminal ends of the cords form the acini of the glands. Secretion by the parotid glands via the parotid duct begins at approximately 18 weeks of gestation. Again the supporting connective tissue of the gland develops from the surrounding mesenchyme.

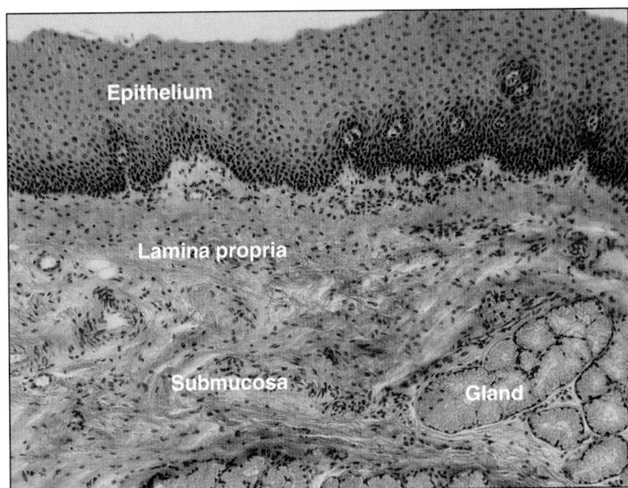

Fig. 11.8 Photomicrograph of a minor salivary gland located in the submucosa deep to the epithelium and lamina propria of the labial mucosa. The gland has mucous acini; most minor salivary glands have mostly mucous acini. The saliva secreted by minor salivary glands reaches the oral cavity through unnamed short ducts that open directly onto oral mucosa surface.

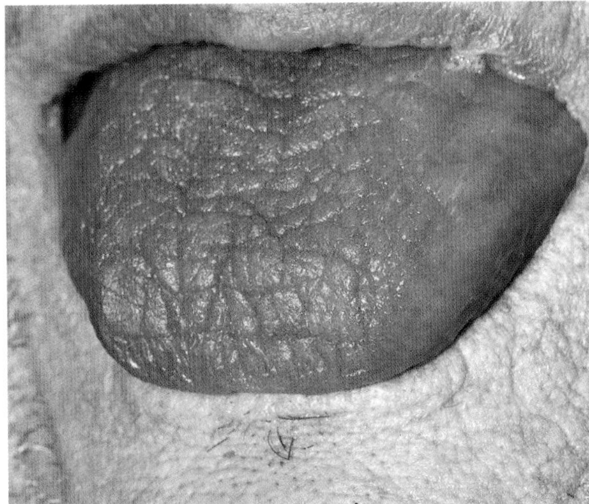

Fig. 11.9 Xerostomia (dry mouth) due to hyposalivation (reduced saliva production) in an aged oral cavity causing inflammation of the oral mucosa, including the tongue and lips. (Courtesy of Margaret J. Fehrenbach, RDH, MS.)

The submandibular glands develop later than the parotid glands and appear late in the sixth week of prenatal development. They develop bilaterally from epithelial buds in the sulcus surrounding the sublingual folds on the floor of the primitive mouth. Solid cords branch from the buds and grow posteriorly, lateral to the developing tongue.

The cords of the submandibular gland later branch further and then become canalized to form the ductal part. The submandibular gland acini develop from the cords' rounded terminal ends at 12 weeks, and secretory activity via the submandibular duct begins at 16 weeks. Growth of the submandibular gland continues after birth with the formation of more acini. Lateral to both sides of the tongue, a linear groove develops and closes over to form the submandibular duct.

The sublingual glands appear in the eighth week of prenatal development, later than the other two major salivary glands. They develop from epithelial buds in the sulcus surrounding the sublingual folds on the floor of the mouth, lateral to the developing submandibular gland. These buds branch and form into cords that canalize to form the sublingual ducts associated with the gland. The rounded terminal ends of the cords form acini.

Much like the major salivary glands, the minor salivary glands arise from both the ectoderm and endoderm associated with the primitive mouth. They then remain after development as small isolated acini and ducts within the oral mucosa or submucosa lining the mouth.

The contractile myoepithelial cells, which are important in the secretion of saliva from each acinus, arise from neural crest cells and thus are ectodermal in origin. They surround the developing acini as well as parts of the ductal system and become active between the 24th and 25th week of prenatal development.

Aging Salivary Glands

With the aging process, there is a generalized loss of salivary gland tissue; up to 30% to 60% loss has been demonstrated. Changes of the duct system have been also noted. Although decreased production of saliva is often observed in mature persons, whether this is related directly to the reduction in tissue has not been shown (discussed next). The process of aging does not seem to influence the production of resting saliva or unstimulated saliva production, but studies show that stimulated saliva production may be less than usual in mature individuals. The glands also contain occasional adipocytes (or fat cells), which increases with aging (see Fig. 11.3).

Clinical Considerations for Salivary Gland Pathology

Certain medications, disease processes, or destruction of salivary tissue may result in decreased production of saliva by salivary glands. The decreased production of saliva is considered **hyposalivation** (hahy-puh-sal-uh-**vey**-shuhn) and can result in or dry mouth or **xerostomia** (zeer-uh-**stoh**-mee-uh) (Fig. 11.9). Xerostomia can result in increased trauma to a nonprotected oral mucosa, increased cervical caries, speech and mastication problems, and bad breath or halitosis. The disease processes causing hyposalivation can include diabetes, Sjögren syndrome, and rheumatoid arthritis. Destruction occurs after radiation therapy for head and neck cancer because the salivary glands often are in the radiation field, and its cells are highly sensitive. Series of chemotherapies for cancer or bone marrow transplantation also may cause reduced salivary function.

Thus, important changes must be made in the dental treatment plan of the patients with xerostomia due to hyposalivation after checking that the source of the disturbance is not related to any disease processes (such as diabetes) that must first be dealt with directly. Such alterations in care include the recommendation of sipping water, artificial saliva use, remineralization products application such as fluoride (possibly silver diamine in the riskiest cases) and casein phosphopeptide-amorphous calcium phosphate (CPP-ACP), avoidance of alcohol-containing products, and increased recare visits. Medications that stimulate salivary production are available for nondrug-related hyposalivation. In addition, a micropressure sensor unit with a capsule to hold artificial salivary substitute can be placed within a dental prosthesis. Transplanting lost salivary tissue is now being performed in some cases of extreme xerostomia with hyposalivation.

The salivary glands may also become blocked, stopping the drainage of saliva from the duct. This blockage can cause glandular enlargement and tenderness resulting from retention of saliva in the gland. The blockage of the duct can result from either stone (or sialolith) formation or trauma to the duct opening on the surface of the oral cavity, such as biting the tissue.

This retention of saliva in the salivary gland can result in a **mucocele** (**myoo**-koh-seel) if it involves a minor salivary gland or a **ranula** (**ran**-yuh-luh) if it involves the sublingual salivary gland (Figs. 11.10 and 11.11). These two salivary gland lesions are treated by removal of the stone if involved or surgical removal of the entire gland in the case of a minor gland with severed duct.

Another oral lesion associated with salivary glands is **nicotinic stomatitis** (nik-uh-**tin**-ik stoh-muh-**tahy**-tis) (Fig. 11.12). With this lesion, the hard palate is whitened by hyperkeratinization caused by chronic heat production from smoking or hot liquid consumption (see **Chapter 9**). This chronic heat production also causes inflammation of the duct openings of the minor salivary glands of the palatal area, which become dilated in response. This inflammation of the ductal epithelium is seen clinically in the red macules scattered on the whiter background of the palatal oral mucosa.

Salivary biomarkers are used for testing, similarly to the secretions of urine and blood, for drug usage, systemic diseases, and changes in physiologic and psychological states, as well as oral cancer. Unlike the other bodily secretions, using saliva is very successful as a screening test because of the ease and low cost with which the sample can be obtained, removing the invasive nature of the diagnostic test.

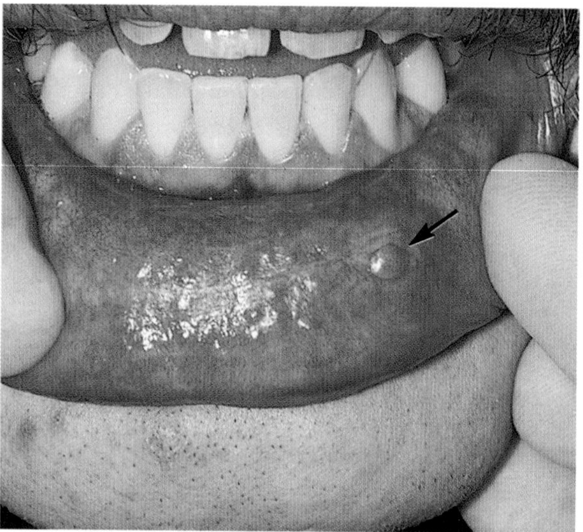

Fig. 11.10 Mucocele *(arrow)* on the lower lip as a bluish translucent enlargement involving the severance of the associated minor salivary gland duct and resulting in blockage of the gland resulting enlargement of the gland. (Courtesy of Margaret J. Fehrenbach, RDH, MS.)

THYROID GLAND PROPERTIES

The thyroid gland is the largest endocrine gland and is located in the anterior and lateral regions of the neck, inferior to the thyroid cartilage (see Fig. 1.13). Because it is ductless, the thyroid gland produces and secretes its products or hormones directly into the blood, such as thyroxine. **Thyroxine** (thahy-**rok**-sin) is a hormone that stimulates the metabolic rate. The gland consists of two lateral lobes connected anteriorly by an isthmus. In a healthy patient, the gland is not visible but can be palpated and should be mobile, moving superiorly with swallowing.

Thyroid Gland Histology

The thyroid gland is covered by a connective tissue capsule that then extends into the gland by way of septa (Fig. 11.13). The septa divide the gland into larger lobes and then smaller lobules. Each lobule is composed of **follicles** (**fol**-i-kuhls), irregularly shaped spheroidal masses that are embedded in a meshwork of reticular fibers. Each follicle consists of a layer of simple cuboidal epithelium enclosing a cavity that is usually filled with **colloid** (**kol**-oid), a stiff material reserved for the future production of thyroxine.

The parathyroid glands typically consist of four to eight small endocrine glands, two on each side, usually close to the thyroid gland or even inside it on its posterior surface. These glands are not visible or palpable during an extraoral examination of a patient. However, the parathyroid glands may alter the physiology of the thyroid gland because of their involvement in a disease process.

Thyroid Gland Development

The thyroid gland is the first endocrine gland to appear in embryonic development and develops from endoderm invaded by mesenchyme. At approximately the 24th day of prenatal development, the thyroid gland develops. It forms from a median downgrowth at the base of the tongue connected by a **thyroglossal duct** (thahy-roh-**gloss**-uhl), a narrow tube that later closes off and becomes obliterated (Fig. 11.14).

The foramen cecum, which is the opening of the thyroglossal duct, is a small pit-like depression located at the apex of the sulcus terminalis points where it points backward toward the oropharynx. This duct shows the origin of the thyroid and the migration pathway of the thyroid gland into the neck region (see Fig. 2.14, *A*).

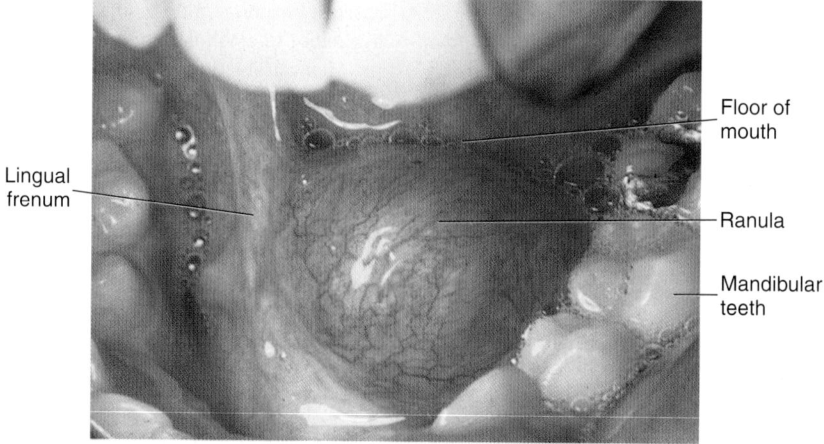

Fig. 11.11 Ranula as an enlargement or type of mucocele on one side of the floor of the mouth that involves the blockage of the sublingual salivary gland duct from stone formation resulting in enlargement of the gland. (Courtesy of Margaret J. Fehrenbach, RDH, MS.)

Clinical Considerations for Thyroid Gland Pathology

During a disease process involving the thyroid gland (such as an endocrine disorder), the gland may become enlarged and may be actually viewed during an extraoral examination. This enlarged thyroid gland is considered a **goiter** (**goi**-ter) (Fig. 11.15). A goiter may be firm and tender when palpated and may contain hard masses. Any patient who has any undiagnosed changes noted in the thyroid gland or complains of related symptoms should have a medical referral.

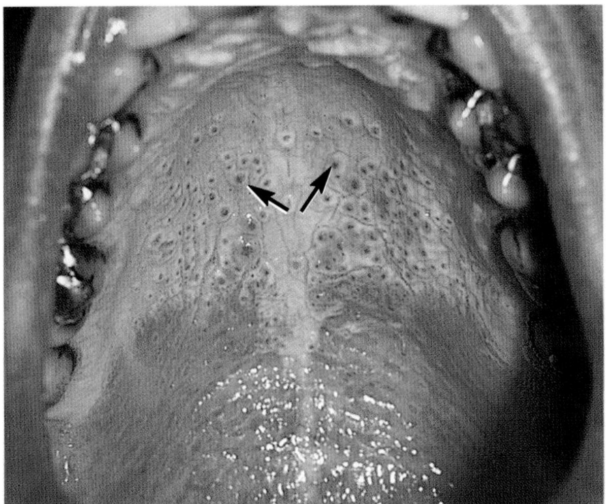

Fig. 11.12 Nicotinic stomatitis with hyperkeratinization of the palatal oral mucosa with its whiter clinical appearance and inflammation of the minor salivary glands ductal openings noted as redder areas *(arrows)*. This lesion can be from chronic heat production from smoking or hot liquid consumption. (Courtesy of Margaret J. Fehrenbach, RDH, MS.)

LYMPHATICS PROPERTIES

The **lymphatics** (lim-**fat**-iks) are a part of the immune system and help fight disease processes. They also serve other functions in the body. The lymphatic system consists of a network of lymphatic vessels linking lymph nodes throughout most of the body. **Tonsillar tissue** located in the oral cavity and pharynx is part of the lymphatic system. This chapter describes only the intraoral tonsillar tissue in detail; the tubal tonsillar tissue is not discussed.

The **lymphatic vessels** are a system of endothelial-lined channels that are mostly parallel to the venous blood vessels in location but are more numerous. Tissue fluid drains from the surrounding region into the lymphatic vessels as **lymph (limf).** Lymph is similar in composition to tissue fluid and plasma (see **Chapters 7 and 8**).

Each lymphatic vessel drains its particular region and all of these vessels communicate with one another. Lymphatic vessels are lined with endothelium similar to blood vessels, but the lymphatic vessels are larger and thicker in diameter than capillaries of the blood system. Lymphatic vessels are found within most of the oral tissue, even within the tooth's pulp.

Smaller lymphatic vessels containing lymph converge into the larger endothelial-lined **lymphatic ducts**, which empty into the venous system of the blood in the chest area. The drainage pattern of the lymphatic vessels into the lymphatic ducts depends on the side of the body involved, either the right or left, because the lymphatic ducts are different on each side.

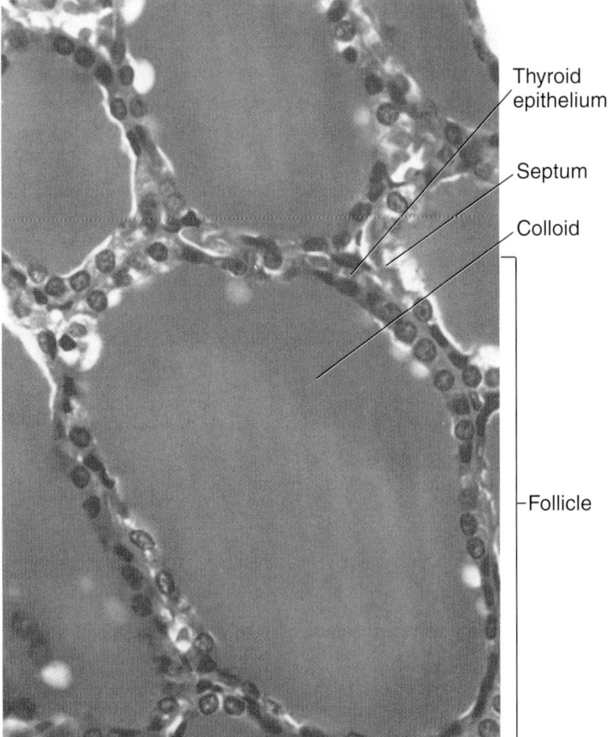

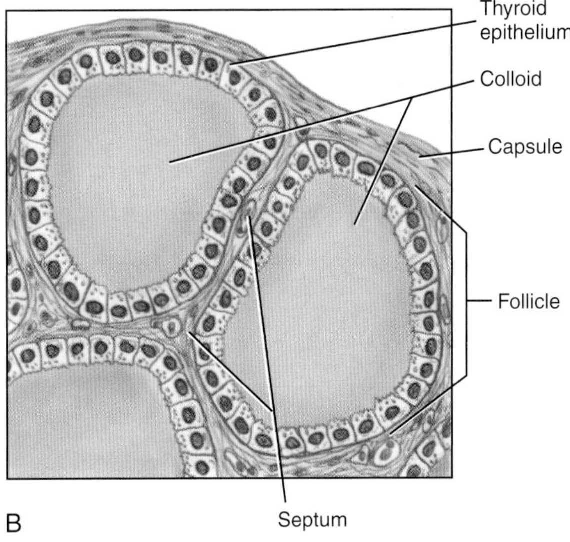

Fig. 11.13 Histology of the Thyroid Gland. **A,** Photomicrograph. **B,** Diagram. (**A,** From Young B, Woodford P, O'Dowd G. *Wheater's Functional Histology*. 4th ed. Edinburgh: Elsevier; 2000.)

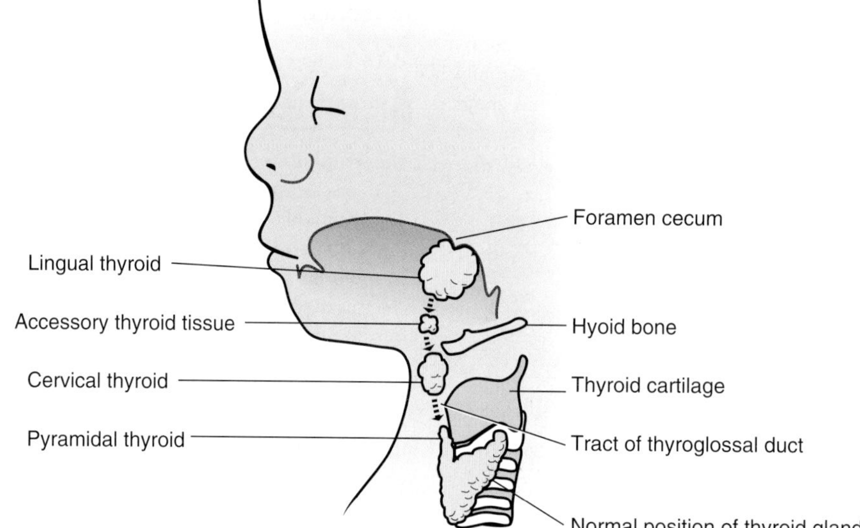

Fig. 11.14 Development of the thyroid gland from a median downgrowth of the tongue *(broken lines with arrows),* connected by a thyroglossal duct. Remnants of thyroid tissue can remain at these original sites and become cystic.

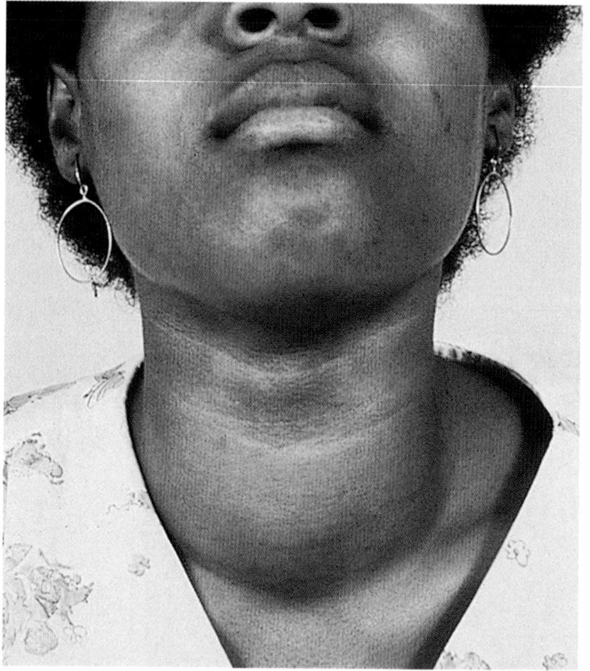

Fig. 11.15 Goiter or Enlarged Thyroid Gland Caused by an Endocrine Disorder. (Courtesy of Margaret J. Fehrenbach, RDH, MS.)

LYMPH NODES

The lymph nodes are bean-shaped bodies grouped in clusters along the connecting lymphatic vessels, positioned to filter toxic products from the lymph to prevent their entry into the blood system (Fig. 11.16, *A*). They are located in various regions of the head and neck area (see Figs. 1.2 and 1.12).

In healthy patients, lymph nodes are usually small, soft, and free or mobile in the surrounding tissue. They can be superficial in position with the smaller blood vessels or deep in the tissue with the larger blood vessels. Usually, lymph nodes cannot be seen or palpated during an extraoral examination of a healthy patient.

The lymph flows into the lymph node through many **afferent vessels**. On one side of the node is a depression or **hilus** (**hih**-luhs) (or hilum) where the lymph flows out of the node through fewer vessels or even a single **efferent vessel**. Lymph nodes can be classified as either primary or secondary nodes. Lymph from a particular tissue region drains into primary nodes (or regional nodes). Primary nodes, in turn, drain into secondary nodes (or central nodes).

Lymph Node Histology

Each lymph node is composed of organized lymphoid tissue and contains lymphocytes that actively filter toxic products from the lymph (see Fig. 8.16). The node itself is surrounded by a capsule with bands of connective tissue, the trabeculae, extending from the capsule into the node. The **trabeculae** (truh-**bek**-yuh-lee) separate the node into masses of lymphocytes, the **lymphatic nodules** (**naj**-oolz) (or lymphatic follicles). The lymph flows between the lymphatic nodules and other tissue spaces or sinuses.

Each lymphatic nodule has a **germinal center** (**jur**-muh-nl) containing many immature lymphocytes (see Fig. 11.16, *B*). As they mature, these lymphocytes enter either the area of the nodule surrounding the germinal center or the lymph. These mature lymphocytes are of the B-cell type and are usually involved in the humoral immune response with immunoglobulin production by the plasma cells (see Fig. 8.16).

Lymph Node Development

Lymphatic vessels develop from the blood vessels by a process of budding and fusion of isolated cell groups of mesenchyme. Peripherally located mesenchymal cells form the lymphatic nodules in the connective tissue associated with the developing lymphatic vessels. The sinuses then surround nodules, which completes the development of a lymph node. Later, a capsule and trabeculae will form around the developing lymphatic nodules from the surrounding mesenchyme.

INTRAORAL TONSILLAR TISSUE PROPERTIES AND HISTOLOGY

Intraoral tonsillar tissue consists of nonencapsulated masses of lymphoid tissue located in the lamina propria of the oral mucosa. It is covered by stratified squamous epithelium that is continuous with the surrounding oral mucosa. Tonsils, like lymph nodes, contain lymphocytes that remove toxic products and then move to the epithelial surface as they mature. Unlike lymph nodes, tonsillar tissue is not located along lymphatic vessels but is situated near airway and food passages to protect the body against disease processes from

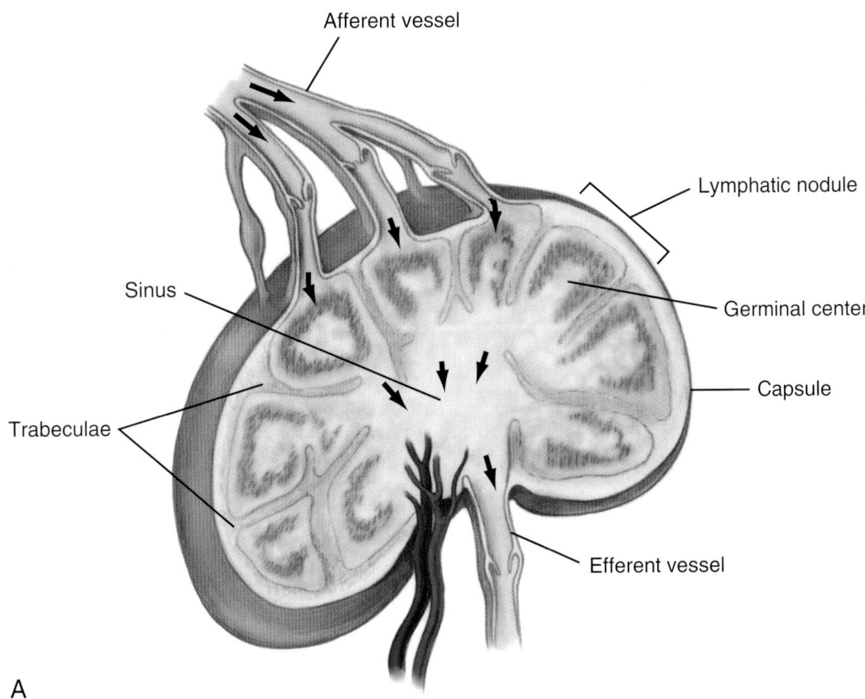

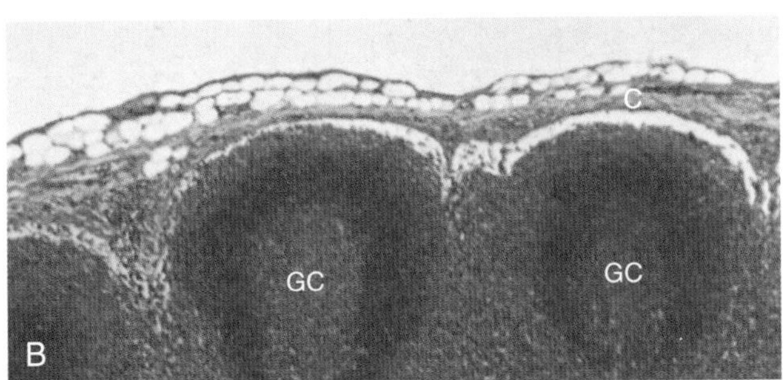

Fig. 11.16 Lymph Node and its Structure. A, Diagram showing entering of lymph by the afferent vessels and exiting by way of the efferent vessel *(arrows)*. **B,** Photomicrograph showing the lymphatic nodule with its germinal center *(GC)* and capsule *(C)*. (**A**, From Fehrenbach MJ, Herring SW. *Illustrated Anatomy of the Head and Neck*. 5th ed. Philadelphia: Elsevier; 2017. **B,** From Young B, Woodford P, O'Dowd G. *Wheater's Functional Histology*. 4th ed. Edinburgh: Elsevier; 2000.)

the related toxins. Tonsillar development is described in **Chapter 4**. The palatine tonsils are two rounded masses of variable size located between the anterior faucial pillar and posterior faucial pillar (see Fig. 2.11).

Microscopically each mass of intraoral tonsillar tissue contains fused-together lymphatic nodules that usually have germinal centers (Fig. 11.17). Each tonsil also has 10 to 20 epithelial invaginations or grooves, which penetrate deeply into the tonsil to form tonsillar crypts. These crypts usually contain shed epithelial cells, mature lymphocytes, and oral bacteria.

The lingual tonsil is an indistinct layer of diffuse lymphoid tissue located on the base of the dorsal surface of the tongue, posterior to the circumvallate lingual papillae (see Fig. 2.14, *A*). The lymphoid tissue consists of many lymphatic nodules, usually each with a germinal center and only one associated tonsillar crypt.

Behind the uvula and on the superior and posterior walls of the nasopharynx are the **pharyngeal tonsils**. When they become enlarged as is common in children, they are considered the *adenoids*. The pharyngeal tonsils along with the palatine and lingual tonsils form an incomplete ring of tissue around the inner pharynx, the **Waldeyer tonsillar ring** (val-**dahy**-er).

Clinical Considerations for Lymphoid Tissue Pathology

When a patient has an active disease process (such as cancer or infection) in a specific region, the region's lymph nodes respond. The resultant enlarged lymph node with its change in the consistency of its lymphoid tissue is from the process of **lymphadenopathy** (lim-fad-n-**op**-uh-thee). Lymphadenopathy is due to both an increase in the size of each individual lymphocyte and the overall cell count in the lymphoid tissue. With more and larger lymphocytes within the lymph node itself, the lymphoid tissue is better able to fight the disease process.

The presence of lymphadenopathy allows the node to now be easily palpated during an extraoral examination. More important, changes in consistency from firm to bony hard may occur. Palpation of an involved node may become painful and the node can as well become fixed and attached to the surrounding tissue.

Lymphadenopathy can also occur in the intraoral tonsillar tissue, causing tissue enlargement that can be viewed on an intraoral examination (Fig. 11.18). The intraoral tonsils may also be tender when swallowing. Severe lymphadenopathy may cause airway obstruction and complications from the infection of the tonsillar tissue. If any lymph nodes are palpable or if there is an enlargement or infection of intraoral tonsillar tissue, these findings should be noted in the patient record and a medical referral should be made.

The immune system with its inflammatory response and the associated lymphatics are also triggered with the development or progression of periodontal disease (see **Chapters 10 and 14**). In addition, during the immune system's response the liver releases nonspecific marker for inflammation, *C (cross)-reactive protein* (CRP), which allows for the recognition of periodontopathogens and damaged cells of the periodontium, attracting other inflammatory mediators to the damaged and infected site. The presence of CRP also marks the periodontopathogens for destruction by white blood cells; the primary white blood cells responsible for killing invading these pathogens are the neutrophils (see **Chapter 8**).

NASAL CAVITY PROPERTIES

The **nasal cavity** (**ney**-zuhl) is the inner space of the nose (Fig. 11.19). It communicates with the exterior by two nares. The nares are separated by the midline nasal septum, which consists of both bone and cartilage (see Fig. 1.4). The nasal septum also divides the internal nasal cavity into two parts.

Each lateral wall of the nasal cavity has three projecting structures or **nasal conchae** (**kong**-kee), which extend inward. Beneath each concha are openings through which the paranasal sinuses or nasolacrimal ducts communicate with the nasal cavity. The posterior part of the nasal cavity communicates with the nasopharynx and then with the rest of the respiratory system. The development of the nasal cavity and septum is described in **Chapter 5**.

NASAL CAVITY HISTOLOGY

The nasal cavity is lined by a respiratory mucosa like the rest of the respiratory system. **Respiratory mucosa** (**res**-per-uh-tawr-ee/**res**-per-uh-tohr-ee) is different from oral mucosa lining the oral cavity but similar to that lining the trachea and bronchi (see Fig. 8.2). It consists of ciliated

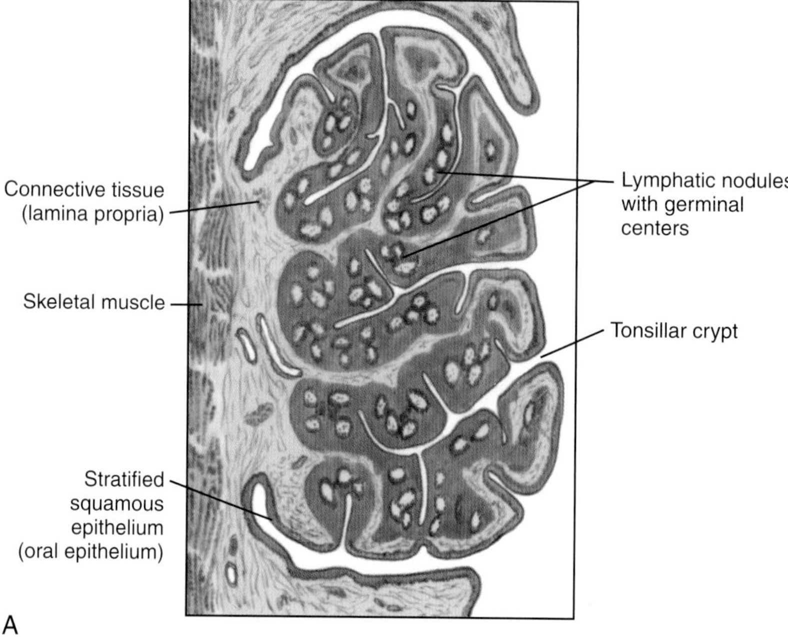

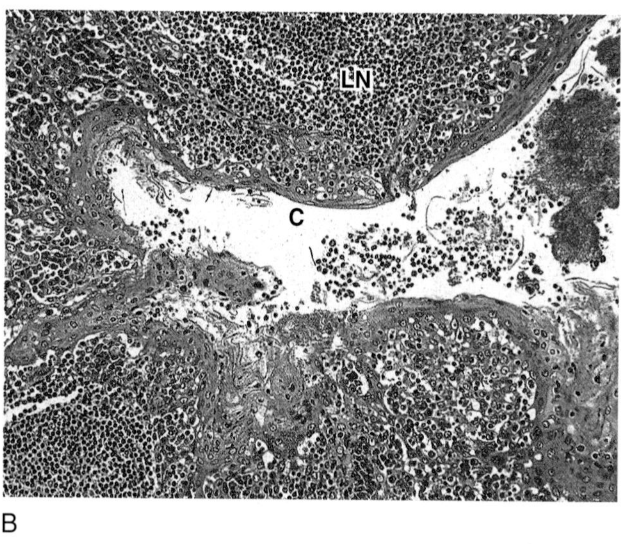

Fig. 11.17 Histology of the Palatine Tonsils. **A,** Diagram. **B,** Photomicrograph showing lymphatic nodule *(LN)* and the crypt *(C)* lined by epithelium. Note that the crypt usually contains oral bacteria. (**B,** From Stevens A, Lowe J. *Human Histology*. 5th ed. St. Louis: Elsevier; 2020.)

pseudostratified columnar epithelium (Fig. 11.20). Within the epithelium and surrounded by mucous and serous glands are **goblet cells** (**gob**-lit), which rest on the basement membrane. Fluids or mucus from the goblet cells and glands keep this mucosa moist, provide humidity, and trap any foreign materials from the inspired air.

The moist mucus forms a superficial coating on the respiratory mucosa. This coating is moved by ciliary action posteriorly to the nasopharynx, where it is either expectorated or swallowed. In this manner, foreign materials are trapped and removed. Because the lamina propria of the mucosa is extremely vascular, it also warms the incoming breathed air. In the roof of each part of the nasal cavity is a specialized region containing the **olfactory mucosa** (ol-**fak**-tuh-ree), which carries the receptors for the sense of smell.

Overlying the conchae is an extensive superficial plexus of large thin-walled vessels termed **erectile tissue** (ih-**rek**-tl). This tissue is capable of considerable engorgement. This engorgement happens at periodic intervals of 30 to 60 minutes, thus closing off the involved side of the nasal cavity to enable the respiratory mucosa to recover from the effects of dryness during respiration. The deepest parts of the lamina propria are continuous with the periosteum of the nasal bone or perichondrium of the nasal cartilage.

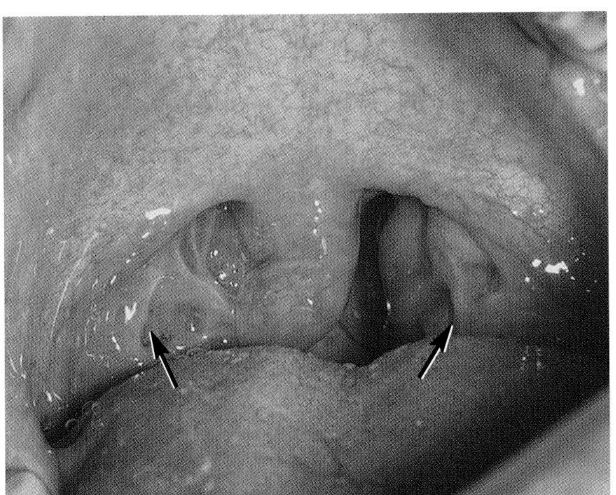

Fig. 11.18 Lymphadenopathy of the Palatine Tonsils *(arrows)* Showing Enlargement. (From Fehrenbach MJ, Herring SW. *Illustrated Anatomy of the Head and Neck.* 5th ed. Philadelphia: Elsevier; 2017.)

The respiratory mucosa of the nasal cavity and septum is continuous and similar to that of the nasopharynx (see Fig. 2.18). The respiratory mucosa of the nasopharynx gives way to the stratified squamous epithelium with the introduction of the oropharynx lining. The stronger stratified squamous epithelium of the oropharynx, with its soft palate and posterior wall of the pharynx, allows the mechanical stress of swallowing.

PARANASAL SINUSES PROPERTIES

The **paranasal sinuses** (pahr-uh-**ney**-zuhl **sahy**-nuhs-ez) are paired air-filled cavities in bone that include the frontal, sphenoidal, ethmoidal, and maxillary sinuses (Fig. 11.21). The sinuses communicate with the nasal cavity through small openings in the lateral nasal wall. The openings mark the outpouchings or evaginations from which the paranasal sinuses develop. The sinuses serve to lighten the skull bones, act as sound resonators, and provide mucus for the nasal cavity.

PARANASAL SINUSES HISTOLOGY

The sinuses are lined with respiratory mucosa consisting of ciliated pseudostratified columnar epithelium continuous with the epithelial lining of the nasal cavity (see Figs. 8.2 and 11.20). The epithelium of the sinuses, although it is similar to that of the nasal cavity, is thinner and contains fewer goblet cells. The respiratory mucosa of the sinuses also shows a thinner underlying lamina propria that is continuous with the deeper periosteum of the bone. It also has fewer associated glands and no erectile tissue is present in the sinuses.

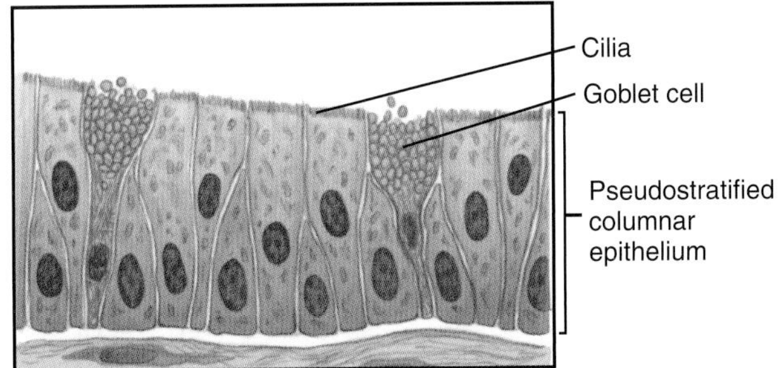

Fig. 11.20 Histology of the Respiratory Mucosa Lining the Nasal Cavity.

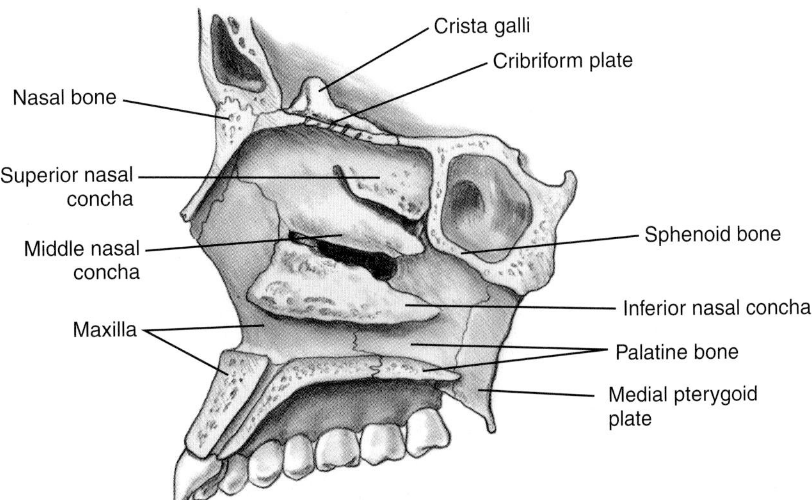

Fig. 11.19 Nasal Cavity and its Nasal Conchae. (From Fehrenbach MJ, Herring SW. *Illustrated Anatomy of the Head and Neck.* 5th ed. Philadelphia: Elsevier; 2017.)

PARANASAL SINUSES DEVELOPMENT

Certain sinuses develop during late fetal life; the rest develop after birth. They form as outgrowths of the wall of the nasal cavity and become air-filled extensions in the adjacent bones. The original openings of the outgrowths persist as orifices of the adult sinuses.

The maxillary sinuses are small at birth and only a few of the ethmoidal sinuses are present. The maxillary sinuses grow until puberty and are not fully developed until all the permanent teeth have erupted in early adulthood. The ethmoidal sinuses do not start to grow until 6 to 8 years of age.

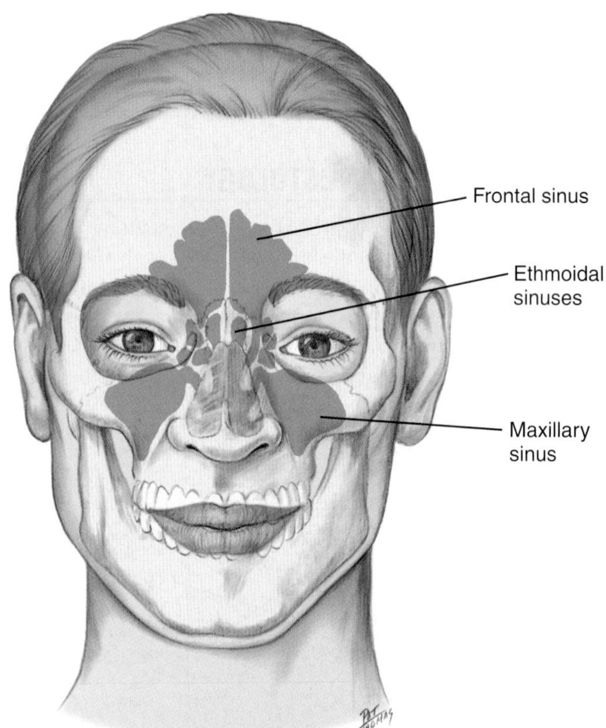

Fig. 11.21 Paranasal Sinuses: Frontal, Ethmoidal, Maxillary. Sphenoidal sinus is not shown in this view because it is deep to the ethmoidal sinuses. (From Fehrenbach MJ, Herring SW. *Illustrated Anatomy of the Head and Neck*. 5th ed. Philadelphia: Elsevier; 2017.)

The frontal sinuses and sphenoidal sinuses are not present at birth. At approximately 2 years of age, the two anterior ethmoidal sinuses grow into the frontal bone, forming the frontal sinus on each side and are visible on radiographs of the region by the seventh year. At the same time, the two posterior ethmoidal sinuses grow into the sphenoid bone and form the sphenoidal sinuses. Growth of sinuses in the size and shape of the face is important during infancy and childhood and adds resonance to the voice during puberty.

 Clinical Considerations for Nasal Cavity and Paranasal Sinus Pathology

The respiratory mucosa of the nasal cavity and paranasal sinuses can become inflamed and the space congested with mucus as a result of allergies or respiratory tract infection. This inflammation can lead to a stuffed-up feeling in the nasal cavity and **sinusitis** (sahy-nuh-**sahy**-tis) within the sinus. The symptoms for both are discomfort caused by the pressure of the increased mucus production with nasal or pharyngeal discharge.

With blocked nasal passages and with sinusitis, medications are used to produce vasoconstriction in the blood vessels while reducing the amount of mucus produced. In cases of chronic sinusitis, surgical treatment may be needed. Patients undergoing these respiratory difficulties may not be able to successfully use nitrous oxide and may feel uncomfortable with the use of a rubber dam. This patient may continually breathe through the mouth instead of their nasal passages, causing chronic gingivitis of the maxillary anterior teeth, from the drying of the tissue. In all cases, a medical consult is needed.

Because the roots of the maxillary posterior teeth are in close proximity to the maxillary sinus, maxillary sinusitis can sometimes result as infection spreads from a periapical abscess associated with one of the roots of a maxillary posterior tooth (Fig. 11.22). As the infection spreads, the sinus floor becomes perforated and the mucosa of the sinus becomes involved in the infection. During an extraction, a contaminated tooth or root fragments can also be surgically displaced into the maxillary sinus. In addition, because of their close proximity, the pain from maxillary sinusitis can sometimes be mistakenly misinterpreted by the patient as involving the maxillary teeth instead of the sinus(es) (see **Chapter 17**). Differential diagnosis of the symptoms and radiographs, including cone-beam computed tomography (CBCT), can aid in determining the correct cause for this facial pain.

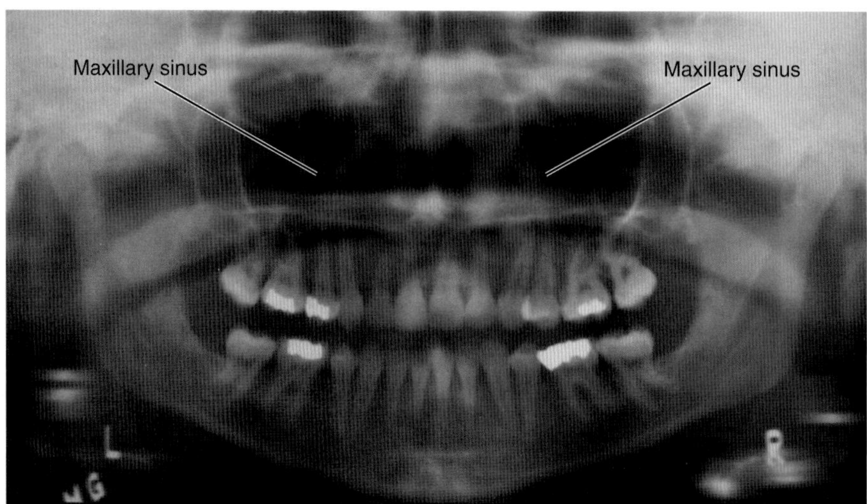

Fig. 11.22 Panoramic radiograph demonstrating that the roots of the maxillary posterior teeth are in close proximity to the maxillary sinuses. (Courtesy of Margaret J. Fehrenbach, RDH, MS.)

12

Enamel

Additional resources and practice exercises are provided on the companion Evolve website for this book: http://evolve.elsevier.com/Fehrenbach/illustrated.

LEARNING OBJECTIVES

1. Define and pronounce the key terms in this chapter.
2. Describe the enamel properties and the clinical considerations concerned with enamel structure, integrating it into patient care.
3. Discuss the processes involved in the apposition and maturation stages of enamel as well as the clinical considerations concerned with enamel formation and pathology, integrating it into patient care.
4. Identify the components of the enamel on a diagram.
5. Discuss the histology of enamel and the clinical considerations for dental procedures concerning enamel, integrating it into patient care.

ENAMEL PROPERTIES

Preservation of the enamel of every tooth during a patient's lifetime is one of the goals of every dental professional because it is not a renewable tissue. Dental professionals must take into consideration the properties and histology of enamel when diagnosing enamel caries, deciding the caries risk for patients, counseling patients and communities on fluoride use, applying enamel sealants as well as restorations, and using and recommending polishing or toothpaste agents (discussed later).

Mature enamel is a crystalline material that is the hardest mineralized tissue in the body (Table 12.1; see Table 6.2). Enamel can endure crushing pressure of around 100,000 pounds per square inch. A layering of the deeper dentin and surrounding periodontium, coupled with the hardness of the enamel, produces a cushioning effect of the tooth's differing structures enabling it to endure the pressures of mastication.

In its mature state, it is noted for its almost total absence of the softer organic matrix; enamel contains no collagen. Enamel in a healthy state, without trauma or disease, can be removed only by rotary cutting instruments or rough files, such as those used in dental practice. Enamel is avascular and has no nerve supply within it. Although enamel is the hardest mineralized tissue in the body, it can be lost forever because it is nonvital and therefore not a renewable tissue. However, it is not a static tissue because it can undergo mineralization changes (discussed later).

Mature enamel is by weight 96% inorganic material or mineralized, 1% organic material, and 3% water. This crystalline formation of mature enamel consists mostly of calcium hydroxyapatite with the chemical formula of $Ca_{10}(PO_4)_6(OH)_2$. The calcium hydroxyapatite is similar to that found in lesser percentages in dentin, cementum, and the alveolar process. On radiographs, the differences in the mineralization of different parts of the tooth and surrounding periodontium can be noted (see Fig. 2.5). Enamel appears more radiopaque (or lighter) than either dentin and pulp or surrounding periodontium because it is denser than the latter structures, both of which appear more radiolucent (or darker).

Other minerals, such as carbonate, magnesium, potassium, sodium, and fluoride, are also present in smaller amounts. Studies have challenged this composition of enamel, and, instead, maintain that it is mostly carbonated hydroxyapatite because of its relationship with fluoride uptake. Whatever the true composition, the ribbon-like crystals of enamel are set at different angles throughout the crown area, each 30% larger than those in dentin. The sheer size difference of enamel and dentinal crystals is a leading factor contributing to enamel's hardness over dentin. Discussion of the elegant crystalline nature of enamel is inadequate at best, but this chapter is an attempt to do justice to this beautiful jewel-like material.

Enamel is usually the only part of a tooth that is seen clinically in a healthy oral cavity because it covers the anatomic crown (see Fig. 15.8). Enamel provides a hard surface for mastication and speech; it is able to withstand the masticatory impact of 20 to 30 pounds of pressure per tooth. Enamel shows a thinner layer in the cervical region and is thicker in masticatory surfaces, such as at the incisal ridge and cusps, where impact can be greater. Thickness can also range per tooth type from 0 to 2 mm for incisors to 2.6 mm for molars.

With this thickness and its crystalline nature, enamel forms an insulating barrier that protects the tooth from physical, thermal, and chemical forces that would otherwise be injurious to the vital tissue in the underlying dentin and pulp.

Enamel also provides the pleasing whiteness of a healthy smile. Enamel alone is various shades of bluish white, which is seen on the incisal ridge of newly erupted incisors, but it turns various shades of yellow-white elsewhere because of the underlying dentin (see Fig. 16.8, *A*). The enamel on primary teeth has an increased level of opaque crystalline form and thus appears whiter than on permanent teeth (see Fig. 15.4).

Because the overall shade of enamel varies in each person and even within a dentition, a shade value is taken when integrating tooth-colored restorative materials or artificial teeth or crowns within an individual dentition. The goal is to match the color of the patient's surrounding natural teeth as closely as possible. This shade value is selected by comparing the patient's natural teeth to a shade guide of plastic model crowns that have been moistened and are viewed in natural light. New technology allows a digital read-out of the color of the enamel (vital whitening process or bleaching is discussed later.)

Clinical Considerations with Enamel Structure

One way that enamel and other hard tissue of the tooth are lost is through **attrition** (uh-**trish**-uhn), which is the wearing of hard tissue as a result of tooth-to-tooth contact (Table 12.2). The wear on masticatory surfaces from attrition increases with aging. Over time, the permanent first molars wear more than seconds; the seconds wear more than thirds. However, attrition can occur at severe levels in a shorter amount of time and involve an excessive loss of enamel, which is discussed further in **Chapter 20** with regard to parafunctional habits (see also Figs. 16.8, *B*, 16.17, 16.24, and 20.8). The relationship between attrition, the loss of the vertical dimension of the face, and related alveolar process loss is discussed in **Chapter 14**.

Occlusal or incisal surfaces worn by attrition are called **wear facets**. When active tooth grinding with bruxism parafunctional habit occurs, the enamel rods are fractured and become highly reflective to light. The angle of the wear facet on the tooth surface is potentially significant to the periodontium. Horizontal facets tend to direct forces on the vertical axis of the tooth to which the periodontium can adapt most effectively. Angular facets direct occlusal forces laterally and increase the risk of periodontal damage.

Enamel loss may also result from friction caused by excessive toothbrushing and abrasive toothpaste. This wear of enamel is considered **abrasion** (uh-**brey**-zhuhn). Dental personnel must keep this in mind when discussing homecare with patients and explain that there is no need to harshly treat the teeth in order to keep them healthy.

Enamel can also be lost by **erosion** (ih-**roh**-zhuhn) through chemical means. Erosion is particularly apparent in patients with the eating disorder of bulimia, in which patients force themselves to vomit to remove their stomach contents in pursuit of weight loss (Fig. 12.1, *A*). The lingual surface of the maxillary anterior teeth and the occlusal surface of maxillary posterior teeth are eroded by the acid content of the vomit; it can also be considered in this case to be *perimolysis*. The yellow underlying dentin is thereby exposed and can undergo attrition because it is less mineralized than enamel. Treatment of bulimia is multifactorial and includes behavior changes. Similar erosion can be caused by gastric reflux as well as certain recreational drug use (e.g., methamphetamine abuse with "meth mouth"). If facial enamel lesions of the anterior teeth are evident, the patient may be overusing acid-containing carbonated drinks (including soft, sport, or health formulations especially "diet" formulations and those containing citric acid).

Another way that enamel can be lost is by **enamel caries.** Caries is a process through which a cavity is created by demineralization or loss of minerals. This demineralization is due to acid production by cariogenic bacteria and occurs to enamel when the pH is less than 5.5 (see later discussion in this chapter).

Finally, enamel can be lost as a result of **abfraction** (ab-**frak**-shuhn) (see Fig. 12.1, *B*). Abfraction is caused by increasing the tensile and compressive forces during tooth flexure, which may occur during parafunctional habits with their occlusal loading (see **Chapter 20**). It consists of cervical lesions that cannot be attributed to any particular cause such as erosion or toothbrush abrasion. Abfraction causes the enamel to actually "pop off" from the dentin layers, starting at the cervical region, thus exposing the lesion to possible further wear, dentinal hypersensitivity, or caries.

The type of tooth surface polishing agent used by dental professionals as well as by patients at home is also a very important consideration

TABLE 12.1 Comparison of Physical Properties of Enamel and Dentin

Physical Property	Enamel	Dentin
Specific gravity	2.9	2.14
Hardness (Knoop number)	296	64
Stiffness (Young modulus)	131 GN/m^2	12 GN/m^2
Compressive strength	76 MN/m^2	262 MN/m^2
Tensile strength	46 MN/m^2	33 MN/m^2

GN, Giganewtons (N × 109); *MN*, meganewtons (N × 106).
From Nanci A. *Ten Cate's Oral Histology*. 9th ed. St. Louis: Elsevier; 2018.

TABLE 12.2 Enamel Structure Loss

Method	Features	Clinical Appearance
Attrition	Loss through tooth-to-tooth contact from mastication with aging or more severely with parafunctional habits	• Matching wear on masticatory surfaces • Shiny facets on amalgam contacts • Enamel and dentin wear at the same rate • May have fracture of cusps or restorations
Abrasion	Loss through friction from toothbrushing and/or toothpaste	• Usually located at facial cervical regions • Lesions more wide than deep • Canines commonly affected because of tooth position
Erosion	Loss through chemical means (via acid) not involving bacteria	• Broad concavities within smooth surface enamel • Cupping of occlusal surface (or incisal grooving) with dentin exposure (with possible dentinal hypersensitivity) • Increased incisal translucency • Wear on nonmasticatory surfaces (exact location depends on acid intake type) • Raised and shiny amalgam restorations • Preservation of enamel cuff in gingival crevice • Pulp exposure and loss of surface characteristics of enamel in primary teeth
Caries	Loss through chemical means (via acid) from cariogenic bacteria by way of dental biofilm	• All surfaces can be affected • Occlusal surfaces more commonly affected, especially in pits and grooves • May have rapid progression of interproximal smooth surface lesions if progress goes unchecked • Cervical lesions sometimes secondary to other forms of hard tissue loss or gingival recession
Abfraction	May have loss through tensile and compressive forces during tooth flexure with parafunctional habits	• Can affect both facial and lingual cervical regions • Deep and narrow V-shaped notch • Commonly affects single teeth that have occlusal loads

in retaining enamel structure. Older toothpastes and professional polishing agents abraded the enamel surface, removing valuable tooth layers to obtain temporary esthetic results (vital whitening of enamel is discussed later). Selective polishing methods by dental professionals are now used only to remove extrinsic stain on natural enamel surfaces; many clinicians use ultrasonic devices for the majority of the removal instead because it is faster and prevents overall enamel removal. However, the use of less abrasive professional and homecare polishing agents, such as with the newer air polishing agents (glycine), helps preserve the limited enamel on the crowns. It is also not necessary to polish the teeth to remove dental biofilm before topical fluoride application or in many cases before enamel sealant placement.

There are models now being tested that can rebuild lost enamel structure in order to replace conventional restorative methods that use artificial materials like composites, ceramics, and amalgam to restore functional properties. These biomimetic methods are designed to rebuild the intricate apatite crystallite structure by application of calcium phosphate chemistry that stimulates the regrowth of the involved tissue and ideally restores the mechanic and optic properties of enamel.

ENAMEL MATRIX FORMATION

Amelogenesis is formation of enamel matrix that occurs during the apposition stage of tooth development. The exact time of the apposition stage for each tooth varies according to the tooth that is undergoing development. Many factors can affect amelogenesis (see Fig. 6.16).

Enamel matrix is produced by ameloblasts during its secretory phase (Fig. 12.2). Each ameloblast is approximately 4 micrometers in diameter, 40 micrometers in length, and is hexagonal or six-sided in a cross section. The ameloblasts are columnar cells that differentiate during the apposition stage in the crown area. Ameloblasts are not differentiated in the root area; therefore the enamel is usually just confined to the anatomic crown.

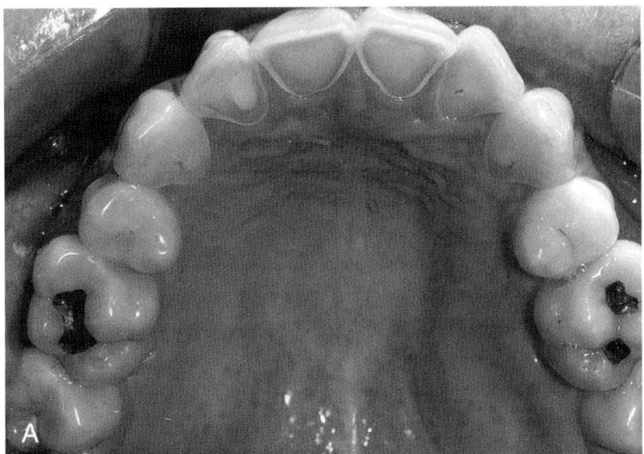

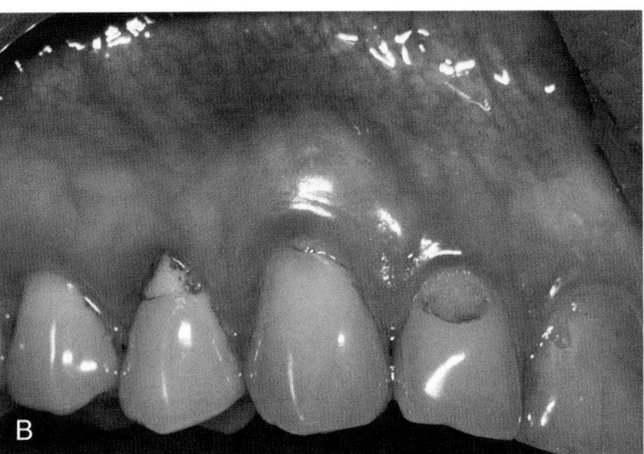

Fig. 12.1 Enamel Loss. **A,** Lingual erosion in a patient with a past history of bulimia. Note that the facial surface of the permanent maxillary central incisors has been restored using veneers because of the amount of hard tissue loss from *perimolysis*, which caused the teeth to look even more transparent and gray in tone. **B,** Abfraction of the maxillary right quadrant, especially on the permanent maxillary lateral incisor, with the permanent maxillary first premolar already restored once but now has secondary enamel caries around the margins. (Courtesy of Margaret J. Fehrenbach, RDH, MS.)

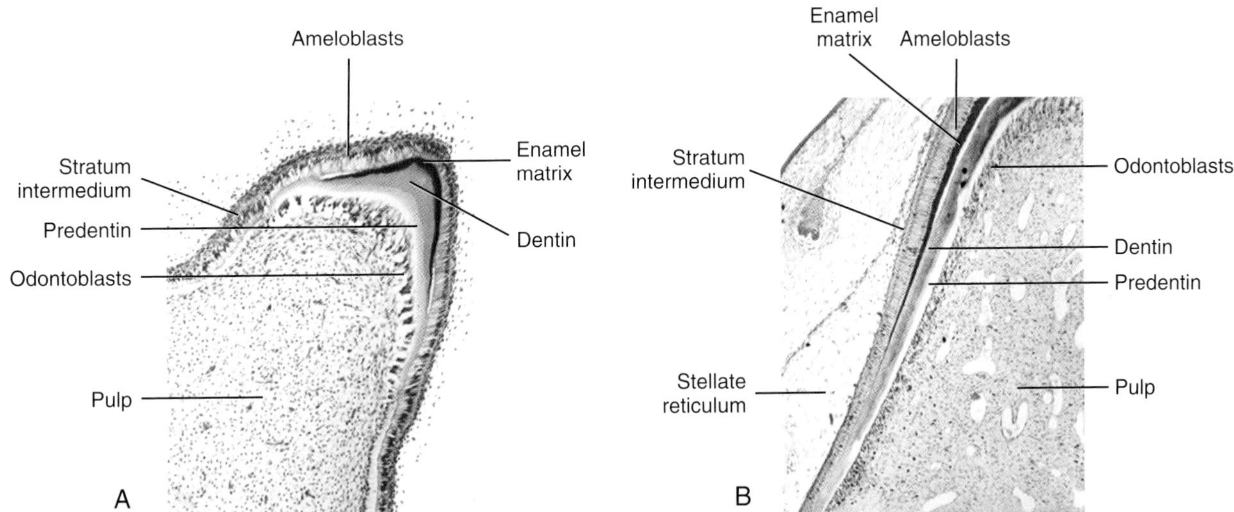

Fig. 12.2 Photomicrographs of a Tooth Undergoing Matrix Formation of Both Enamel and Dentin. **A,** Dentin already showing maturation. **B,** Close-up view shows ameloblasts producing enamel matrix from their Tomes processes. (Courtesy of P. Tambasco de Oliveira, PhD.)

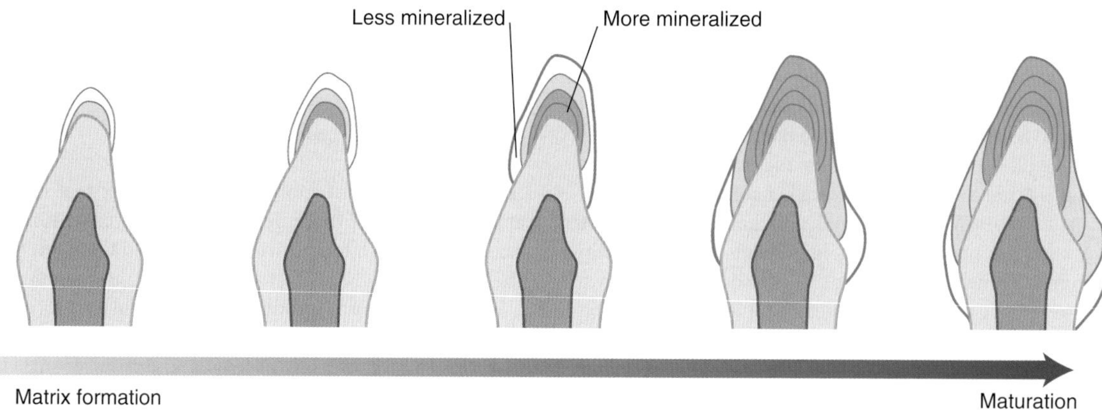

Fig. 12.3 Wave Patterns in the Crown from the Time of Enamel Matrix Formation to Maturation of Enamel.

The enamel matrix is secreted from each ameloblast from its own Tomes process with its "picket-fence" microscopic structure (see Figs. 6.12 and 12.2, *B*). Tomes process is not a true separate process, but instead it is a projection of the basal or secretory end of each ameloblast that faces the dentinoenamel junction (DEJ). This is unlike the process associated with the odontoblast, which is a true cytoplasmic process separate from a cell body. However, like the odontoblasts on the other side of the DEJ, ameloblasts produce approximately 4 micrometers of enamel matrix daily during tooth development.

Tomes process is responsible for the way the enamel matrix is laid down; it is the guiding factor similar to a snowplow going through a snowy parking lot. First, the body of the cell located between the processes deposits its enamel matrix between the ameloblasts, which will become the periphery of the enamel rods, forming an outside mold for the enamel between the enamel rods, the interrod enamel or interprismatic region, which is discussed later with the rods. Secondly, the Tomes process of individual ameloblasts will infill the future main body of the enamel rod. Thus there is a one-to-one relationship between the secretory face of Tomes process and each enamel rod produced. However, multiple ameloblasts contribute to the enamel between the enamel rods at the interrod enamel or interprismatic region.

Enamel matrix is an ectodermal product because ameloblasts are derived from the inner enamel epithelium of the enamel organ, which was originally derived from the ectoderm of the embryo. Initially, enamel matrix is composed of proteins, carbohydrates, and only a small amount of calcium hydroxyapatite crystals. Unlike dentin, cementum, and the alveolar process that are mesodermal products, enamel does not contain collagen protein. Instead, it has two unique classes of proteins, amelogenins and ameloblastin, as well as enamelins, the latter being very similar to keratin.

Because it only has a small amount of calcium, the initial enamel matrix is therefore only partially mineralized as compared with fully matured or mineralized enamel (discussed later). Ameloblasts are also responsible for this partially mineralized state of the enamel matrix; they actively pump calcium into the enamel matrix in order to form hydroxyapatite as matrix is secreted. Enamel matrix is first formed in the incisal or occlusal part of the future crown nearer to the forming DEJ (Fig. 12.3). This is the first wave of enamel appositional growth on the masticatory surface and later moves to the nonmasticatory surface. The second wave of enamel appositional growth overlaps the first wave with the entire process moving cervically to the cementoenamel junction (CEJ). This is discussed in more detail in the next section in regards to enamel matrix maturation. The morphology of the CEJ is discussed further in **Chapter 14.**

Clinical Considerations During Enamel Formation

Certain developmental disturbances, such as an enamel pearl and enamel dysplasia, can occur in enamel during the apposition stage for enamel (see Box 6.1, *O-P*). Another common developmental disturbance is the deepened **pit and groove patterns** on the lingual surface of anterior teeth and on the occlusal surface of posterior teeth (see **Chapters 16 and 17**; Figs. 16.10 and 17.8). These are created when ameloblasts back into one another during the apposition stage, cutting off their source of nutrition. This loss of nutritional support causes incomplete maturation of enamel matrix, making it weak or even absent in that area. These areas of incompletely matured enamel can lead to enamel caries with the presence of a supporting environment (discussed later in this chapter).

ENAMEL MATRIX MATURATION

During the maturation stage of tooth development, enamel matrix completes its mineralization process to its full level of 96% after the apposition stage when it is only partially mineralized at approximately 30%. Thus, mineralization of enamel matrix to a fully matured tissue actually covers two stages of tooth development—the apposition and maturation stages. Enamel mineralization also continues after eruption of the tooth (discussed next).

During the maturation of enamel matrix, ameloblasts move from production to actively transporting materials for mineralization by undergoing cellular modulation in cycles that correspond to mineralization waves that travel across the crown of a developing tooth from least mature regions to most mature regions of the enamel (discussed next). First the cells accomplish the removal of water and organic material from the enamel. This allows introduction of additional inorganic material next into the already partially mineralized enamel. Thus the ameloblasts are specifically responsible for maturation of enamel matrix into mature enamel.

Two waves of enamel mineralization during the maturation stage follow the same pattern as that of the apposition stage (see Fig. 12.3). The first wave of enamel mineralization occurs in the incisal or occlusal part of the future crown nearer to the DEJ and moves to the nonmasticatory surface. The second wave of enamel mineralization overlaps the first wave as the process moves cervically to the forming CEJ.

After the ameloblasts are finished with both enamel appositional growth and maturation, they become part of the reduced enamel epithelium (REE) along with the other tissue types within the compressed enamel organ (see Figs. 6.23 and 6.24). The ameloblasts undergo a reduction in height and a decrease in their volume and

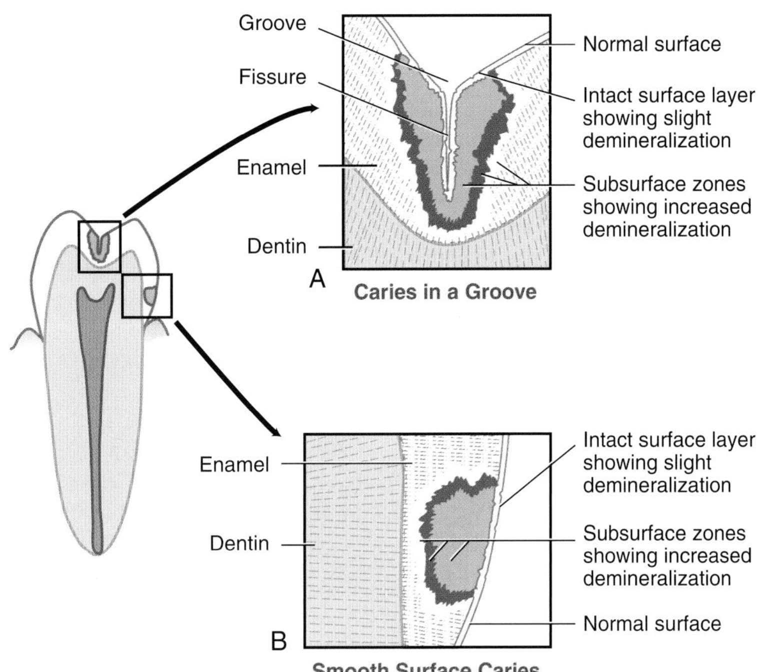

Fig. 12.4 Process of Enamel Caries Demonstrating the Different Zones for the Two Main Types of Caries. **A,** Caries in a groove. **B,** Smooth surface caries. Note that both types initially have an intact surface layer with slight demineralization and that the increased demineralization of caries occurs mostly in the subsurface zones.

organelle content. The REE will later fuse with the oral mucosa, creating a protective tunnel to allow the enamel cusp tip to erupt through the oral mucosa into the oral cavity (see Fig. 6.25, *D*). Unfortunately, the ameloblasts are lost forever as the fused tissue disintegrates during tooth eruption, preventing any further enamel appositional growth. The entire tissue can later become part of Nasmyth membrane (see Fig. 6.29).

Enamel is not a renewable tissue because there is no way to retrieve the lost ameloblasts and then have them become involved in tissue regeneration of enamel. Research now involves the study of **amelogenins** (am-uh-loh-**jen**-inz), which comprise the principal extracellular matrix protein component involved in the process of mineralizing enamel. Amelogenins may play a substantial role in controlling the growth and organization of enamel crystals, which may be able to be harnessed for enamel replacement after enamel loss through caries or other pathology (discussed next).

After the tooth erupts into the oral cavity, however, the mineralization of enamel continues. This posteruptive maturation is due to the deposition of minerals, such as fluoride and calcium, from saliva into hypomineralized areas of enamel (see discussion of fluoride next). And a forced type of enamel mineralization through therapeutic means is also helpful to the preservation of the tooth.

Clinical Considerations with Enamel Pathology

A **noncavitated lesion** (nohn-kav-i-**tey**-ted) refers to initial (or incipient) caries lesion development before cavitation occurs. Noncavitated lesions are characterized by a change in color, glossiness, or surface structure as a result of demineralization before there is a macroscopic breakdown in surface tooth structure. In the pits and grooves and on smooth surfaces these noncavitated lesions are first noted clinically in many cases as a *white-spot lesion*, with the involved enamel appearing whiter and rougher as a result of slight surface demineralization of the enamel.

These lesions represent areas with net mineral loss due to an imbalance between demineralization and remineralization. Remineralization is the deposition of minerals into mature enamel from salivary minerals and fluoride or other therapies (discussed later). Reestablishing a balance between demineralization and remineralization may stop the caries disease process while leaving a visible clinical sign of past disease.

As discussed earlier, the weak areas of deepened pits and grooves are targets for enamel caries (Fig. 12.4, *A*). Dental biofilm can become sheltered in these irregular areas or anatomic niches that cannot even be reached by careful homecare. The dental biofilm produces acids that slowly demineralize the weakened enamel areas, producing caries. There is a constant "tug-of-war" between demineralization and remineralization at the enamel surface; when demineralization outweighs remineralization, enamel caries results with subsequent cavitation.

With the cariogenic process, the surface enamel of the pit or groove (also known as a fissure) remains intact as the subsurface zones become further demineralized. Thus enamel caries remains in the subsurface, enlarging its pathway to the connected dentin and/or pulp area to form dentinal caries, or pulpitis, if the acidic and/or bacterial assault continues.

Similar to the enamel caries that occurs in deepened pits and grooves, smooth surface caries that tends to occur interproximally, also does not involve the breakdown or demineralization of the surface layers of enamel (see Fig. 12.4, *B*). Zones are also present with smooth surface caries as they are with caries of pits and grooves. In the past, enamel caries predominated on smooth surfaces interproximally on the teeth. However, with the widespread use of fluoride and homecare, the very nature of tooth decay has changed; the outer enamel surfaces of teeth are strengthened and more resistant and thus pit and groove cavities are now more prevalent than smooth surface cavities.

Pit and groove caries are traditionally the most difficult to detect using radiographs due to the direction from which the images are taken. However, a cavitated lesion may also be detected through the use of a "sticky" explorer for both types of enamel caries. The enamel surface having been finally undermined the explorer falls into the already destroyed subsurface.

It is important to remember that early subsurface lesions cannot be detected on radiographs until they spread at least 200 micrometers into the dentin, a process that can take more than 3 to 5 years and usually only for smooth surface caries. Light induced devices that measure changes in laser fluorescence of hard tissue allow dental professionals to better diagnose early carious lesions involving the enamel in a pit and groove before involving the deeper and more extensive dentin layers. However, clinicians should not rely on device readings alone to determine the extension of incipient pit and groove caries; instead clinical evidence must also be considered.

If caries is only present in the enamel, it does not cause pain to the patient because the enamel has no nerves within it. For the same reason, initial cavity preparation is usually painless during removal of enamel only. Pain occurs only when the deeper layers of dentin and then the associated pulpal tissue are involved (see Fig. 13.12). Thus, it is important to emphasize to patients the need for recall examinations for early detection of decay before pain is involved. Pain is a late finding in caries and the risk of tooth loss increases while waiting for this symptom to appear.

Fluoride can enter the enamel systemically through the blood supply of developing teeth before eruption by ingestion of fluoride in drops, tablets, or treated water, all of which are considered preeruptive methods. With systemic fluoride, the fluoride ions are incorporated into the hydroxyapatite (Hap) molecular structure through substitution for hydroxide or carbonate ions creating fluoride-enriched Hap.

Fluoride is not uniformly distributed throughout the dental crown and is most abundant in the outer layers of enamel compared with the enamel closer to the dentin. As the fluoride level in enamel increases and the carbonate level decreases, the enamel becomes less acid soluble, making it more caries resistant.

In contrast, studies have shown that topical fluoride use, as opposed to systemic use, has a more important role in caries control than previously thought, especially for adult patients. Topical use results in an increased level of remineralization of any demineralized regions at the enamel surface, which can actually reverse the carious process. Remineralization is the deposition of minerals into enamel in a way that resembles that of posteruptive maturation, although the minerals are now being deposited into previously demineralized enamel.

Fluoride can also enter enamel topically by direct contact on exposed teeth surfaces by ingestion of fluoridated water or professional application or by directed use of prescription or over-the-counter rinses, gels, foams, chewable tablets, and fluoridated toothpastes, all of which are considered posteruptive methods. Fluoride in prophylaxis pastes provided for use in the dental office provides only brief action and must not take the place of topical fluoride applications.

In addition to its direct mineralizing effect on enamel, fluoride may affect oral bacteria by interfering with the actual microbial acid production, reducing potential enamel destruction. Thus the need for daily topical fluoride exposure through a combination of fluoride therapies has been demonstrated for all age groups. In addition, other noninvasive caries management system therapies such as casein phosphopeptide-amorphous calcium phosphate (CPP-ACP) are being used for tooth remineralization.

The latest topical introduced is silver diamine fluoride (SDF), which is a metal ammine complex of silver fluoride. It is used to arrest and prevent dental caries as well as relieve dentinal hypersensitivity, especially with cases of chronic serious xerostomia, multiple carious lesions, or behavioral management patients, as well as the presence of anatomic niches for the caries process (e.g., furcations, restoration margins, partially erupted molars). The use of SDF will stain most oxidizable surfaces black such as demineralized enamel and dentin but esthetics are not the main concern in these higher risk caries cases.

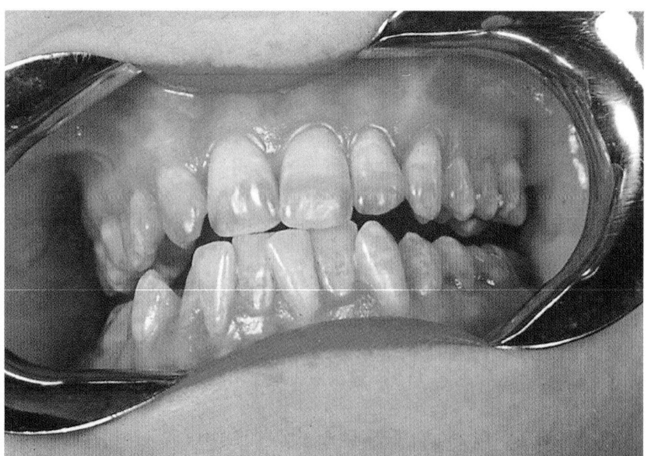

Fig. 12.5 Dental fluorosis with its intrinsic staining of the enamel caused by ingestion of excess amounts of fluoride that in this case occurred naturally in the water system. (From Ibsen OAC, Phelan JA. *Oral Pathology for Dental Hygienists.* 7th ed. Philadelphia: Elsevier; 2018.)

Just as important clinically to situations with reduced fluoride levels is that of excess systemic fluoride intake during tooth development, which can occur in areas where the water naturally has a higher than usual level of fluoride. This can cause a type of enamel dysplasia, dental fluorosis or mottled enamel (Fig. 12.5; see also **Chapter 6**). This type of dysplasia can involve both enamel hypoplasia with pitting and also enamel hypocalcification with intrinsic staining of the enamel, giving affected teeth a spotty discoloration. Dental fluorosis can also occur in lesser amounts in younger children who ingest too much flavored fluoridated toothpaste or inappropriate prescription of systemic fluoride. Vital whitening (or bleaching) may be able to even out the tooth color or esthetic restorations can be placed (discussed later in this chapter).

Protection against enamel caries is provided by the use of enamel sealants that cover the deepened pit and groove patterns on the teeth, including noncavitated lesions so as to arrest the caries (see **Chapters 16 and 17**). Educating patients about the importance of enamel sealants in caries prevention of the permanent dentition for children is an important responsibility for dental professionals and many clinicians are also sealing primary teeth that have an increased caries risk. The American Dental Association and Centers for Disease Control and Prevention now also recommend enamel sealants for adults because of the increased risk of future caries at these unrestored sites or nearby restored margins.

ENAMEL HISTOLOGY

The **enamel rod** (or enamel prism) is the crystalline structural unit of enamel; thus, enamel is composed of millions of enamel rods (Fig. 12.6). Enamel rods and associated structures should be viewed under a microscope to best understand them. The crystals that make up the rod are long ribbons of crystallites that start off thin and become thicker as enamel matures through mineralization. Each enamel rod becomes hexagonal in cross section with the enamel crystals in the rod being usually oriented parallel to its long axis. However, when fully matured, the enamel rods are no longer perfectly hexagonal but instead have an irregular outline because of crowding, flattening each other during the final part of their mineralization. In most areas of enamel, the mature rod is 4 micrometers in diameter and up to 2.5 mm in length. And each enamel rod is usually cylindrical in longitudinal section.

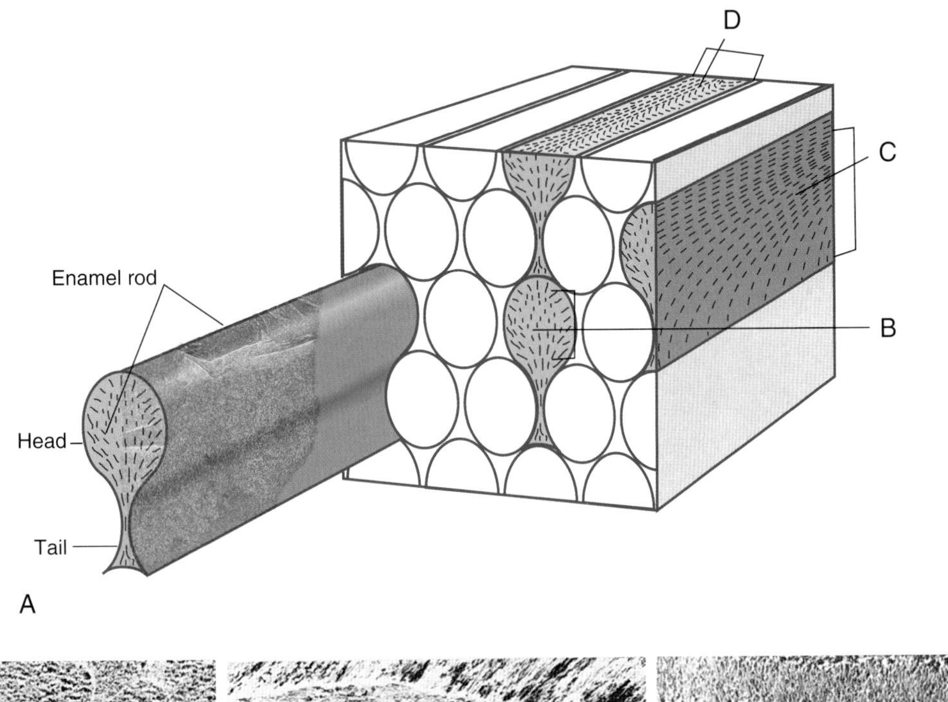

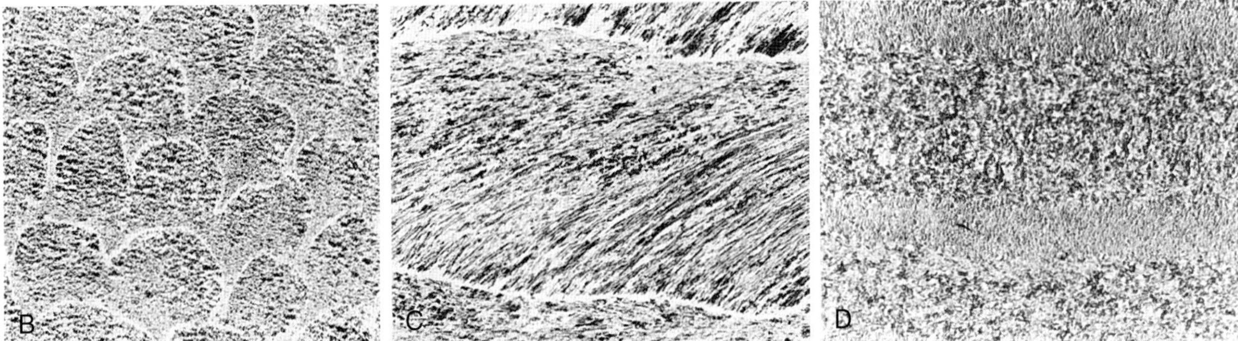

Fig. 12.6 A, Diagram of an enamel rod produced by an ameloblast with its surrounding region of interrod enamel (or interprismatic region) created by surrounding ameloblasts. Note the interdigitation of the rod with other adjacent rods in a block of enamel with varying crystal orientations *(B, C, D)* depending on the exposed facets of the rod. **B,** Electron micrograph in cross section. **C** and **D,** Crystal orientation along the other two cut facets of the block of enamel, all crystals showing the bending of adjacent crystals of the rod core in comparison to interrod enamel (or interprismatic region). (**B, C,** and **D,** Courtesy of A.H. Meckel.)

It is important to note that there are many variations in the structural arrangement of the enamel components and the crystals within each enamel rod are highly complex as a result, with each ameloblast and their own Tomes process affecting the crystal pattern. Also the orientations of similar structured crystals in the adjacent area between the rods (the interrod enamel or interprismatic region, discussed next in this section) diverge slightly from the long axis of the rod core, which is noted as different planes in enamel sections because they have these different orientations.

In addition, the crystals in the rod groups bend sinusoidally to the right or left at a slightly different angle than do adjacent groups, increasing the enamel's strength (see Fig. 12.6). This is shown in the **Hunter-Schreger bands (HSB)** (**hun**-ter-**shray**-ger), alternating light to dark lines noted in certain sections of enamel using reflected rather than transmitted light (see Fig. 12.8, *D*).

The arrangement of enamel rods is understood more clearly than their internal structure. Enamel rods are found in rows along the tooth and within each row the long axis of the enamel rod is usually perpendicular to the underlying dentin as well as the DEJ with a slight inclination toward the cusp as they pass outward, thus preventing enamel fracture. Near the cusp tip they run more vertically; and in cervical enamel, they run mostly horizontally. However, in permanent dentition, the enamel rods near the CEJ tilt slightly toward the apex of the tooth.

Most rods extend the width of the enamel from the DEJ to the outer enamel surface. Thus, each rod varies in length because the width of enamel varies in different locations of the crown area. Those near the cusps or incisal ridges, where the enamel is the thickest, are quite long compared with those near the CEJ. However, the course of the rods from these two end points is not an overall straight course. Rather, the rods show varying degrees of curvature from the DEJ to the outer enamel surface. This curved course of the enamel rods reflects the movements of the ameloblasts during enamel production.

Enamel rods interdigitate at each cusp tip to form a complex known as *gnarled enamel.* This format reduces most of the occlusal stress on enamel, especially at the pronounced cusp tips of posterior teeth. If enamel was not stacked as a spiraling lattice of rod direction in these high-use areas, it would shatter with occlusal stress. The rods also interlock in other areas of the crown and this contributes to the stiffness and hardness of enamel.

Surrounding the outer part of each enamel rod is the **interrod enamel**, creating an interprismatic region that has been secreted by

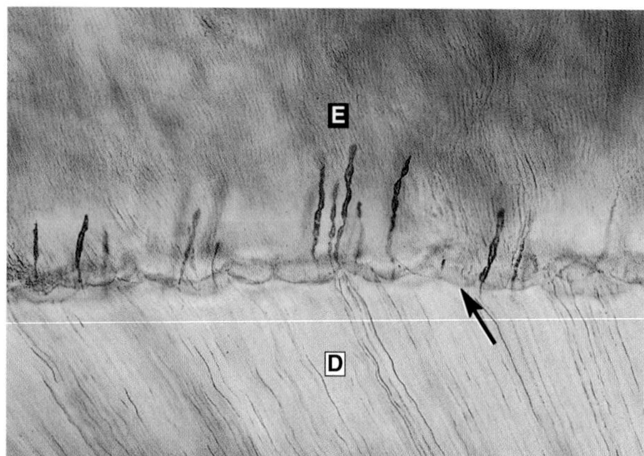

Fig. 12.7 Microscopic section of the dentinoenamel junction demonstrating its scalloped interface *(arrow)*, having its concave side toward the enamel *(E)* and its convex side toward the dentin *(D)*. (From Bernhard Gottlieb Collection, courtesy of James McIntosh, PhD, Assistant Professor Emeritus, Department of Biomedical Sciences, Baylor College of Dentistry, Dallas.)

surrounding ameloblasts (see Fig. 12.6). Even though similar in structure to the enamel rod, this interrod enamel (or interprismatic region) appears different from the rod core on cross sections because of its divergent crystalline orientation. At these boundaries, the crystallites are oriented in different directions and fractures form easily at this interface. Whether an organic rod sheath or lesser-mineralized interprismatic substance exists between the enamel rods remains controversial.

The DEJ between mature enamel and dentin appears scalloped on a cross section of a tooth (Fig. 12.7). The convex side of the DEJ is toward the dentin and the concave side is toward the enamel. This difference in the length of the enamel rods and corresponding dentinal tubules occurs during the appositional growth of the two tissue types (see **Chapter 6**).

The DEJ was formerly the basement membrane between the enamel organ and the dental papilla. In reality, the DEJ is simply a ridge between the two tissue types that allows increased adherence between them, adding to the strength of the junction when the teeth are in function during mastication so as to prevent shearing of the enamel during function. Thus the presence of the DEJ is most pronounced in the coronal region, where occlusal forces are the greatest.

The **lines of Retzius** (ret-**zee**-us) are the incremental lines (or striae) that appear in a microscopic section of mature enamel (Fig. 12.8, *A-C*). These lines are composed of bands or cross striations on the enamel rods that, when combined in longitudinal sections, seem to traverse the enamel rods. In contrast, the lines of Retzius appear as concentric rings on transverse sections of enamel, similar to the growth rings in a tree.

Associated with the lines of Retzius are the raised **imbrication lines** (im-bri-**key**-shuhn) and grooves of **perikymata** (per-i-**key**-maht-uh) noted clinically on the nonmasticatory surfaces of teeth in the oral cavity (Fig. 12.9). The imbrication lines and perikymata are usually lost through tooth wear, except on the protected cervical regions of some teeth. This is especially true for the permanent maxillary central incisors, canines, and first premolars; the surface texture of the enamel in these areas may be confused as calculus near the CEJ.

The exact mechanism that produces the imbrication lines in enamel is still being debated. Some researchers hypothesize that the lines are a result of the *diurnal* or 24-hour metabolic rhythm of the ameloblasts producing the enamel matrix, which consists of an active secretory work period followed by an inactive rest period during tooth development. Thus each band on the enamel rod demonstrates the work/rest pattern of the ameloblasts that generally occurs over a span of a week.

The **neonatal line** (nee-oh-**neyt**-l) is a pronounced incremental line of Retzius (Fig. 12.10). The neonatal line marks the trauma experienced by the ameloblasts during birth, again illustrating the sensitivity of the ameloblasts as they form enamel matrix. Even minor physiologic changes affect them and elicit changes in enamel structure that can be seen only microscopically such as these lines. The darker line marks the border between the enamel matrix formed before and after birth.

As one would expect, the neonatal line is noted in all the crown enamel of the primary dentition and in the larger cusps of the permanent first molars. They contain irregular structures of enamel crystals with disordered arrangements, which are formed by the abrupt bending of the crystals toward the root during enamel formation; usually the crystals gradually bend back again to regain their previous orientation as they move to the crown. Accentuated incremental lines also are produced by systemic disturbances (e.g., fevers) that affect amelogenesis.

The **enamel spindles** are another microscopic feature of mature enamel and represent short dentinal tubules near the DEJ (Fig. 12.11). Enamel spindles are especially noted beneath the cusps and incisal ridges or tips of the teeth. Enamel spindles result from odontoblasts that crossed the basement membrane before it mineralized into the DEJ. Thus, these dentinal tubules become trapped during the appositional growth of enamel matrix, which becomes mineralized around them. Clinical implications of enamel spindles are unknown at this time and it is doubtful that these dentinal tubules contain any live odontoblastic processes as do the other elongated tubules within dentin.

The **enamel tufts** are another microscopic feature and are noted as small dark brushes with their bases near the DEJ (Fig. 12.12). Enamel tufts are best seen on transverse sections of enamel in the inner one-third of enamel. They represent areas of less mineralization from an anomaly of crystallization and have no known clinical importance at this time.

The **enamel lamellae** are partially mineralized vertical sheets of enamel matrix that extend from the DEJ near the tooth's cervix to the outer occlusal surface (see Fig. 12.12). Enamel lamellae are best seen on transverse sections of enamel. Enamel lamellae are narrower and longer than enamel tufts. This is another anomaly of crystallization that has unknown clinical importance at this time. Both enamel tufts and enamel lamellae may be likened to "geologic faults" within mature enamel.

Finally, microscopic images of primary teeth enamel show smooth enamel surface where few areas of irregularity or linear structures are apparent. In contrast, similar images of permanent enamel show a not perfectly smooth surface; there are furrows and irregularities of variable depth and width. It is not known if this difference in dentitions is related to any clinical importance.

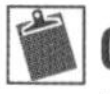 Clinical Considerations for Dental Procedures Involving Enamel

The microscopic features of enamel must be taken into consideration during clinical treatment involving enamel. Enamel resembles a steel product with a moderate level of hardness, which also makes it brittle; therefore, an underlying layer of more break-resistant dentin must be present to preserve its integrity (see earlier discussion and Table 12.1). This property, along with the direction of the enamel rods, is taken into consideration during cavity preparation as well as the dentinal tubule direction (discussed later).

First, the decay and adjacent parts of the enamel are removed in a way that allows all the enamel rods to remain supported by other rods and the underlying dentin. An isolated enamel rod is extremely brittle and breaks away easily. If enamel rods are undercut during cavity preparation, they may break, thus rendering the margin of restoration

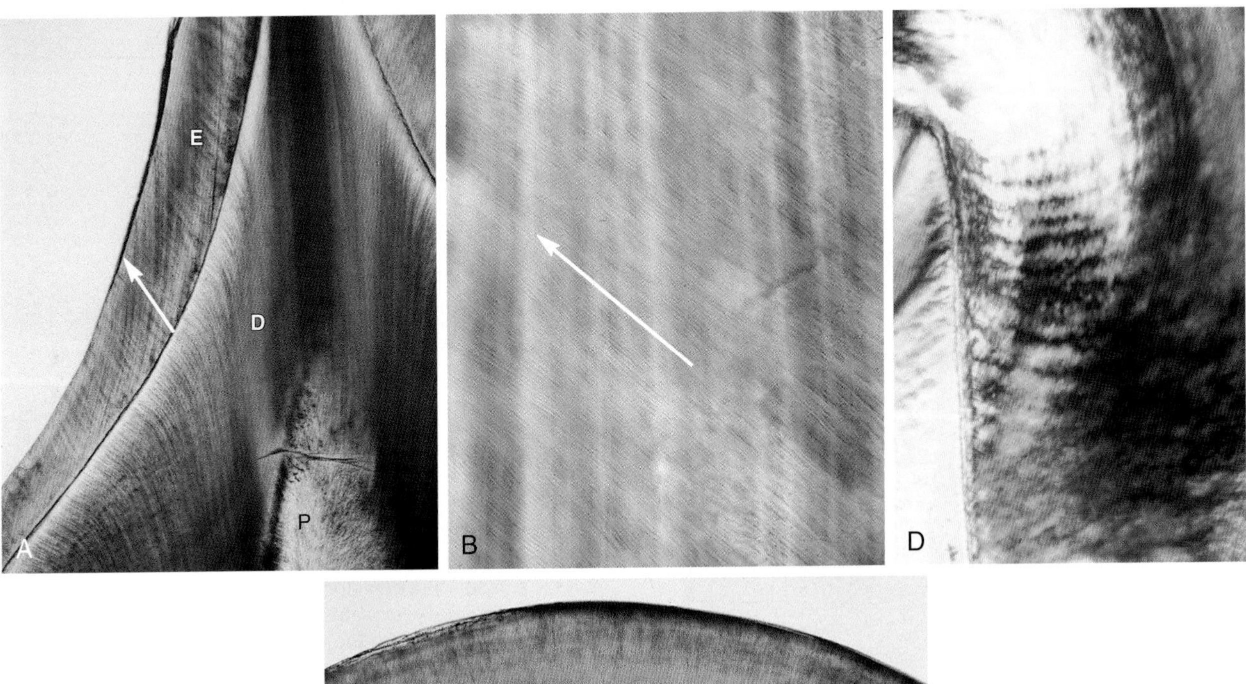

Fig. 12.8 Microscopic Sections of the Lines of Retzius that Traverse the Rods of the Enamel. **A,** Long section of rods *(E)* demonstrating their direction *(arrow)* overlying dentin *(D)* and pulp *(P)* in the crown. **B,** Close-up view of long section of rods demonstrating their direction *(arrow)*. **C,** Cross section of rods overlying dentin *(D)* with the lines of Retzius resembling growth rings of a tree. **D,** Alternating light to dark Hunter-Schreger bands demonstrated using reflected rather than transmitted light (in this case polarized light). (From Bernhard Gottlieb Collection, courtesy of James McIntosh, PhD, Assistant Professor Emeritus, Department of Biomedical Sciences, Baylor College of Dentistry, Dallas.)

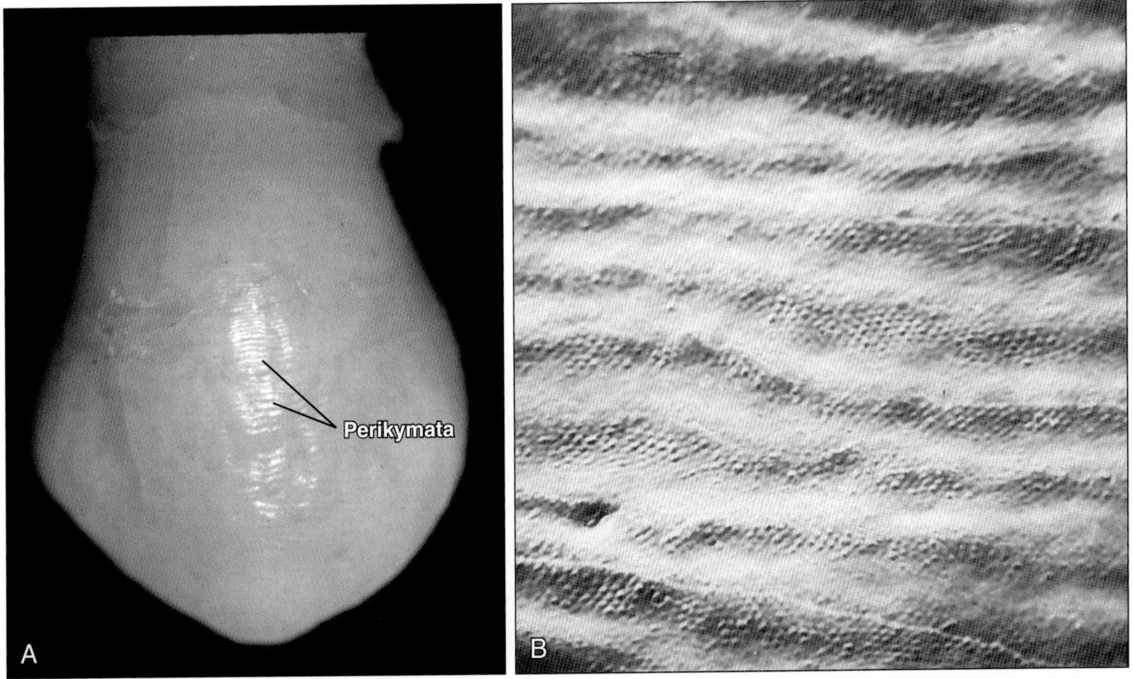

Fig. 12.9 Raised Imbrication Lines and Grooves of the Perikymata. **A,** Labial view of the permanent maxillary canine. **B,** Scanning electron micrograph of the labial surface of the tooth. (Courtesy of D. Weber.)

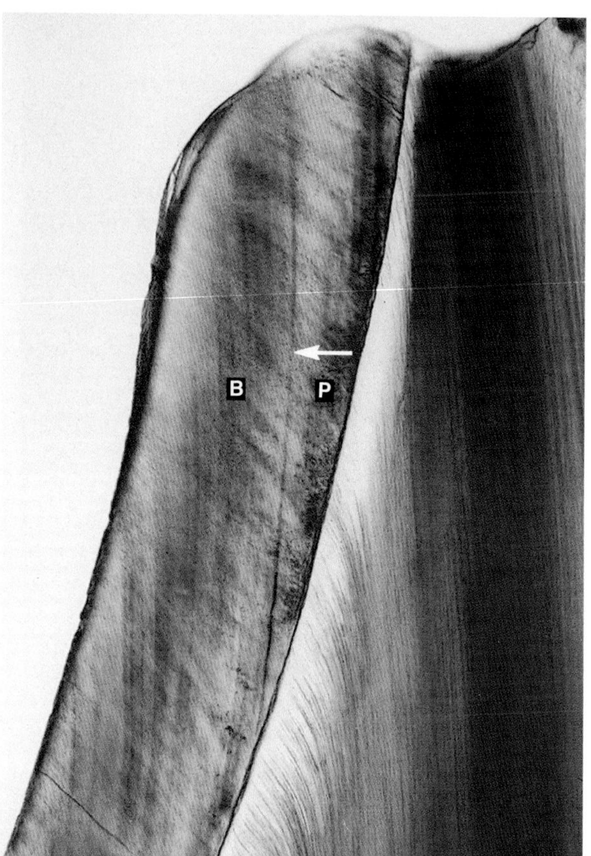

Fig. 12.10 Microscopic section of the neonatal line *(arrow)*, a pronounced line of Retzius that corresponds to the birth of the individual. Thus, it demarcates the enamel formed prenatally *(P)* and after birth *(B)*. (From Bernhard Gottlieb Collection, courtesy of James McIntosh, PhD, Assistant Professor Emeritus, Department of Biomedical Sciences, Baylor College of Dentistry, Dallas.)

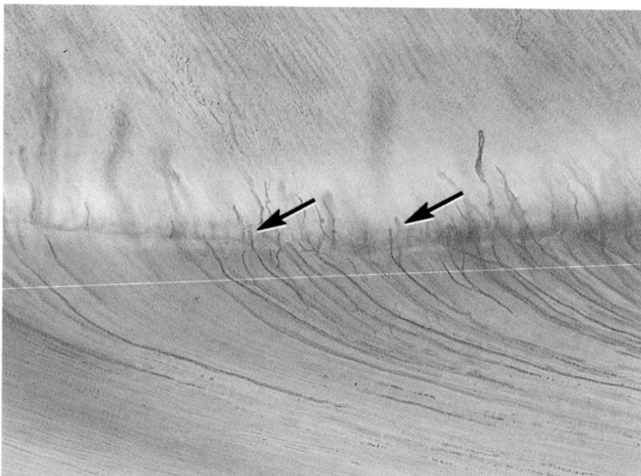

Fig. 12.11 Microscopic section of enamel spindles *(arrows)* within the enamel and near the dentinoenamel junction. (From Bernhard Gottlieb Collection, courtesy of James McIntosh, PhD, Assistant Professor Emeritus, Department of Biomedical Sciences, Baylor College of Dentistry, Dallas.)

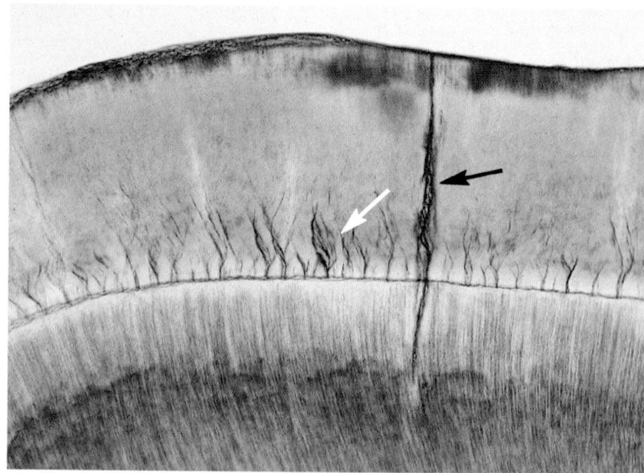

Fig. 12.12 Transverse section of enamel showing enamel tufts *(white arrow)* and enamel lamella *(black arrow)*. (From Bernhard Gottlieb Collection, courtesy of James McIntosh, PhD, Assistant Professor Emeritus, Department of Biomedical Sciences, Baylor College of Dentistry, Dallas.)

possibly leaky as well as defective. This brittleness of unsupported enamel also is noted during the progression of caries since the enamel breaks away easily as the supporting dentin is undermined beneath it.

In the case of an amalgam Class I cavity preparation, the walls of the cavity should be perpendicular or 90° to the cavosurface, which will then expose the rods with its crystals. However, when using a bonding resin, it is important to prepare the same type of cavity preparation with a 45° bevel to the cavosurface to expose the enamel rods and its crystal for subsequent acid etching in order to significantly increase the bond strength.

Acid etching is briefly used to remove some of the organic parts of the enamel crystals in the interrod enamel (or interprismatic region), increasing porosity, enabling a bonding resin or an enamel sealant to flow into the newly created gaps, and thus offer more surface area for better adherence (Fig. 12.13). It also removes the smear layer of the adherent dental biofilm debris.

This demineralization by acid etching is clinically apparent as the surface of enamel whitens. The arrangement of enamelin (discussed earlier) between and around the crystallized rods contributes to enamel's permeability (or microporosity) to these materials as well as fluids, bacteria, and the acid byproducts of dental biofilm. When placing certain enamel sealants (hydrophobic types), dental professionals must be careful to protect the demineralized enamel surface from being contaminated and remineralized by saliva, thereby reducing sealant uptake; luckily, new sealants are more resistant to this situation. The difference in surface smoothness or roughness (as discussed earlier) between the primary and permanent dentitions will also have an impact on a clinician's approach when acid etching the tooth surface for restorations or sealants.

Vital whitening of the teeth (referred to as *bleaching* by patients) is performed externally to remove the gross levels of intrinsic staining that has occurred due to the process of aging of enamel as well as lifestyle choices (e.g., ingestion of dark drinks and foods, as well as tobacco use; see **Chapter 13** about staining of dentin). Staining occurs in the interrod enamel (or interprismatic region) internally on the tooth, which causes the tooth to appear darker or less white overall.

First, the shade of the tooth is taken and recorded (as discussed earlier with dental restorations and replacement) to gauge the changes in whiteness over time during the whitening procedure. Certain natural shades of teeth are more easily whitened than others (yellow tones are more compliant than gray tones). This procedure can be a lifesaver for patients with intrinsic stains to even out the overall tooth color, such as with tetracycline and dental fluorosis. Secondly, the dental professional then supervises the use of whitening agents within the context of a comprehensive, appropriately sequenced treatment plan.

In a perfect state, enamel is colorless, but it does reflect underlying tooth structure with any gross stains because light reflection properties

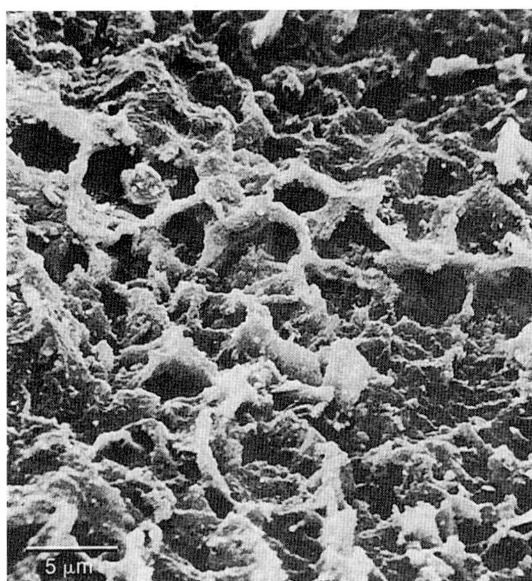

Fig. 12.13 Photomicrograph showing the enamel rods after acid etching, which demineralizes the interrod enamel (or interprismatic region) to allow the flow of the enamel sealant or other restorative materials into the enamel for greater strength. (Courtesy of L. Silverstone.)

of the tooth are low. Oxygen radicals from the peroxide in the whitening agents contact the stains in the interrod enamel within the enamel layer. When this occurs, stains will be removed with the teeth now appearing whiter in color. Teeth not only appear whiter but also reflect light in increased amounts, which makes the teeth appear brighter as well. Additional studies show that patients who have whitened their teeth take better care of them and have a more positive oral health-related quality of life.

After whitening, the tooth is left with dehydration of the enamel surface and possibly dentinal hypersensitivity in areas of exposed dentin such as on the root surface or unrestored caries. This may be tempered by the application of a remineralization agent such as fluoride either along with the whitening agent or afterwards (see **Chapter 13** concerning dentinal hypersensitivity). As the surface of the tooth rehydrates over the next few weeks, there may also be a lowering of the teeth's whiteness by a couple of shades.

Most studies at this time show that tooth whitening when used as a neutral preparation and in the recommended time limits does not produce any ultrastructural or microhardness changes in the enamel; however, the whitening procedure continues to be a controversial issue that needs further study including its effect on tooth restorations. In all cases, supervision by dental health professionals is recommended by the American Dental Association Council on Scientific Affairs to achieve a successful and safe whitening outcome.

13

Dentin and Pulp

Additional resources and practice exercises are provided on the companion Evolve website for this book: http://evolve.elsevier.com/Fehrenbach/illustrated.

LEARNING OBJECTIVES

1. Define and pronounce the key terms in this chapter.
2. Discuss the dentin-pulp complex.
3. Describe the properties of dentin and the clinical consideration for dentin structure, integrating it into patient care.
4. Describe the processes involved in the stages of apposition and the maturation of dentin.
5. Outline the types of dentin and discuss the clinical considerations for dentin pathology, integrating it into patient care.
6. Discuss the histology of dentin.
7. Describe pulp properties, including its anatomic components.
8. Identify the components of both the dentin and the pulp on a diagram.
9. Discuss the histology of pulp and the clinical considerations for pulp pathology and repair, integrating it into patient care.

DENTIN-PULP COMPLEX

Unlike enamel, both dentin and pulp cannot be viewed clinically if the teeth and associated periodontium are healthy. That is because both dentin and pulp make up the inner parts of the tooth and are not exposed to the oral environment except when certain dental pathology exists. In addition, due to their shared developmental background from the dental papilla, close proximity in the tooth, and tissue interdependence, both dentin and pulp form a dentin-pulp complex. This chapter discusses these two types of tissue together as one developmental and functioning unit.

Dental professionals must have a clear understanding of the histology of these two types of tissue. In the past, these two inner types of dental tissue were thought of as being analogous to a "black box" that was opened only during restorative treatment or endodontic therapy and hidden the rest of the time. With the advent of expanded responsibilities and increased preventive concerns for patients, all dental professionals must be able to know about these two interesting and challenging dental tissue types.

DENTIN PROPERTIES

Mature dentin is a crystalline material that is less hard than enamel but slightly harder than bone (see both Tables 6.2 and 12.1). Mature dentin is by weight 70% inorganic or mineralized material, 20% organic material, and 10% water. This crystalline formation of mature dentin consists mostly of calcium hydroxyapatite with the chemical formula of $Ca_{10}(PO_4)_6(OH)_2$. The calcium hydroxyapatite found in dentin is similar to that found in a higher percentage in enamel and in lower percentages in both cementum and bone tissue, such as the alveolar process. In addition, the crystals in dentin are plate-like in shape and 30% smaller in size than those in enamel. Small amounts of other minerals, such as carbonate and fluoride, are also present.

Dentin is covered by enamel in the crown and cementum in the root as well as enclosing the innermost pulp. Thus dentin makes up the bulk of the tooth and protects the pulp. Dentin also has great tensile strength, providing an elastic basis for the more brittle enamel.

Because of the translucency of overlying enamel, the dentin of the tooth gives the white enamel crown its underlying yellow hue, which is a deeper tone in permanent teeth. When the pulp undergoes infection or even dies, there is discoloration of the dentin, which causes darkening of the clinical crown. On a radiograph, the differences in the mineralization levels of different parts of the tooth can be noted (see Fig. 2.5). Dentin appears more radiolucent (or darker) than enamel because it is less dense but more radiopaque (or lighter) than pulp, which has the least density of these three types of dental tissue.

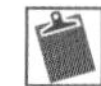

CLINICAL CONSIDERATIONS FOR DENTIN STRUCTURE

If the outer layers of enamel are lost with aging, such as with attrition from mastication, the newly exposed dentin on the crown is various shades of yellow-white and appears rougher in surface texture than enamel (see Fig. 16.17). Attrition, which is the wearing of a tooth surface through tooth-to-tooth contact, can also occur in the newly exposed dentin as well as enamel (see Fig. 20.8). In contrast to hard enamel, this attrition can occur at a more rapid rate when dentin is exposed because its mineralized content is lower. Coronal dentin can be exposed after attrition of the enamel and also with certain enamel dysplasias. Coronal dentin can also become exposed on the incisal ridge of anteriors when trauma causes it to become chipped or worn (see Fig. 16.9, *C*).

Root dentin can be exposed when the thin layer of cementum is lost due to gingival recession with its lower margin of the free gingival crest (Fig. 13.1) (see **Chapter 10**). It also appears various shades of yellow-white and appears rougher in surface texture than enamel. When hand instruments are used on the root to remove deposits such as calculus, there can be improper removal of dentin changing the overall root shape and function. Dentin that is lost externally on either the crown or root is not fully replaced by the possible addition of secondary dentin on the inside of the tooth along the outer pulpal wall (discussed later in this chapter).

Another way that dentin can become exposed and then lost is through dentinal caries, the demineralization resulting from cariogenic

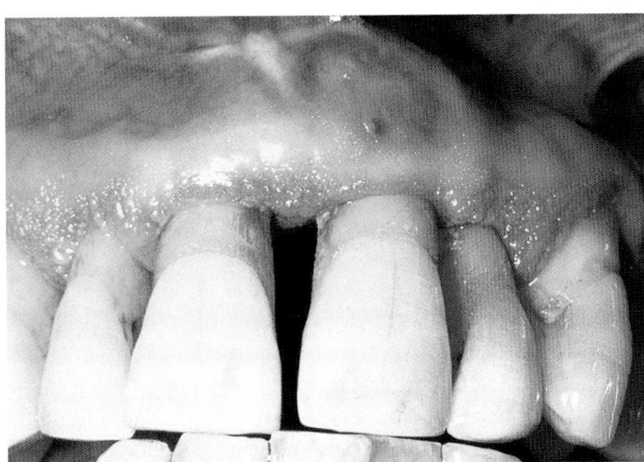

Fig. 13.1 Clinical Facial View of Gingival Recession Exposing Root Dentin. Note the difference in color between the whitish enamel and the more yellowish dentin, which has also undergone additional staining of the root surfaces due to exposure. (Courtesy of Margaret J. Fehrenbach, RDH, MS.)

bacteria (discussed later in this chapter). Dentin demineralizes when the pH is less than 6.8. Finally, cavity preparation during restorative treatment exposes and then removes any carious dentin in order to prevent further deeper decay.

Dentinal hypersensitivity can also occur when instruments expose dentin, such as on root surfaces; this can be prevented with certain mineralizing products or temporarily reduced with the use of local anesthetic injections during dental procedures (discussed later in this chapter).

Removal of extrinsic stains by hand instrumentation can also remove even more dentin; thus ultrasonic devices or air polishing using glycine that remove no hard tooth tissue when used correctly may be better choices for extrinsic stain removal (as discussed in **Chapter 12**).

When dentin remains exposed, it can also pick up intrinsic beverage, food, and tobacco stains over time, becoming more yellow or even brown to black (see Figs. 13.1 and 16.17). It absorbs these stains because it is more permeable or porous than intact enamel. Dentin is permeable due to both its high organic content and the presence of dentinal tubules, acting as a sponge to contain these staining products and causing esthetic concerns for patients. Vital whitening (referred to as *bleaching* by patients) can be performed either at the office or in the home to remove some of the intrinsic stains within dentin to even out the overall tooth color, including those related to tooth development such as tetracycline stain (see Fig. 3.19).

However, whitening at home must be done with appropriate supervision because it may also lead to dentinal hypersensitivity and many over-the-counter products can contain acidic preparations. Vital whitening is discussed further in **Chapter 12**. Most studies at this time show that tooth whitening when used as a neutral preparation in recommended time limits does not produce ultrastructural or microhardness changes in the dentin and pulp; however, the whitening procedure continues to be a controversial issue that needs further study including its effect on tooth restorations.

DENTIN MATRIX FORMATION

Dentinogenesis is the formation of the initial dentin matrix or predentin during the apposition stage of tooth development (Fig. 13.2). The exact time of the apposition stage varies according to the tooth that is undergoing development. Many factors can affect dentinogenesis when it is occurring (see **Chapter 6**).

Predentin is a mesenchymal product consisting of nonmineralized collagen fibers produced by the odontoblasts. Predentin consists of mostly Type I collagen and also small amounts of Type III and V, along with

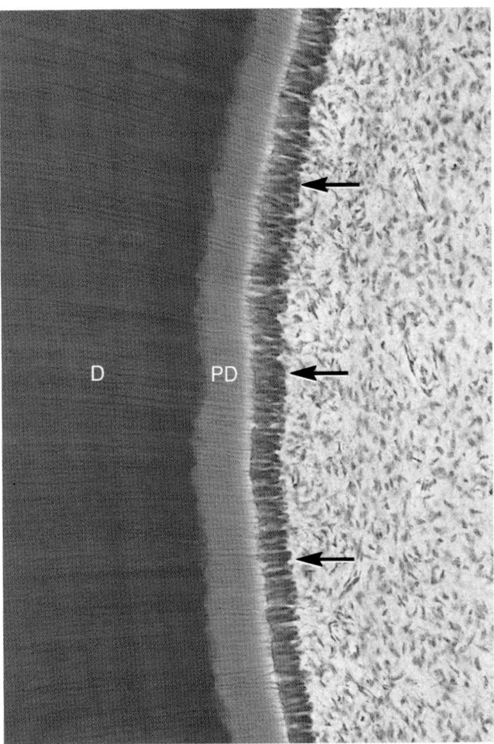

Fig. 13.2 Microscopic section of odontoblasts *(arrows)* producing predentin *(PD)* that will mature into dentin *(D)*. (From Bernhard Gottlieb Collection, courtesy of James McIntosh, PhD, Assistant Professor Emeritus, Department of Biomedical Sciences, Baylor College of Dentistry, Dallas, TX.)

dentin phosphoprotein. The latter acidic protein is important in the regulation of mineralization of dentin because it is highly attractable to calcium.

Originally odontoblasts were the outer cells of the dental papilla before the apposition stage of tooth development. Thus dentin and pulp have similar developmental backgrounds because both are originally derived from the dental papilla of the tooth germ. These newly formed odontoblasts are induced by the equally newly formed ameloblasts to produce predentin in layers, moving away from the dentinoenamel junction (DEJ). Unlike cartilage and bone as well as cementum, the odontoblast's cell body does not become entrapped in the product; rather, one long cytoplasmic attached extension remains behind within the formed dentin. Odontoblasts produce approximately 4 micrometers of predentin daily during tooth development, similar to the amount of enamel matrix produced daily by the ameloblasts on the other side of the DEJ.

However, the appositional growth of dentin, unlike enamel, occurs throughout the life of the tooth, filling in the pulp chamber of both the crown and root (discussed later in this chapter). The wave pattern of dentin development follows the same format as that of enamel but on the opposite side of the DEJ (see Figs. 12.2 and 12.3). It starts at the incisal or occlusal part of the future crown and then spreads down as far as the adjacent cervical loop of the enamel organ. Although ameloblasts are lost after the eruption of the tooth and enamel production ceases, production of dentin continues because of the retention of the odontoblasts. These tall bowling pin–shaped cells remain within the tooth lined up along the outer pulpal wall.

DENTIN MATRIX MATURATION

Maturation of dentin or mineralization of predentin occurs soon after its appositional growth. The process of dentin maturation takes place in two

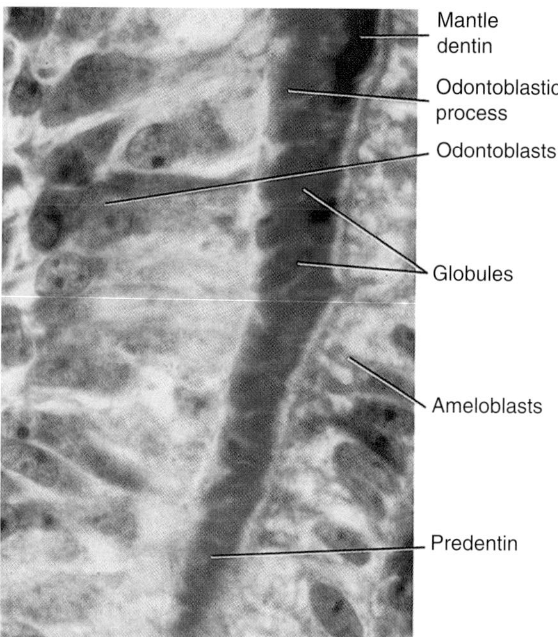

Fig. 13.3 Photomicrograph of dentin maturation showing the odontoblasts producing predentin that contains odontoblastic processes with the ameloblasts located on the opposite side of the dentinoenamel junction. The predentin matures by forming globules, which undergo mineralization into mantle dentin because it is near the dentinoenamel junction. (From Nanci A. *Ten Cate's Oral Histology*. 9th ed. St. Louis: Elsevier; 2018.)

phases: primary and secondary (Fig. 13.3). Initially, the calcium hydroxyapatite crystals form as globules or *calcospherules* in the collagen fibers of the predentin, which allows both the expansion and fusion during the primary mineralization phase. This process is analogous to the wash of watercolor paint placed on wet paper for a background as the blobs of color run into each other, although within dentin it is a fully three-dimensional process.

Later, new areas of mineralization occur as globules form in the partially mineralized predentin during the secondary mineralization phase. These new areas of crystal formation are more or less regularly layered on the initial crystals allowing them to expand, although the globules tend to fuse incompletely. This process is analogous to additional blobs of paint placed in specific areas over a fuzzy painted background, but the colors of this additional layer do not run into each other to cover the page because the paper is no longer wet.

This incomplete fusion of globules during the secondary mineralization phase results in differences noted in the microscopic appearance of the crystalline form of dentin. In areas where both primary and secondary mineralization have occurred with complete crystalline fusion, these appear as lighter rounded areas on a microscopic section of dentin and are considered **globular dentin** (**glob**-yuh-ler) (Fig. 13.4).

In contrast, the darker arclike areas in a microscopic section of dentin are considered **interglobular dentin** (in-ter-**glob**-you-ler). In these areas, only primary mineralization has occurred within the predentin and the globules of dentin do not fuse completely. Thus, interglobular dentin is slightly less mineralized than globular dentin. Interglobular dentin is especially evident in coronal dentin, near the DEJ, and in certain dental anomalies, such as in dentin dysplasia (see Fig. 6.17).

MATURE DENTIN COMPONENTS

Within mature dentin, certain components (such as dentinal tubules and their contents) are present (Figs. 13.5 and 13.6). Dentinal tubules are long tubes in the dentin that extend from the DEJ in the crown area or dentinocemental junction (DCJ) in the root area to the outer wall of the pulp in both cases. After appositional growth of predentin and maturation into dentin, the cell bodies of the odontoblasts remain in the pulp inside the tooth along its outer wall (discussed later). The tubules are also tapered with their width being thinner near the DEJ or DCJ and then wider as they near the pulp.

Like enamel, dentin is avascular. Instead of its own blood vessels supplying its nutrition, odontoblasts within the dentin receive it by way of tissue fluid in the dentinal tubules that originally traveled from the blood vessels located in the adjacent pulp. Within each dentinal tubule is a space of variable size containing dentinal fluid, an odontoblastic process, and may also include a part of an afferent axon.

The **dentinal fluid** in the tubule also presumably includes the tissue fluid surrounding the cell membrane of the odontoblast, which is continuous from the cell body in the pulp. The odontoblastic process is a long cellular extension located within the dentinal tubule that is still attached to the cell body of the odontoblast within the pulp. In a microscopic section of a tooth, odontoblastic processes within the dentinal tubule sometimes are not found at the periphery of dentin near the DEJ or DCJ. This absence may or may not be an artifact given that live cell structures are difficult to preserve in dead mineralized tissue. Studies suggest that the process occupies the full length of the tubule from the DEJ or DCJ to the pulp during only the early stages of odontogenesis. In mature dentin, however, the process may or may not run the full length of the dentinal tubule to extend near either the outlying DEJ or DCJ.

An afferent nerve axon (or sensory nerve axon) is associated with part of the odontoblastic process in some dentinal tubules (see **Chapter 8** discussion of nerves). The myelinated axon may not extend farther than the process and thus may not be located along either the DEJ or DCJ. Yet, the nerve cell body associated with the axon is located in the pulp along with the odontoblastic cell body. This axon is mostly involved in registration of the sensation of pain and not usually any other sensations, even when triggered by other sensations such as heat (discussed later).

Three types of nerve fibers are found within dentin, including A (both delta and beta) and C fibers. They are classified according to their diameter and their conduction velocity. The A fibers are mostly stimulated by an application of cold, producing sharp pain, whereas stimulation of the C fibers produce a dull aching pain. Because of their location and arrangement, the C fibers are also responsible for referred pain.

The direction of the tubule reflects the pathway of the odontoblast during appositional growth of predentin. There are two types of curvature established by the direction of the dentinal tubules: primary and secondary (Fig. 13.7). The *primary curvature* of the dentinal tubules reflects the overall tubule course over time, which resembles a large S-shaped curve. The *secondary curvature* of the tubule consists of small delicate curves noted in the primary curvature, reflecting the smaller daily changes in odontoblast direction during the appositional growth of dentin.

Dentinal tubules are not interrupted by the formation of the interglobular areas of dentin but pass right through them. Tubules can branch at any point along the way from the DEJ or DCJ to the pulp. Dentinal tubules are also crowded near the pulp because of the narrowing of this region (see Fig. 13.5). Finally, dentin tubules are responsible for permeability of material across the dentinal surface if exposed. The quantity and diameter of these dentinal tubules affect the permeability of dentin and may enhance the carious process (see later discussion in this chapter).

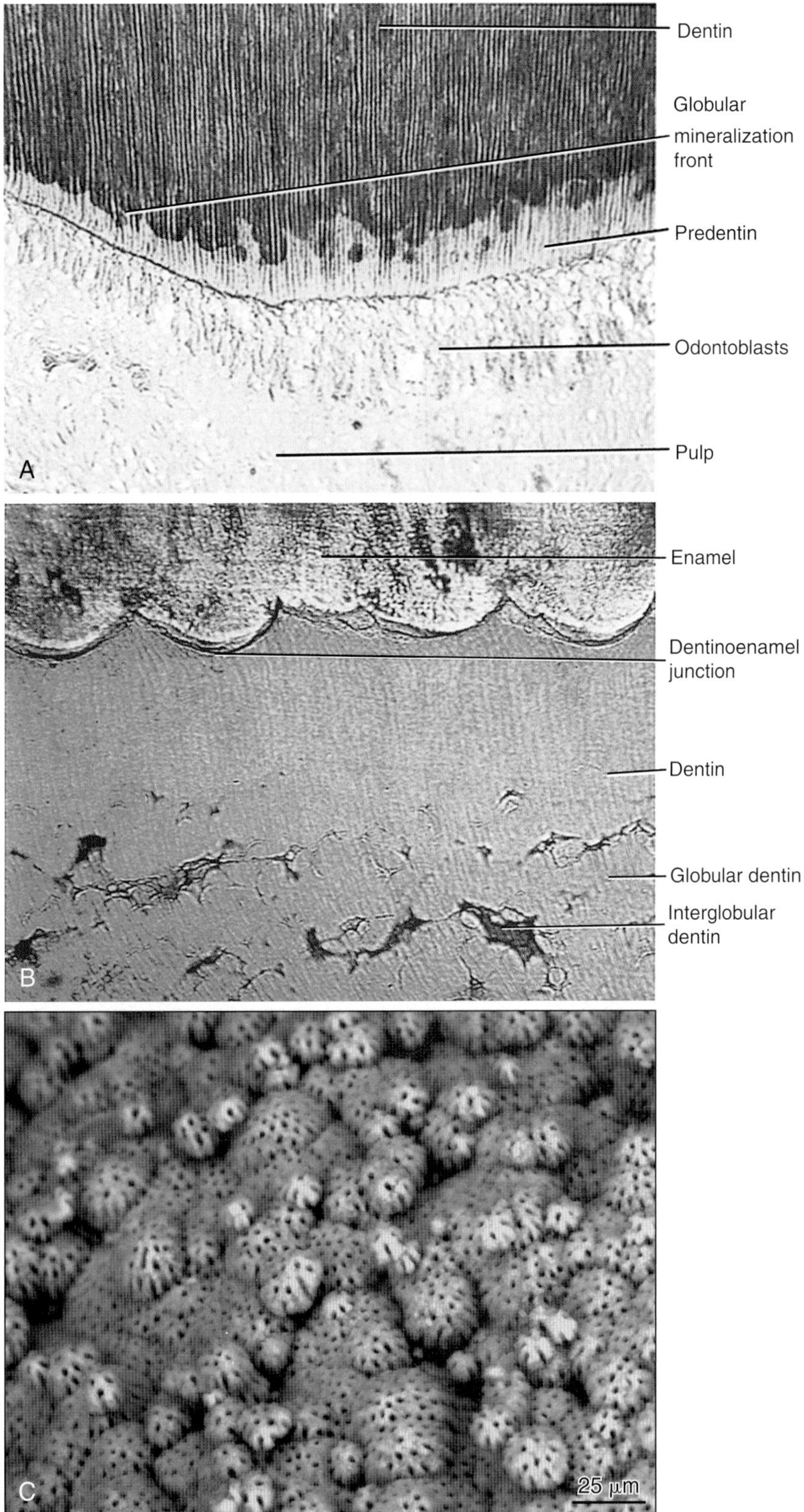

Fig. 13.4 Photomicrographs of Globular and Interglobular Dentin. A, Section of the globular mineralized front near the outer pulpal wall during primary mineralization. **B,** Ground section near the dentinoenamel junction with its highly mineralized globular dentin (lighter) and less mineralized interglobular dentin (darker) after both primary and secondary mineralization. **C,** Scanning electron micrograph of globular dentin. (From Nanci A. *Ten Cate's Oral Histology*. 9th ed. St. Louis: Elsevier; 2018.)

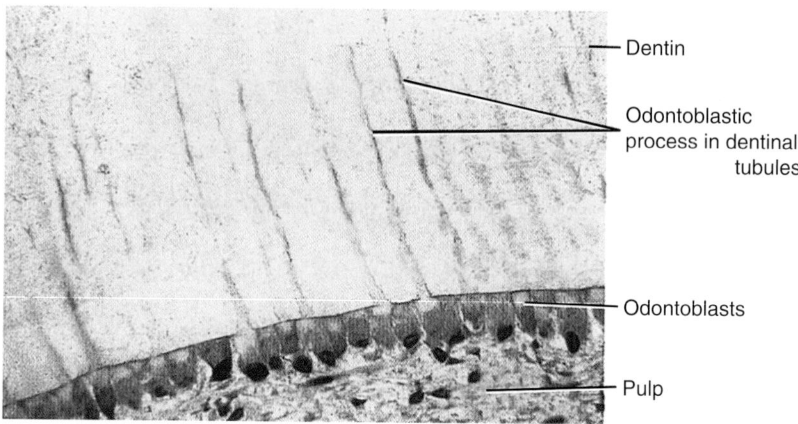

Fig. 13.5 Photomicrograph of the Dentinal Tubules in Dentin with the Odontoblastic Processes Entering the Tubules from the Pulp. The pulp contains an outer layer of the cell bodies of odontoblasts to which the odontoblastic processes are still attached. (From CD-ROM from Nanci A. *Ten Cate's Oral Histology.* 6th ed. St. Louis: Elsevier; 2003.)

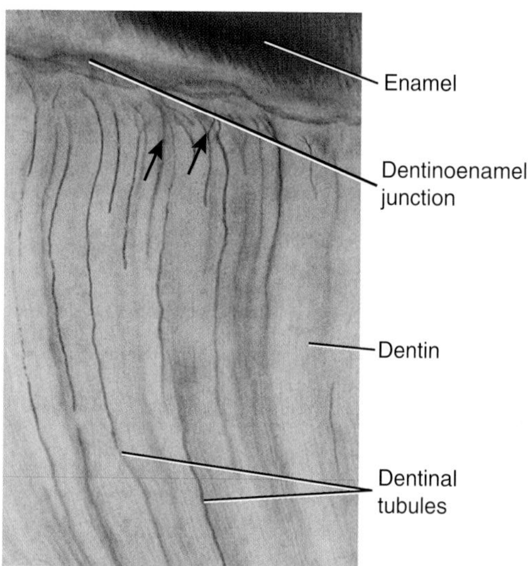

Fig. 13.6 Microscopic Section of the Components of the Dentinal Tubule. The dentinal tubules contain odontoblastic processes *(arrows)* as well as dentinal fluid. (From CD-ROM from Nanci A. *Ten Cate's Oral Histology.* 6th ed. St. Louis: Elsevier; 2003.)

DENTIN TYPES

Dentin is not a uniform tissue within the tooth but differs from region to region (Table 13.1). Different types of dentin can be designated by their relationship to the dentinal tubules (Fig. 13.8; see also Fig. 13.5). Dentin that creates the wall of the dentinal tubule is **peritubular dentin** (per-ee-**too**-byuh-ler) (or intratubular dentin). Peritubular dentin is highly mineralized after dentin maturation. The dentin that is found between the tubules is **intertubular dentin** (in-ter-**too**-byuh-ler). Intertubular dentin is highly mineralized but less so than peritubular dentin.

Dentin can also be categorized by its relationship to the enamel and pulp (Fig. 13.9). **Mantle dentin** is the first predentin that forms and matures within the tooth near the DEJ and underneath the enamel. Mantle dentin shows a difference in the direction of the mineralized collagen fibers compared with the rest of the dentin, having fibers that are perpendicular to the DEJ. Large diameter collagen fibers, the *von Korff fibers,* are associated with this type of dentin. Mantle dentin also has more peritubular dentin than the later formed inner dentin and thus has higher levels of mineralization.

Deep to the mantle dentin is the layer of dentin around the outer wall of pulp, the **circumpulpal dentin** (sur-kuhm-**pul**-puhl), which makes up the bulk of the dentin in a tooth. This type forms and matures after mantle dentin. The collagen fibers of circumpulpal dentin are mostly parallel to the DEJ compared with those of mantle dentin.

Dentin can also be categorized according to the time that it was formed within the tooth (Fig. 13.10). **Primary dentin** is formed in a tooth before the completion of the apical foramen or foramina of the root, which is the opening(s) in the root's pulp canal. Most of the dentin in the tooth was formed during this time period. Primary dentin is characterized by its regular pattern of dentinal tubules.

Secondary dentin is formed after the completion of the apical foramen or foramina and continues to form throughout the life of the tooth. Secondary dentin is formed more slowly than primary dentin; thus it makes up less of the dentin in the tooth. As it is being formed by the odontoblasts lined up along the dentin-pulp interface, the secondary dentin fills in the pulp chamber along its outer wall. This secondary time period of dentinogenesis is noted for its only slightly irregular pattern of tubules but it has the same mineral content.

Microscopically a dark line shows the junction between the primary and secondary dentin that results from an abrupt change in the course of the odontoblasts during appositional growth as the tooth's apex or apices are completed (see Fig. 13.10). Most of the secondary dentin fills in on the roof and floor of the pulp chamber, causing pulp recession (discussed later in this chapter).

One type of dentin, **tertiary dentin** is formed quickly in local regions in response to a localized injury to the exposed dentin (see Fig. 13.10) (discussed next).

Clinical Considerations for Dentin Pathology

Apart from dentin that is resorbed during the shedding of primary teeth, the dentin formed is mostly stable during the life of the tooth. However, in a few cases dentin can become resorbed in permanent dentition, but the cause is idiopathic (or unknown) and can involve either an internal or external resorption process. It can be noted radiographically but it is hard to discern between the two processes. In contrast, when the process begins on the external surface of the root and then penetrates through the cementum into dentin (usually not into the pulp) it can lead to a pinkish crown color noted clinically from the granulation tissue seen beneath the translucent enamel so it is now considered a "pink tooth."

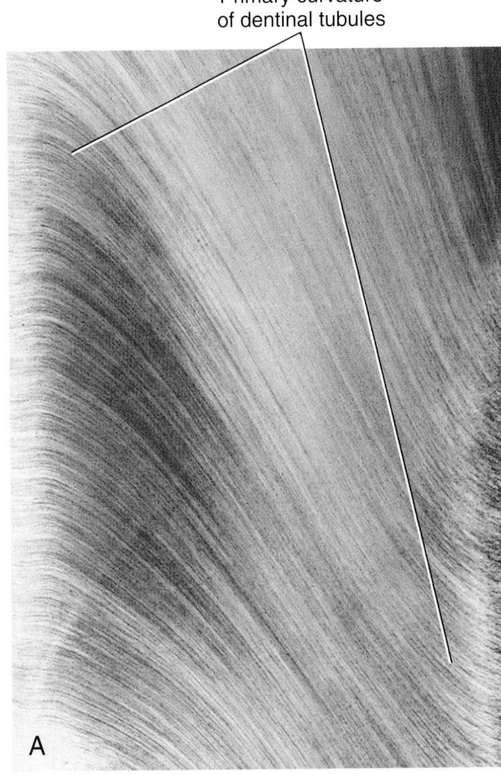

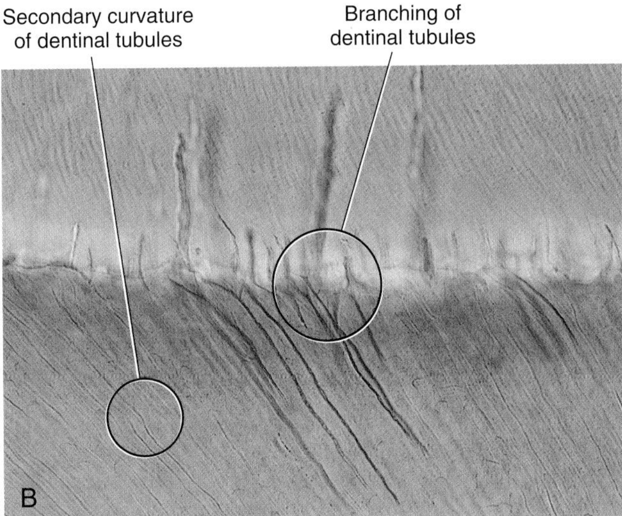

Fig. 13.7 Curvature of the Dentinal Tubules in Dentin. A, Primary curvature. **B,** Secondary curvature *(smaller circle)* with branching noted near the dentinoenamel junction *(larger circle)*. (From Bernhard Gottlieb Collection, courtesy of James McIntosh, PhD, Assistant Professor Emeritus, Department of Biomedical Sciences, Baylor College of Dentistry, Dallas.)

Similar but much more serious than the resorption process in dentin is when the dentinal tubules serve as an entry mechanism for cariogenic microorganisms as the carious process begins to extend from the enamel to form **dentinal caries** (Fig. 13.11). Microscopically the microorganisms can be seen actually using the dentinal tubules as chutes that allow them to move toward the inner placed pulp due to their connection with the odontoblasts in the outer pulpal wall. When caries extends into the dentin from enamel (see enamel caries

TABLE 13.1 Dentin Types

Type	Location and Chronology	Histologic Features
Peritubular dentin	Wall of tubules	Highly mineralized
Intertubular dentin	Between tubules	Highly mineralized
Mantle dentin	Outermost layer near dentinoenamel junction underneath enamel	First dentin formed
Circumpulpal dentin	Layer around outer pulpal wall	Dentin formed after mantle dentin
Primary dentin	Formed before completion of apical foramen	Formed more rapidly; more mineralized than secondary
Secondary dentin	Formed after completion of apical foramen	Formed more slowly; less mineralized than primary
Tertiary dentin	Formed as result of localized injury to exposed dentin	Irregular course of tubules

discussion in **Chapter 12**), the carious process moves more rapidly because of the increased organic composition of dentin as compared with enamel.

In addition, because of the primary curvature of the dentinal tubules, the pulp may be affected at a more apical level than the level at which the external injury (such as caries) occurred. The cavity preparation process during restorative treatment considers this curvature of the tubules when carious dentin is removed. Light-induced devices that measure changes in laser fluorescence of hard tissue can now allow dental professionals to better diagnose early carious lesions.

Tertiary dentin forms quickly in local regions in response to a localized injury to the exposed dentin (see Fig. 13.10). The dentinal injury could be due to caries, cavity preparation, attrition, or gingival recession. Tertiary dentin thus forms underneath the exposed dentinal tubules along the outer pulpal wall, trying to seal off the injured area. Odontoblasts in the area of the affected tubules may perish because of the injury but neighboring undifferentiated mesenchymal cells of the pulp can move to the area and become odontoblasts (discussed further later in this chapter). This type of tertiary dentin is considered to be *reparative dentin.*

If the tertiary dentin is formed by existing odontoblasts, it is considered to be *reactive dentin.* For both types, if there is a more rushed timetable for dentin formation the tubules in tertiary dentin may assume a more irregular course than in secondary dentin as noted microscopically.

A certain type of tertiary dentin, **sclerotic dentin** (skli-**rot**-ik), is often found in association with the chronic injury of caries, attrition, and abrasion as well as in an aging tooth. The process produces a denser radiopaque (or lighter) primary dentin. In this type of dentin, the odontoblastic processes die and leave the dentinal tubules vacant; that is why it also referred to as *transparent dentin.* These hollow dentinal tubules then become retrofilled and finally occluded by a mineralized substance similar to peritubular dentin. In fact, this type of dentin may be involved with prolonging pulp vitality because it reduces the permeability of dentin. Clinically, this is noted with presence of arrested caries in mature dentitions: it appears as a dark, smooth, and shiny region on the tooth surface.

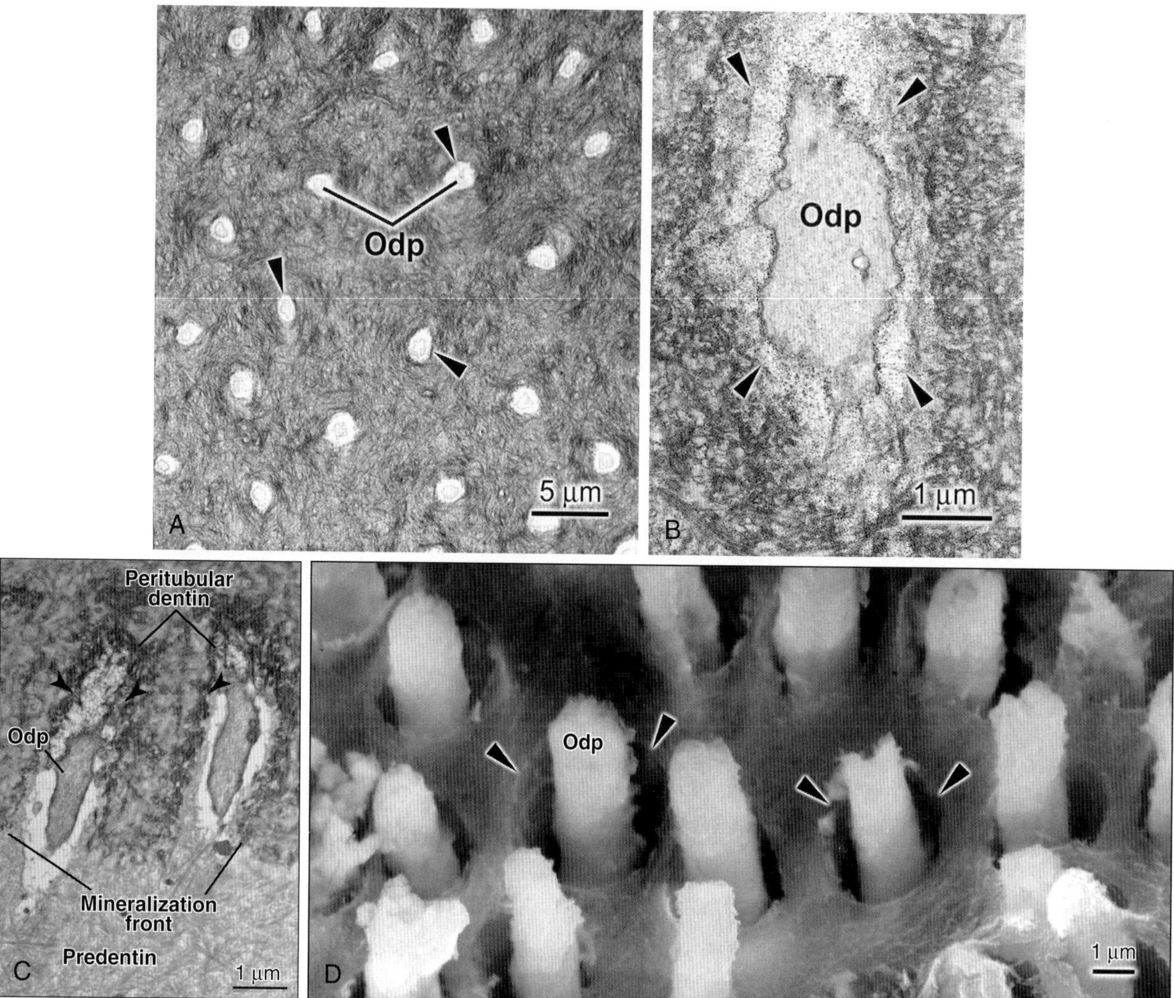

Fig. 13.8 Cross sections of dentinal tubules composed of peritubular dentin *(arrowheads)* containing odontoblastic processes *(Odp)* and surrounded by intertubular dentin. **A,** Light micrograph. **B, C,** Transmission electron micrographs showing close-up view of the process and then a more global view starting at the mineralization front and extending to predentin. **D,** Scanning electron microscope. (From Nanci A. *Ten Cate's Oral Histology*. 9th ed. St. Louis: Elsevier; 2018.)

Certain medications placed during cavity preparation with restorative treatment can promote secondary dentin formation and thus help protect the underlying pulp after outer dentin is lost due to caries or even from cavity preparation. During cavity preparation, the dental tubules are also usually sealed with certain preparations for less sensitivity post restoration.

When cutting dentin during cavity preparation there is production of a **smear layer**, which is composed of adherent dental biofilm debris. It is about 1 micrometer thick and its composition reflects the underlying dentin, although different quantities and qualities of smear layer can be produced by the various instrumentation techniques. Its function is presumed to be protective as it lowers dentin permeability. However, it masks the underlying sound dentin and interferes with attempts to bond dental restorative material to the dentin.

When dentin is exposed as a result of caries, cavity preparation, gingival recession, or attrition, the open dentinal tubules may be painful for the patient as discussed earlier causing **dentinal hypersensitivity** (hahy-per-sen-si-**tiv**-i-tee). However, in some cases it is the microscopic anatomy of the tooth that is the culprit; the enamel and cementum do not meet, leaving a gap with dentin exposed at the cementoenamel junction (CEJ) interface area a third of the time (see Fig. 14.7). In addition, the protective layers of both cementum and dentin can be inadvertently removed as a result of scaling with hand instruments, initiating sensitivity that may or may not be temporary. Branching of the dentinal tubules containing the live odontoblastic processes throughout dentin adds to the overall level of exposure.

Certain additional situations may additionally trigger the short sharp pain of dentinal hypersensitivity. This includes stimuli such as thermal changes (cold water spray or ice); mechanical irritation (vibrations from instrumentation, dental handpieces, or ultrasonics); dehydration (stream of air or heat during cavity preparation); or chemical exposure (foods such as thick or hypertonic sweet, salty, or sour fluids; tooth-colored restorative materials or vital whitening agents). By contrast, the pain from other tooth-related situations (such as from caries and pulpal or gingival infections) is usually dull and chronic in nature.

However, dentinal hypersensitivity is often a type of diffuse pain, making localization to a specific tooth difficult for the dental

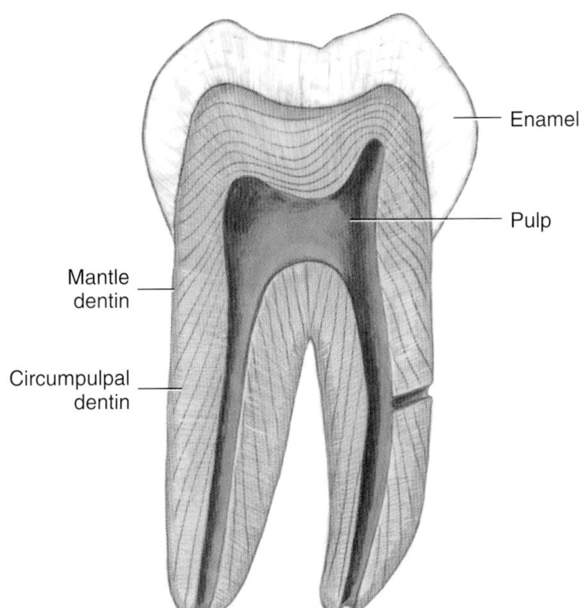

Fig. 13.9 Main Types of Dentin and Relationship to the Enamel and Pulp: Mantle Dentin and Circumpulpal Dentin.

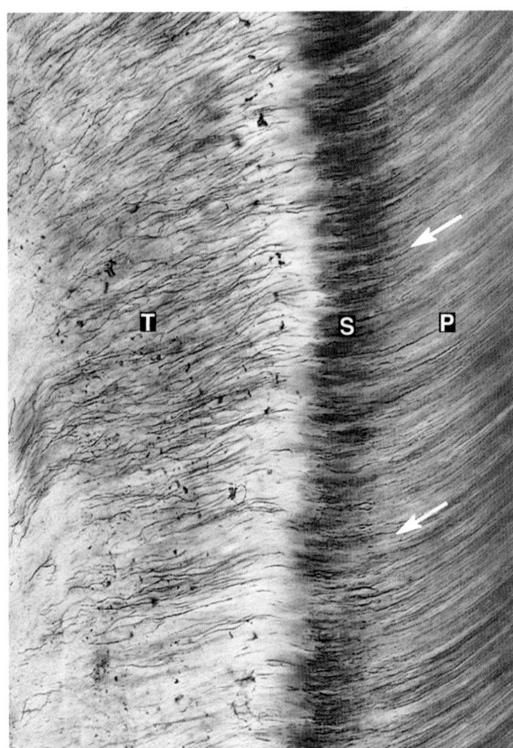

Fig. 13.10 Microscopic section of various types of dentin showing the relationship to the time of formation (from early to late): primary *(P)*, secondary *(S)*, and tertiary *(T)*, with a dark line at the junction of the primary and secondary dentin *(arrows)* caused by an abrupt change in the course of the odontoblasts during appositional growth. Note also the more irregular course of dentinal tubules in tertiary dentin than in secondary dentin. (From Bernhard Gottlieb Collection, courtesy of James McIntosh, PhD, Department of Biomedical Sciences, Baylor College of Dentistry, Dallas.)

professional as well as for the patient. This pain may wrongly be interpreted as caries, pulpal or gingival infections, or soft tissue inflammation. Because of the chronic nature of attrition and gingival recession, the pain present may not be as painful as other forms of dentinal

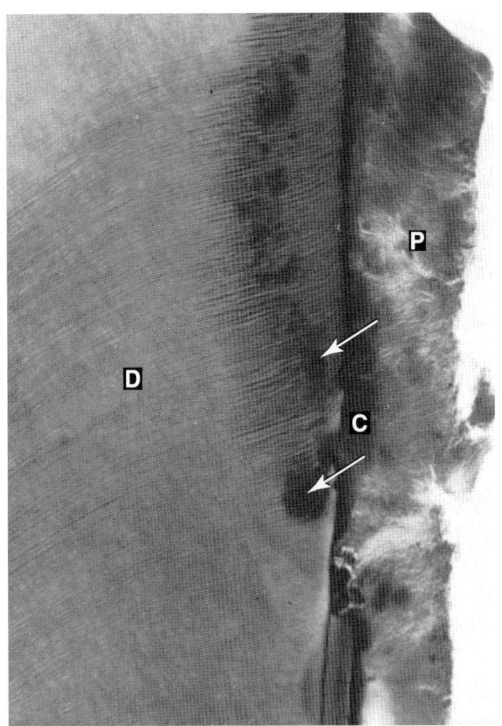

Fig. 13.11 Photomicrograph of the dentinal caries showing the cariogenic microorganisms entering the deeper dentin *(D)* through the dentinal tubules *(arrows)*. Note that cementum *(C)* has already been invaded by the cariogenic microorganisms from the dental biofilm or plaque *(P)* covering the root area. (From Carranza, FA, Perry DA. *Periodontology for the Dental Hygienist*. Philadelphia: Saunders; 1986.)

exposure because both of these are gradual processes, allowing time for subtle changes to occur in the dentinal tubules to close them off from the stimulation (discussed later). Dentinal hypersensitivity can occur within both of the dentitions and associated tooth types as well as all their surfaces but is especially evident in premolars and canines, usually on the facial and cervical regions.

The still controversial but widely accepted hydrodynamic theory of dentinal hypersensitivity suggests that it is due to changes in the dentinal fluid associated with the processes (Fig. 13.12). This mechanism may be due to one or more of the following: evaporation and loss of dentinal fluid, movement of the fluid, and ionic changes in the fluid. These changes in the dentinal fluid then stimulate the small myelinated A-delta fibers present in some dentinal tubules near the dentin-pulp interface, thus transmitting the sensation of a sharp localized pain to the pulp and then on to the brain (see later discussion of pulp innervation). That may be the reason the previously mentioned painful stimuli are present with dentinal hypersensitivity since they are involved with dentinal fluid movement within the tubule and because local anesthetics do not block sensation when they are placed on the surface of exposed dentin as they would with a fully innervated tissue. However, in the future more than one theory may be used to fully explain surface dentinal hypersensitivity.

Dentinal hypersensitivity can be treated successfully in some cases with solutions applied either by professionals or within over-the-counter products available to patients. These desensitizing agents, many of which are also used for caries control, remineralize the tooth (fluoride and casein phosphopeptide-amorphous calcium phosphate [CPP-ACP]), temporarily block the exposed open ends of the dentinal tubules (similar to the process of tooth staining) or interfere with nerve transmission to stop it completely such as with local anesthesia of the

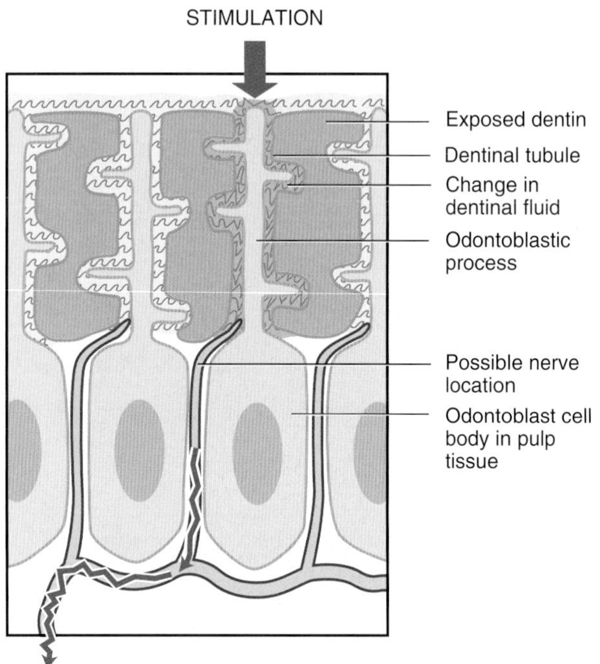

Fig. 13.12 Possible Mechanisms Involved in the Hydrodynamic Theory of Dentinal Hypersensitivity. Stimulation of the exposed dentinal tubules such as with cold water *(top arrow)* causes changes in the dentinal fluid, which is then transmitted to the nerves associated with the odontoblast cell bodies in the pulp.

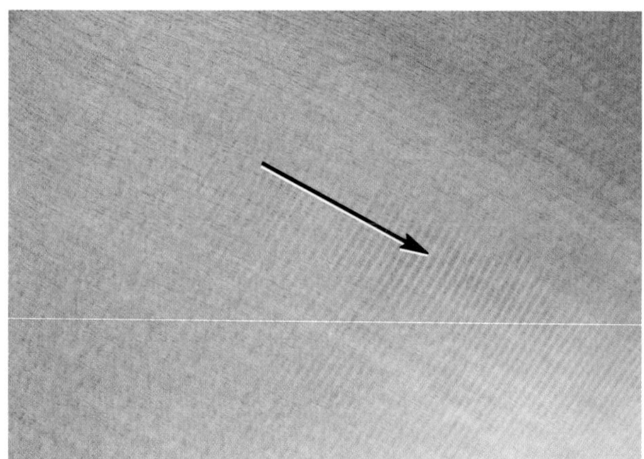

Fig. 13.13 Imbrication lines of von Ebner that transverse the dentinal tubules in dentin, with their direction noted *(arrow)*. Note the regular pattern of dentin formation. (From Bernhard Gottlieb Collection, courtesy of James McIntosh, PhD, Assistant Professor Emeritus, Department of Biomedical Sciences, Baylor College of Dentistry, Dallas.)

pulp. However, restorations sometimes are the only permanent method to reduce hypersensitivity of the exposed dentinal surface in severe cases. Methods that will fully seal the exposed dentinal tubules and thus prevent any dentinal hypersensitivity are being studied.

DENTIN HISTOLOGY

When mature dentin is examined microscopically, certain features (such as dentinal tubules and most types of dentin) are easily noted. However, the dentinal process within tubules is hard to discern microscopically. Other microscopic features are also noted and will be discussed further. These features can occur in both primary and secondary dentin.

The **imbrication lines of von Ebner** are incremental lines or bands in a microscopic section of dentin that can be likened to the growth rings of trees; they are also similar to the incremental lines of Retzius noted in enamel (Fig. 13.13). These lines show the incremental nature of dentin during the apposition stage of tooth development and run at 90° to the dentinal tubules. With each daily 4-micrometers increment of dentin by the odontoblasts, the orientation of the deposited collagen fibers differs slightly. More severe changes occur every fifth day, giving rise at every 20 micrometers to an imbrication line as noted.

The **contour lines of Owen** are a number of adjoining parallel imbrication lines that are also present in a microscopic section of dentin. These specific imbrication lines demonstrate a disturbance in body metabolism that affects the odontoblasts by altering their formation efforts, appearing as a series of dark bands. The most pronounced contour line is the neonatal line that occurs during the trauma of birth (Fig. 13.14). Other contour lines can occur in conjunction with the clinically visible tetracycline stain of the teeth in which the antibiotic

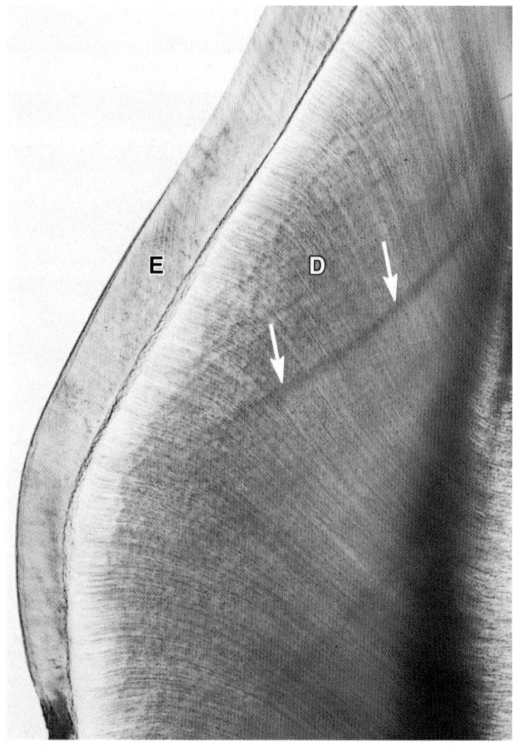

Fig. 13.14 Pronounced neonatal line, the contour line of Owen *(arrows)*, as well as other parallel adjacent contour lines in dentin *(D)* underlying enamel *(E)*. Note that they tend to appear together as a series of dark bands. (From Bernhard Gottlieb Collection, courtesy of James McIntosh, PhD, Assistant Professor Emeritus, Department of Biomedical Sciences, Baylor College of Dentistry, Dallas.)

taken systemically during tooth development becomes chemically bound to the dentin in varying amounts (see Fig. 3.19). Most of this intrinsic stain can be lightened with vital whitening to even out the tooth color or dental restorations can be used.

Another feature of dentin is **Tomes granular layer**, which is most often found in a microscopic section of dentin in the peripheral part beneath the root's cementum, adjacent to the DCJ (Fig. 13.15). However, the area only looks granular because of its spotty

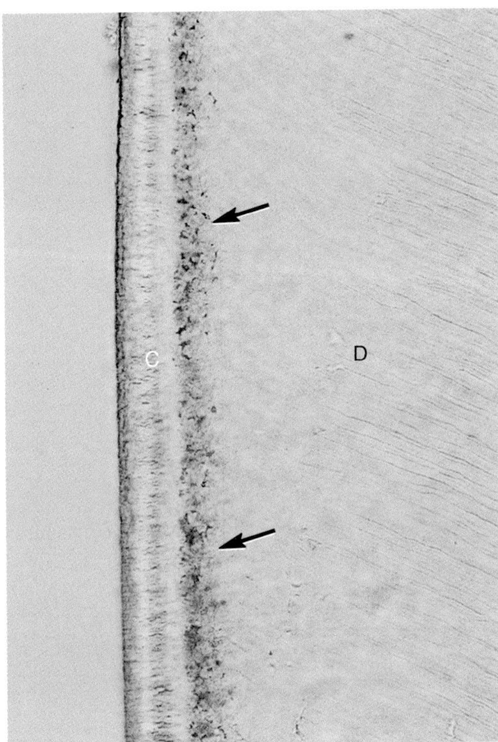

Fig. 13.15 Tomes granular layer *(arrows)* in dentin *(D)* near the dentinocemental junction and beneath layers of cementum *(C)*. (From Bernhard Gottlieb Collection, courtesy of James McIntosh, PhD, Assistant Professor Emeritus, Department of Biomedical Sciences, Baylor College of Dentistry, Dallas.)

microscopic appearance; the cause of the visible change in this region of dentin is unknown. It may be due to less mineralized areas of dentin having an increased level of interglobular dentin or the presence of branching of the terminal parts of dentinal tubules found near the DCJ, similar to that noted near the DEJ. It is unknown if it has any clinical significance. The DCJ itself is a less distinct junction than the DEJ because these two types of tissue intermingle in the root of the tooth.

AGING DENTIN

With aging, the diameter of the dentinal tubule narrows because of deposition of peritubular dentin on the inner wall. This narrowing may be related to the decreased ability of pulp to react to various stimuli with age. In addition, the passageways of the tubules to the pulp are not as wide open at a younger age; thus the stimuli are not transmitted as rapidly and in as large amounts as they were previously (discussed further in regard to pulp). Studies show the complete obliteration of older tubules with mineralization of the associated odontoblastic processes.

With age odontoblasts also undergo cytoplasmic changes, including a reduction in organelle content. As discussed previously, dentin becomes more exposed as a result of both attrition and gingival recession, which may or may not lead to dentinal hypersensitivity (discussed earlier). Assessing age from the dentition constitutes an important step in constructing an identity profile of a decedent. However, instead of microscopic features related to the aging process, dentinal translucency is one of the best morphohistologic parameters to use for dental age estimation, not only in terms of accuracy but also simplicity, along with use of related software and digital devices.

PULP PROPERTIES

The pulp is the innermost soft tissue of the tooth and appears radiolucent (dark) because it is less dense than the radiopaque (or lighter) hard tissue of the tooth (see Fig. 2.5). The pulp of a tooth is a connective tissue with all the components of such tissue (discussed later in this chapter). During tooth development, the pulp forms from the central cells of the dental papilla (see Fig. 6.7). During odontogenesis, when the predentin forms around the dental papilla, the innermost tissue is considered pulp (see Figs. 6.10 and 6.11). Thus pulp has a background similar to that of dentin because both are derived from the dental papilla of the tooth germ.

One important consideration that relates to the dentin-pulp complex is that the pulp is involved in the support, maintenance, and continued formation of dentin because the cell bodies of the odontoblasts remain along the outer pulpal wall (discussed later). Another function of the pulp is sensory because the cell bodies associated with the afferent axons in the dentinal tubules are located among this layer of odontoblasts. All sensations directed to the pulp are perceived by the brain as only the sensation of pain. Therefore, extreme temperature changes and response to touch such as vibrations that affect the pulp or dentin by way of the pulp's nerves are perceived only as painful stimuli. Thus the pulp being a sensory organ dictates that local anesthesia needs to be administered for pain control during many dental procedures.

Pulp also serves a nutritional function for itself as well as dentin because the dentin contains no blood supply of its own. Dentin depends on the pulp's vascular supply and associated tissue fluids for its nutrition. Nutrition is obtained through the dentinal tubules and their connection to the odontoblasts' cell bodies that line the outer pulpal wall.

Finally, the pulp has a protective function because it is involved in the formation of secondary dentin or tertiary dentin, which increases the coverage of the pulp. In addition, if the pulp suffers any injury that also involves the odontoblasts its undifferentiated mesenchyme contains cells that can differentiate into fibroblasts, which then create fibers and intercellular substances as well as odontoblasts to create more dentin. The pulp also has white blood cells (WBCs) within its vascular system and surrounding tissue; these allow triggering of inflammatory and immune responses.

PULP ANATOMY

The large mass of pulp is contained within the **pulp chamber** of the tooth (Fig. 13.16). The shape of each pulp chamber corresponds directly to the overall shape of the tooth and thus is individualized for every tooth (see **Chapters 16 and 17**). The pulpal tissue in the pulp chamber has two main divisions: coronal pulp and radicular pulp.

The **coronal pulp** (**kuh**-rohn-nl) is located in the crown of the tooth. Smaller extensions of coronal pulp into the cusps of posterior teeth form the **pulp horns**. These pulp horns are especially prominent in the permanent dentition under the buccal cusp of premolars and in the primary dentition under the mesiobuccal cusp of molars. In contrast, pulp horns are not found on anterior teeth and all pulp horns recede with age. To prevent exposure of the pulpal tissue, these regions must be taken into consideration during cavity preparation with restorative treatment, such as the use of radiographs to locate them.

The **radicular pulp** (or root pulp) is the part of the pulp located in the root of the tooth within the pulp canal, which is also considered the "root canal" by patients. The radicular pulp extends from the cervical part of the tooth to each apex of the tooth. This part of the pulp canal has openings from the pulp through the cementum into the surrounding periodontal ligament (PDL). These openings include each apical foramen as well as any accessory canals.

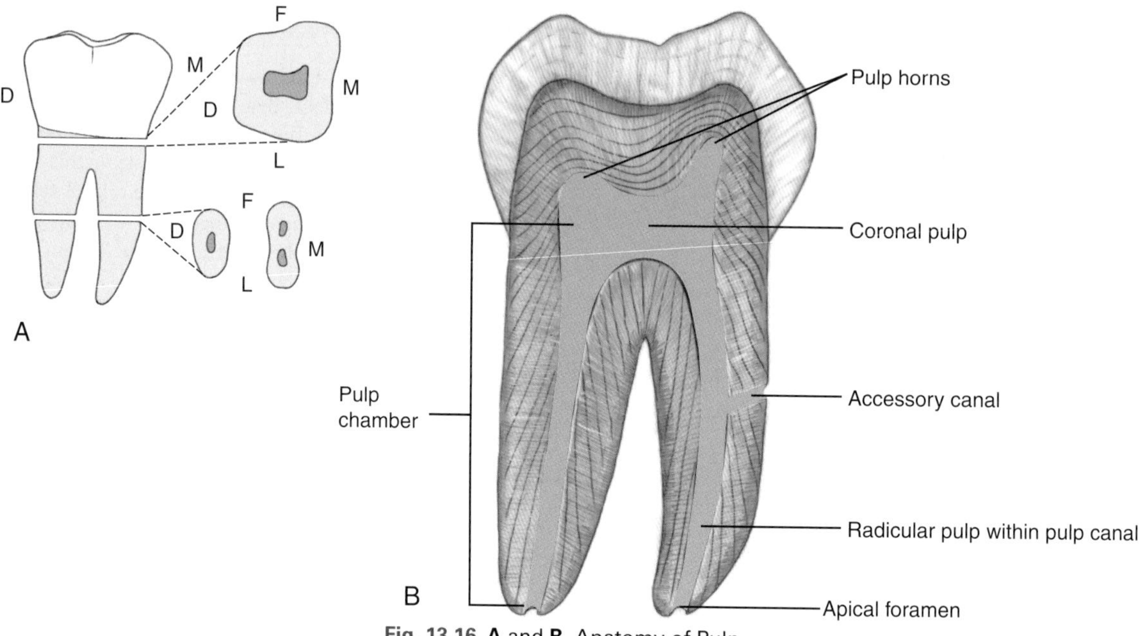

Fig. 13.16 A and **B,** Anatomy of Pulp.

TABLE 13.2 Arterial Supply to Permanent Teeth and Periodontium

Teeth and Associated Periodontium	Major Branches of Maxillary Artery
Posterior maxillary and periodontium	Posterior superior alveolar artery
Anterior maxillary and periodontium	Infraorbital artery
Mandibular and periodontium	Inferior alveolar artery

From Fehrenbach MJ, Herring SW. *Illustrated Anatomy of the Head and Neck.* 5th ed. St Louis: Elsevier; 2017.

TABLE 13.3 Nerve Supply to the Permanent Teeth and Periodontium

Teeth and Associated Periodontium	Branches of Trigeminal Nerve or Fifth (V) Cranial Nerve
Maxillary anterior teeth, maxillary anterior facial periodontium	Anterior superior alveolar nerve from maxillary nerve (V_2)
Maxillary anterior lingual periodontium	Nasopalatine nerve from maxillary nerve (V_2)
Maxillary posterior teeth, maxillary posterior buccal periodontium	Middle superior alveolar and posterior superior alveolar nerve from maxillary nerve (V_2)
Maxillary posterior lingual periodontium	Greater palatine nerve from maxillary nerve (V_2)
Mandibular teeth and facial periodontium of the mandibular anterior teeth and premolars	Inferior alveolar nerve from mandibular nerve (V_3)
Mandibular posterior buccal periodontium	Long buccal nerve from mandibular nerve (V_3)
Mandibular lingual periodontium	Lingual nerve from mandibular nerve (V_3)

From Fehrenbach MJ, Herring SW. *Illustrated Anatomy of the Head and Neck.* 5th ed. St Louis: Elsevier; 2017.

The **apical foramen** (**ey**-pi-kuhl) is the opening from the pulp into the surrounding PDL near each apex of the tooth. If more than one foramen is present on each root, the largest one is designated as the apical foramen and the rest are considered accessory foramina.

This opening is surrounded by layers of cementum but still permits arteries, veins, lymphatics, and nerves to enter and exit the pulp from the PDL allowing the tooth to remain vital (Tables 13.2 and 13.3). Thus communication between the pulp and the PDL is possible because of the apical foramen. Each apical foramen is the last part of the tooth to form; it forms after the crown erupts into the oral cavity. In developing teeth, each foramen is large and centrally located. As the tooth matures, each foramen becomes smaller in diameter and is offset in position. Each foramen may be located at the anatomic apex of each of the roots but is usually located slightly more occlusal from each apex.

Accessory canals may also be associated with the pulp and are extra openings from the pulp to the PDL (Fig. 13.17; see Fig. 13.16). Accessory canals are also called *lateral canals* because they are usually located on the lateral surface of the roots of the teeth, but this is not always the case because they can be found anywhere along the root surface. Accessory canals form when Hertwig epithelial root sheath encounters a blood vessel during root formation. Root structure then forms around the blood vessel, forming the accessory canal. Not all teeth have these canals and they are present in differing amounts in the various tooth types.

Thus teeth have a variable number of these canals, which sometimes poses problems during endodontic therapy or root canal treatment (discussed later). Radiographs do not always indicate the number or position of these canals, unless they are examined with instruments using radiopaque materials during this therapy. Gingival recession may expose the opening of an accessory canal, especially in the furcation

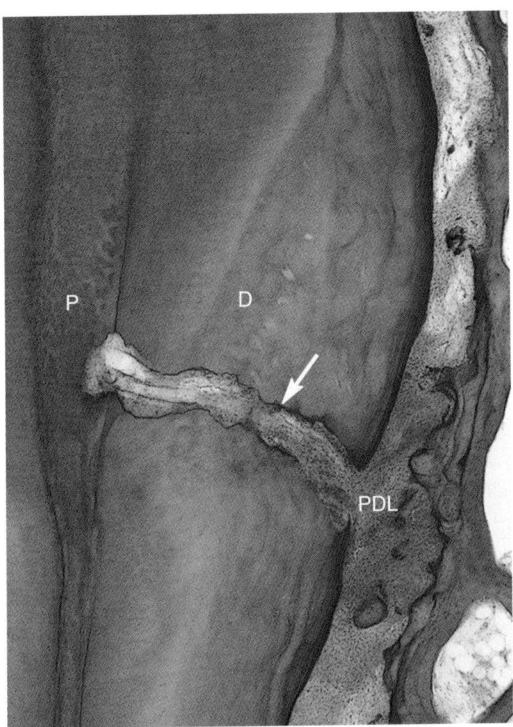

Fig. 13.17 Accessory canal *(arrow)* located in the root, which is composed of pulp *(P)* and dentin *(D)* covered by cementum. Note that the accessory canal is open to the periodontal ligament *(PDL)*. (From Bernhard Gottlieb Collection, courtesy of James McIntosh, PhD, Assistant Professor Emeritus, Department of Biomedical Sciences, Baylor College of Dentistry, Dallas.)

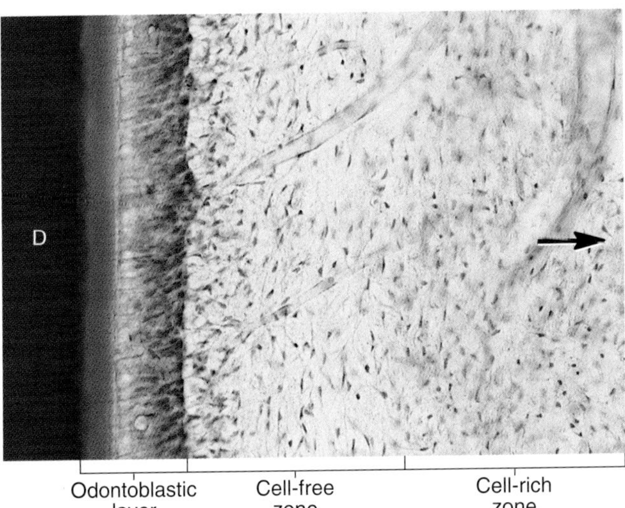

Fig. 13.18 Zones of pulp deep to the dentin *(D)* from the outer three zones to inner zone of the pulpal core *(arrow)*. (From Bernhard Gottlieb Collection, courtesy of James McIntosh, PhD, Assistant Professor Emeritus, Department of Biomedical Sciences, Baylor College of Dentistry, Dallas.)

area, which may cause the spread of infection into the pulp from caries or periodontal disease.

PULP HISTOLOGY

Because pulp is a connective tissue, it has all the components of such tissue: intercellular substance, tissue fluid, certain cells, lymphatics, vascular system, nerves, and fibers (Fig. 13.18). As in all forms of connective tissue, the fibroblasts are the largest group of cells in the pulp (see Fig. 8.5). The odontoblasts are the second largest group of cells in the pulp, but only their cell bodies are located in the pulp. The odontoblasts are located only along the outer pulpal wall.

In addition to fibroblasts and odontoblasts, the pulp contains an undifferentiated mesenchyme type of stem cells, **dental pulp stem cells (DPSCs).** These cells are a rich resource for the dentin-pulp complex because they can transform into fibroblasts or odontoblasts if either cell population is reduced after injury (discussed further at the end of this chapter).

The pulp also contains WBCs in its tissue and vascular supply, but levels are usually low unless the cells are ready to be triggered by an inflammatory or immune reaction. The red blood cells are located in the extensive vascular supply. The fibers present in the pulp are mostly collagen fibers and some reticular fibers since the pulp contains no elastic fibers. Additionally present is an extensive vascular supply and rudimentary lymphatics.

Two types of nerves are associated with the pulp, including both myelinated nerves (20% to 30%) and unmyelinated nerves (70% to 80%) (see **Chapter 8**). They are mostly nociceptors, relatively unspecialized nerve cell endings that mostly relay the sensation of pain, such as can occur with injuries to the pulp. This can include mechanical or chemical injury and temperature extremes, all which can occur with cavity preparation (see earlier discussion with dentin). The myelinated nerves are the axons of sensory or afferent neurons that are located in the dentinal tubules in dentin. The associated nerve cell bodies are located between the odontoblasts' cell bodies in the odontoblastic layer of the pulp. The unmyelinated nerves are associated with the blood vessels. The nerve fibers originate from the mandibular and maxillary branches of the trigeminal nerve and have their cell bodies in the trigeminal ganglion.

TABLE 13.4 Microscopic Zones in Pulp

Zones (From Outer to Inner Zones)	Microscopic Features
Odontoblastic layer	Lines outer pulpal wall and consists of cell bodies of odontoblasts, which may form secondary dentin, causing cell bodies to realign themselves; cell bodies of afferent axons from dentinal tubules located between cell bodies of odontoblasts
Cell-free zone	Contains fewer cells than odontoblastic layer; nerve and capillary plexus located here
Cell-rich zone	Contains increased density of cells compared with cell-free zone and more extensive vascular supply
Pulpal core	Located in center of pulp chamber; similar to cell-rich zone with many cells and extensive vascular supply

PULP ZONES

Four zones are evident when the pulp is viewed microscopically: odontoblastic layer, cell-free zone, cell-rich zone, and pulpal core (Table 13.4; see Fig. 13.18). This chapter discusses these zones in order from the outermost zone closest to the dentin to the center of the pulp.

The first zone of pulp closest to the dentin is considered the *odontoblastic layer.* This zone lines the outer pulpal wall. It consists of a layer of the cell bodies of odontoblasts, whose odontoblastic processes are located in the dentinal tubules in the adjacent dentin. The odontoblasts are capable of forming secondary or tertiary dentin along the outer

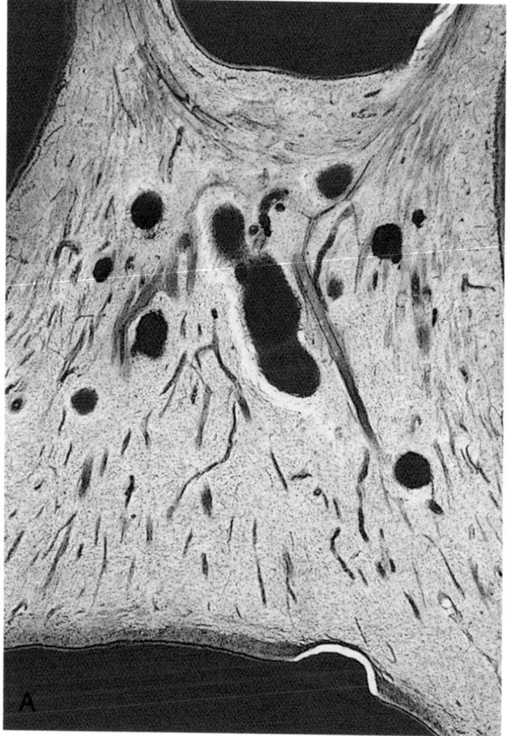

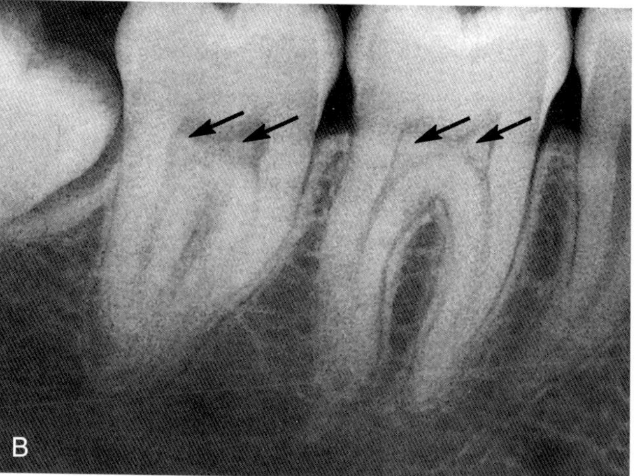

Fig. 13.19 Pulp Stones in Multirooted Teeth. **A,** Microscopic section. **B,** Radiograph *(arrows)*. (**A,** From Bernhard Gottlieb Collection, courtesy of James McIntosh, PhD, Assistant Professor Emeritus, Department of Biomedical Sciences, Baylor College of Dentistry, Dallas. **B,** Courtesy of Margaret J. Fehrenbach, RDH, MS.)

pulpal wall. If this occurs, the odontoblasts realign on the pulpal side next to this newly-formed dentin. In addition, the cell bodies of the afferent axons from the dentinal tubules in dentin are located between the cell bodies of the odontoblasts.

The next zone, nearest to the odontoblastic layer and inward from the dentin, is considered the *cell-free zone*. This refers to the zone appearing to be virtually free of a cell population, but this is only true when using lower-power magnification. In reality, this zone consists of fewer cells in contrast to the odontoblastic layer, but it is not entirely cell free. A nerve and capillary plexus are also located in this zone. No secondary or tertiary dentin is formed here initially, but newly formed dentin may encroach upon this zone.

The next zone after the cell-free zone is considered the *cell-rich zone*, inward from dentin. The cell-rich zone as its reference implies has an increased density of cells compared with the cell-free zone but still does not contain as many cells as the odontoblastic layer. This zone also has a more extensive vascular supply than does the cell-free zone.

The final zone of pulp is considered the *pulpal core*, which is in the center of the pulp chamber. This zone consists of many cells and an extensive vascular supply. Except for its location, it is very similar to the cell-rich zone.

AGING PULP

The pulp horns recede with aging. Also with increased age, the pulp undergoes a decrease in intercellular substance, water, and cells, which are replaced with an increased amount of collagen fibers. This decrease in cells is especially evident in the reduced number of undifferentiated mesenchymal cells. Thus the pulp becomes more fibrotic with increased age, leading to a reduction in the regenerative capacity of the pulp due its loss of these cells.

Also the overall pulp cavity may be smaller by the addition of secondary or tertiary dentin, thus clinically causing **pulp recession**. This is especially noted in molar teeth and is important in determining the form of cavity preparation for certain restorative treatment. The lack of sensitivity associated with mature teeth is due to receded pulp horns, pulp fibrosis, addition of secondary or tertiary dentin, or may involve all of these age-related changes. Now restorative treatment can proudly be performed without local anesthesia on mature dentitions in many cases.

The pulp's apical foramen may also become obliterated with deposits of cementum over time, leading to blockage of blood vessels serving the tissue, especially the veins (see **Chapter 14**). This can result in vascular congestion and then pulpal necrosis, resulting slowly in painless tooth death without any evidence of caries, periodontal disease, or endodontic infection.

Clinical Considerations for Pulp Pathology and Repair

Pulp stones (or denticles) are sometimes present in the pulp (Fig. 13.19). These can be mineralized masses of dentin complete with dentinal tubules and odontoblastic processes (also known as true); in other cases, they are amorphous in structure (also known as false). They can be free or unattached to the outer pulpal wall or they can be attached to the dentin at the dentin-pulp interface. Pulp stones are formed during tooth development and also later as the pulp ages and they may be due to microtrauma. They are quite common and may fill most of the pulp chamber. They are detected as radiopaque masses in radiographs and may be a problem during endodontic therapy.

However, when the pulp is injured by cavity preparation through mechanical or chemical injury and even by extensive caries or other types of injury, it may undergo inflammation with **pulpitis** (pul-**pahy**-tis). This inflammation of pulpitis initially remains localized within the confines of the dentin. However, the pressure from this confined pulpitis can result in extreme pain as the inflammatory edema presses on the afferent nerves contained in the pulp (see earlier discussion). New studies also show that nicotine use by cutting vascularity also weakens the ability for the pulp to fight illness and disease; the risk of endodontic therapy is increased over 70%.

Knowing the exact anatomy of a tooth's pulp chamber using radiographs, especially the extension of the pulp horns into the overlying cusps, is important when practicing proper restorative dentistry. Research now shows that when a caries lesion encroaches pulp that is diagnosed as healthy or with *reversible pulpitis*, only the coronal portion of the pulpal tissue (immediately adjacent to the caries) has signs of inflammation but not the entire pulp tissue as was previously thought. Therefore, the clinician can treat the carious exposed or indirect exposed pulp tissue with a pulp cap or pulpotomy—without the need for a pulpectomy (see discussion next). Calcium hydroxide has now been replaced with a bioceramic material for coverage of exposed or indirectly exposed pulpal tissue. A permanent restoration is then completed over the area to prevent any infection.

Irreversible pulpitis can later cause a pulpal infection in the form of a periapical abscess or cyst in the surrounding periodontium, spreading through the apical foramen or any accessory canal. This is an example of the communication between the pulp and the surrounding periodontium, where disease states can extend between the tissue types, which ends up involving both. However, rarely does infection or other diseases of the periodontium involve the pulp.

If the pulp dies from the infection with *irreversible pulpitis* due to bacterial invasion of the pulp tissue, it must be surgically removed by a pulpectomy. An inert radiopaque rubbery material (gutta-percha) is then placed within the pulp chamber, including into the radicular pulp within each pulp canal during endodontic (or vital pulp) therapy. This is also referred to as "root canal treatment" by the patient.

When the pulp is removed by this treatment, the tooth is no longer vital because its nutritional source from the vascular pulpal tissue has been removed. Thus the endodontically treated tooth may darken and become brittle and break during mastication. The darkening is due to leftover degradative products from pulpal necrosis with the death of the pulp tissue that were passed along the dentinal tubules.

A permanent full-coverage restorative crown is placed on the treated natural crown to protect it from breaking and to prolong retention of the tooth as well as to improve its appearance if tooth colored. Internal or external nonvital whitening may also be necessary to reduce darkening with certain esthetic restorations or if coverage is deferred. If an abscess or cyst formation develops in the periodontium as a result of pulpitis, further surgery (apicoectomy) must be performed to remove the apical lesion.

Dental professionals must try to prevent injury to the pulp during preventive procedures and restorative treatment. Such iatrogenic injury to the pulp can result from the heat or vibrations emitted by an older dental handpiece during cavity preparation as well as excessive coronal polishing, causing mechanical injury. The pulp can also undergo chemical injury by various restorative materials placed during cavity preparation (see earlier discussion). Newer water-cooled handpieces with rapid rotation, which minimize the heat and vibrations on the tooth as well as selective polishing techniques, are now used successfully to reduce the incidence of pulpal damage.

Liners are also currently placed over dentin when using toxic chemical restorative materials to prevent future pulpal damage. Then cement bases are placed after the liner to protect the pulp from restorations that can serve as thermal conductors, such as gold inlays/crowns or silver amalgams. Tertiary types of dentin will also fill in around the sensitive pulp after the restoration has been placed within 6 months to a year, thereby reducing future pulpal pain.

The vitality of the dentin-pulp complex during health and after injury depends on pulpal tissue cell activity and the signaling processes that regulate the cell's behavior. This is especially true regarding the DPSCs present within the cell-rich zone of the pulp. Research has led to a better understanding of the molecular control of cellular behavior. Growth factors play a pivotal role in signaling the events of tissue formation and repair in the dentin-pulp complex.

Harnessing these growth factors can provide exciting opportunities for biologic approaches to dental tissue repair and the blueprint for replacement tissue engineering of the tooth. These approaches offer significant potential for improved clinical management of dental disease and maintenance of tooth vitality.

In addition, work is continuing directly with the DPSCs because this particular type of stem cell has the future potential to differentiate into a variety of other cell types that were originally derived from the embryonic mesenchyme, including muscle, bone, cartilage, and fat as well as dental tissue, such as dentin, cementum, PDL, and lamina propria. This embryonic origin of DPSCs from neutral crest cells (NCCs) explains their multipotency.

The viable DPSCs are very simple to collect, without any mortality and morbidity. This is a noncontroversial topic since they can be collected without the involvement of any ethical issues. Being an autologous transplant, they also do not possess any risk of immune reaction or tissue rejection and hence immunosuppressive therapy is not required. And they may also be useful for close relatives of the donor such as grandparents, parents and siblings. Apart from these considerations, banking is more economical when compared to cord blood and may be complementary to cord cell banking.

The DPSCs are most viable in primary teeth; permanent molars (such as thirds) also have the cells, though fewer. Processing has to be quick after removal and the freezing process is the same as used to store cord blood stem cells using cryopreservation. The dental pulp can be easily cryostored for long periods and it can be used to form a cryobank for adult tissue regeneration. The DPSCs retain their potential after cryopreservation; the cryopreservation of the whole dental pulp leads to a safe recovery.

Teeth that merely fall out may have damaged pulp and may not be a useful source, especially if viability standards are not set. Studies strongly support the use of telomere length and CD271 expression as viable markers of high proliferative capacity and multipotent DPSCs populations. Consequently, if such superior DPSC populations are to be fully exploited for regenerative medicine, studies must use these and other potential markers of DPSC proliferation and senescence.

In the latest research studies, the DPSCs have also shown great potential to be used in regenerative medicine for dental-related problems including the treatment of various human diseases, including brain, eye, heart, liver, bone, skin, and muscle diseases. Regenerative medicine is the emerging field of using stem cells to repair, replace, or enhance biologic function lost to injury, disease, congenital abnormalities, or aging.

In addition, identification of the genes controlling odontoblast differentiation might lead to development of methods enabling induction of tertiary dentin formation under carious lesions. Identification of the genes active during dentinogenesis might lead to recognition of regulatory factors, which would cause secondary dentinogenesis to proceed at the rate of primary dentinogenesis filling in any cavity formed, so that present-day restorations would become a thing of the past.

14

Periodontium: Cementum, Alveolar Process, and Periodontal Ligament

Additional resources and practice exercises are provided on the companion Evolve website for this book: http://evolve.elsevier.com/Fehrenbach/illustrated.

LEARNING OBJECTIVES

1. Define and pronounce the key terms in this chapter.
2. Give an overview of periodontium properties, including its components.
3. Identify each individual component of the periodontium on a diagram.
4. Discuss cementum properties and the clinical considerations with cementum structure, integrating it into patient care.
5. Discuss cementum development, histology, types, and repair as well as the clinical considerations for cementum pathology, integrating it into patient care.
6. Discuss alveolar process properties, including jaw anatomy and histology.
7. Discuss the clinical considerations with the alveolar process, integrating it into patient care.
8. Describe periodontal ligament properties.
9. Identify the fiber groups of the periodontal ligament on a diagram and discuss the functions assigned to each of them.
10. Discuss the clinical considerations for periodontal ligament pathology and repair, integrating it into patient care.

PERIODONTIUM PROPERTIES

To understand the pathologic changes that occur during the disease states involving the **periodontium** (per-ee-oh-**don**-shuhm), dental professionals must first appreciate the histology of the healthy periodontium. Thus, the underlying histologic features of these components provide a clue to the clinical appearances noted with the periodontium, whether in a healthy or diseased state.

The periodontium consists of both the supporting soft and hard dental tissue between the tooth and the alveolar process as well as parts of the tooth and alveolar process (Fig. 14.1). The periodontium serves to support the tooth in its ongoing relationship to the alveolar process. Thus, the periodontium includes the cementum, alveolar process, and periodontal ligament (PDL), as well as each of the individual components of each type of tissue. Some clinicians may include various types of gingival tissue in the category of the periodontium, but it has only a minor role in the support of the tooth (see **Chapter 10**).

CEMENTUM PROPERTIES

The cementum is the part of the periodontium that attaches the teeth to the alveolar process by anchoring the PDL (Fig. 14.2). However, in a healthy patient the cementum is not clinically visible because it usually covers the entire root, overlying Tomes granular layer in dentin, a region which is not usually exposed in a healthy oral cavity. Cementum helps provide a protective cover over the open dentinal tubules within the root dentin if exposure occurs.

Cementum is a hard tissue that is thickest at the tooth's apex or apices and in the interradicular areas of multirooted teeth (50 to 200 micrometers) and thinnest at the **cementoenamel junction (CEJ)** (si-**men**-toh-ih-**nam**-uhl) at the cervix of the tooth (10 to 50 micrometers). Unlike bone, cementum has no nerve supply and is also avascular (without blood vessels) exhibiting little turnover, receiving its nutrition through its own embedded cells from the surrounding vascular PDL. However, like the other dental hard tissue of both dentin and the alveolar process, cementum can be deposited throughout the life of the tooth, including after eruption if not exposed (see Table 6.2).

Mature cementum is by weight 65% inorganic or mineralized material, 23% organic material, and 12% water. This crystalline formation of mature cementum consists mostly of calcium hydroxyapatite with the chemical formula of $Ca_{10}(PO_4)_6(OH)_2$. The calcium hydroxyapatite found in cementum is similar to that found in higher percentages in both enamel and dentin, but more closely resembles the percentage found in bone tissue, such as the alveolar process. Other forms of calcium are also present. The organic components include collagen, glycoproteins, and proteoglycans with mostly Type I collagen as well as lesser amounts of other types.

Because of its mineral level, cementum appears more radiolucent (or darker) than either enamel or dentin, but it appears more radiopaque (or lighter) than pulp when viewed on radiographs; however, any cemental layer(s) near the CEJ may not be viewable on radiographs due to its thinness (see Fig. 2.5).

Clinical Considerations with Cementum Structure

In certain situations, when cementum is initially exposed from gingival recession (such as occurring during chronic advanced periodontal disease), it is a dull pale yellow, lighter than dentin but darker than enamel's whitish shade (discussed later). When instruments are used against its surface, the exposed cementum feels grainy compared with the harder dentin and the even harder and smoother enamel surfaces. However, when cementum is exposed through gingival recession, it quickly undergoes abrasion by mechanical friction because of its low mineral content and thinness, exposing the underlying dentin (see Fig. 13.1). The exposure of the deeper dentin can lead to extrinsic staining and dentinal hypersensitivity (see **Chapter 13**).

Studies are showing that such histologic features may result in an increased risk of **cemental caries** (si-**men**-tuhl). The incidence of cemental caries increases in mature adults as gingival recession occurs from either trauma or periodontal disease. It is a chronic condition that forms a large shallow lesion and slowly invades first the root's cementum and then dentin to cause a chronic infection of the pulp (Fig. 14.3). Because dental pain is a late finding, many lesions are not detected early, resulting in restorative challenges and increased tooth loss. Xerostomia (or dry mouth), poor manual dexterity for adequate homecare, and poor nutrition in mature adults can complicate cemental caries; all of these issues must be addressed during dental treatment of mature patients.

Increased controversy surrounds treatment of periodontal disease that involves the removal of the outer layers of cementum during root scaling performed during nonsurgical periodontal therapy. Dental biofilm and the related hardened calculus are associated with the cemental surface of the root deep inside an active periodontal pocket (Figs. 14.4 and 14.5; see also **Chapter 10**). In the past, it was believed that bacterial toxins (or endotoxins) could be absorbed into the outer part of cementum from the adjacent dental biofilm and that these outer layers of "toxic" cementum must be removed by manual scaling for the dentogingival junctional tissue to heal and form a more occlusal epithelial attachment. Now it is believed that these toxins are

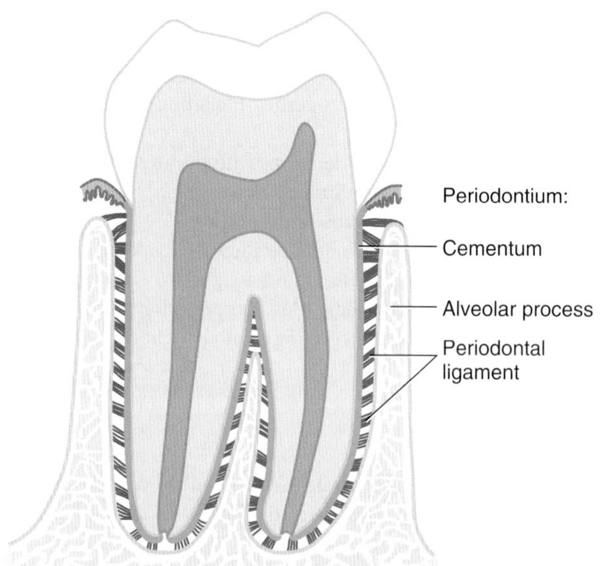

Fig. 14.1 Periodontium with its Components.

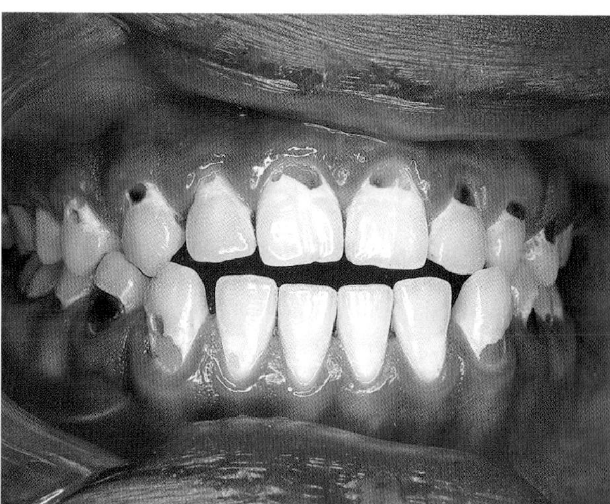

Fig. 14.3 Cemental Caries with Invasion Into the Adjacent Dentin. Pulpal involvement is a late finding due to the initial shallowness of the lesions. (Courtesy of Margaret J. Fehrenbach, RDH, MS.)

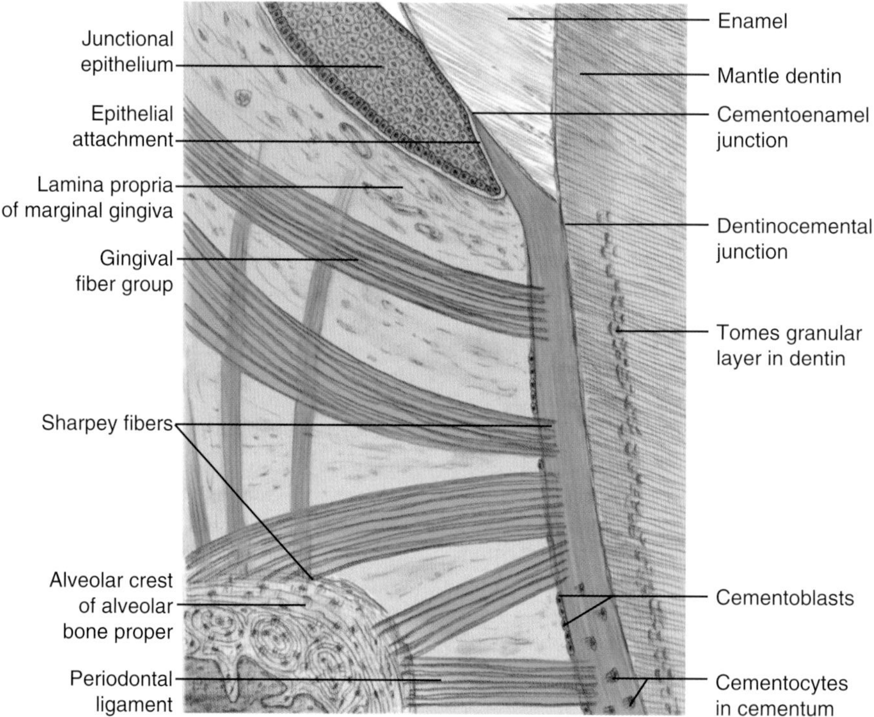

Fig. 14.2 Cementum and its relationship to both the tooth and the alveolar bone proper with Sharpey fibers from the periodontal ligament inserting into both tissue types. Note the Tomes granular layer in the adjacent underlying dentin.

loosely adherent to the cementum and that the cementum does not need to be mechanically removed by scaling, but instead, the use of ultrasonic devices can flush these toxins from the cementum without removing any of the associated hard tissue. Root scaling performed during nonsurgical periodontal therapy is only to be used to remove hardened calculus. More ultrastructural studies in this area are necessary as more evidence-based therapies of periodontal disease are considered.

CEMENTUM DEVELOPMENT

The development of cementum has been subdivided into a prefunctional stage, which occurs throughout root formation, and a functional stage, which starts when the tooth comes into occlusion and continues throughout life.

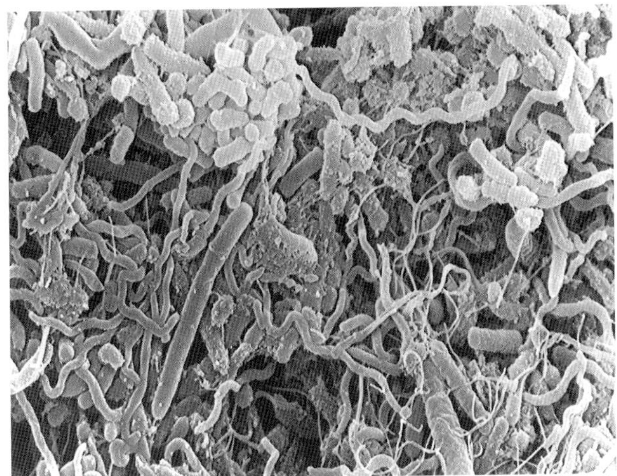

Fig. 14.4 Scanning electron micrograph of subgingival dental biofilm on the cemental root surface in a deep periodontal pocket. (Courtesy of Jan Cope, RDH, MS.)

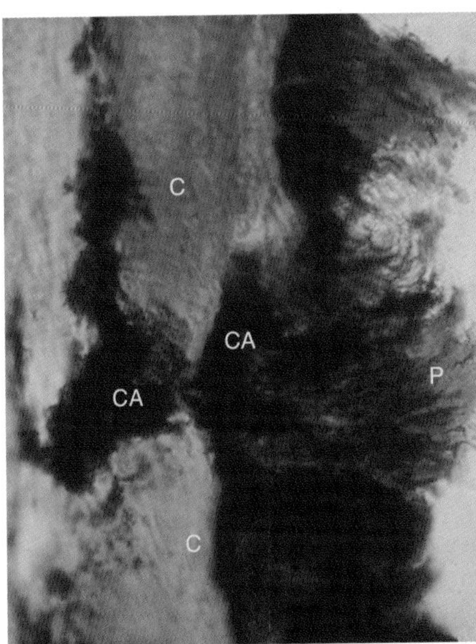

Fig. 14.5 Calculus *(CA)* penetrates the tooth surface and is embedded within the cementum *(C)*. Note that dental biofilm or plaque *(P)* also is attached to the rough calculus *(CA)*. In some cases, the calculus on the root is more mineralized than the underlying cementum or even dentin. (From Newman MG, Takei HH, Klokkevold PR, Carranza FA. *Carranza's Clinical Periodontology*. 13th ed. Philadelphia: Elsevier; 2020.)

Cementum, which develops from the dental sac, forms on the root dentin after the disintegration of Hertwig epithelial root sheath (see Fig. 6.20). This disintegration allows the undifferentiated cells of the dental sac to come into contact with the newly formed surface of root dentin, inducing these cells to become cementoblasts. The cementoblasts then disperse to cover the root dentin area and undergo cementogenesis, laying down cementoid. Unlike ameloblasts and odontoblasts, which leave no cellular bodies in their secreted products during the later steps within the apposition stage, many of the cementoblasts become entrapped by the cementum they produce, becoming cementocytes (Fig. 14.6). Again the cementum is more similar to the alveolar process with its osteoblasts becoming entrapped osteocytes.

When the cementoid reaches the full thickness needed, the cementoid surrounding the cementocytes becomes mineralized or matured and is then considered cementum. As a result of the appositional growth of cementum over the dentin, the dentinocemental junction (DCJ) is formed. This interface is not as defined either clinically or microscopically as that of the dentinoenamel junction (DEJ), given that cementum and dentin are derived from a common type of tissue during development since both the dental sac and the dental papilla were originally derived from ectomesenchyme; therefore both are of mesenchymal origin. This is unlike enamel derived from the dental lamina with its ectodermal origin.

CEMENTUM HISTOLOGY

Cementum is composed of a mineralized fibrous matrix and cells. The fibrous matrix consists of both Sharpey fibers and intrinsic nonperiodontal fibers (see Fig. 14.2). **Sharpey fibers** (**shar**-pee) are collagen fibers from the PDL that are partially inserted into the outer surface of the cementum at 90° or perpendicular. They are inserted on the other

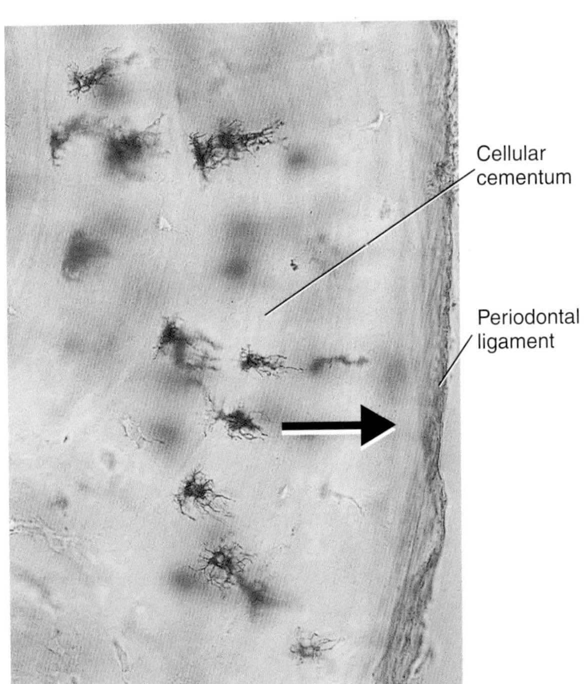

Fig. 14.6 Microscopic section of cellular cementum with its cementocytes within their lacunae and the canaliculi oriented toward the periodontal ligament for nutrition *(arrow)*. (From Bernhard Gottlieb Collection, courtesy of James McIntosh, PhD, Assistant Professor Emeritus, Department of Biomedical Sciences, Baylor College of Dentistry, Dallas.)

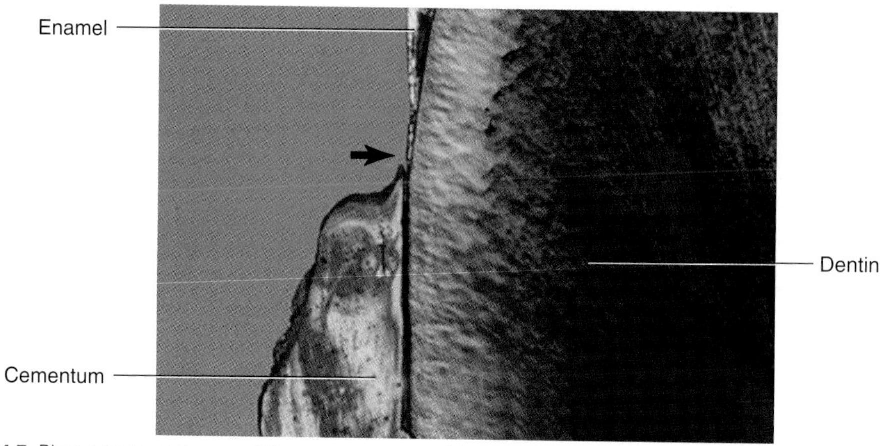

Fig. 14.7 Phase-contrast image of the cementoenamel junction interface where cementum and enamel do not meet, leaving a gap where dentin is exposed *(arrow)*, which may lead to dentinal hypersensitivity. (Courtesy of P. Tambasco de Oliveira, PhD.)

end into the alveolar process at the same angulation. These fibers are organized to function as a ligament between the tooth and alveolar process. The intrinsic non-PDL fibers of the cementum are collagen fibers made by the cementoblasts and laid down in a nonorganized pattern, yet all these fibers still run parallel to the DCJ.

The cells of cementum are the entrapped cementoblasts, now considered cementocytes (see Fig. 14.6). Each cementocyte lies in its lacuna (plural, lacunae), similar to the pattern noted in bone. These lacunae also have canaliculi or canals. Unlike those in bone, however, these canals in cementum do not contain nerves, nor do they radiate outward. Instead, the canals are oriented toward the PDL and contain cementocytic processes that exist to diffuse nutrients from the vascularized PDL; however, cementocytes far away in the deeper layers may no longer be vital.

After the appositional growth of cementum in layers, the cementoblasts that do not become entrapped in cementum line up along the cemental surface for the entire length of the outer covering of the PDL. These cementoblasts can form subsequent layers of cementum if the tooth is injured (discussed later).

There are three types of transitional interfaces that may be present at the CEJ. Therefore, the relationship of the cementum to the apical enamel border is variable. The traditional view was that certain interfaces dominated in certain oral cavities. Newer studies with the scanning electron microscope indicate that the CEJ may exhibit all of these interfaces in an individual's oral cavity and there is even considerable variation when one tooth is traced circumferentially so that these variable relationships may co-exist on a single tooth (Figs. 14.7 and 14.8).

In some cases, the cementum may overlap the enamel at the CEJ so that the cementum on the root may be continuous with a patch of coronal cementum (but less frequently than previously thought since at less than 15% of the cases). Thus the novice clinicians may have difficulty discerning the CEJ from calculus deposits around the cervix with this situation. However, compared with the usually spotty placement and roughness of calculus, cementum exhibits a more uniform placement and continual roughness when using an explorer.

Another type of interface that can occur with the CEJ is that the cementum and enamel may meet end-to-end forming a butt joint, presenting no problems for either the clinician or patient and it is the most common finding at about 52% of cases. Finally, another type of interface at the CEJ is that a gap may exist between the cementum and enamel, exposing dentin in about 33% of cases. Thus these patients may experience dentinal hypersensitivity (see Fig. 13.12).

CEMENTUM TYPES

Two basic types of cementum are formed by cementoblasts: acellular and cellular (Fig. 14.9, *A* and Table 14.1). **Acellular cementum** consists of the first layers of cementum deposited at the DCJ and thus is also referred to as *primary cementum*. It is formed at a slower rate than other types and contains no embedded cementocytes. At least one layer of acellular cementum covers the entire outer surface of each root with many more layers covering the cervical one-third near the CEJ (see Fig. 14.3). The width of acellular cementum never changes over time since no additions can be made to its inner placement.

The other type of cementum is **cellular cementum**, which is sometimes referred to as *secondary cementum* because it is deposited later than the primary type (see Figs. 14.6 and 14.9, *B*). Cellular cementum consists of the last layers of cementum deposited over the acellular cementum, mostly in the apical one-third of each root. It is formed at a faster rate than acellular type, catching the cementoblasts during production and thus many embedded cementocytes are found within it. Lining up at its periphery are cementoblasts located in the PDL, which allow the future production of more cellular cementum in response to tooth wear and movement and is also associated with repair of periodontal tissue.

Thus the width of cellular cementum can change during the life of the tooth, especially at the apex or apices of the tooth (discussed next). This type of cementum is also common in interradicular areas. It is important to note that Sharpey fibers in the inner acellular cementum are fully mineralized; those in cellular cementum at the periphery are usually mineralized only partially.

CEMENTUM REPAIR

Similar to bone tissue such as the alveolar process, cementum can undergo removal within the tissue as a result of trauma (Fig. 14.10). This removal involves resorption of cementum by the odontoclast, resulting in reversal lines. When viewed in a microscopic section of cementum, these reversal lines appear as scalloped lines, just as in bone such as the alveolar process. However, cementum is less readily resorbed than bone, an important consideration during orthodontic tooth movement (discussed later).

At the same time, there can be repair of traumatic resorption area by involving the appositional growth of cementum by cementoblasts in the adjacent PDL. Appositional growth of this recently formed protective cementum is noted by the arrest lines. These arrest lines when

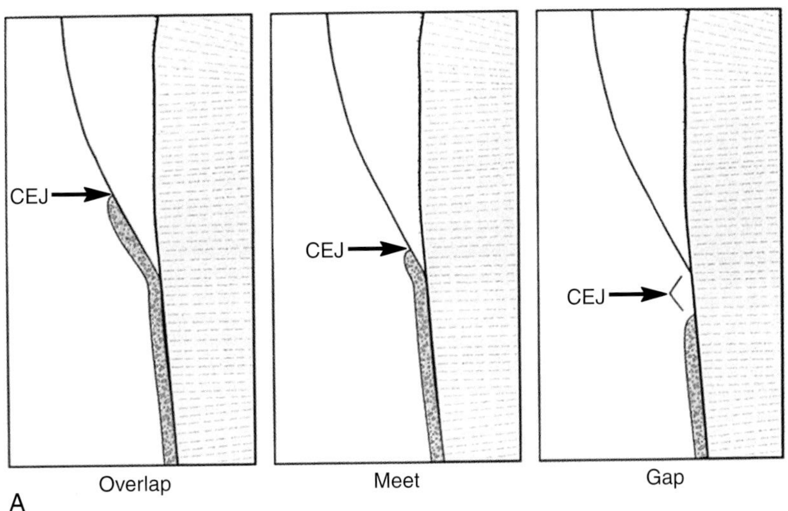

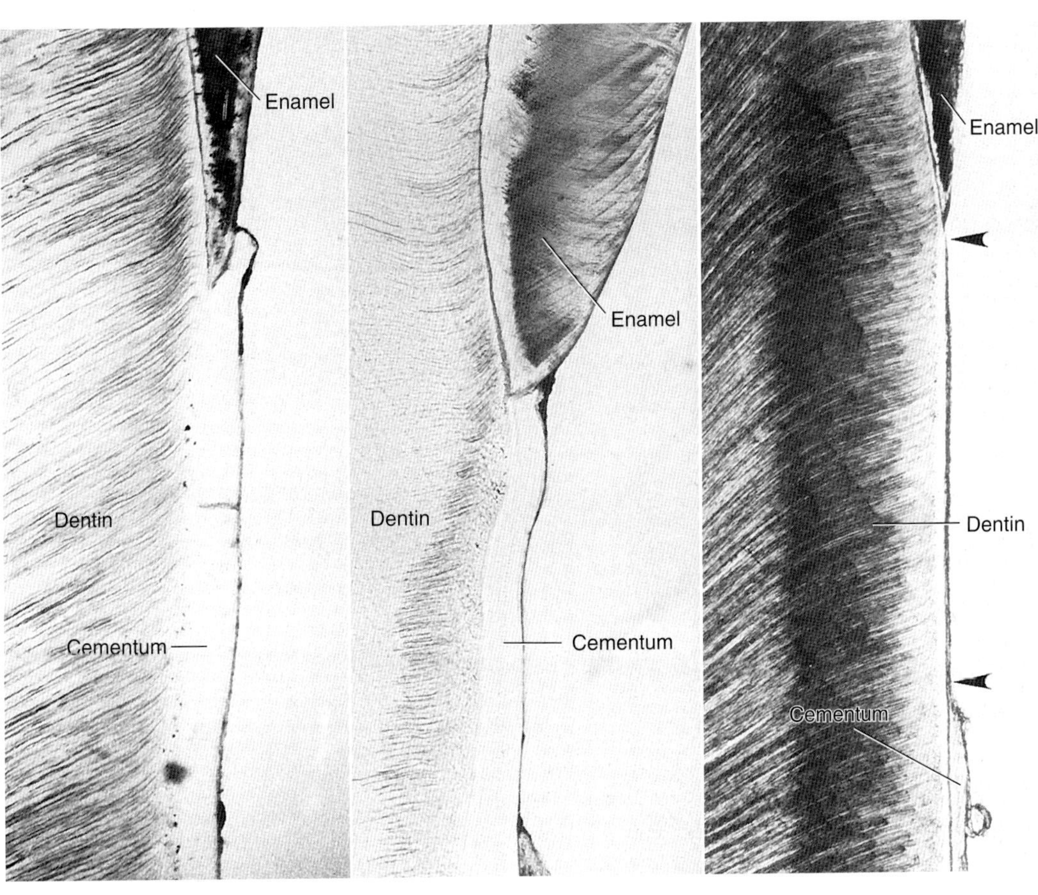

Fig. 14.8 Three types of interfaces (overlap, meet, and gap) present at the cementoenamel junction *(CEJ)* throughout a dentition as well as points along the way *(arrows)*. **A,** Cementum may overlap enamel *(overlap)*; may meet end-to-end *(meet)*; may be a gap between enamel and cementum, leaving dentin exposed *(gap)*. **B,** Ground sections of the same three interfaces with gap exposing dentin highlighted in last section *(arrowheads)*. (**B,** From Nanci A. *Ten Cate's Oral Histology*. 6th ed. St. Louis: Elsevier; 2003.)

viewed in a microscopic section, look like smooth growth rings in a cross section of a tree. This is similar to what occurs in bone tissue, such as the alveolar process. Both reversal and arrest lines are prominent in cementum subjected to occlusal trauma or to orthodontic tooth movement, as well as during the shedding of primary teeth and eruption of the permanent tooth. However, unlike bone, cementum does not continually undergo remodeling or repair as part of its history and will do so only when severely traumatized. Additionally, aging does not result in a change in mineral content of cementum like bone, but its permeability may lessen.

Finally, there is accumulating histologic evidence that cementum is critical for appropriate maturation of the periodontium, both during development as well as with regeneration of periodontal tissue. And since cementum is a matrix rich in adhesion molecules (especially

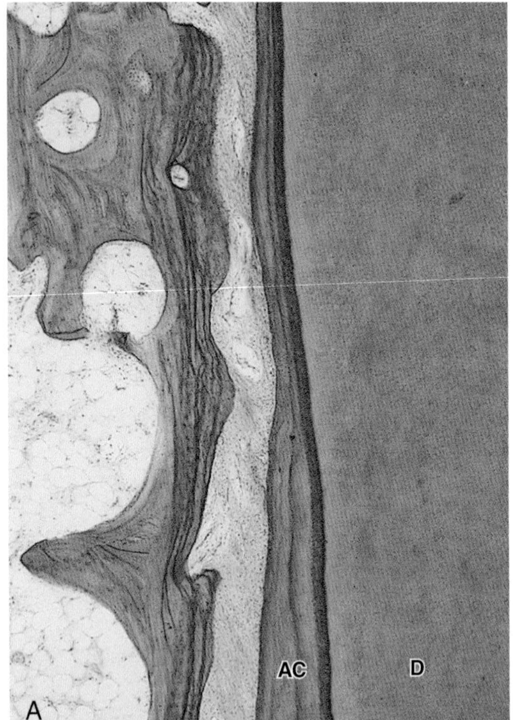

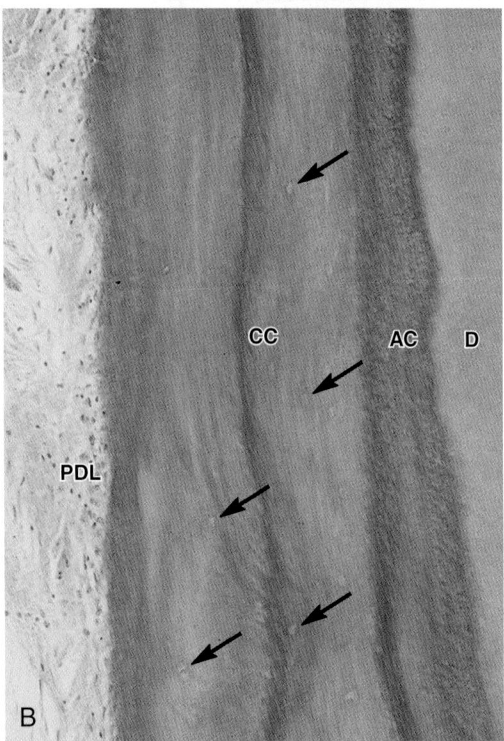

Fig. 14.9 Two Types of Cementum on the Root Surface. **A,** Acellular cementum *(AC)* without cementocytes makes up the first layers deposited at the dentinocemental junction over the dentin *(D)*. **B,** Cellular cementum *(CC)* that contains embedded cementocytes *(arrows)* is the last of the layers deposited over the thin layer of acellular cementum *(AC)* adjacent to the dentin *(D)*. Cells adjacent to the periodontal ligament *(PDL)* are cementoblasts. (From Bernhard Gottlieb Collection, courtesy of James McIntosh, PhD, Assistant Professor Emeritus, Department of Biomedical Sciences, Baylor College of Dentistry, Dallas.)

TABLE 14.1 Cementum Types

Acellular	Cellular
First layer(s) deposited	Formed after acellular layer(s)
At least one layer over entire root with many layers near cervical one-third	Layered over acellular, mostly in apical one-third, especially in interradicular region
Formed at slower rate	Formed at faster rate
No embedded cementocytes	Embedded cementocytes
Width constant over time	Can widen over time; layers can be added

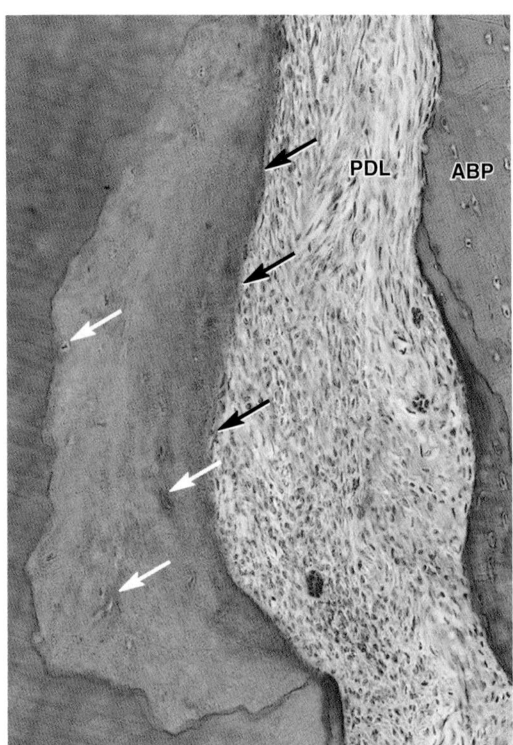

Fig. 14.10 Reversal lines and arrest lines in cementum with embedded cementocytes *(white arrows)* that has undergone repair due to severe trauma. On the surface of the cementum are the cementoblasts *(dark arrows)* within the surrounding periodontal ligament *(PDL)*. Note that the alveolar bone proper *(ABP)* has similar lines noted as a result of bone remodeling. (From Bernhard Gottlieb Collection, courtesy of James McIntosh, PhD, Assistant Professor Emeritus, Department of Biomedical Sciences, Baylor College of Dentistry, Dallas.)

cementum attachment protein, CAP) and growth factors during the process of cementogenesis (especially cementum protein-1 from cementoblasts, CEMP1), these factors may have potential usefulness for regeneration of the periodontal structures in a more predictable therapeutic manner after periodontitis than procedures used presently.

Clinical Considerations for Cementum Pathology

Cementicles (si-**men**-tih-kuhlz) are mineralized spherical bodies of cementum found either attached to the cemental root surface or lying free in the PDL (Fig. 14.11). They form from the appositional growth of cementum around cellular debris in the PDL, possibly as a result of microtrauma to Sharpey fibers. They become attached or fused from the continued appositional growth of cementum and may be large enough to be noted on radiographs.

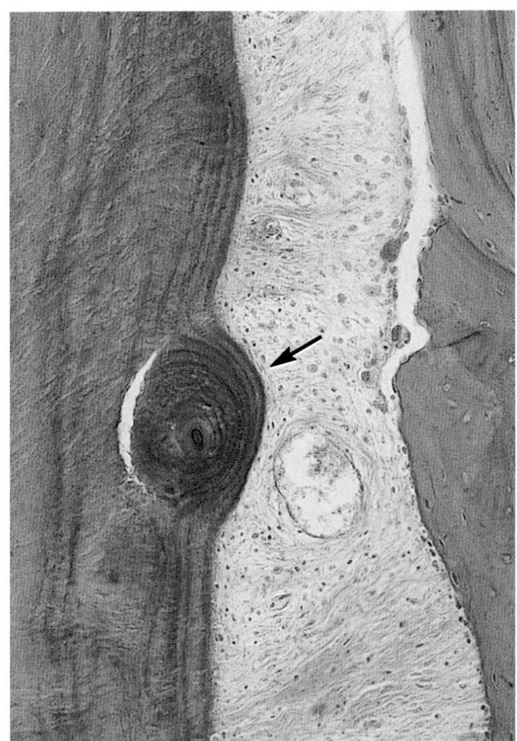

Fig. 14.11 Cementicle attached to the cemental surface within the periodontal ligament *(arrow)*. (From Bernhard Gottlieb Collection, courtesy of James McIntosh, PhD, Assistant Professor Emeritus, Department of Biomedical Sciences, Baylor College of Dentistry, Dallas.)

Cemental spurs can be found at or near the CEJ. These are symmetrical spheres of cementum attached to the cemental root surface similar to enamel pearls. Cemental spurs result from irregular deposition of cementum on the root and may be noted on radiographs. Both cementicles and cemental spurs can present some clinical problems in differentiating them from calculus; however, because they are hard, they are not easily removed. Therefore the spurs may also interfere with periodontal therapy and homecare; they may need to be removed by bur reduction during periodontal surgery.

Hypercementosis (hahy-per-si-mehn-**toh**-sis) is the excessive production of cellular cementum, which mostly occurs at the apex or apices of the tooth but could occur anywhere on the apically third of one or more teeth (Fig. 14.12). It may be present on radiographs as a radiopaque (or lighter) mass at each root apex. This condition may have resulted from occlusal trauma caused by excessive occlusal forces and during certain pathologic conditions (such as with chronic periapical inflammation), as well as systemic conditions (generalized level noted with Paget disease). It may also be a compensatory mechanism in response to attrition to increase occlusal tooth height, keeping the dentition in functional occlusion. However, such overgrowth of deposits forms into bulbous enlargements on the roots and may interfere with extractions, especially if adjacent teeth become fused, such as with concrescence (see Box 6.1, *Q*). It may also result in pulpal necrosis if at a severe level by blocking blood supply via the apical foramen (see **Chapter 13**).

In contrast, an unwanted side effect of rapid orthodontic therapy can be root apex resorption, reducing the overall length of the tooth, which is especially noted with permanent maxillary incisors (discussed later). The risk of tooth mobility is also increased. However, with new

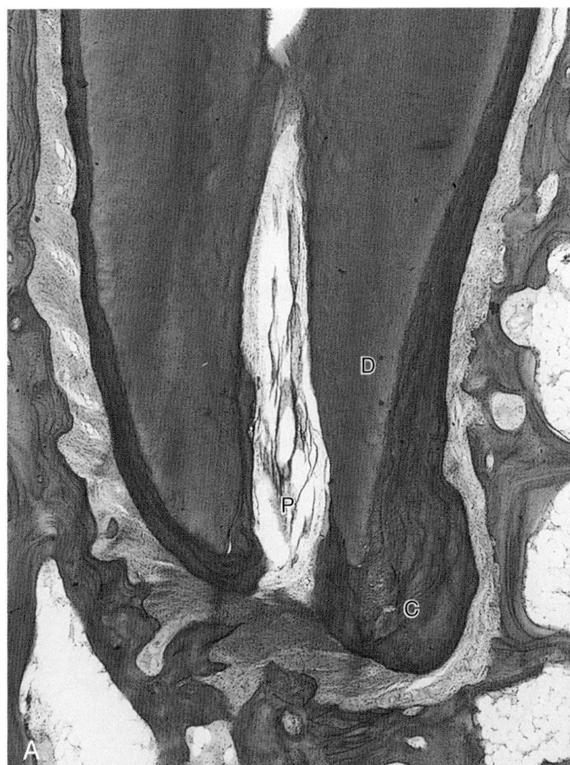

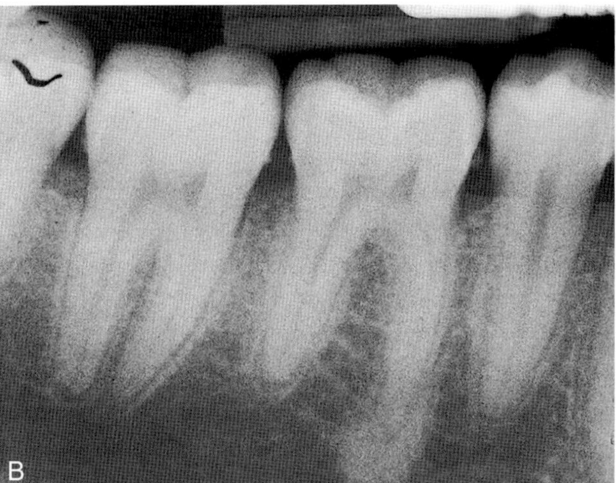

Fig. 14.12 Hypercementosis at the Root Apices Due to Traumatic Occlusal Forces on Permanent Mandibular Molar Teeth. **A,** Microscopic section with tooth components identified: dentin *(D)*, cementum *(C)*, and radicular pulp *(P)*. **B,** Radiograph. (**A,** From Bernhard Gottlieb Collection, courtesy of James McIntosh, PhD, Assistant Professor Emeritus, Department of Biomedical Sciences, Baylor College of Dentistry, Dallas; **B,** Courtesy of Margaret J. Fehrenbach, RDH, MS.)

bioefficient orthodontic therapy being utilized, this effect has been minimized. In addition, thankfully cementum is resistant to resorption in a younger dentition during orthodontic therapy, unlike the alveolar process.

ALVEOLAR PROCESS PROPERTIES

The **alveolar process** is that part of either the maxilla or mandible that supports and protects the teeth. The alveolar process is also that part of the periodontium to which the cementum of the tooth is attached through the PDL (Fig. 14.13). The term *alveolar process* will be used mostly in this textbook since it has a clinical connotation; whereas the other term that could be used, *alveolar bone,* has more of a histologic background instead.

The alveolar process is a hard mineralized tissue with all the components of other bone tissue (see Fig. 8.9). It is important to note that alveolar process is more easily remodeled than cementum, thus allowing orthodontic tooth movement (discussed later). When viewing a microscopic section, the remodeled alveolar process shows arrest lines and reversal lines as does all bone tissue.

Like all bone, mature alveolar process is by weight 60% inorganic material or mineralized, 25% organic material, and 15% water. This crystalline formation consists mostly of calcium hydroxyapatite with the chemical formula of $Ca_{10}(PO_4)_6(OH)_2$. The calcium hydroxyapatite in the alveolar process is similar to that found in higher percentages in both enamel and dentin but is most similar to the levels in cementum (see Table 6.2). The minerals of potassium, manganese, magnesium, silica, iron, zinc, selenium, boron, phosphorus, sulfur, chromium, and others are also present but in smaller amounts.

JAW DEVELOPMENT

Both the maxilla and mandible develop from tissue of the first pharyngeal or branchial arch (or mandibular arch). The maxilla forms within the fused maxillary processes of the mandibular arch and the mandible forms within the fused mandibular processes of the mandibular arch. Both jaws also start as small centers of intramembranous ossification located around the stomodeum. These centers then increase in diameter, growing into the mature jaws (see **Chapter 8**). In addition, both jaws also have several skeletal units during development that are related to the overall morphology or form of the bones. Each of these units is influenced in its growth pattern by some adjacent structure that acts on the developing bone.

The maxilla's primary center of intramembranous ossification for each half of the maxilla appears around the seventh week of prenatal development. It is located at the termination of the infraorbital nerve, just superior to the dental lamina of the primary maxillary canine tooth in each maxillary process. Secondary ossification centers, the zygomatic, orbitonasal, nasopalatine, and intermaxillary, then appear and fuse rapidly with the primary centers. The two intermaxillary centers generate the alveolar process and primary palate region.

The subsequent growth of the maxilla can be subdivided into several skeletal units: the basal body unit that develops beneath the infraorbital nerve surrounding it to form the infraorbital canal; the orbital unit that responds to the growth of the eyeball; the nasal unit that depends on nasal septal cartilage for its growth; the alveolar unit that forms in response to the maxillary teeth; and the pneumatic unit that reflects maxillary sinus expansion. The primary bone initially formed in the maxilla is soon replaced by secondary bone as the face and oral cavity develop.

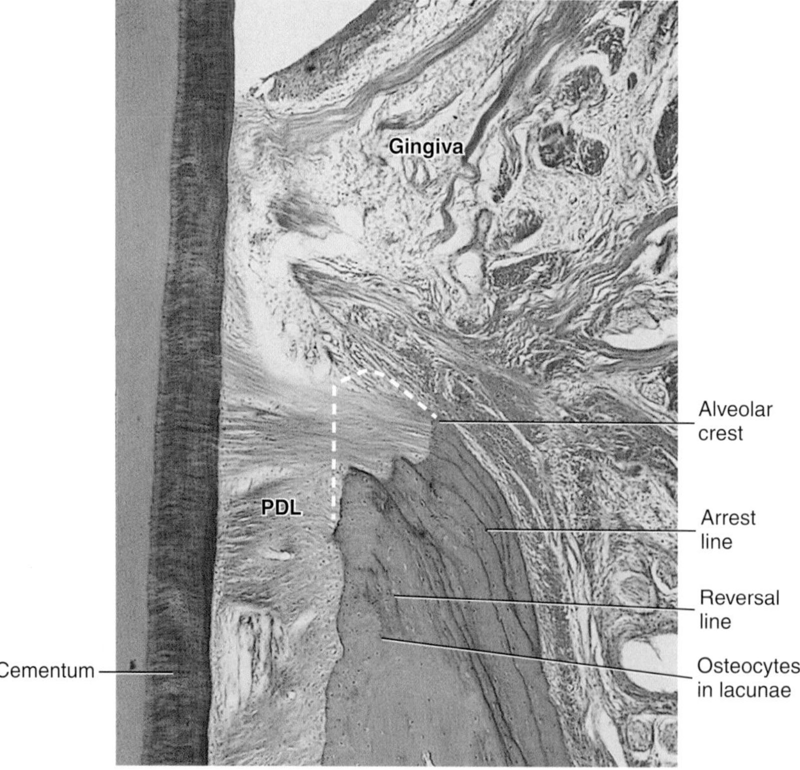

Fig. 14.13 Alveolar process with its microscopic components is identified, including osteocytes in lacunae as well as arrest and reversal lines, deep to the gingiva and adjacent to the periodontal ligament *(PDL)* and deeper cementum. Note that there has been a slight resorption of the alveolar crest *(dashed lines)* showing the beginning of periodontitis as well as disruption of the superior part of the alveolar crest group fibers. (From Bernhard Gottlieb Collection, courtesy of James McIntosh, PhD, Assistant Professor Emeritus, Department of Biomedical Sciences, Baylor College of Dentistry, Dallas.)

During the sixth week of prenatal development on each side of the embryo's mandibular arch, a primary ossification center appears in the angle formed by the division of the inferior alveolar nerve and its incisive and mental branches; it appears as a rod derived from the first pharyngeal or branchial arch (or mandibular arch) on the lateral aspect of Meckel cartilage (see Figs. 4.11 and 5.3).

In the seventh week, the first bone tissue in the body of the mandible forms. Bone development spreads rapidly from the angle anterior to the midline. The anterior bone forms around Meckel cartilage to produce a trough with medial and lateral plates that unite inferiorly around the incisive nerve. This trough extends to the midline on the embryo, where it comes into close approximation with a similar trough from the other side.

These two separate bilateral centers of ossification of the mandibular arch remain separated at the mandibular symphysis until shortly after birth. The trough turns into the mandibular canal as bone is formed over the incisive nerve joining the lateral and medial plates of initial bone.

Bone development in the mandibular arch also spreads posteriorly toward the point where the mandibular nerve is divided into its lingual and inferior alveolar branches. This ossification initially forms a gutter, which later evolves into a canal that contains the inferior alveolar nerve, the mandibular canal.

The mandible subsequently develops as several skeletal units: a condylar unit that forms the articulation with the temporal bone; the body of the mandible that is the center of all growth of the mandible; the angular unit that forms in response to the lateral pterygoid and masseter muscles; the coronoid unit that forms in response to the temporalis muscle development; and the alveolar unit that forms in response to the development of the mandibular teeth.

Because it acts as a temporary supporting structure in the embryonic mandible, most of Meckel cartilage disappears as the mandible develops. The primary bone formed along Meckel cartilage is soon replaced by secondary bone. Secondary cartilage appears between the tenth and fourteenth weeks of prenatal development to form the head of the condyle, part of the coronoid process, and the mental protuberance.

Separate from Meckel cartilage, the coronoid cartilage becomes incorporated into the expanding intramembranous bone of the mandibular ramus and disappears before birth. In the mental region, a similar situation occurs as the cartilage there disappears when the mandibular processes fuse at the mandibular symphysis (see Fig. 1.9).

The condylar cartilage appears initially as a cone-shaped structure and is the primordium of the condyle. Chondrocytes differentiate in the center and increase by interstitial and appositional growth. By the middle of fetal life, most of the condylar cartilage is replaced with bone as a result of endochondral ossification, but its superior end persists into puberty. Thus, the condylar cartilage acts as a *growth center* for the temporomandibular joint until puberty is over (see **Chapter 8** and Figs. 8.13 and 19.4).

Clinical Considerations During Jaw Development

The developmental dental anomaly of anodontia in which tooth germ(s) are congenitally absent may affect the development of the alveolar processes of the associated jaw (see Box 6.1, *A-B*). This occurrence of anodontia can prevent the alveolar processes of either the maxilla or the mandible from developing locally. Proper development is impossible because the alveolar unit of each dental arch only forms in response to the tooth germs that will erupt later in the area. Instead only basal bone will be present in each one of the involved areas of the jaws (discussed next).

JAW ANATOMY AND HISTOLOGY

Each mature jaw, either the maxilla or mandible, is composed of two types of bone tissue with differing physiologic functioning (Fig. 14.14). The part that contains the roots of the teeth is the alveolar process, which is also referred to as the *alveolar bone* as discussed earlier or also *alveolar ridge*. The part apical to the roots of the teeth is the **basal bone,** which then forms the body of the maxilla or body of the mandible and thus is not part of the periodontium. Both the alveolar process and basal bone are covered by periosteum.

The alveolar process (or alveolar bone) is divided into the alveolar bone proper and the supporting alveolar bone. Microscopically both the alveolar bone proper and the supporting alveolar bone have the same components: fibers, cells, intercellular substances, nerves, blood vessels, and lymphatics but the arrangement of these components is different (see **Chapter 8**; see Fig. 14.13).

The **alveolar bone proper (ABP)** is the lining of the tooth socket or alveolus (plural, alveoli) (see Fig. 14.14). Although the ABP is composed of compact bone, it may be referred to as the *cribriform plate* because it contains numerous holes where Volkmann canals with its nerves and blood vessels pass from the ABP into the PDL. The ABP is also considered *bundle bone* because Sharpey fibers, a part of the fibers of the PDL, are inserted here (Fig. 14.15). Similar to those of the cemental surface, Sharpey fibers in ABP are each inserted at 90° or perpendicular to the alveolar process to mediate the anchorage of the tooth These fibers are fewer in number, although thicker in diameter than those present in cementum. As in cellular cementum, Sharpey fibers in bone are usually mineralized only partially at their periphery. The attached gingiva along with the periosteum of the ABP serves as a mucoperiosteum (see **Chapter 9**).

The ABP consists of plates of compact bone that surround the tooth and assume the shape of the tooth. The ABP varies in thickness from 0.1 to 0.5 mm. The part of the ABP that is present on radiographs is considered the **lamina dura** (**door**-uh), which is uniformly radiopaque (or lighter) (Fig. 14.16). The integrity of the lamina dura is important when studying radiographs for pathologic lesions.

The **alveolar crest** is the most cervical rim of the ABP (Fig. 14.17). In a healthy situation, the alveolar crest is slightly apical to the CEJ by approximately 1 to 2 mm. The alveolar crests of neighboring teeth are also uniform in height along the jaw in a healthy jaw.

A part of the alveolar crest that is between neighboring teeth is present on periapical and bitewing radiographs as a radiopaque (or lighter) triangle at the most coronal part of the interdental septum or bone (see Fig. 14.16, *A*). This anatomic representation can be used for educating patients about bone loss levels occurring with periodontal disease; however, a bitewing radiograph shows only the levels of ABP interproximally, limited to being within only two dimensions. In reality, bone loss occurs in three dimensions and at any surface adjacent to the tooth root and in varying amounts around it.

The **supporting alveolar bone (SAB)** consists of both cortical bone and trabecular bone. The **cortical bone** (**kawr**-ti-kuhl) consists of a plate of compact bone on both the facial and lingual surfaces of the alveolar process; thus *cortical plate* is also used to describe this part of the alveolar process (see Fig. 14.15). These cortical plates are usually about 1.5 to 3 mm thick over posterior teeth, but the thickness is highly variable around anterior teeth. The cortical bone is not visible on periapical or bitewing radiographs but only on occlusal radiographs as a uniformly radiopaque (or lighter) bony sheet, both facial and lingual to the teeth (see Fig. 14.16, *B*).

The **trabecular bone** (truh-**bek**-yuh-ler) consists of cancellous bone (or spongy bone) that is located between the ABP and the plates of cortical bone (see Fig. 14.15). Only the parts of trabecular bone between the

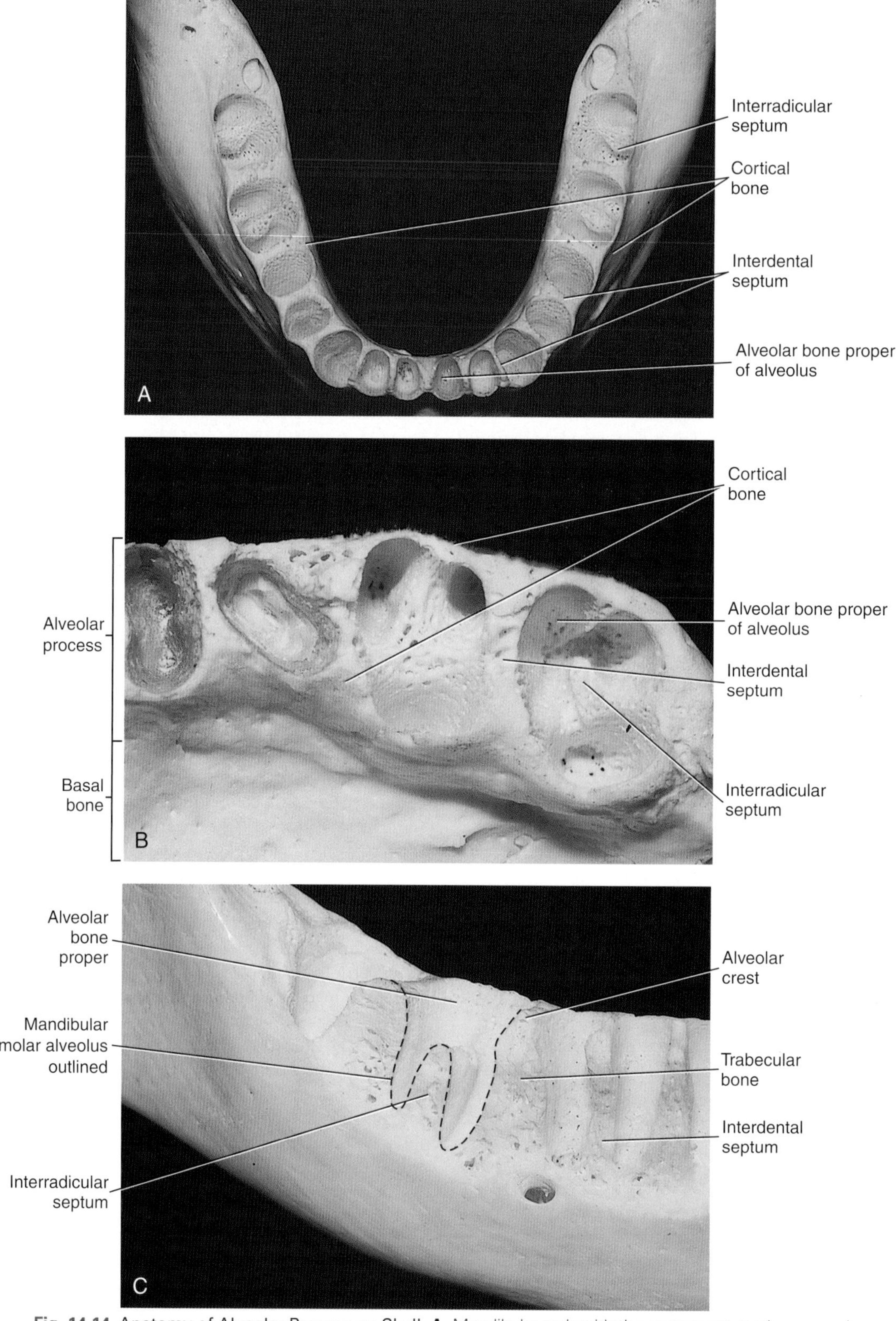

Fig. 14.14 Anatomy of Alveolar Process on Skull. **A,** Mandibular arch with the permanent teeth removed. **B,** Part of the maxilla with the teeth removed demonstrating the surrounding cribriform plate of the alveolar bone proper of the alveolus. **C,** Cross section of the mandible with the teeth removed and a mandibular molar alveolus highlighted *(dashed lines)*. (Courtesy of Margaret J. Fehrenbach, RDH, MS.)

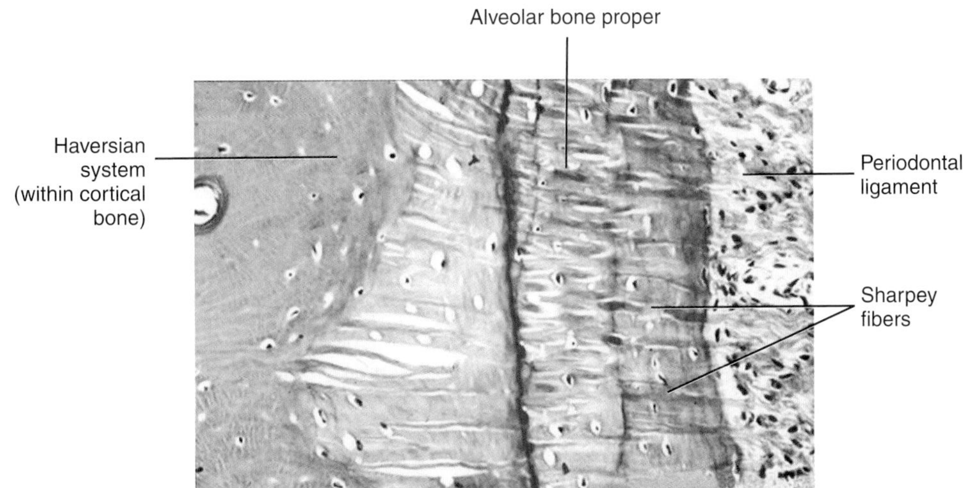

Fig. 14.15 Microscopic section of the insertion of Sharpey fibers from the periodontal ligament into the alveolar bone proper in the root area. Note the Haversian system within the cortical bone as well as the alveolar bone proper. (Courtesy of P. Tambasco de Oliveira, PhD.)

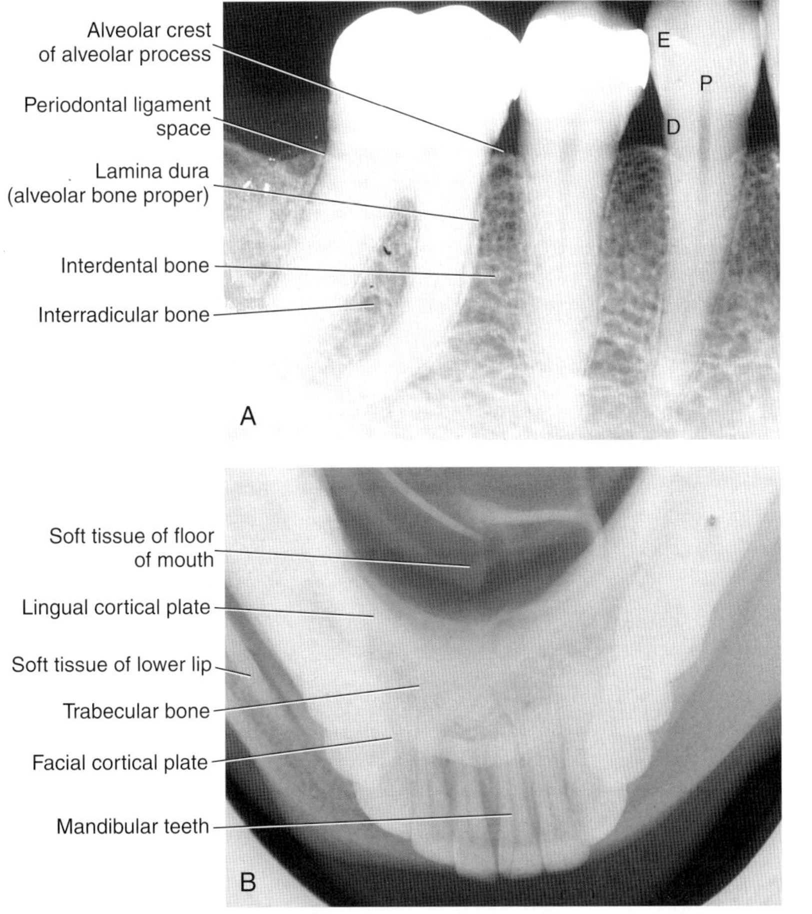

Fig. 14.16 Radiographic Landmarks of the Alveolar Process of the Mandible. **A,** Periapical radiograph. **B,** Occlusal radiograph. Tooth components are also identified: enamel *(E)*, dentin *(D)*, and pulp *(P)*. (Courtesy of Margaret J. Fehrenbach, RDH, MS.)

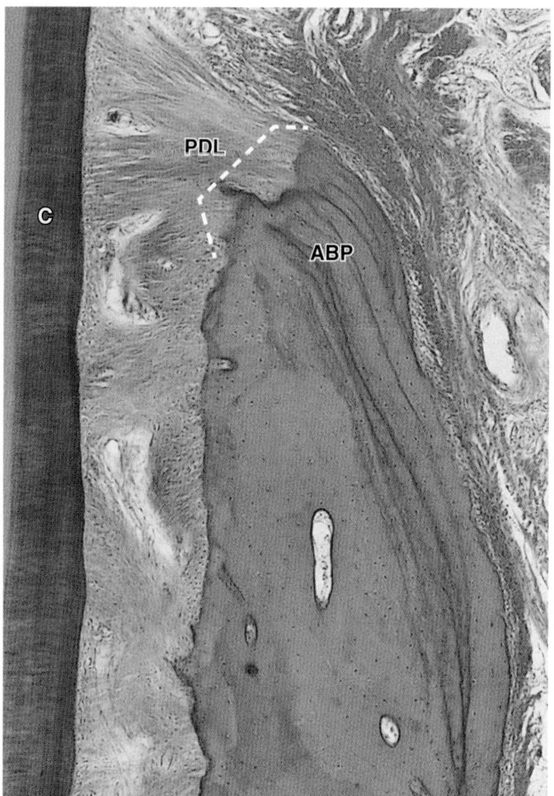

Fig. 14.17 Photomicrograph of the alveolar crest of the alveolar bone proper *(ABP)* and its relationship to the root covered by cementum *(C)* with the alveolar crest fibers of the periodontal ligament *(PDL)* inserting Sharpey fibers into both tissue types. Note that there is slight resorption of the alveolar crest *(dashed lines)* showing the beginning of periodontitis. (From Bernhard Gottlieb Collection, courtesy of James McIntosh, PhD, Assistant Professor Emeritus, Department of Biomedical Sciences, Baylor College of Dentistry, Dallas.)

teeth and between the roots are ever present on any type of radiographs; this trabecular bone appears less uniformly radiopaque and more porous than the uniformly radiopaque lamina dura of the ABP.

The alveolar process that separates two neighboring teeth is the **interdental septum** (or interdental bone) (Fig. 14.18). It is present on both periapical and bitewing radiographs (see Fig. 14.17). The interdental septum consists of both the compact bone of the ABP and cancellous bone of the trabecular bone. The alveolar process that separates the roots of the same tooth is the **interradicular septum** (in-ter-**ra**-dik-you-ler) (or interradicular bone) (Fig. 14.19). The interradicular septum consists of both ABP and trabecular bone; however, only a part of the interradicular septum is ever present on periapical or bitewing radiographs (see Fig. 14.17).

Clinical Considerations with Dental Procedures and Pathology Involving Alveolar Process

Bone remodeling can be forced with orthodontic therapy to produce tooth movement for repositioning (Fig. 14.20). The bands, wires, or appliances put pressure on one side of the tooth and adjacent alveolar process, creating a *compression zone* in the PDL. This compression in the PDL leads to bone resorption. On the opposite side of the tooth and bone, a *tension zone* develops in the PDL and causes the deposition of new bone. Thus the tooth or teeth are slowly moved along the jaw to achieve a more ideal dentition that works in harmony (see **Chapter 20**). In this way, the width of the space between the alveoli and the root is kept about the same.

Mesial drift (**mee**-zee-uhl) (or physiologic drift) is the natural movement phenomenon in which all the teeth move slightly toward the midline of the oral cavity over time (see Fig. 20.21). This can cause crowding late in life of a once-perfect dentition. It occurs quite slowly, depending mostly on the degree of wear of the contact points between adjacent teeth and on the number of missing teeth. Overall, the amount of movement may total no more than 1 cm over a lifetime. However, this crowding may lead to poor homecare in the region as well as less than optimal esthetics.

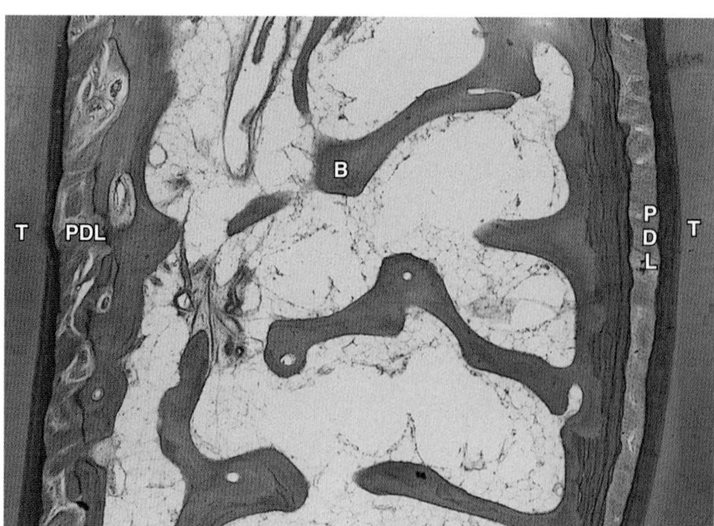

Fig. 14.18 Microscopic section of interdental septum or bone *(B)* found between the roots of two neighboring teeth *(T)* and surrounded on each side by the horizontal group of the periodontal ligament *(PDL)*. (From Bernhard Gottlieb Collection, courtesy of James McIntosh, PhD, Assistant Professor Emeritus, Department of Biomedical Sciences, Baylor College of Dentistry, Dallas.)

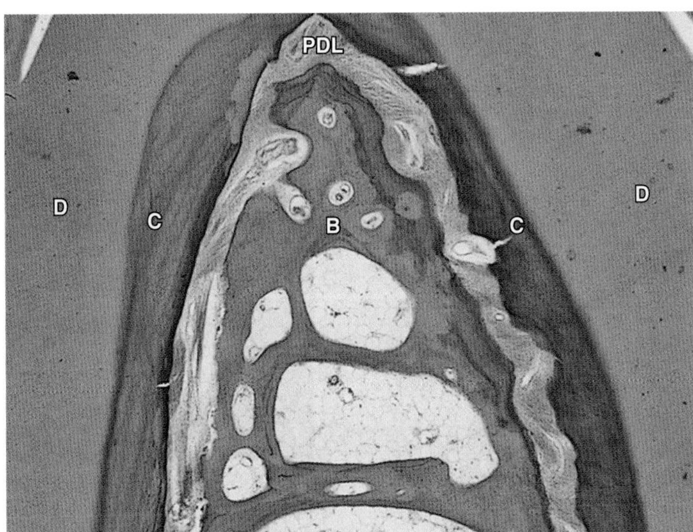

Fig. 14.19 Microscopic section of interradicular septum or bone between two roots *(B)* of a mandibular molar and surrounded on each side by the interradicular group of the periodontal ligament *(PDL)*. The molar's roots are composed of dentin *(D)* and cementum *(C)*. (From Bernhard Gottlieb Collection, courtesy of James McIntosh, PhD, Assistant Professor Emeritus, Department of Biomedical Sciences, Baylor College of Dentistry, Dallas.)

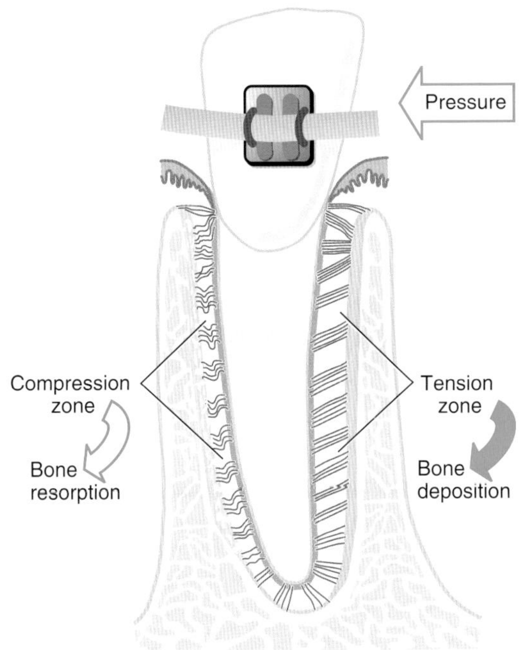

Fig. 14.20 Process of Tooth Movement During Orthodontic Therapy. Appliances put pressure on one side creating a *zone of compression* in the periodontal ligament on the opposite side, which leads to bone resorption. On the same side, a *zone of tension* develops causing deposition of new bone. Thus the tooth or teeth are slowly moved along the jaw.

After extraction of a tooth, the clot in the alveolus fills in with primary bone, which later is remodeled into mature secondary bone. However, with the loss of teeth a patient becomes **edentulous** (ee-**den**-chuh-luhs), either partially or completely and the surrounding alveolar process progressively undergoes resorption (Fig. 14.21). The bony trabeculae supporting the alveoli also decrease in number and in thickness as the alveolar process itself becomes thinner. In contrast, the underlying basal bone of the body of the maxilla or mandible remains less affected becomes the major constituent of each jawbone because it does not need the presence of teeth to remain viable. Thus, the alveolar process depends on the functional stimulation from retained teeth during mastication and speech for preservation of its structure.

Overeruption (or *super-eruption*) within the alveolar process can also occur with loss of teeth, especially if involved with the permanent posterior teeth (see Figs. 17.43 and 17.56). **Overeruption** is the physiologic movement of a tooth lacking an opposing partner within the occlusion. Exposure of root surface may also precipitate dentinal hypersensitivity, root caries, and create esthetic compromise as well as compromise the tooth's periodontal health. Treatment planning is key to preventing undesirable vertical tooth movement such as with the restoration of the edentulous space to allow for opposing occlusion or interceptive orthodontics. The exact mechanism that causes this movement of the dentition is still controversial; it may be an adjustment process to retain balance among the various components of the masticatory apparatus or may just be related to the wear of both the proximal and occlusal tooth surfaces.

The loss of the alveolar process due to aging, coupled with attrition of the teeth, causes also a progressive loss of height of the lower third of the vertical dimension of the face when the teeth are in maximum intercuspation (Fig. 14.22; see Figs. 1.3 and 1.10 for comparison and **Chapter 20**). The extent of this loss is determined based on clinical judgment using the Golden Proportions. This part of the vertical dimension is important in determining the way in which the teeth and jaws function. In addition, a proper amount of height in the lower third of the face reduces the level of facial wrinkles and lines around the mouth as the skin ages, sags, and loses its resilience (see **Chapter 8**). With the loss of vertical dimension in the lower third, mature patients can take on a cartoon "Popeye" facial appearance that is esthetically displeasing and more importantly results in poor functioning of the teeth and jaws.

Resorption of the alveolar process can occur in higher levels in postmenopausal women who experience a shortage of estrogen, which usually helps maintain bone density; however, severe bone loss levels may occur with the onset of osteoporosis. The placement of a denture, either partial or full, or a bridge, as well as a dental implant (discussed next) may provide the stimulation of the teeth in the alveolar process. Over time, however, some amounts of the alveolar process are lost even with these types of tooth replacements, especially if the prosthesis

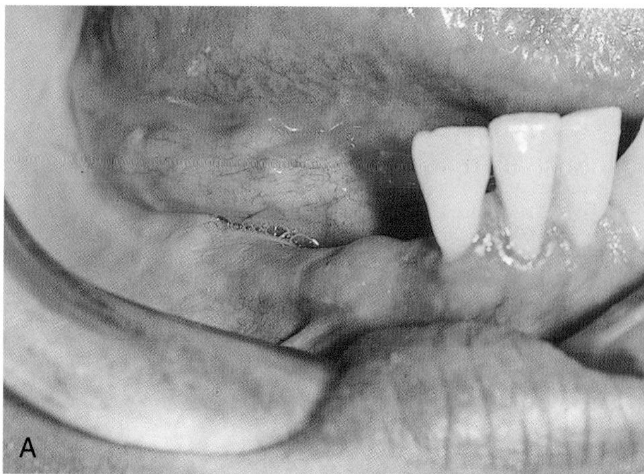

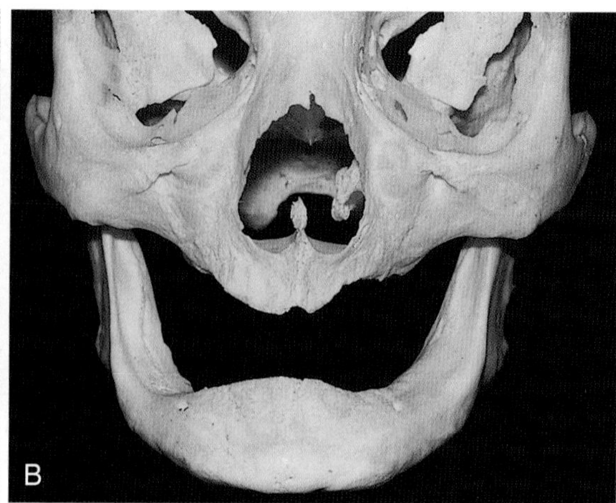

Fig. 14.21 Edentulous States with Resultant Changes in the Alveolar Process. A, Partially edentulous case from the extraction of the posterior teeth with loss of the alveolar process of the mandibular posterior sextant with only the basal bone remaining. **B,** Complete edentulous skull from a past full mouth extraction of the teeth with the bone loss of both the alveolar processes with only basal bone remaining. (Courtesy of Margaret J. Fehrenbach, RDH, MS.)

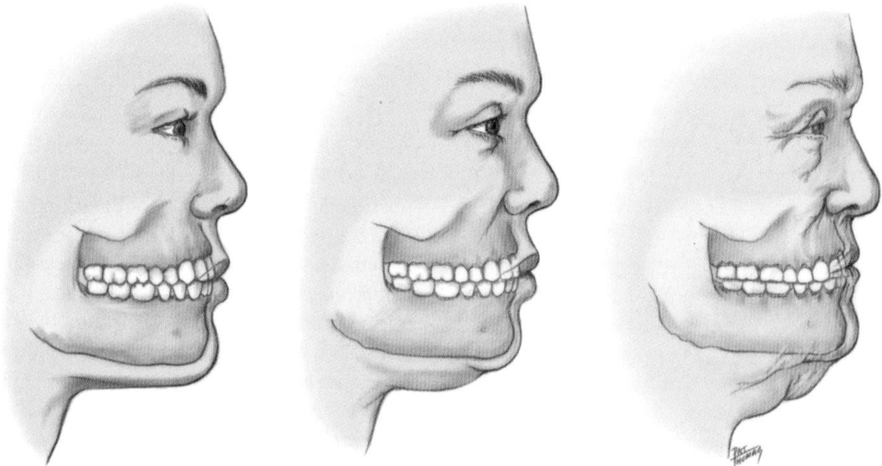

Fig. 14.22 Loss of vertical dimension in the inferior third of the face in 20-year increments (age 20, age 40, and age 60) as the bone from alveolar process is lost from the jaws. The permanent teeth themselves have also undergone a reduction in height by slight attrition, the mechanical wear of the masticatory surface. Note the increase in level of facial wrinkles and lines around the mouth caused by these orofacial changes and more importantly the loss of full function of the dentition. This amount due to aging can be dramatically increased with tooth loss, severe periodontal disease, or increased levels of attrition.

produces excessive compression of the underlying bone. Loss of the alveolar process also accompanies aging but this loss is also increased in clinical conditions where blood supply is compromised and hypoxia (or reduced oxygen) occurs, such as following severe inflammation, radiation trauma, or bone fracture.

Ideally, a dental implant is placed in an edentulous area, which preserves the integrity of the bone, provides adequate stimulation, and serves as a permanent replacement for a lost tooth or teeth, preventing further loss of vertical dimension (Fig. 14.23). However, there needs to be a certain level of the alveolar process present for this to be successful. A basic dental implant has a core part made of titanium that is surgically implanted in the alveolar process of either jaw with an attached prosthetic superstructure of a tooth or denture; the high success rate of these current implants has now been demonstrated.

The deeper core of the basic dental implant has an open structure, allowing bone to bond to it over a short time, so as to undergo osseointegration of the implant to the surrounding alveolar process. However, unlike natural teeth having an insertion of the principal fiber groups of the PDL into the alveolar process via Sharpey fibers that allows supported tooth movement, an implant has no movement. Instead, the implant makes direct contact with the alveolar process as well as with the surrounding connective tissue and its more superficial epithelium, the *periimplant tissue.* Research has shown that a sulcular epithelium consisting of the circular fibers of the gingival tissue surrounds and also attaches to the superior part of the implant by hemidesmosomes in tissue that structurally resembles a junctional epithelium. After osseointegration and healing of the tissue, a prosthetic superstructure of a tooth or denture is then attached to the surgical part of the implant.

Studies have shown that failure to obtain and maintain this cellular junction may lead to apical migration of the epithelium on the bone-implant interface, possible soft tissue encapsulation of the

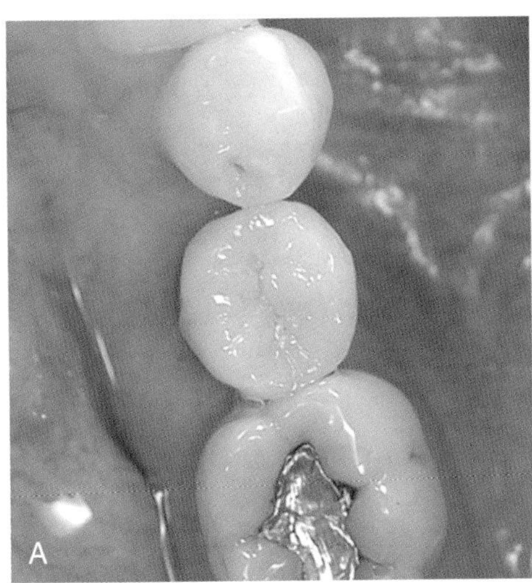

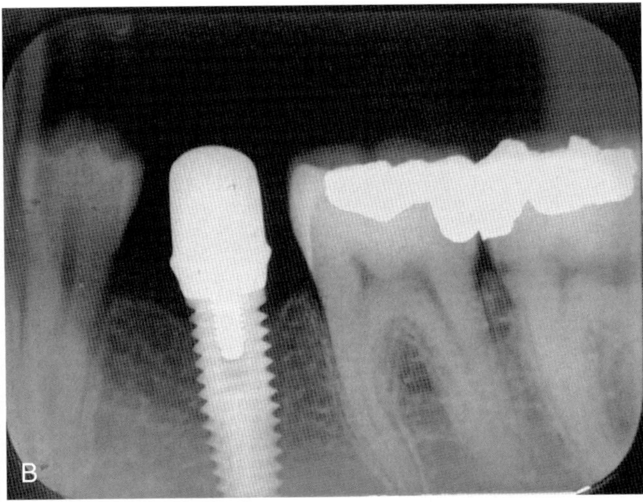

Fig. 14.23 Basic Single-Tooth Dental Implant Placed in the Mandible. **A,** Clinical photograph after prosthetic replacement. **B,** Previous radiograph. Note that the implant had successfully undergone osseointegration of the titanium core and the prosthetic suprastructure could then be placed to replace a missing permanent mandibular second premolar due to partial anodontia. (**A** and **B,** From Newman MG, Takei HH, Klokkevold PR, Carranza FA. *Carranza's Clinical Periodontology*. 13th ed. Philadelphia: Elsevier; 2020.)

implant, and eventual implant failure resulting from mobility. Thus, the need exists for special devices for professional care and homecare of an implant's prosthetic superstructure to remove any deposits and prevent periimplant disease. Sadly, most patients with implants have a history of inadequate homecare that led to the initial tooth loss and tend to repeat their negative behavior.

In addition, the placement of an immediate load implant upon extraction of a noninfected tooth or teeth is now available. For this placement to be considered successful adequate bone must exist and a sufficiently large implant must be placed; once placed, the implant must be able to resist occlusal forces. The temporary prosthetic superstructure must be adjusted so that no forces are placed on it during function; meeting all of these criteria allows osseointegration. After a period of 9 weeks, a permanent prosthetic superstructure can be placed, shortening treatment time by 4 to 6 months.

During the chronic advanced periodontal disease of periodontitis, the localized alveolar process is also lost at varying levels depending on the length and amount of disease involved (Fig. 14.24; see Fig. 10.12 and discussion in **Chapter 10**). This bone loss may be due to an overresponse of the immune system and the activation of certain osteoclast populations; among the bioactive agents implicated are cytokines and prostaglandins. Cytokines are small proteins that function as signaling compounds for the white blood cells, which are necessary to the inflammatory response (see **Chapter 8**). Examples of cytokines include the various interleukins (ILs), such as IL-1, IL-6, and IL-1β. along with tumor necrosis factor-alpha (TNF-α).

When periodontitis initially develops or as it progresses, hard and soft tissue destruction is by both collagen and extracellular matrix (ECM) degradation. This degradation is primarily by proteinases, protein-degrading enzymes. There are many types of proteinases, including *matrix metalloproteinase (MMP);* more than 25 MMPs have currently been identified and broadly categorized into six groups. Several of these degrade collagen, including MMP-1, MMP-8, and MMP-13, thereby being classified as collagenases.

Assessment of MMP in the tissue of periodontium, gingival cervical fluid, or saliva may serve as an important future biomarker in diagnosis of periodontal diseases and also for prognostic follow-up. Targeted therapy aimed at reducing effects of MMP may serve as a useful adjunct for treatment of periodontitis. At this critical time, a subantimicrobial dose (SD) of doxycycline may be used during periodontal therapy to inactivate collagenase. This use of SD of the doxycycline can be locally by placement of fibers into the gingival sulcus or systemically by oral dosage. This antibiotic is broad spectrum and is active against most of the periodontal pathogens due to its low minimum inhibitory concentration (MIC).

The bone loss is first evident in the most coronal part of the ABP, the alveolar crest, which looks moth-eaten both microscopically and radiographically (see Figs. 14.13 and 14.24). As the loss of the alveolar process slowly progresses apically, the tooth becomes increasingly mobile, also increasing the risk of future tooth loss. **Mobility** is the movement of tooth because of loss of support by periodontium. Prevention of further loss of the alveolar process and thus management of the periodontal disease is important in the dental treatment plan for these patients and may include the homecare removal of oral deposits, surgical procedures to increase self-cleansing, and the use of SD level of antibiotics. Studies now also show that chronic periodontitis represents a co-morbidity that contributes to a "gerovulnerability" within the aging population.

Bone grafting may be included during surgical periodontal therapy especially during implant placement. The bone graft is sourced from either the alveolar process or other bone (such as the patient's chin) and even from other sources (such as cadavers) with the use of **guided tissue regeneration (GTR)**. GTRs are surgical procedures that utilize barrier membranes to direct the growth of new bone and soft tissue at sites having insufficient volumes or dimensions for proper function, esthetics, or prosthetic restoration. The use of GTR is based on the long-recognized concept that fibroblasts from the PDL as well as undifferentiated mesenchyme have the potential to re-create the original periodontal attachment.

Using GTR to treat narrow intrabony defects and class II mandibular furcations has been very successful as has its use to support bone growth on an alveolar process and to allow stable placement of the dental implant. However, GFR offers limited benefits in the treatment of other types of periodontal defects. Bone repair is also being enhanced by the use of platelet-rich plasma (PRP) within the alveolus along with both bone defect treatment such as a tissue graft and with implant placement (see **Chapter 8**). Treatments for the management of osteoporosis involving the jaws may be used in the future with more localized bone loss within the alveolar process.

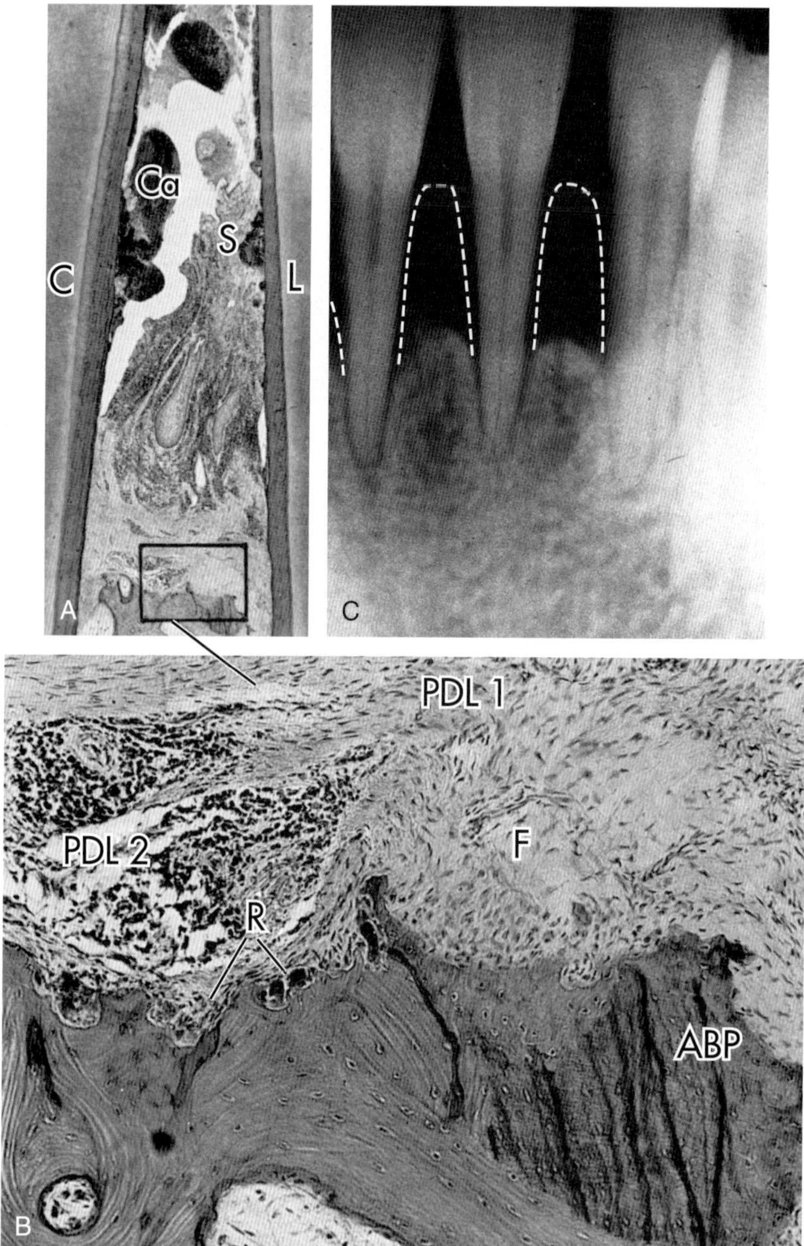

Fig. 14.24 Bone Loss Caused by the Chronic Advanced Periodontal Disease of Periodontitis. A, Microscopic section of periodontitis occurring between a lateral incisor *(L)* and a canine *(C)* demonstrating calculus *(Ca)* and a periodontal pocket with suppuration *(S)*. **B,** Close-up view showing bone resorption *(R)* from the alveolar bone proper *(ABP)* due to osteoclast activity beneath the inflammation in the periodontal ligament *(PDL 2)* but the superior area with the interdental ligament remains intact *(PDL 1)*; areas of fibrosis *(F)* are also noted in reaction. **C,** Radiograph showing severe bone loss from previously healthy levels *(dashed lines)* on permanent mandibular incisors. This bone loss initially involved the alveolar crest and moved apically as the periodontitis progressed. (**A** and **B,** From Newman MG, Takei HH, Klokkevold PR, Carranza FA. *Carranza's Clinical Periodontology*. 9th ed. Philadelphia: Saunders; 2002. **C,** Courtesy of Margaret J. Fehrenbach, RDH, MS.)

The density of the alveolar process in a given area also determines the route that dental infection takes with abscess formation as well as the efficacy of local infiltration of the agent during the administration of local anesthesia. In addition, the differences in alveolar process density determine the easiest and most convenient areas of bony fracture to be used if needed during tooth extraction of impacted teeth (see Fig. 17.62).

Finally, with occlusal trauma the part of the ABP present on radiographs as the lamina dura may become thickened in response, along with the widening of the PDL space (discussed later and see **Chapter 20**). Thus the ABP becomes thicker with the individual bony trabeculae supporting the alveoli also increasing in number and in thickness as well.

There can also be loss of integrity of the lamina dura when studying radiographs for pathologic lesions such as with bone cancer, giving various aggressive radiolucent presentations that appear "moth-eaten" with an ill-defined zone of multiple small radiolucencies that may coalesce or instead be permeated with numerous tiny radiolucencies in between the residual bone trabeculae.

PERIODONTAL LIGAMENT PROPERTIES

The PDL is that part of the periodontium that provides for the attachment of the teeth to the surrounding ABP by way of the root cementum (see Fig. 14.1). The width of the PDL ranges from 0.15 to 0.38 mm, with its thinnest part around the middle third of the root. The PDL appears on radiographs as the **periodontal ligament space** that is a radiolucent (or darker) area located between the denser radiopaque (or lighter) lamina dura of the ABP and the similar radiopaque (or lighter) cementum (see Fig. 14.16).

The PDL is an organized fibrous connective tissue that also maintains the gingival tissue in proper relationship to the teeth. In addition, the PDL transmits occlusal forces from the teeth to the bone, allowing for a small amount of movement and acting as a shock absorber for the soft tissue structures around the teeth, such as the nerves and blood vessels (see **Chapter 20**). Other functions of the PDL are discussed in detail later in this chapter. In general, these other functions include serving as the periosteum for both the cementum and the alveolar process. Cells in the PDL also participate in the development and resorption of the hard tissue of the periodontium allowing for the remodeling of all of tissue types present. Additionally, it has blood vessels that provide nutrition for the cells of the ligament and surrounding cells of the cementum and the alveolar process.

Finally, the PDL and its nerve supply provide a most efficient proprioceptive mechanism, allowing us to feel even the most delicate forces applied to the teeth and any displacement of the teeth resulting from these forces (such as metal foil in candy wrappers). Unlike the soft connective tissue of the pulp, the PDL not only transmits pain, but also touch, pressure, and temperature sensations.

Even after patients have endodontic (or vital pulp) therapy (also referred to as "root canal treatment" by patients) and the tooth becomes nonvital, they may feel some level of discomfort when biting down or when the clinician taps the teeth when measuring tooth percussion sensitivity. This discomfort is not due to sensations from the removed pulp tissue but from sensations coming from the still present PDL; this comes from the pressure from even the slightest intrusive movements of the tooth during mastication. In some cases, the inflammation associated with the pulp (or pulpitis) travels through the apical foramen to involve the periodontium, thus causing apical inflammation and destruction (see **Chapter 13**). Surgery may have to be performed to remove the resultant apical lesion (apicoectomy).

Similar to the alveolar process, the PDL develops from the dental sac of the tooth germ and thus is a mesodermally derived tissue (see Fig. 6.20). Unlike other connective tissue of the periodontium, however, the PDL does not show any overwhelming histologic changes related to aging but its width does decrease with age.

Because the PDL is a connective tissue, it has all the components of a connective tissue, such as intercellular substance, cells, and fibers (Fig. 14.25; see **Chapter 8**). It has mostly Type I collagen as well as lesser amounts of other types.

The PDL also has a vascular supply, lymphatics, and nerve supply, which enter the apical foramen of the tooth to supply the pulp (see **Chapter 13**). Two types of nerves are found within the PDL. One type is afferent (or sensory), which is a myelinated nerve and transmits sensations that occur within the PDL (as discussed earlier); the other type is an autonomic sympathetic nerve, which regulates the blood vessels (see **Chapter 8**).

PERIODONTAL LIGAMENT CELLS

The PDL has all the cells that are found in most connective tissue, such as the cells of blood and endothelium (Fig. 14.26). And like all connective tissue, the fibroblast is the most common cell in the PDL, producing fibers and intercellular substance (see Fig. 8.5). Studies have demonstrated that these fibroblasts further appear to function as mechanosensing entities that regulate collagen-secretory and collagen-remodeling activities according to the level of strain within the ligament. Mechanical challenge also plays an important role during the activation of periodontal fibroblasts in response to injury.

The PDL also has cells that are not present in other connective tissue, such as a line of cementoblasts along the cemental surface of the root. Osteoblasts are also present in the PDL at the periphery of the adjacent ABP. In addition, the PDL has osteoclasts as well as odontoclasts. Each

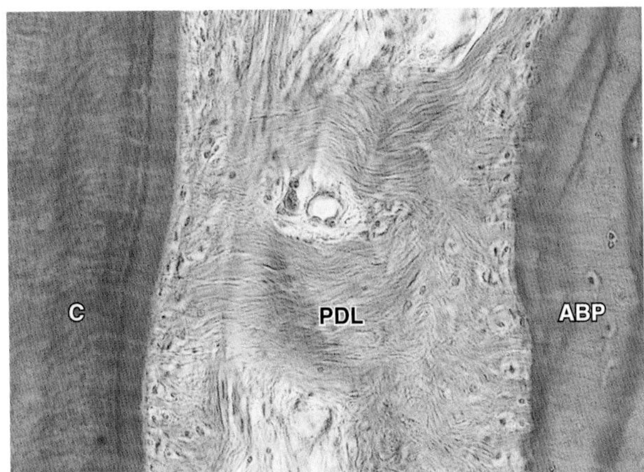

Fig. 14.25 Microscopic section of the periodontal ligament *(PDL)*, which is located between the alveolar bone proper *(ABP)* and cementum *(C)*, inserting Sharpey fibers into both tissue types. (From Bernhard Gottlieb Collection, courtesy of James McIntosh, PhD, Assistant Professor Emeritus, Department of Biomedical Sciences, Baylor College of Dentistry, Dallas.)

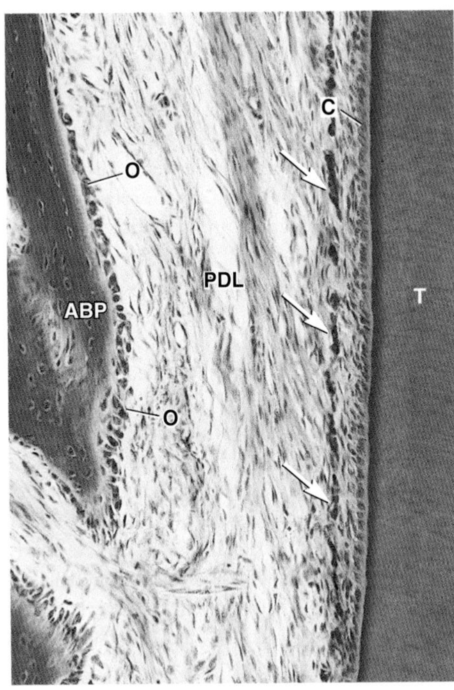

Fig. 14.26 Microscopic section of the periodontal ligament *(PDL)* that includes a layer of osteoblasts *(O)* on the periphery of the alveolar bone proper *(ABP)* with a line of cementoblasts *(C)* on the cemental surface of the tooth *(T)*. Note the epithelial rests of Malassez within the periodontal ligament *(white arrows)*. (From Bernhard Gottlieb Collection, courtesy of James McIntosh, PhD, Assistant Professor Emeritus, Department of Biomedical Sciences, Baylor College of Dentistry, Dallas.)

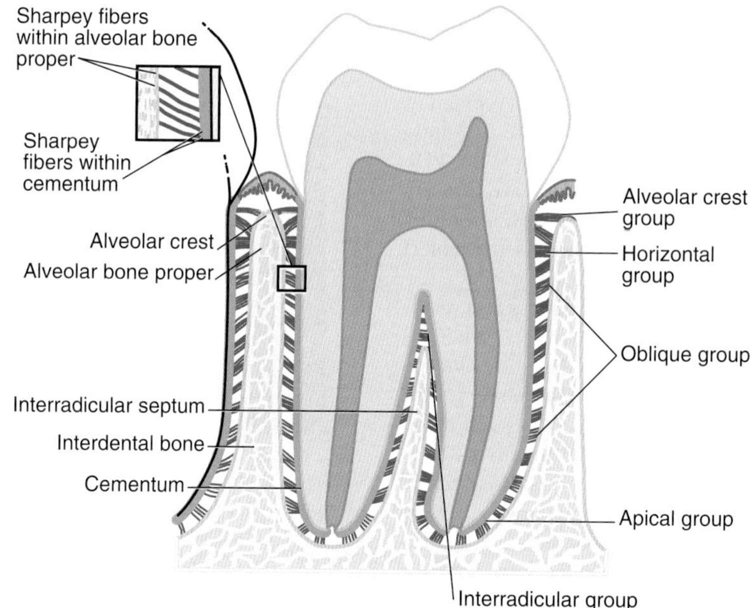

Fig. 14.27 Diagram of a Sagittal Section of a Multirooted Tooth and Periodontal Ligament. Fiber subgroups of the alveolodental ligament are identified: alveolar crest group, horizontal group, oblique group, apical group, and interradicular group. Note Sharpey fibers located within both the alveolar bone proper and cementum.

of these specific cell types can form either cementum or bone; they can even resorb either tissue, depending on the need of the periodontium or the demands of the adjacent environment. Also present are undifferentiated mesenchymal cells, which can differentiate into any of these cells if any of these cell populations are injured. Thus, the PDL serves as a protective periosteum for both the root cementum and adjacent ABP.

In addition, the epithelial rests of Malassez (ERM) are present within the PDL (see Fig. 14.26). These groups of epithelial cells are stranded in mature PDL after the disintegration of Hertwig epithelial root sheath during the formation of the root (see Figs. 6.19 and 6.20). Studies are now demonstrating that these cell rests that are the descendants of HERS and are an unique odontogenic epithelium in the adult periodontium. The ERM also play a more active role and can be activated to participate in PDL repair and regeneration. In addition, there have been recent advances regarding the characterization of the cytokine profile of the ERM which validate their important function in PDL homeostasis with an emphasis on their role in alveolar process remodeling. Studies involving dental procedures from dental implant placement to orthodontic therapy are looking at the potential of the ERM.

The ERM can also become cystic, usually forming nondiagnostic radiolucent apical lesions. This occurs as a result of chronic periapical inflammation after pulpitis occurs. These cysts must be surgically removed and then observed for recurrence on follow-up visits.

PERIODONTAL LIGAMENT FIBER GROUPS

The PDL is wider near the apex and cervix of the tooth and narrower between these two end points of cementum and bone. All the fibers in the PDL are collagen in structure. Most of the fibers are considered **principal fibers**. The principal fibers are not found as individual fibers but are organized into groups or bundles according to their orientation to the mature tooth and related function; these bundles overall resemble spliced ropes working together. Each is approximately 5 micrometers in diameter. Histologists refer to these groups by various names, but this textbook uses the most commonly used names by the dental community.

During mastication and speech certain forces are exerted on a tooth, such as rotational, tilting, extrusive, or intrusive forces. The principal fibers of the PDL distribute these forces, protecting its soft tissue and allowing some give when they occur, similar to a rubber band attached at both ends to two hard objects. Studies show that the fiber bundles go the length of the PDL space and then branch along the two end points of cementum and bone, increasing the strength of the ligament. In addition, the fibers can accomplish this task because the ends of each fiber are anchored within both cementum and the ABP or in cementum alone from adjacent roots or teeth. These fibers are of a wider diameter on the bone (or alveolar process) side than the cementum (or tooth) side but are less numerous.

The ends of the principal fibers that are within either cementum or ABP are considered Sharpey fibers (see Fig. 14.17). Sharpey fibers are each partially inserted into the hard tissue of the periodontium at 90° or perpendicular to either cemental or bony surface as discussed earlier. Over time, they become mineralized and become part of the mineralized tissue. Whether they originate from bone or cementum, they initially unravel into smaller fibers, which join up with those of adjacent fibers to produce a meshwork of interconnected fibers oriented between bone and cementum. Thus, the periodontal fibers do not stretch cable-like from cementum to bone but form a meshwork of interconnected fibers.

In addition to the collagen fibers, the PDL also contains oxytalan fibers that are related to the microfibrillar component of elastic fibers. These generally run parallel to the root surface, although they can occasionally insert into cementum and may be part of the vascular support within the ligament.

Alveolodental Ligament

The main principal fiber group is the **alveolodental ligament** (al-**vee**-uh-loh-**dent**-uhl), which consists of five fiber subgroups classified into several groups on the basis of their anatomic location: alveolar crest, horizontal, oblique, apical, and interradicular on multirooted teeth (Fig. 14.27; Table 14.2). If viewed on sagittal section or from both a facial or lingual view of the PDL, the fiber subgroups have different orientations from the cervix to the apex or apices. If the alveolodental

TABLE 14.2 **Alveolodental Ligament Fiber Subgroups**

Fiber Subgroups	Location	Function
Alveolar crest group	Attached to cementum just below cementoenamel junction and runs in inferior and outward direction to insert into alveolar crest of alveolar bone proper	To resist tilting, intrusive, extrusive, and rotational forces
Horizontal group	Just apical to alveolar crest group and runs 90° to long axis of tooth from cementum to alveolar bone proper, just inferior to alveolar crest	To resist tilting forces and rotational forces
Oblique group	Runs from cementum in oblique direction to insert into alveolar bone proper more coronally	To resist intrusive forces and rotational forces
Apical group	Radiates from cementum around root apex to surrounding alveolar bone proper, forming base of alveolus	To resist extrusive forces and rotational forces
Interradicular group (only on multirooted teeth)	Runs from the cementum of one root to cementum of other root(s) superficial to interradicular septum and thus has no bony attachment superficial to interradicular septum	To resist intrusive, extrusive, tilting, and rotational forces

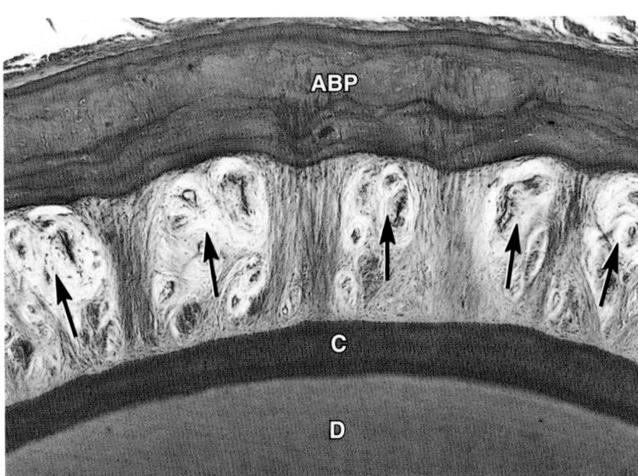

Fig. 14.28 Cross section of the tooth composed of cementum *(C)* and dentin *(D)*, highlighting the spokelike arrangement of the fibers subgroups of alveolodental ligament *(arrows)*, in most cases running between the cementum and alveolar bone proper *(ABP)* of the surrounding alveolus. (From Bernhard Gottlieb Collection, courtesy of James McIntosh, PhD, Assistant Professor Emeritus, Department of Biomedical Sciences, Baylor College of Dentistry, Dallas.)

ligament is viewed on cross section, the fiber subgroups appear as spokes of a wheel around the tooth (Fig. 14.28). Thus, the overall function of the alveolodental ligament is to resist rotational forces or twisting of the tooth in its alveolus. Each of the five fiber subgroups also has its own specific function related to its differing orientation to the tooth.

The **alveolar crest group** of the alveolodental ligament is attached to the cementum just below the CEJ and runs in an inferior and outward direction to insert into the alveolar crest of the ABP. Its function is to resist tilting, intrusive, extrusive, and rotational forces.

The **horizontal group** of the alveolodental ligament is just apical to the alveolar crest subgroup and runs at 90° to the long axis of the tooth from cementum to the ABP, just inferior to its alveolar crest. Its function is to resist tilting forces, which work to force the tooth to tip mesially, distally, lingually, or facially, and to resist rotational forces.

The **oblique group** (oh-**bleek**) of the alveolodental ligament is the most numerous of the fiber subgroups and covers the apical two-thirds of the root (Fig. 14.29). This subgroup runs from the cementum in an oblique direction to insert into the ABP more coronally. Its function is to resist intrusive forces, which try to push the tooth inward as well as rotational forces.

The **apical group** of the alveolodental ligament radiates from cementum around the apex of the root to the surrounding ABP, forming the base of the alveolus. Its function is to resist extrusive forces, which try to pull the tooth in an outward manner, and rotational forces.

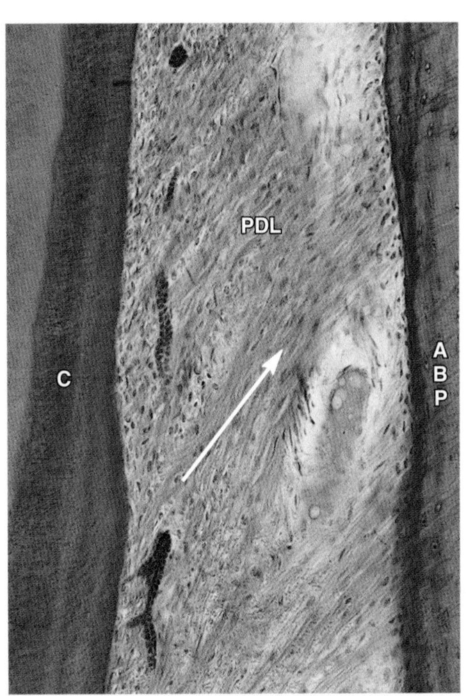

Fig. 14.29 Photomicrograph of a tooth at the location of the oblique group of the periodontal ligament *(PDL)* that runs from the cementum *(C)* in an oblique direction *(arrow)* to insert more coronally into alveolar bone proper *(ABP)*; this fiber group makes up the bulk of the alveolodental ligament. Having both cemental and bony attachments, its function is to resist intrusive forces, which try to push the tooth inward as well as rotational forces. (From Bernhard Gottlieb Collection, courtesy of James McIntosh, PhD, Assistant Professor Emeritus, Department of Biomedical Sciences, Baylor College of Dentistry, Dallas.)

The **interradicular group** of the alveolodental ligament is found only between the roots of multirooted teeth. This subgroup runs from the cementum of one root to the cementum of the other root(s) superficial to the interradicular septum and thus has no bony attachment. This subgroup works together with the alveolar crest and apical subgroups to resist intrusive, extrusive, tilting, and rotational forces.

Interdental Ligament

Another principal fiber other than the alveolodental ligament is the **interdental ligament** (or transseptal ligament) (Figs. 14.30 and 14.31).

This principal fiber inserts mesiodistally or interdentally into the cervical cementum of neighboring teeth at a height coronal to the alveolar crest of the ABP and apical to the base of the junctional epithelium. Thus the fibers traverse from cementum to cementum without any bony attachment, connecting all the teeth of the arch. Its function is to resist rotational forces and thus to hold the teeth in interproximal contact.

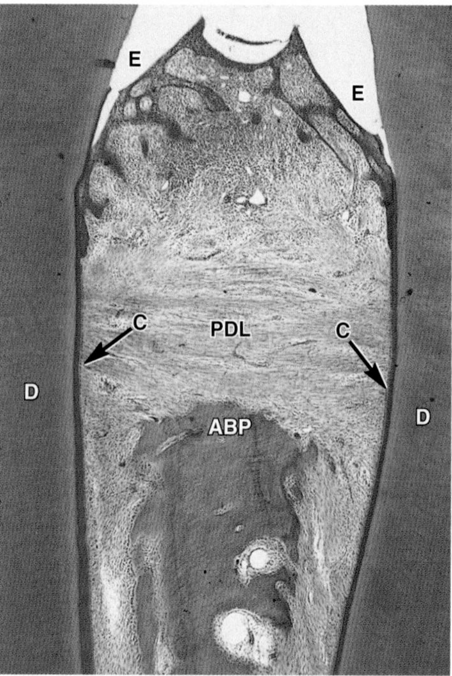

Fig. 14.30 Microscopic section of interdental ligament of the periodontal ligament *(PDL)*, which is located between the cementum *(C with arrow)* of two neighboring teeth with their dentin *(D)* and enamel (space, *E*) and coronal to the alveolar crest of the alveolar bone proper *(ABP)*. (From Bernhard Gottlieb Collection, courtesy of James McIntosh, PhD, Assistant Professor Emeritus, Department of Biomedical Sciences, Baylor College of Dentistry, Dallas.)

Gingival Fiber Group

Some histologists also consider the **gingival fiber group** to be part of the principal fibers of the PDL and so it will be discussed here for completeness (Fig. 14.32). These are a separate but adjacent group that is found within the lamina propria of the marginal gingiva (see Fig. 10.1). These include the fiber subgroups of the circular and dentogingival ligament, as well as the alveologingival and dentoperiosteal ligaments, but other terms may also be used for referencing these fiber groups. They do not support the tooth in relationship to the jaws such as the principal fibers of the PDL, which resist any forces of mastication or speech; instead the gingival fiber group supports only the marginal gingiva in an effort to maintain its relationship to the tooth.

The circular ligament encircles the tooth as shown on a cross section of a tooth, interlacing with the other gingival fiber subgroups. Like "pulling the purse strings" of the gingiva, it helps to only maintain gingival integrity.

The dentogingival ligament is the most extensive of the gingival fiber group. It inserts in the cementum on the root apical to the epithelial attachment and extends into the lamina propria of the marginal and attached gingiva. Thus the dentogingival ligament has only one mineralized attachment to the cementum. The dentogingival ligament works with the circular ligament to maintain gingival integrity mostly of the marginal gingiva.

The alveologingival ligament radiates from the alveolar crest of the ABP and extend coronally into the overlying lamina propria of the marginal gingiva. It helps to attach the gingiva to the ABP because of its one mineralized attachment to bone. The dentoperiosteal ligament courses from the cementum near the CEJ and then across the alveolar crest. The dentoperiosteal ligament anchors the tooth to the bone and protects the deeper PDL.

Clinical Considerations for Periodontal Ligament Pathology and Repair

To a lesser extent, orthodontic therapy also affects the PDL similar to the alveolar process (discussed earlier, see Fig. 14.20). On the side within the *tension zone*, the PDL space will become wider; on the side within the *compression zone* under pressure, it will become narrower. The interdental ligament is also responsible for the memory of tooth positioning within each dental arch. Therefore, a sufficiently prolonged

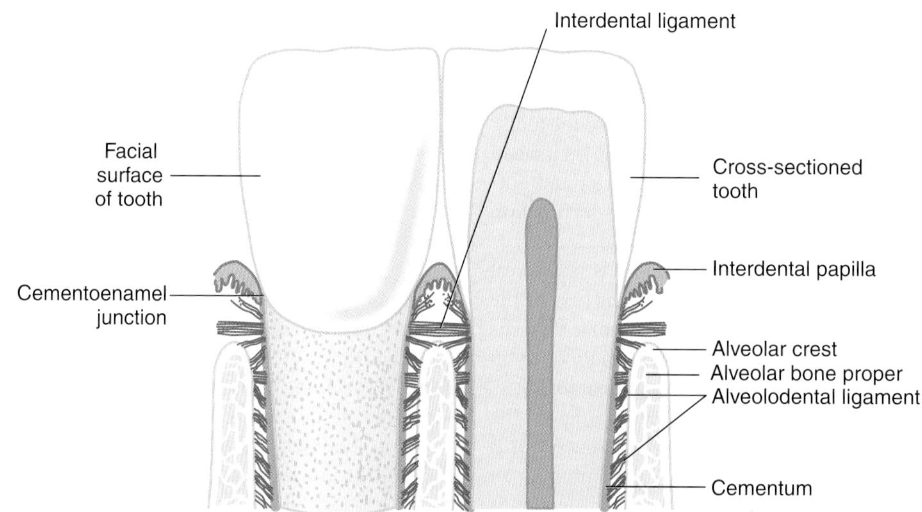

Fig. 14.31 Interdental ligament, which inserts mesiodistally or interdentally into the cervical cementum of neighboring teeth coronal to the alveolar crest of the alveolar bone proper; thus it does not have any bony attachment. Its function is to resist rotational forces and thus hold the teeth in interproximal contact.

retention period must be allowed to reattach the interdental ligament fully to its new position and thereby ensure the maintenance of the clinical stability of tooth position established during orthodontic therapy. This is because the turnover time for the interdental ligament is not as rapid as the alveolodental ligament. Retainers, removable and permanent, are used to establish and then maintain this desirable alignment.

Occlusal trauma involves trauma to periodontium from occlusal disharmony. It is important to note that occlusal trauma does not cause periodontal disease but can accelerate the progression of existing disease with certain changes noted in the PDL. When traumatic forces of occlusion are placed on a tooth, the PDL widens to take the extra forces (see **Chapter 20**). The width of the ligament can even double in size as the individual principal fiber bundles become thicker. Thus, early occlusal trauma can be viewed on radiographs as a widening of the radiolucent (or darker) PDL space between the radiopaque (or lighter) lamina dura of the ABP and the similar radiopaque (or lighter) cementum (Fig. 14.33). Thickening of the lamina dura, which represents the ABP, is also possible with occlusal trauma in response to the overall loss of the alveolar process (see earlier discussion).

Advanced occlusal trauma is additionally noted by the late manifestation of increased mobility of the tooth and may allow for the occurrence of pathologic tooth migration (PTM) (Fig. 14.34). This mobility and migration are due to the further weakened periodontium when even the occlusal forces need not be at abnormal levels if the periodontal support is reduced; the width is compensated for by the deposition of cementum.

Changes can also be noted microscopically in the PDL as a result of advanced occlusal trauma: thrombosis, dilation, and edema of the blood supply; hyalinization of the collagen fibers; the presence of an inflammatory infiltrate; and nuclear changes in the osteoblasts, cementoblasts, and fibroblasts. However, no microscopic changes are noted in the gingival collagen fibers or in the adjacent junctional epithelium with occlusal trauma. Studies also show that microscopic changes distinct from existing early periodontal disease are reversible if the causes of trauma are eliminated. Conversely, a reduction in function leads to narrowing of the ligament and a decrease in number and thickness of the fiber bundles compounding the initial trauma.

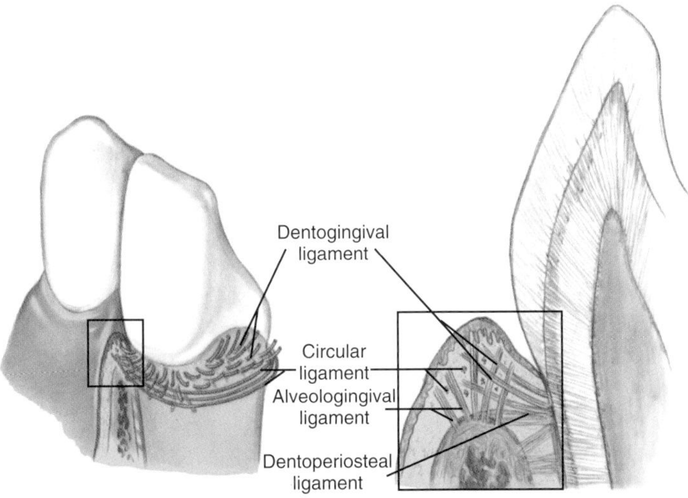

Fig. 14.32 Fiber subgroups of the gingival fiber group: circular ligament, dentogingival ligament, alveologingival ligament, and dentoperiosteal ligament. These are located in the lamina propria of the marginal gingiva and support only the gingival tissue in order to maintain its relationship to the tooth.

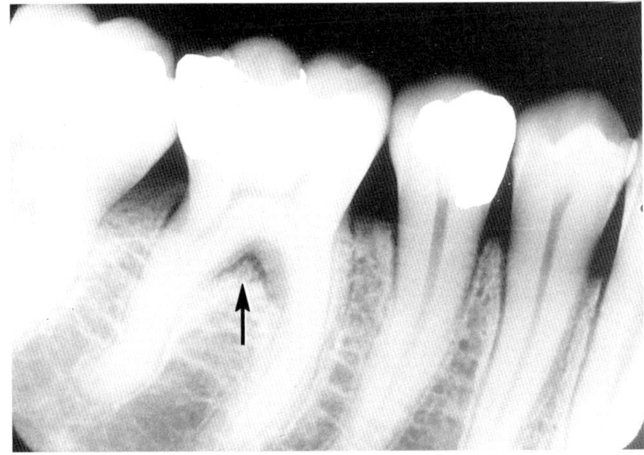

Fig. 14.33 Early occlusal trauma noted radiographically with a widening of the radiolucent periodontal ligament space *(arrow)* between the radiopaque lamina dura of the alveolar bone proper and the similarly radiopaque cementum; thickening of the lamina dura in response is also possible. (Courtesy of Margaret J. Fehrenbach, RDH, MS.)

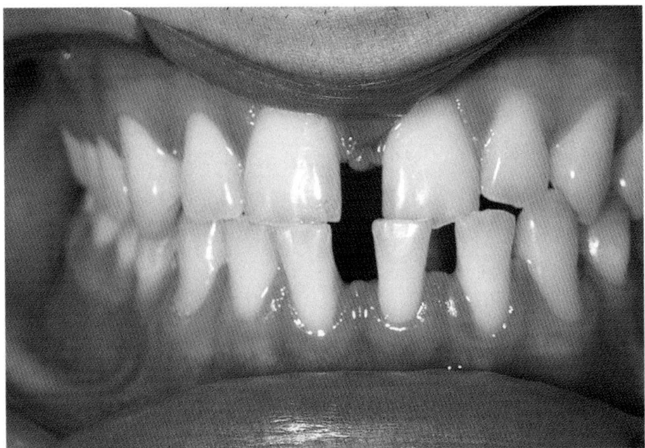

Fig. 14.34 Pathologic tooth migration caused by the weakened periodontium in which the occlusal forces need not be at an abnormal level if the periodontal support is already reduced by periodontal disease. (Courtesy of Margaret J. Fehrenbach, RDH, MS.)

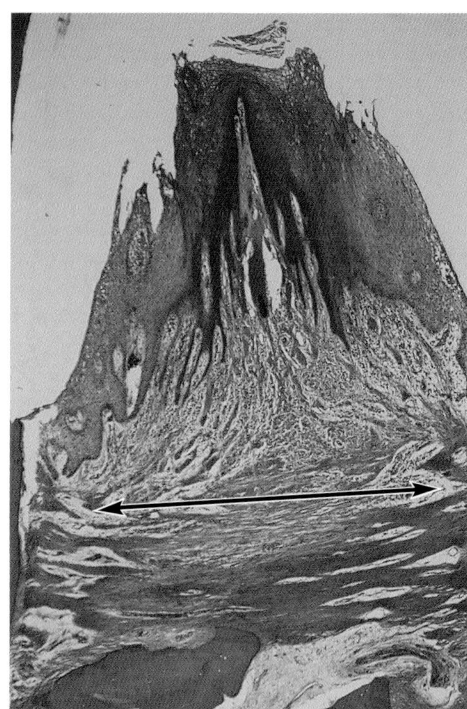

Fig. 14.35 Microscopic section of two adjacent suprabony periodontal pockets in an interdental space. Note the horizontal arrangement of the interdental ligament even with the presence of active periodontitis *(arrow)*. (From Newman MG, Takei HH, Klokkevold PR, Carranza FA. *Clinical Periodontology*. 13th ed. Philadelphia: Elsevier; 2020.)

The PDL also undergoes drastic changes with the chronic advanced periodontal disease of periodontitis that involves the deeper structures of the periodontium. The fibers of the PDL become disorganized and their attachments to either the ABP or cementum through Sharpey fibers are lost because of the resorption of these two hard dental tissue types (see Figs. 10.12 and 14.24). The first fibers involved with periodontitis are the alveolar crest group of the alveolodental ligament, which is located at the most coronal level to the adjacent alveolar process.

The destruction of the PDL with periodontitis then progresses further in an apical manner similarly to the destruction of the alveolar process, affecting (in order) the horizontal, then oblique, then apical fiber groups, and then finally the interradicular subgroups, if present. The teeth involved in advancement of periodontal disease become increasingly mobile, moving in directions that indicate the amount and type of fiber group lost, such as buccal to lingual or with downward pressure as the periodontitis progresses inward to the apices of the teeth.

Thus, the principal fiber group that remains the longest in the presence of active periodontitis, despite the previous destruction of the entire adjacent alveolodental ligament, is the interdental ligament (Fig. 14.35). The interdental ligament keeps reattaching itself in a more apical manner as the periodontitis proceeds apically so that the teeth have at least the support of interproximal contact. Thus, when teeth become severely mobile interproximally (from mesial to distal) after mobility in other directions is already present, the prognosis is poor because now there is the further destruction of the still remaining interdental ligament. Mobility and its amount and direction per tooth should be charted in the patient record to achieve an overall prognosis for a dentition with periodontitis.

The use of GTR is not only involved in the treatment of the loss of the alveolar process (as discussed earlier) but also will assist with the repair of the resultant disorganization of the PDL caused by periodontitis. Using this method to both increase alveolar process levels and strengthen the PDL, a membrane of various materials allows only osteoblasts and fibroblasts to produce either bone or PDL fibers at the diseased site. The use of GTR is becoming even more successful because the membrane type now being used results in less reactive inflammation at the site.

15

Overview of Dentitions

Additional resources and practice exercises are provided on the companion Evolve website for this book: http://evolve.elsevier.com/Fehrenbach/illustrated.

LEARNING OBJECTIVES

1. Define and pronounce the key terms in this chapter.
2. Describe the two dentitions and the relationship to each other.
3. Recognize tooth types and outline the tooth numbering systems.
4. Assign the correct universal or international number for a tooth and its correct dentition period on a diagram or a skull and for a tooth model or a patient.
5. Define each dentition period and discuss the clinical considerations concerning each dentition period, integrating it into patient care.
6. Use the correct dental anatomy terminology and discuss the clinical considerations concerning tooth anatomy, integrating it into patient care.
7. Use the correct orientational tooth terms and discuss the clinical considerations concerning tooth surfaces, integrating it into patient care.
8. Identify tooth forms and discuss the clinical considerations concerning them, integrating it into patient care.

DENTITIONS

The *dentition* is the natural teeth in the jaws. As described in **Chapter 6** in relationship to tooth development, a person has two dentitions during a lifetime: a primary dentition and a permanent dentition.

The first dentition present is the primary dentition (Fig. 15.1). Child patients and their supervising adults refer to the primary teeth as *baby teeth*. An older term for the primary dentition is the *deciduous dentition*. This reference is derived from the concept that the primary dentition is shed (just as a deciduous tree sheds leaves) and replaced entirely by the permanent dentition. The permanent dentition is the second dentition to develop; therefore the permanent dentition is sometimes considered the *secondary dentition* (Fig. 15.2). The permanent teeth are referred to as the *adult teeth* by patients. By recent convention (or convenience), clinicians seem to prefer to mix and match terms when referring to the two dentitions as in *primary dentition* and *permanent dentition*.

However, the permanent dentition is also sometimes mistakenly considered the *succedaneous dentition* because most of these permanent teeth succeed primary predecessors. Dental professionals must remember that the molars of the permanent dentition are nonsuccedaneous because they are without any primary predecessors; only the anteriors and premolars of the permanent dentition are truly succedaneous. Development of the primary dentition, eruption and shedding of the primary teeth, and development of the permanent dentition were discussed further in **Chapter 6**, which can be reviewed before the discussion of specific tooth anatomy.

TOOTH TYPES

Teeth comprise around 20% of the surface area of the oral cavity—maxillary more so than mandibular teeth. Tooth types of both arches within the primary dentition include 8 incisors, 4 canines, and 8 molars, for a total of 20 teeth (see Fig. 15.1). The anatomy of the primary dentition is discussed further in **Chapter 18**.

Tooth types of both arches within the permanent dentition include 8 incisors, 4 canines, 8 premolars, and 12 molars, for a total of 32 teeth (see Figs. 2.4 and 15.2). Note that only the permanent dentition has premolars; in contrast, the primary dentition does not have premolars. The detailed anatomy of the permanent dentition is discussed further in **Chapter 16** (anterior teeth) and **Chapter 17** (posterior teeth).

TOOTH DESIGNATION

The primary teeth and the permanent teeth are both designated by the **Universal Numbering System (UNS)** (Fig. 15.3). This system is the most widely used in the United States for the designation of both dentitions because it is adaptable to electronic data. With the UNS, the primary teeth are designated from each other in a consecutive arrangement by using capital letters, *A* through *T*, starting with the maxillary right second molar, moving clockwise and ending with the mandibular right second molar (see Fig. 15.1).

The permanent teeth are designated from each other in the UNS in consecutive arrangement as the patient is observed from in front by using the digits *1* through *32*, starting with the maxillary right third molar, moving clockwise and ending with the mandibular right third molar (see Fig. 15.2). The clockwise convention also is also used when

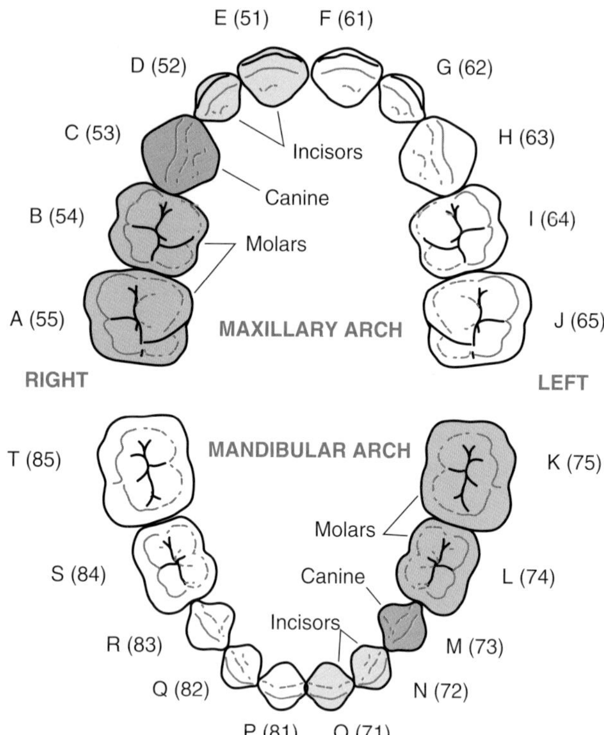

Fig. 15.1 Primary dentition during the primary dentition period with tooth types and Universal Numbering System identified (with International Numbering System identified in parentheses).

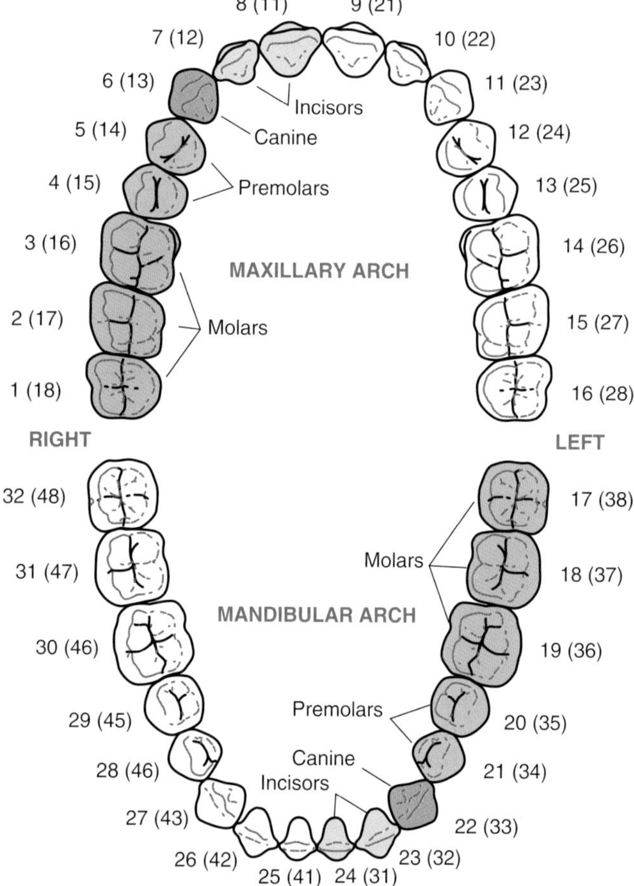

Fig. 15.2 Permanent dentition during the permanent period with tooth types and Universal Numbering System identified (with International Numbering System identified in parentheses).

charting restorations or periodontal conditions in the oral cavity for a patient. When speaking about a certain tooth such as the permanent maxillary right central incisor, the clinician calls it "number eight."

However, the need for a system that can be used internationally as well as by electronic data transfer is recognized; thus the acceptance of the **International Numbering System (INS)** (or International Designation System) by the International Standards Organization (ISO) and the World Health Organization (WHO) (see Fig. 15.3). With this system, the teeth are designated from each other by using a two-digit code. The first digit of the code indicates the quadrant (see later discussion under general dental terms) and the second indicates the tooth's position in this quadrant. This is based on the system of the Fédération Dentaire Internationale (FDI).

Thus with the INS, the digits 1 through 4 are used for quadrants in a clockwise manner in the permanent dentition, and digits 5 through 8 are used in a clockwise manner for those quadrants of the primary dentition. For the second digit, which indicates the tooth, the digits 1 through 8 are used for the permanent teeth, starting at the midline and numbering in a distal direction; sometimes with a period placed between the digits. The digits 1 through 5 are then used for the primary dentition, again starting at the midline and numbering in a distal direction. When speaking about a certain tooth such as the permanent maxillary right central incisor, the clinician calls it "tooth one–one."

Another system that is can be used during orthodontic therapy is the **Palmer Notation Method**, which is also known as the *Military Numbering System* (see Fig. 15.3). It is helpful with this dental specialty because it allows immediate discussion of the teeth that require prompt treatment and it can produce an easy to view graphic mapping of the dentitions. In this system, the teeth are designated from each other with a right-angle symbol indicating the quadrants and arch, with the tooth number placed inside, similar in numbering to INS that superseded it.

DENTITION PERIODS

Although there are only two dentitions, there are three **dentition periods** throughout a person's lifetime because the two dentitions overlap in time: primary, mixed, and permanent (Table 15.1). Each patient should be assigned a dentition period to allow the most effective dental treatment for that period. This specificity is especially important with the consideration of orthodontic therapy because growth during certain dentition periods can be maximized to allow expansion of the jaws and movement of the teeth.

PRIMARY DENTITION PERIOD

The first dentition period is the **primary dentition period** (see Fig. 15.1). This period begins with the eruption of the primary mandibular central incisors. Thus this period occurs between approximately 6 months and 6 years of age (see Fig. 6.22, *A*, for chronologic order, Table 18.1 for approximate ages and Fig. 20.5 for sequence). Only the primary teeth are present during this time, with their full eruption completed at 30 months, usually when the primary second molars are in occlusion. The jaws are beginning to also grow further during this period to accommodate the coming larger and more numerous permanent teeth. This period usually ends when the first permanent tooth erupts—the permanent mandibular first molar.

MIXED DENTITION PERIOD

The **mixed dentition period** follows the primary dentition period (Fig. 15.4; see **Chapter 6**). This period occurs between approximately 6 and 12 years of age. Both primary and permanent teeth are present during this transitional stage. During this time, both shedding of primary teeth and eruption of permanent teeth begin after their crowns are completed. Thus this period begins with eruption of the first permanent tooth, a permanent mandibular first molar, which is guided by the distal surface of the primary second molar. This period usually ends with shedding of the last primary tooth, which usually occurs from age 11 to 12.

The color differences between the primary and permanent teeth become apparent during this middle phase as any supervising adult has noticed in the child and routinely and enviously points it out to the dental professionals. The primary crowns are lighter in color than the darker permanent crowns owing to the fact that the permanent teeth have less opaque enamel and thus the underlying yellow dentin is more visible (see Fig. 18.4). Also more evident is the difference in the crown size and root length between the smaller and shorter primary teeth and the larger and longer permanent teeth.

The jaws undergo the fastest and most noticeable growth during this period of transition consistent with the onset of puberty to accommodate the larger size and number of permanent teeth. Women shed their primary teeth and receive their permanent teeth slightly earlier than men, which may reflect their earlier overall physical maturation level.

PERMANENT DENTITION PERIOD

The final dentition period is the **permanent dentition period** (see Fig. 15.2). This period begins with shedding of the last primary tooth. Thus this dentition period begins approximately after 12 years of age. Included is the eruption of all the permanent teeth, except for teeth that are congenitally missing or impacted and cannot erupt, usually involving the third molars (see Fig. 6.22, *B,* for chronologic order; Table 15.2 and **Appendix D** for approximate ages; and Fig. 20.6 for sequence).

The permanent teeth are usually the only teeth present during this period. Growth of the jaws is not as noticeable because it slows and then eventually stops. Thus there is little growth of the jaws overall during this period given that puberty has passed. Tooth types tend to erupt in pairs so that if any change in this pattern exists in a patient, a radiograph of the area may be required. When a child patient is unusually early or late regarding the usual sequential eruption of teeth, the biologic family dental history should be reviewed for developmental anomalies.

Clinical Considerations for Dentition Periods

The clinical considerations associated with both the primary and the permanent dentition periods are discussed later in each appropriate chapter. However, the mixed dentition period also has characteristic

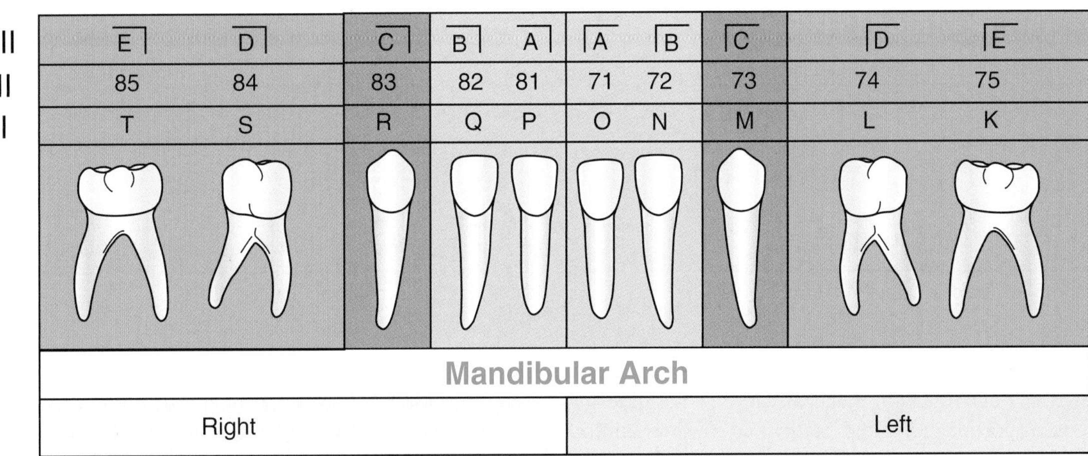

Fig. 15.3 Tooth designation systems including Universal Numbering System, International Numbering System, and Palmer Notation Method. **A,** For the primary teeth. **B,** For the permanent teeth.

Continued

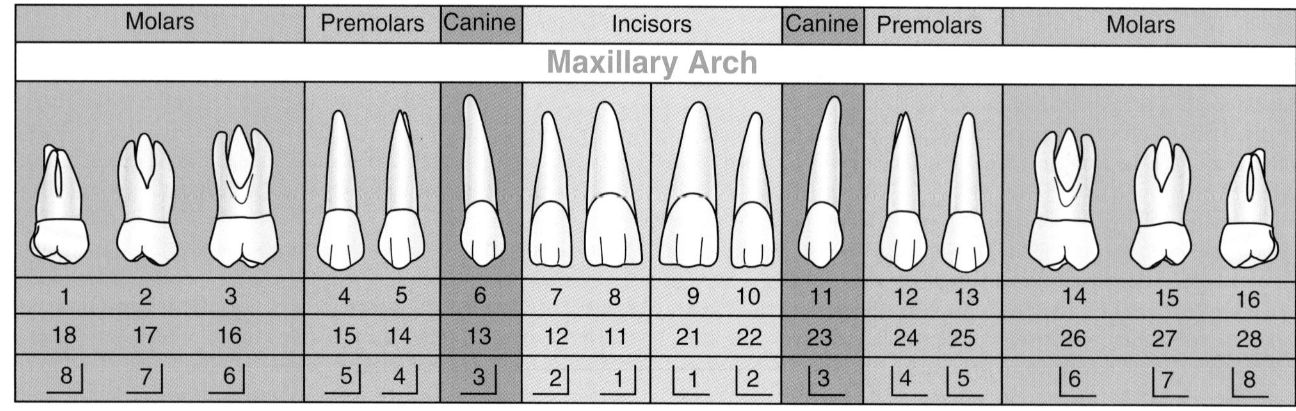

Fig. 15.3 cont'd.

TABLE 15.1 Dentition Periods with Clinical Considerations

	Primary Dentition Period	Mixed Dentition Period	Permanent Dentition Period
Approximate time span	~6 months to ~6 years	~6 years to 12 years	After ~12 years
Teeth marking start of period	Eruption of primary mandibular central incisor	Eruption of permanent mandibular first molar	Shedding of last primary tooth
Dentition present	Primary	Primary and permanent	Usually permanent
Growth of jaws	Beginning	Fastest and most noticeable	Slowest and least noticeable

Data from Nelson S. *Wheeler's Dental Anatomy, Physiology and Occlusions.* 10th ed. Philadelphia: Elsevier; 2015.

physiologic and psychological effects. This dentition period is sometimes considered an "ugly duckling stage" because of the differing tooth colors, disproportionately sized teeth, and various clinical crown heights. The patient's smile shows temporary edentulous areas and crowding. In many cases, the surrounding gingiva responds to all these changes as well as hormonal fluctuations by becoming inflamed.

Homecare may be difficult for patients during the mixed dentition period because these changes, such as crowding, may promote dental biofilm retention. Child patients and supervising adults must be reminded to be especially diligent about homecare and be reassured that this stage is only temporary. Early interceptive orthodontic therapy may also be initiated during this dentition period; a series of panoramic radiographs is important for monitoring tooth development (see Fig. 6.27, *A* and **Chapter 20**).

If in the primary and/or mixed dentition gingival inflammation is only slight with little dental biofilm formation but bone loss around the newly erupted permanent first molars and mandibular anteriors is severe early aggressive periodontitis (previously referred to as *juvenile periodontitis*) may be suspected. Early intervention in this serious periodontal disease can prevent further bone loss.

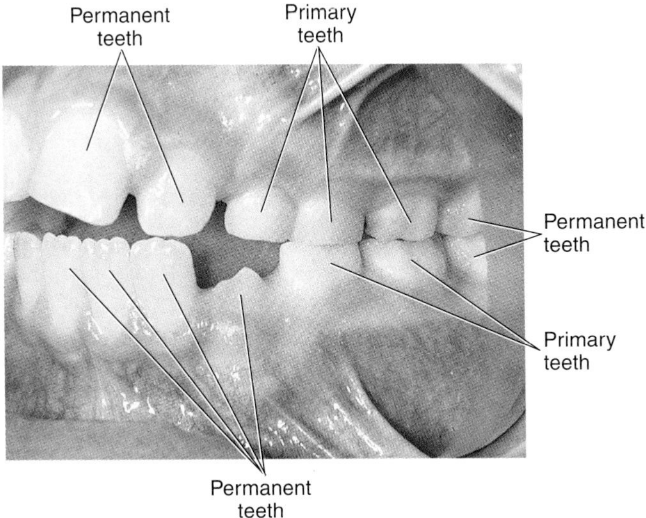

Fig. 15.4 Mixed Dentition Period with its Primary and Permanent Teeth Identified. (Courtesy of Margaret J. Fehrenbach, RDH, MS.)

TABLE 15.2 Approximate Eruption and Root Completion Ages for Permanent Teeth (in Years)

Tooth Type	Eruption	Root Completion
Maxillary Teeth		
Central incisor	7 to 8	10
Lateral incisor	8 to 9	11
Canine	11 to 12	13 to 15
First premolar	10 to 11	12 to 13
Second premolar	10 to 12	12 to 14
First molar	6 to 7	9 to 10
Second molar	12 to 13	14 to 16
Third molar	17 to 21	18 to 25
Mandibular Teeth		
Central incisor	6 to 7	9
Lateral incisor	7 to 8	10
Canine	9 to 10	12 to 14
First premolar	10 to 12	12 to 13
Second premolar	11 to 12	13 to 14
First molar	6 to 7	9 to 10
Second molar	11 to 13	14 to 15
Third molar	17 to 21	18 to 25

Data from Nelson S. *Wheeler's Dental Anatomy, Physiology and Occlusions.* 10th ed. Philadelphia: Elsevier; 2015.

DENTAL ANATOMY TERMINOLOGY

Dental professionals must be able to understand and correctly use dental anatomy terminology. **Dental anatomy** is the area of the dental sciences dealing with the morphology or form of the teeth for both the crown and root. Restorative dentistry uses many specific dental anatomy terms when discussing treatment and pathology. Periodontal therapy of the teeth also necessitates using many of these detailed terms, such as *line angles,* when performing procedures such as probe readings of the gingival sulcus that surrounds each tooth.

GENERAL DENTAL TERMS

As noted earlier, each tooth is surrounded and supported by the bone of the tooth socket or alveolus (plural, alveoli) (Fig. 15.5). Each alveolus is located in the alveolar process or tooth-bearing part of each jaw. Each alveolar process of the jaws is also considered a dental arch—either the maxillary arch or the mandibular arch.

The teeth in the maxilla are the maxillary teeth; the teeth in the mandible are the mandibular teeth (see Fig. 15.5). Occlusion is the method by which the teeth of the mandibular arch come into contact with those of the maxillary arch. The term *occlusion* is also used to describe the anatomic alignment of the teeth and the relationship to the rest of the masticatory system (see **Chapter 20**).

Each dental arch has a midline, an imaginary vertical plane that divides the arch into two approximately equal halves, a right and a left (see Fig. 15.6). The midline is similar to the median or midsagittal plane of the body. The midline is an important consideration in the evaluation of a patient's smile.

Teeth can also be described according to the position in each dental arch and in relationship to the midline (Fig. 15.6). The incisors and canines are considered anterior teeth because they are closer to the midline. In contrast, the molars (and premolars, if present) are considered posterior teeth because they are farther from the midline.

Each dental arch can be further divided into two **quadrants (kwod-ruhnts)**, with four quadrants in the entire oral cavity. Thus teeth are described as being located in one of the four quadrants: maxillary right quadrant, maxillary left quadrant, mandibular right quadrant, and mandibular left quadrant. This designation is useful when planning a course of dental treatment for a patient because it allows the treatment of one or more oral regions at a time.

The correct sequence of words when describing an individual tooth using a **D-A-Q-T System** is based on the tooth within its quadrant: ***D*** for dentition, ***A*** for arch, ***Q*** for quadrant, and ***T*** for tooth type. An example of this would be the written description of the permanent *(D)* mandibular *(A)* left *(Q)* first premolar *(T)*.

Some dental treatment plans also include the use of **sextants (sek-stuhnts)**, which further divide each dental arch into three parts according to the relationship to the midline: right posterior sextant, anterior sextant, and left posterior sextant (see Fig. 15.6). An example is that the permanent maxillary right central incisor is in the maxillary anterior sextant of the permanent dentition. This division follows the mapping of oral nerve pathways, especially in the maxillary arch. Thus the use of sextants can be useful in dental treatment plans for regions, such as those that use local anesthesia for patient pain control like periodontal therapy.

To prevent miscommunication globally, the ISO also includes the designation of areas in the oral cavity (used also in the tooth designation system). A two-digit number designates these areas and at least one of the two digits is zero (Table 15.3). An example of this system is that *00* designates the entire the oral cavity and *01* designates the maxillary arch only.

TOOTH ANATOMY TERMS

Each tooth consists of a crown and one or more roots (Fig. 15.7; see Fig. 2.5). The crown has dentin covered by enamel and each root has dentin covered by cementum. The inner part of the dentin of both crown and root also covers the pulp cavity of the tooth. The pulp cavity has a pulp chamber, pulp canal (or canals) with an apical foramen (or foramina) and may have pulp horn (or horns).

In this textbook the illustrations of the head and neck as well as any structures related to them are oriented according to the patient's head

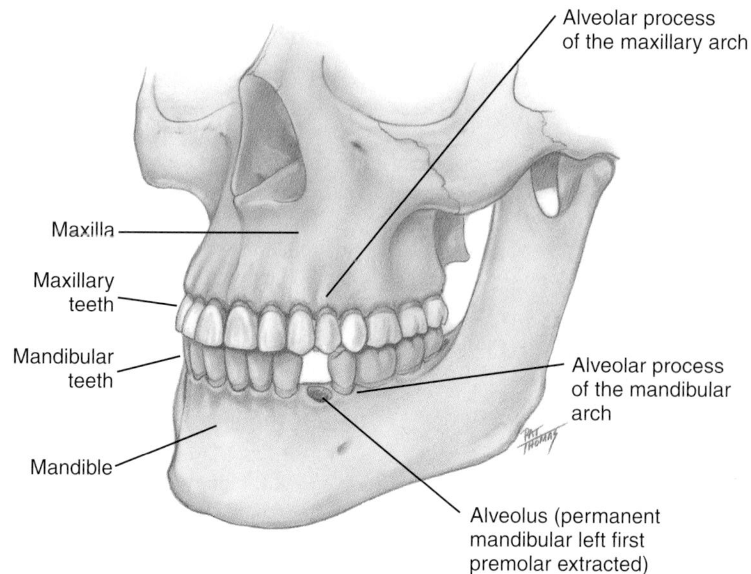

Fig. 15.5 Permanent Dentition with the Maxillary Arch and Mandibular Arch as well as Associated Structures Identified.

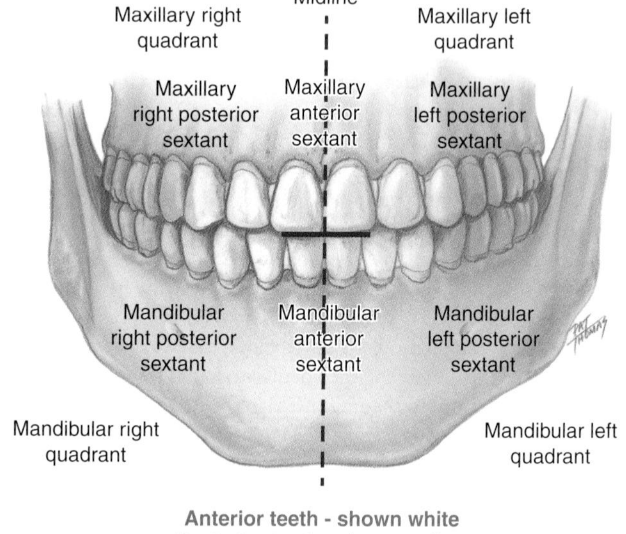

Fig. 15.6 Permanent Dentition with the Anterior and Posterior Teeth, Midline, Quadrants, and Sextants Identified.

TABLE 15.3 International Standards Organization Designation of Areas of Oral Cavity

Area	Number
Oral cavity	00
Maxillary arch	01
Mandibular arch	02
Maxillary right quadrant	10
Maxillary left quadrant	20
Mandibular left quadrant	30
Mandibular right quadrant	40
Maxillary right sextant	03
Maxillary anterior sextant	04
Maxillary left sextant	05
Mandibular left sextant	06
Mandibular anterior sextant	07
Mandibular right sextant	08

being in anatomic position unless otherwise noted (see **Appendix A**). This is the same as if the patient were being viewed straight on while sitting upright in the dental chair. Thus maxillary teeth show the root superior to the crown; mandibular teeth show the root inferior to the crown (see Fig. 15.3).

Orientation of the dental chart is traditionally from the dental professional's view (i.e., the patient's right corresponds to the notation chart's left). The designations "left" and "right" on the chart, however, nonetheless correspond to the patient's left and right, respectively. Other dental charts may show each of the teeth "unfolded" so that the facial, occlusal or incisal, and lingual surfaces of the teeth can be noted.

The enamel of the crown and cementum of the root usually meet close to the cementoenamel junction (CEJ), an external line at the neck or cervix of the tooth (see Fig. 14.8). There are three types of interfaces at the CEJ and multiple situations are possible on one tooth or even one surface of the tooth. At the CEJ, the cementum over the neck of each tooth may overlap the enamel, the enamel may meet the cementum edge to edge, or a small area of underlying dentin may be exposed because there is a gap between the enamel and cementum. The CEJ usually feels smooth or evenly grainy or has a slight groove when explored.

Parts of the crown and root of a tooth can also be designated using more specific terms in order to assist the clinician during patient dental charting (Fig. 15.8, *B*). The **anatomic crown** is the part covered by enamel. It remains mostly constant throughout the life of the tooth, except for presence of attrition and other physical wear. In contrast, the **clinical crown** is only that part of the anatomic crown that is visible and not covered by the gingiva. Its height is determined by the location of the marginal gingiva. The clinical crown of a tooth can change over time, especially with gingival recession as the marginal gingiva recedes toward the root (see Fig. 13.1). This textbook when discussing the crown of a tooth refers to the anatomic crown of a healthy tooth unless designated otherwise.

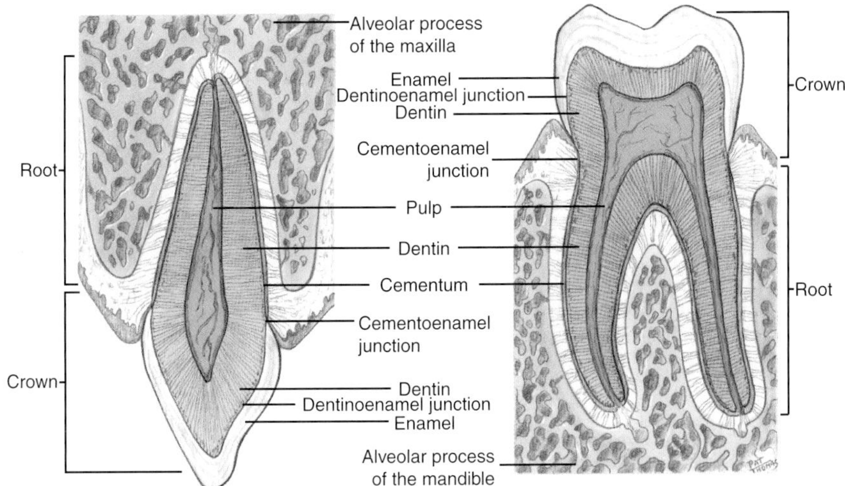

Fig. 15.7 Anterior and Posterior Tooth Identifying the Dental Tissue Types.

Similarly, the **anatomic root** is that part of the root covered by cementum. The **clinical root** of a tooth is that part of the anatomic root that is visible, subject to variability over time, again related to gingival recession (see Fig. 10.10). This textbook when discussing the root of a tooth, refers to the anatomic root of a healthy tooth unless designated otherwise.

Some clinicians describe features of a tooth related to the **root axis line (RAL)**, which is an imaginary line representing the long axis of a tooth drawn in a way to bisect the root (and thus the crown) into two halves (see Fig. 20.9). When viewing the root axis lines of the teeth overall, it is important to note that the tooth's crown and root are never strictly vertically placed within the alveolar process but have some degree of angulation as discussed in **Chapter 20**. The long axis of a tooth is used when taking radiographs with the paralleling technique.

Teeth may have one or more roots, but all the roots of both dentitions have common traits. All roots are widest at the CEJ and taper toward the apex of the tooth. There are three basic shapes to the roots on cervical cross section: triangular, oval (as in ovoid or egg-shaped), or elliptical (or elongated oval) (Fig. 15.8, *B*). In midroot sections, root shapes are generally the same as in cervical sections, although smaller.

Many surfaces of the roots have depressions or **root concavities**. These indentations in the root surface commonly occur on the proximal root surfaces of anteriors and posteriors and the buccal and lingual surfaces of molars. An area between two or more of these roots is a furcation; see further discussion in **Chapter 17** and see Table 17.1. Cervical cross section root shapes may be altered by the presence of root concavities.

 Clinical Considerations with Tooth Anatomy

Certain restorations may cover the entire anatomic crown area; these are full artificial crowns (or what patients call "*caps*"). Post and core may be placed within the crown and root to help with the buildup of restorative materials to support an individual restoration.

A full artificial crown should ideally cover the entire prepared anatomic crown but enlarged gingival tissue or loss of anatomic crown structure may require a surgical periodontal procedure of *crown lengthening* to increase the amount of the clinical crown and reduce the surrounding gingival tissue by removal. However, many clinicians feel that a restored artificial crown should be partial if possible, avoiding the CEJ region that is in contact with the gingival tissue in order to preserve tissue health. In a dentition case with poorer prognosis, a root (or roots) may be retained without the crown(s) if there is enough structure and periodontal attachment to support a removable prosthesis, such as an overdenture.

Historically in dental education, the importance of clinical crown anatomy was emphasized with limited emphasis on clinical root anatomy. Subsequently, dental professionals have seen an increased educational emphasis placed on detailed knowledge of root anatomy. This change in emphasis is due to a new recognition of the importance of precise periodontal root instrumentation to achieve oral health in cases of disease as well as preserving of the crown of the teeth by restorations. Initially, pocket analysis using periodontal probes yields the situational root morphology and deposit level in a patient with periodontal disease. Once root morphology is understood and the patient's periodontal needs ascertained, the dental professional can also choose the most effective treatment plan, including instrumentation. In addition, the awareness of root morphology will prevent the destruction of the root by overinstrumentation by hand.

Root concavities should be carefully explored during instrumentation appointments and charted in the patient's record. These concavities can become exposed to the oral environment due to periodontal disease but still be hidden to the clinician under a periodontal pocket, presenting complications during periodontal or even endodontic instrumentation and homecare. Treatment failures have been linked to deposits remaining either after therapy or with continued poor homecare because these deposits contribute to the continuation of the disease process. However, a significantly greater attachment loss occurs for root surfaces with proximal root grooves as compared with those that lack proximal root grooves.

Whereas these concavities can act as predisposing factors in the periodontal disease process, the depressions also increase the attachment area producing a root shape more resistant to damaging occlusal forces. Thus root contours present both harmful and protective effects that must be considered individually in the patient's periodontal prognosis.

Performing periodontal debridement of roots and associated furcations involves a set instrumentation treatment plan; the best approach is to treat each root as a separate tooth when access permits, with a combination of strokes using hand instruments, air polisher, or ultrasonic device.

Until recently, clinicians were not able to visualize the root surface unless access was gained by periodontal flap surgery to fold back the overlying oral mucosa. Instead they had to rely only on tactile sense and resultant mental picture to understand the subgingival topography. However, with the recent development of endoscopic technology, with its small camera that can fit within a deepened sulcus, clinicians today are able to see the root surface in real time. When incorporated into more clinical practice settings in the future, such devices may change the way many dental procedures are performed.

ORIENTATIONAL TOOTH TERMS

Each tooth has five surfaces: facial, lingual, masticatory, mesial, and distal surfaces. Thus each tooth is like a box with sides. Some of the surfaces of the tooth are identified by the orientational relationship to other orofacial structures, similar to the designation of the soft tissue of the oral cavity (Fig. 15.9; see Fig. 2.1). The tooth surface closest to the surface of the face is facial. The facial tooth surface closest to the lips is labial. Those facial tooth surfaces closest to the inner cheek are buccal. Therefore, the anterior teeth have a labial surface, and posterior teeth have a buccal surface.

The tooth surface closest to the tongue is lingual. Those lingual surfaces closest to the palate on the maxillary arch are sometimes also considered palatal. The **masticatory surface** is the chewing surface on the most superior surface of the crown. This is the **incisal surface** (in-sahy-zuhl) for anterior teeth and the **occlusal surface** for posterior teeth.

The masticatory surfaces of both anterior and posterior teeth have linear elevations or **ridges**, which are named according to location. The masticatory surfaces of both canines and posterior teeth also have at

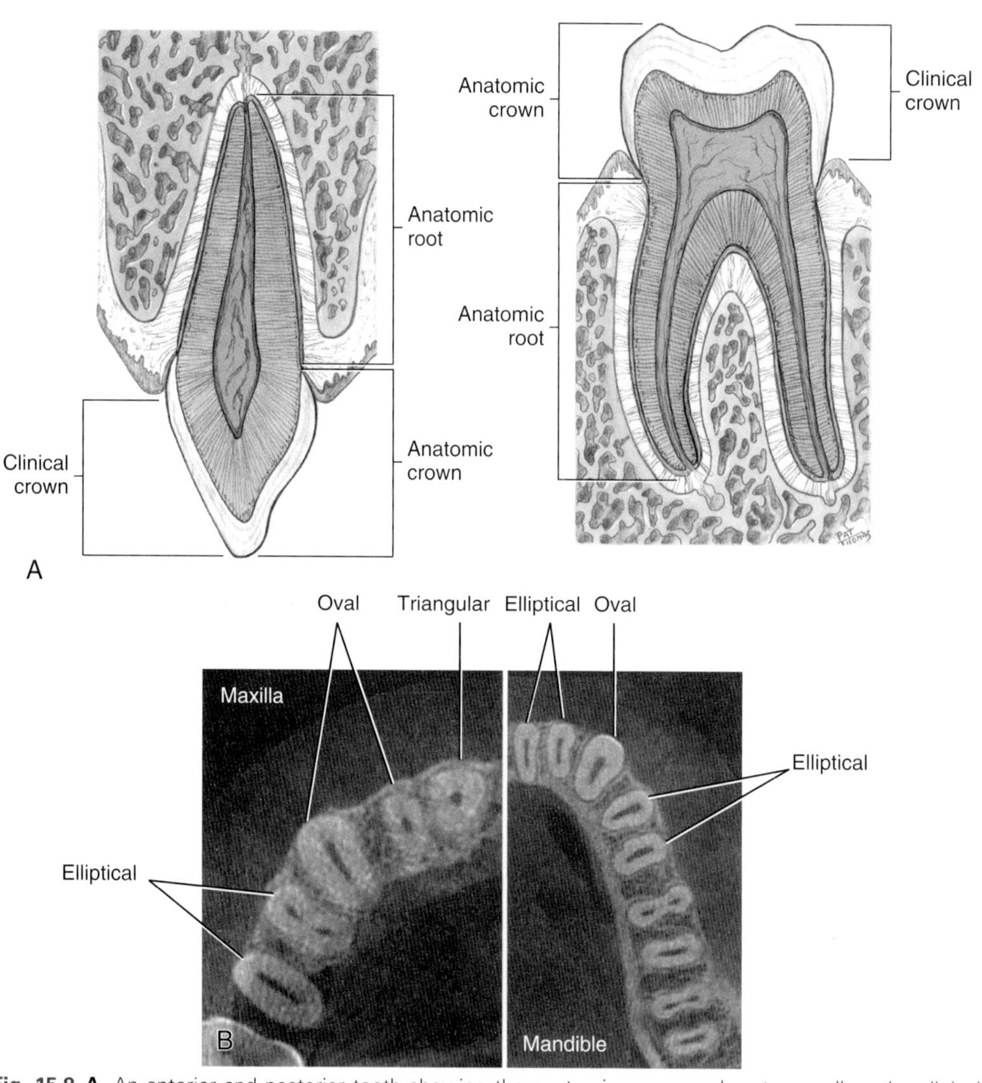

Fig. 15.8 A, An anterior and posterior tooth showing the anatomic crown and root as well as the clinical crown. The clinical root is not shown because this is a healthy periodontal situation without gingival recession; with gingival recession there may be an exposed clinical root visible. **B,** Cone-beam computed tomography of axial views of a quadrant of the maxilla and the mandible showing cervical cross sections of the adult dentition. Note the three basic shapes to the roots on cervical cross section: triangular, oval (or ovoid), or elliptical (or elongated oval). (**B,** From Metzger Z. The self-adjusting file [SAF] system: An evidence-based update. *J Conserv Dent.* 2014;17[5]:401–419.)

least one major elevation, the **cusp**; cusps contribute to a significant part of the tooth's surface. Maxillary and mandibular canines both have one cusp and the maxillary premolars and the mandibular first premolars usually have two cusps. Mandibular second premolars frequently have three cusps: one buccal and two lingual. Maxillary molars have two buccal cusps and two lingual cusps; a minor fifth cusp may form on these teeth (cusp of Carabelli). In contrast, mandibular molars may have five or four cusps.

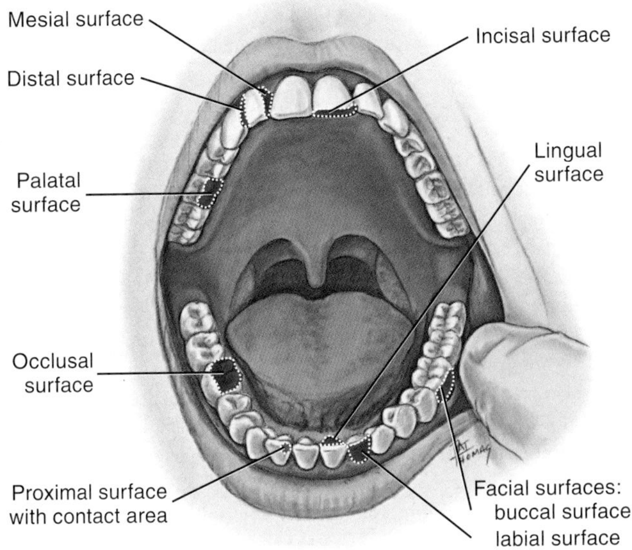

Fig. 15.9 Surfaces of the teeth highlighted *(red)* with the orientational relationship to other oral cavity structures noted as related to the midline and to other teeth.

Surfaces of both the crown and the root are also defined by the relationship to the midline (see Fig. 15.9). The surface closest to the midline is termed the **mesial**; the surface farthest away from the midline is termed the **distal** (**dis**-tl).

Together, both the mesial and the distal surfaces between adjacent teeth are termed the **proximal** (**prok**-suh-muhl). In other words, either surface of a tooth that is next to an adjacent tooth is referred to as a proximal surface, which may therefore be either the mesial or the distal surface. The area between adjacent tooth surfaces is the **interproximal space** (in-ter-**prok**-suh-muhl).

It is noted when viewing teeth overall that the proximal CEJ curvature is greatest on the anterior and the least on the posterior teeth. However, this curvature is approximately similar on mesial and distal surfaces of the two teeth that face each other. In addition, on any given tooth, the height of the CEJ curvature is greater on the mesial aspect of that tooth than it is on the distal aspect.

The area where the crowns of adjacent teeth in the same arch physically touch each adjacent proximal surface is the **contact area** or as referred to by clinicians, the *contact* (see Fig. 15.9). Its presence is checked when dental floss is passed between two teeth and some resistance is felt. The proper contact relation between neighboring teeth in each arch serves to keep food impaction between the teeth and it helps stabilize the dental arches by the combined anchorage of all the teeth having contact within each arch. Except for the third molars, each tooth in the arch is supported in part by its contact with two neighboring teeth, one mesial and one distal. The third molars (and the second molars if not third molar is present) are kept from drifting distally by the angulation of their occlusal surfaces with their roots and by the direction of the occlusal forces.

The contact areas on the mesial and distal surfaces are usually also considered the location of the height of contour on the proximal surfaces when in an ideal alignment (Fig. 15.10). Thus the **height of contour** (or crest of curvature) is the greatest elevation of the tooth

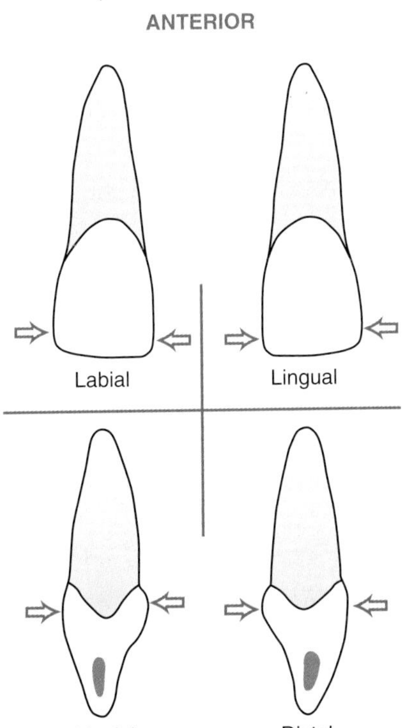

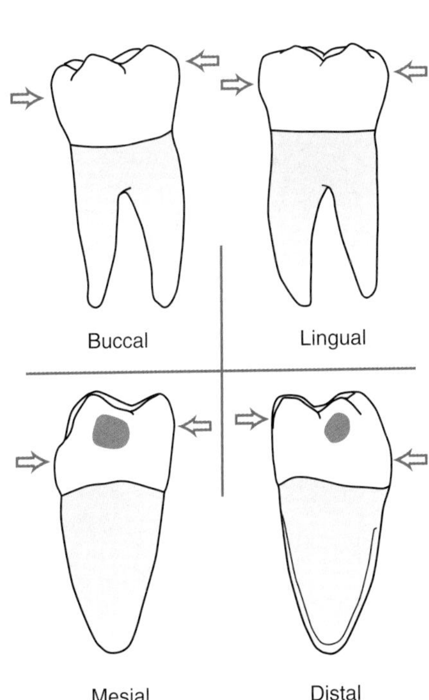

Fig. 15.10 Anterior and posterior teeth with the height of contour for each surface noted *(open arrows)* and contact areas highlighted *(red)*.

either incisocervically or occlusocervically on a specific surface of the crown when viewing its profile from the labial or buccal and the lingual. The crown also has a facial or lingual height of contour that is easily seen when viewing the crown's profile from the mesial and the distal. The facial and lingual surfaces of a tooth also have a height of contour that is easily seen when viewing the tooth's profile from the proximal aspect.

When two teeth in the same arch come into contact, the curvatures next to the contact areas form spaces considered **embrasures** (em-**bray**-zhuhrs) (Fig. 15.11). These consist of triangular-shaped spaces between two teeth, created by the sloping away of the mesial and distal surfaces and may diverge facially, lingually, occlusally, or apically with

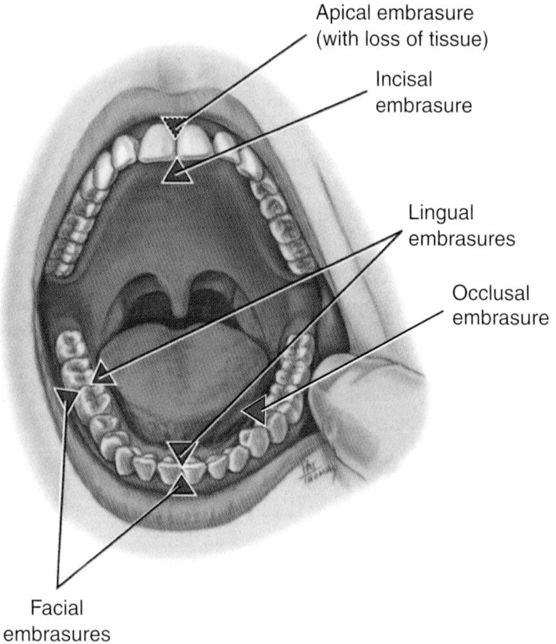

Fig. 15.11 Embrasures highlighted *(red triangles)* that form between two teeth created by the sloping away of the mesial and distal surfaces, which may diverge facially, lingually, incisally/occlusally, or apically with loss of tissue.

loss of tissue. The embrasures are continuous with the interproximal spaces between the teeth and there is an increasing angle of the occlusal embrasures anteroposteriorly. They form spillways between teeth to direct food away from the gingiva. Also they provide a mechanism for teeth to be more self-cleansing. Finally, the embrasures protect the gingiva from undue frictional trauma but still provide the proper degree of stimulation to the tissue.

All these tooth contours (such as contact areas, heights of contour, and embrasures) are important in the function and health of the masticatory system (see **Chapter 20**). These specific forms and alignments of the teeth serve to shelter the vulnerable gingivosulcular area from damage and help to stabilize the position of the teeth within each dental arch.

Each tooth can also be divided by imaginary lines to designate specific crown areas of the tooth. A **line angle** is formed by the lines that are created at the junction of two crown surfaces, with the name being derived by combining the names of those two surfaces (Fig. 15.12). When combining terms such as *mesial* and *labial,* the *al* from the end of the first surface is dropped and an *o* is added and combined with the second surface, thus creating *mesiolabial.* If the first letter of the second word results in doubling a vowel, a hyphen is placed between the words, such as *mesio-occlusal.* An example of line angle designation would be the mesiolabial line angle, which is the junction of the mesial and labial surfaces.

Posterior teeth have eight line angles per tooth: mesiobuccal, distobuccal, mesiolingual, distolingual, mesio-occlusal, disto-occlusal, bucco-occlusal, and linguo-occlusal. Anterior teeth have only six line angles per tooth: mesiolabial, distolabial, mesiolingual, distolingual, labioincisal, and linguoincisal. Anteriors have fewer line angles than posteriors because the mesial and distal incisal line angles are rounded; thus the mesioincisal and distoincisal line angles are practically nonexistent.

A **point angle** is another way to determine a specific area of the crown (Fig. 15.13). The junction of three surfaces of the crown, the point angle, takes its name from those three surfaces. Each tooth has four point angles. Examples of point angle designations are mesiolabioincisal for an anterior tooth or mesiobucco-occlusal for a posterior tooth.

Finally, a crown surface can be divided both horizontally and vertically into three parts or **thirds** to designate specific tooth areas (Fig. 15.14). An example is the middle third of the labial surface of an anterior tooth's crown. However, the root can be divided into thirds only

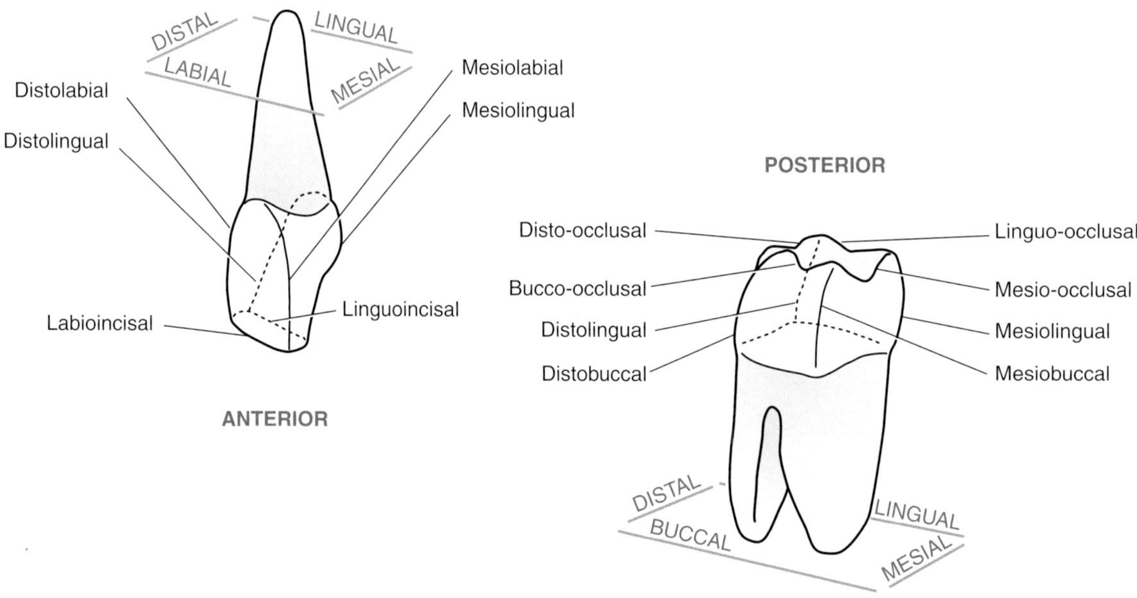

Fig. 15.12 Anterior and Posterior Tooth with the Designation of Line Angles of the Crown.

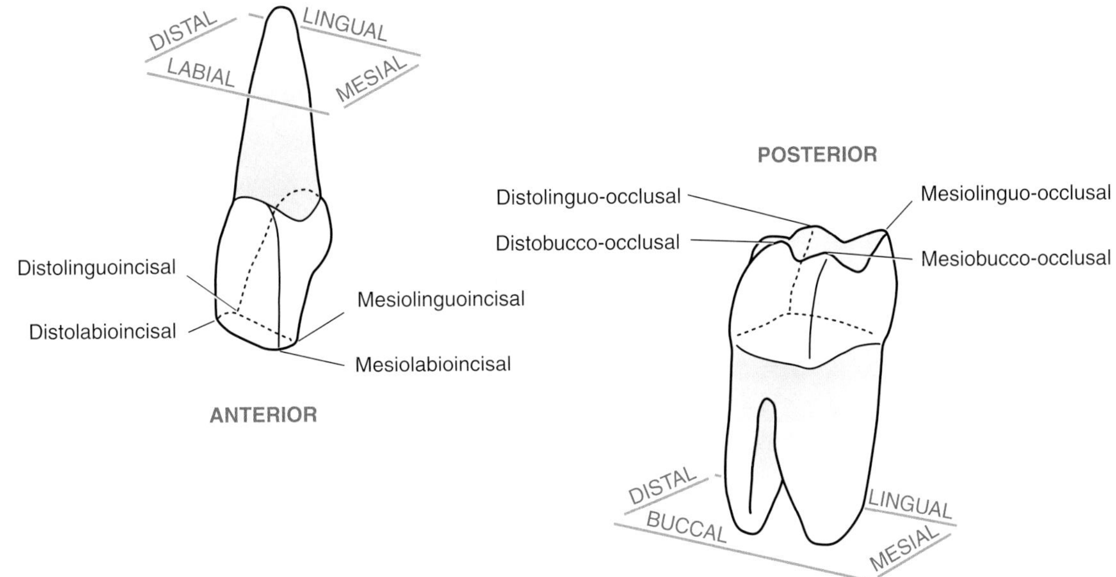

Fig. 15.13 Anterior and Posterior Tooth with the Designation of Point Angles of the Crown.

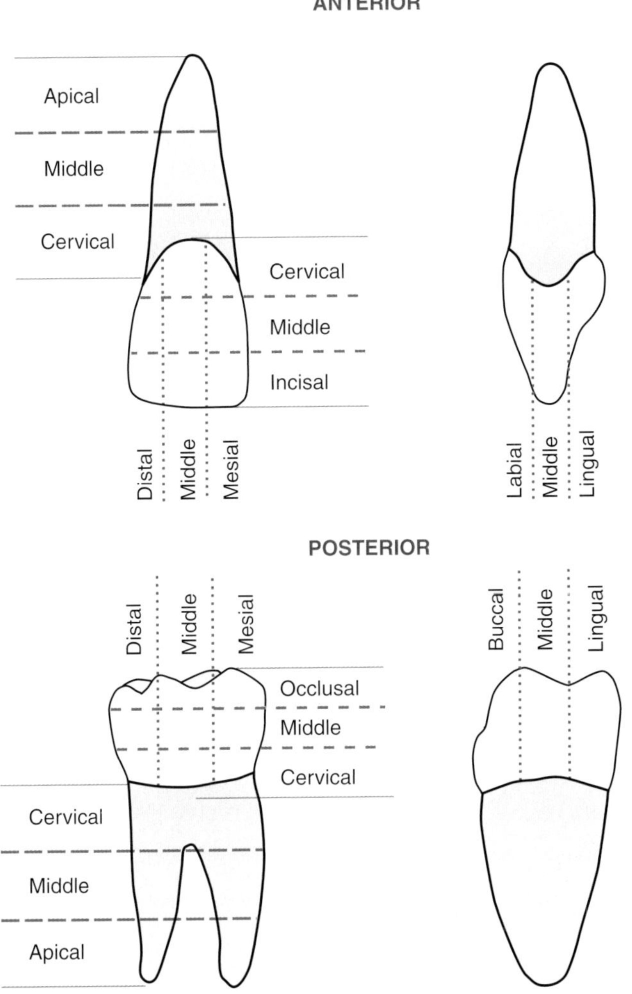

Fig. 15.14 Anterior and Posterior Tooth with the Designation of Crown and Root Thirds. Note that the root can only be divided into thirds horizontally.

horizontally. An example of designating a third area on a tooth root is the cervical third of the buccal surface of a posterior tooth's root. In comparison, the root can only be divided vertically into halves by the RAL as discussed earlier, such that the halves when viewing the tooth from the mesial or distal are designated as labial or buccal and lingual; the halves when viewing the tooth from the labial or buccal are designated as mesial and distal.

Note that in reference to line angles, point angles, thirds, or even a direction, there is an accepted sequencing of combined names of the involved surfaces. The accepted sequence allows that the one term *mesial* precedes the term *distal* and also that both *mesial* and *distal* precede all other terms. The terms *labial, buccal,* and *lingual* follow *mesial* or *distal* but precede *incisal* or *occlusal* in any combination.

Clinical Considerations for Tooth Surfaces

The tooth's angles, height of contour, and surrounding negative spaces (dark areas) define the front or face of a tooth when the design of a patient's smile is considered because these features are noted first when contemplating someone's smile. Altering placement and shape of these features changes the face of a tooth and its perceived size and the appearance of the smile. Note that ideally the mesial part of the face and silhouette of a tooth is more angled vertically than the distal part of the face of a tooth.

After studying the surfaces of a tooth, dental professionals must be careful to note that access to the proximal surfaces and the interproximal space is more difficult than access to facial and lingual surfaces, although line angles can also present difficulties. These access challenges may occur during homecare as well as for the clinician during instrumentation and restorative treatment.

TOOTH FORM

Each tooth type as already discussed has a specific form, no matter which dentition it is in (Table 15.4). This tooth form is related to the function during mastication for the tooth type as well as to its role in speech and esthetics. The form and function of each tooth type are similar for both the primary and permanent dentitions.

TABLE 15.4 Tooth Forms

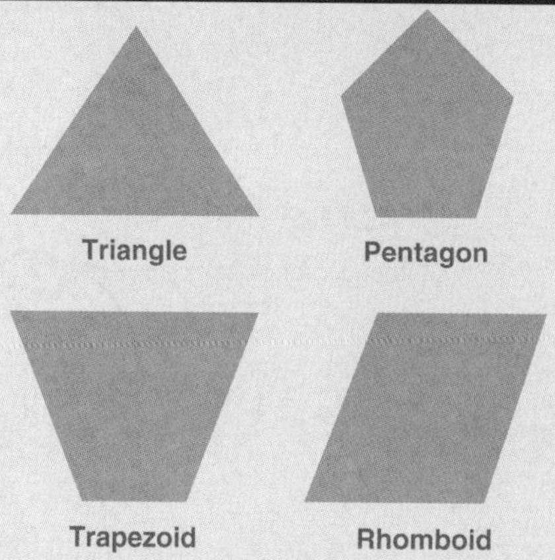

Triangle
Pentagon
Trapezoid
Rhomboid

TOOTH TYPE	TOOTH FORMS OF CROWNS WITH GEOMETRIC SHAPES	FUNCTION DURING MASTICATION
Incisors	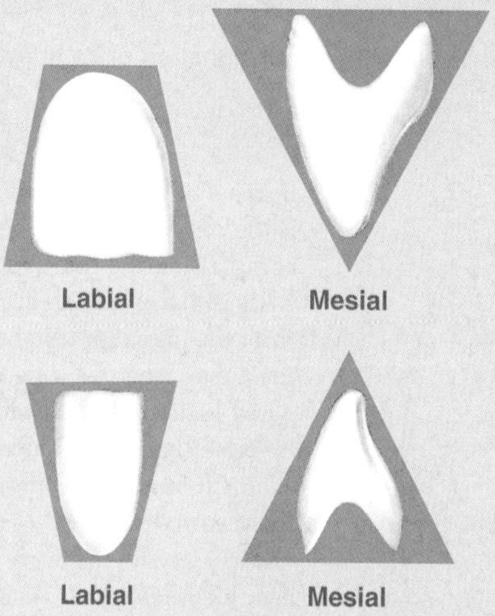 Labial, Mesial; Labial, Mesial PERMANENT MAXILLARY AND MANDIBULAR RIGHT INCISORS	Biting and cutting because of triangular proximal form
Canines	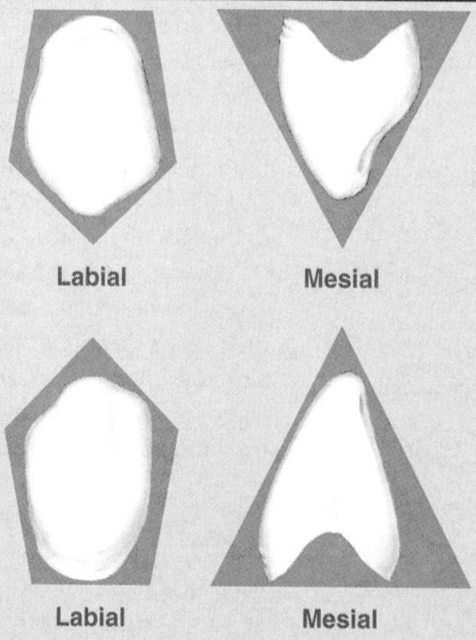 Labial, Mesial; Labial, Mesial PERMANENT MAXILLARY AND MANDIBULAR RIGHT CANINES	Pierce or tear food because of tapered shape and prominent cusp

TABLE 15.4 **Tooth Forms—cont'd**

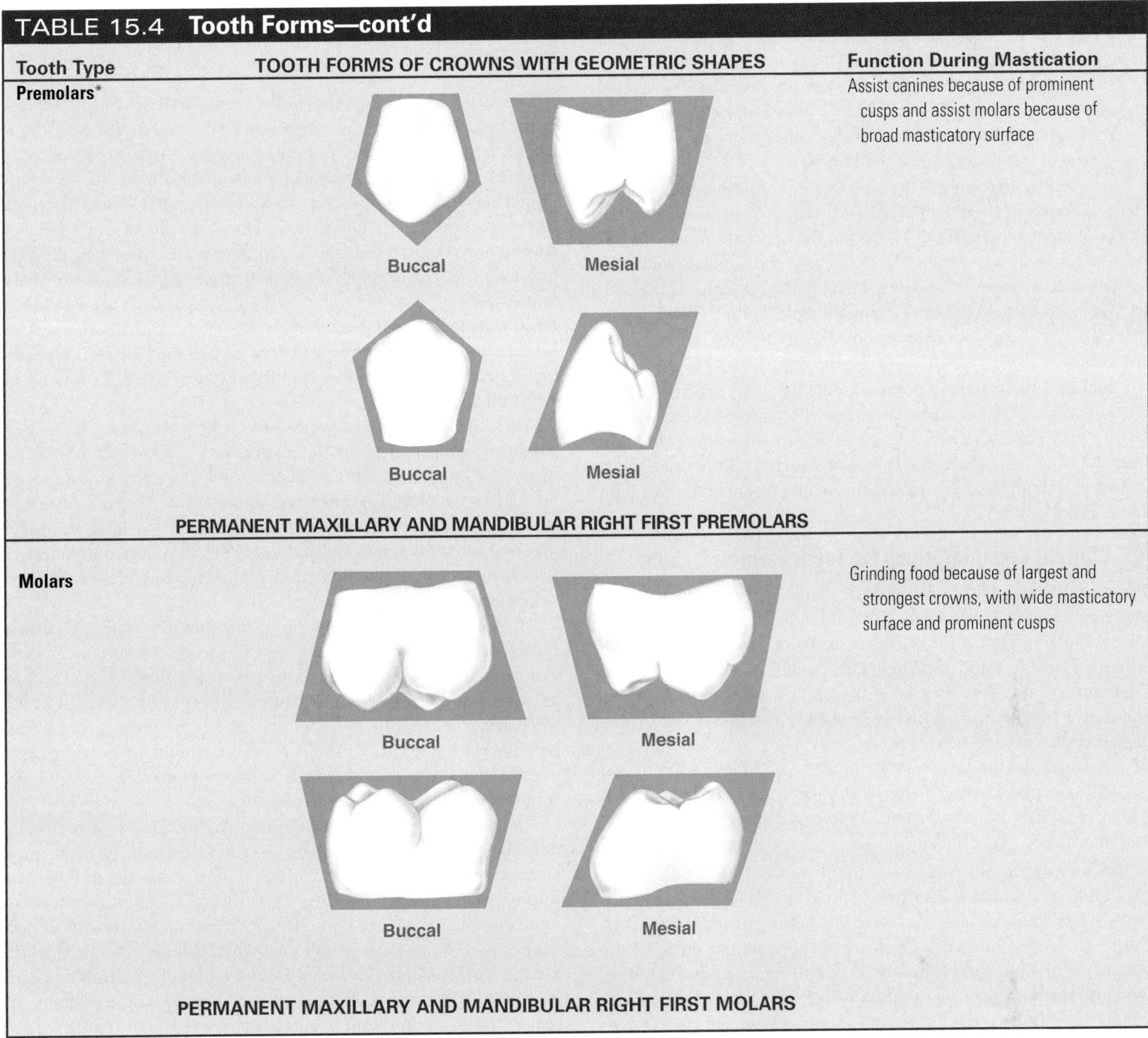

*Premolars are only found in the permanent dentition.

The incisors function as instruments for biting and cutting food during mastication because of the triangular proximal form of their crowns. The canines because of their tapered shape and the prominent cusp of their crowns function to pierce or tear food during mastication.

The premolars, which are found only in the permanent dentition, assist the canines in piercing and tearing food because of prominent cusps of their crowns during mastication. The premolars also assist the molars in grinding food during mastication because of the crown's wide masticatory surface, the occlusal surface. Finally, as the teeth with the largest and strongest crowns, the molars function in grinding food during mastication, assisted by the premolars. The wide masticatory surface, the occlusal surface of the molars with their prominent cusps, function during mastication.

Tooth types also have tooth forms of the crown that usually follow a rough outline of specific geometric shapes. Certain general shapes of the crown outline can be seen for each tooth type when viewing from each of the four perspectives; these specific shapes will be discussed in more detail in **Chapters 16 and 17** with each individual tooth type. As already discussed, the crowns of the incisors are triangular from both mesial or distal views with the apex of the triangle at the masticatory surface of the tooth, the incisal surface, with its base at the cervix. From both labial and lingual views, the crown outline of incisors is trapezoidal or four-sided with only two parallel sides; the longer of the two parallel sides is toward the incisal surface.

Morphologically canines can be considered a transitional tooth between incisors and premolars in the permanent dentition. Similar to the incisors, the crowns of canines are triangular from both mesial and distal views as are all anteriors but are pentagonal or five-sided from both labial or lingual views.

Only found in the permanent dentition, premolars are considered also morphologically to be a transitional tooth between canines and molars. From both buccal and lingual views, the premolars' crowns are pentagonal or five-sided, similar to canines.

For maxillary premolars, the crown outline from mesial or distal views is trapezoidal, or four-sided with only two parallel sides; the longer of the two parallel sides is toward the occlusal surface. In contrast, the mandibular premolars' crowns are rhomboidal from both mesial or distal views or four-sided having the opposite sides parallel. The rhomboidal outline is inclined lingually, thus allowing correct intercuspal contact of the mandibular tooth with the maxillary antagonists.

Similar to the maxillary premolars, the maxillary molars' crowns are trapezoidal in shape when viewed from both mesial or distal as are all maxillary posteriors while the mandibular molars are rhomboidal from the same views as are all mandibular posteriors. In contrast, when viewed from both buccal or lingual, the molars' crown outline for both arches is trapezoidal.

 Clinical Considerations for Tooth Form

Variation of teeth within a particular tooth type is a given and is always of interest to clinicians. The individual tooth form and its related function can be lost as a result of attrition, caries, and trauma or even extraction and shedding with complete loss of the tooth. Functional tooth form that has been lost can be approximated by restorative treatment in many cases using artificial crowns as discussed earlier or replacement bridges, partial or complete and fixed or removable dentures, as well as implants (see Fig. 14.23). If not restored or replaced, this change in form over time can affect mastication, especially in older patients, who may change to a softer diet that may be poor nutritionally.

Because the specific shape of a tooth varies in each person and may even vary within a dentition, a mold of the restored crown is made when integrating artificial crowns within an individual dentition. The goal is to match as closely as possible the shape of the patient's teeth on the opposite side so that the arch appears symmetrical and the crowns fit the space provided. This mold is selected by comparing it with a mold guide of white plastic model crowns provided by various manufacturers. The shade of the tooth is also a consideration (see **Chapter 12**).

CONSIDERATIONS FOR DENTAL ANATOMY STUDY

It is important to note that **Appendix C** in this textbook includes charts of the measurements of the permanent dentition. Student dental professionals should note that the values are mean values of ideal teeth; real teeth vary in size among patients and do not always directly reflect proportionate jaw size. Student dental professionals should also note that most of the descriptions in this textbook are also of ideal teeth. For consistency, the professionally drawn figures are larger than life-size; however, size relationships among teeth are retained, similar to those to be drawn and also illustrated in the flashcards from the ***Workbook for Illustrated Dental Embryology, Histology, and Anatomy.*** Also included are directions on how to draw each of the teeth, which allows the student dental professional to further study each of the features of each individual tooth.

These drawn ideal teeth within the figures also have no wear or pathology, similar to plastic or plaster teeth. Extracted tooth specimens may be real but have detractions too. The detailed features on most extracted tooth specimens are sometimes harder to see because of signs of wear on both the crown and even the root apex. The teeth may also show the trauma related to caries and restorative treatment. Examining a healthy dentition in a dental setting does present the teeth to best advantage.

However, many of the specific distinguishing features of a tooth can be seen only when holding an extracted tooth specimen. Thus extraction allows both the anatomic crown and the anatomic root to be viewed at once. In contrast, fewer features can be seen clinically when parts of the CEJ and root are covered by gingival tissue and only the clinical crown is visible. However, clinical views of the teeth are still important for observation of overall tooth arrangements and relationships.

Thus extracted teeth provide a more realistic form of dental anatomy than plastic or plaster teeth because they have more clearly formed cusps, ridges, fossae, and pits; variations of the ideal tooth form can thus be seen. Extracted teeth can also provide an opportunity to view rarer as well as more common dental anomalies. However, infection control procedures must be followed when handling extracted teeth; see the ***Workbook for Illustrated Dental Embryology, Histology, and Anatomy*** for detailed procedures. When studying dental anatomy, all opportunities for observation must be considered for the most effective level of expertise to be achieved: extracted tooth specimens, plastic or plaster teeth, and dentitions in a clinical setting.

16

Permanent Anterior Teeth

Additional resources and practice exercises are provided on the companion Evolve website for this book: http://evolve.elsevier.com/Fehrenbach/illustrated.

LEARNING OBJECTIVES

1. Define and pronounce the key terms in this chapter.
2. Identify the permanent anterior teeth and discuss their properties and the clinical considerations concerning them, integrating it into patient care.
3. Assign the correct names and universal or international tooth number for each permanent anterior tooth on a diagram or a skull and for a tooth model or a patient.
4. Demonstrate the correct location of each permanent anterior tooth on a diagram, a skull, and a patient.
5. Identify the permanent incisors and their general features and discuss their clinical considerations, integrating it into patient care.
6. Describe the general and specific features of the permanent maxillary incisors and discuss the clinical considerations concerning them, integrating it into patient care.
7. Describe the general and specific features of the permanent maxillary canines and discuss the clinical considerations concerning them, integrating it into patient care.
8. Describe the general and specific features of the permanent mandibular canines and discuss the clinical considerations concerning them, integrating it into patient care.
9. Assign the correct names and universal or international tooth number for each permanent anterior tooth on a diagram or a skull and for a tooth model or a patient.
10. Demonstrate the correct location of each permanent anterior tooth on a diagram, a skull, and a patient.

PERMANENT ANTERIOR TEETH PROPERTIES

Permanent anterior teeth include the incisors and canines (Fig. 16.1; see Figs. 2.4 and 15.2). They are usually visible when the dental patient smiles. These teeth are aligned to form a smooth curving arc from the distal of canine on one side of the arch to the distal of the canine on the opposite side.

All anterior teeth are thought to be composed of four developmental lobes, three labial lobes (mesiolabial, middle labial, and distolabial), and one lingual lobe (Fig. 16.2). Two vertical labial **developmental depressions** outline the separations between the labial developmental lobes: the mesiolabial and distolabial developmental depressions. Lobe discussion as was noted in **Chapter 6** is controversial but is included for completeness when discussing in detail the various tooth types.

All permanent anterior teeth are succedaneous, which means that each one replaces the primary tooth of the same type. The development and shedding of the primary dentition as well as the development of the permanent dentition can be reviewed in **Chapter 6**.

The long crown of an anterior tooth has an incisal surface that is considered the **incisal ridge**, which is its masticatory surface (Fig. 16.3). The crown outline of anteriors is triangular when viewed from the proximal with the apex at the incisal ridge and the base of the triangle at the cervix (Fig. 16.4; see Table 15.4). These teeth are wider mesiodistally than labiolingually when compared with posteriors. For anteriors, the height of contour for both the crown's labial and lingual surfaces is in the cervical third. Each contact area of anteriors is usually centered labiolingually on their proximal surfaces and has a smaller area than the contacts of posterior teeth (see Fig. 15.10). On each proximal surface, the cementoenamel junction (CEJ) curvature of all anteriors is greater than that of the posteriors.

The lingual surfaces of all anteriors have a **cingulum** (**sing**-gyuh-luhm), which is a raised rounded area on the cervical third of the lingual surface in varying degrees of prominence or development (Fig. 16.5). The cingulum corresponds to the lingual developmental lobe. Ridges may also be present on the lingual surface. The lingual surface on anteriors is bordered mesially and distally on each side by a rounded raised border, the **marginal ridge**.

Some anteriors have a more complex lingual surface with a **fossa** (**fos**-uh) (plural, **fossae** [**fos**-ee]), which is a shallow and wide depression (Fig. 16.6). Some may also have **developmental pits**, which are located in the deepest part of each fossa. Other anteriors may have on their lingual surface a **developmental groove** (or primary groove), which is a sharp deep V-shaped linear depression that marks the junction between the developmental lobes.

In addition, a **supplemental groove** (or secondary groove) may also be present on the lingual surface of anteriors, which is a shallower and more irregular linear depression than the developmental groove (see Fig. 16.6). Supplemental grooves branch from the developmental grooves but are not always present in the same pattern on each different tooth type. In general, the more anterior the tooth is located in the arch, the fewer supplemental grooves are present and the less pronounced or smoother the lingual surface.

Anteriors usually have a single root, with some exceptions. When considering anterior roots, these roots appear either triangular, oval (as in ovoid or egg-shaped), or elliptical (or elongated oval) on cervical cross section, which give them narrower lingual surfaces, an important consideration with clinical procedures. Each root of the maxillary anterior teeth has great lingual and slight distal inclination (see Fig. 20.9). Each root of the mandibular anterior teeth varies in angulation from an almost vertical surface to a strong lingual inclination, with the canines possibly having a slight distal root inclination.

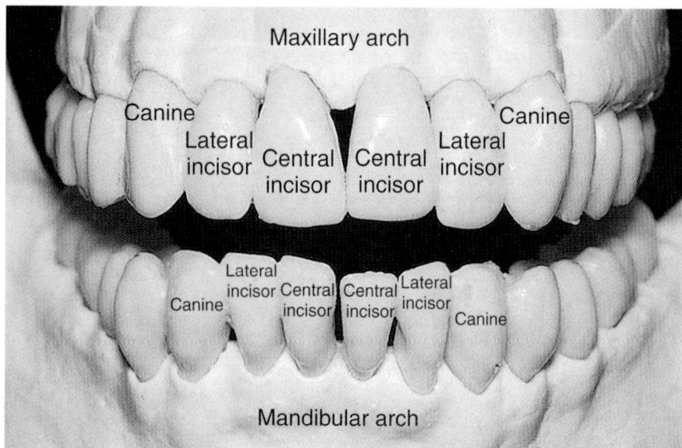

Fig. 16.1 Permanent Anterior Teeth Identified, Which Include the Incisors and Canines. (Courtesy of Margaret J. Fehrenbach, RDH, MS.)

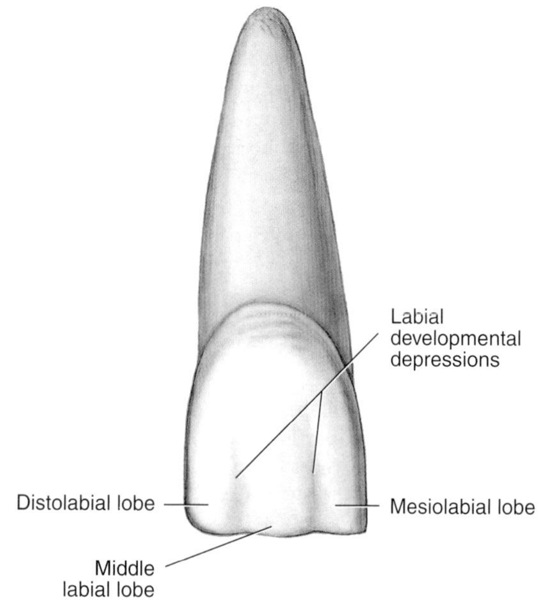

Fig. 16.2 Example of Lobe Development in a Permanent Anterior Tooth.

Clinical Considerations with Permanent Anterior Teeth

Patients may have difficulty in maintaining homecare of anteriors because their dental arch position naturally may allow the lips to overhang the teeth. Thus patients may provide care only to the incisal two-thirds of the labial surface of the crowns of anteriors, especially noted is the missing the associated cervical area and labial gingival tissue; this may also make instrumentation or restoration difficult. Mouth breathing may also dry the maxillary labial gingival tissue, causing localized inflammation.

Instrumentation and restorative treatment may also be compromised in the area where the greater curvature of the CEJ is present interproximally on anteriors and where accessibility is limited as well as having the teeth in close proximity. The grooves on the lingual surface of anteriors may present areas for dental biofilm retention if they extend to the root and are near the adjacent gingival tissue; for this reason the grooves may need to be reduced with minor odontoplasty.

When the anterior teeth are restored or undergo orthodontic therapy, the Golden Proportions can be useful guidelines to balance the size of the teeth with one another (see Fig. 1.10). These guidelines designate the ideal width of the maxillary lateral incisor as a factor of 1.0×, the width of the central incisors as 1.618× and the width of the canines as 0.168× as observed in two dimensions from the labial aspect. Other formulas state that the maxillary central should be 60% wider than the lateral and the lateral should be 60% wider than the canine as measured from the midline to the mesial aspect. In addition, each incisor should also ideally have an 8:10 width-to-length ratio.

Consideration of smile design may involve the drawing of a line following the ideal outline formed by the incisal ridges of the maxillary anterior teeth; the ideal line should be 1 to 3 mm parallel or equidistant to the lower lip line. Straight smiles are perceived as more masculine and more curved smiles are perceived as more feminine. In addition, if the upper lip line appears convex instead of concave compared with the lower lip line, the smile will be perceived as more youthful (see Fig. 14.22). Some variation of one's smile will occur with aging due to a noticeable loss of elasticity in the lips, which results in sagging, prominence of the mandibular anterior teeth, and diminution of the maxillary anterior teeth.

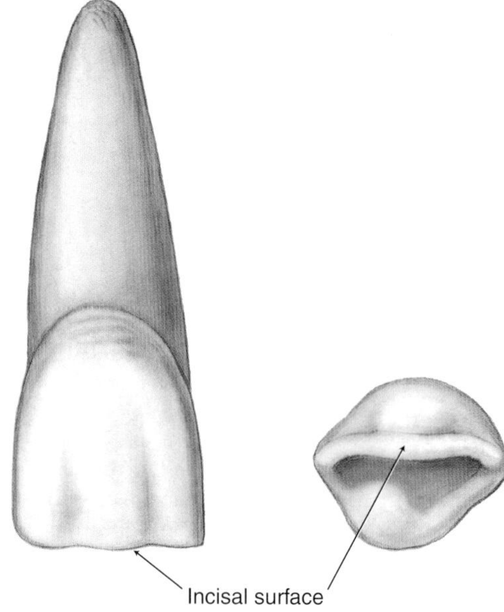

Fig. 16.3 Example of an Incisal Surface on a Permanent Anterior Tooth.

PERMANENT INCISORS

GENERAL FEATURES OF PERMANENT INCISORS

Permanent incisors are the eight most anterior teeth of the permanent dentition with four in each dental arch (Table 16.1). The two types are the central incisors and the lateral incisors. The centrals are closest to the midline and the laterals are the second teeth from the midline. One of each type is present in each quadrant of each dental arch. Both types are mesial to the permanent canines when the permanent dentition is fully erupted. The permanent incisors are succedaneous and replace the primary incisors of the same type. On occasion, the permanent incisors seem to spread out across the arch as a result of open spacing during initial eruption, especially in the maxillary arch but with the eruption of the permanent canines, these spaces often close (see Fig. 15.4).

The incisors' masticatory surface functions as instruments for biting and cutting food during mastication because of their incisal

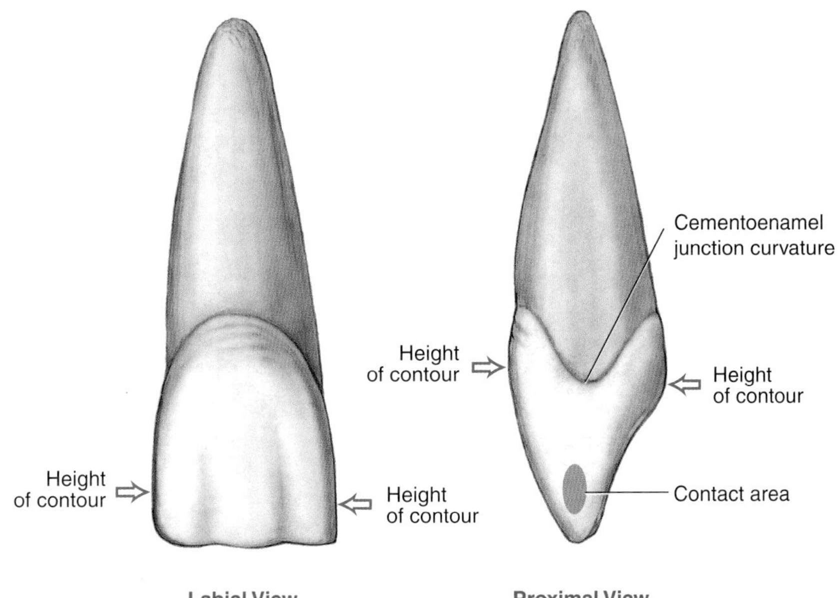

Fig. 16.4 Example of a Permanent Anterior Tooth with the Various Heights of Contour and Contact Area Identified.

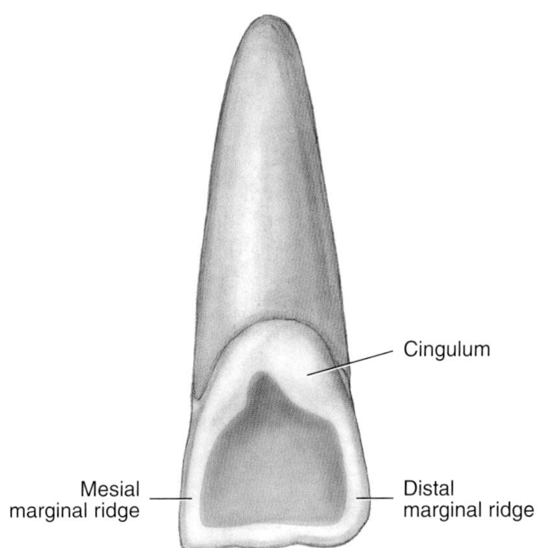

Fig. 16.5 Example of Lingual Surface Features on a Permanent Anterior Tooth.

ridge, triangular proximal form, and arch position (see Table 15.4). Their lingual surface is shaped like a shovel to help guide food into the mouth. They also support the lips and facial muscles as well as maintain vertical dimension of the face. Additionally, they contribute to overall arch appearance. Finally, they are involved during the articulation of speech and assist in guiding jaw closure as the teeth come together.

From both the labial and lingual, the crown outline of incisors is trapezoidal or four-sided with only two parallel sides. The longer of the two parallel sides is toward the incisal surface (see Table 15.4).

When newly erupted, each incisor also has three **mamelons** (**mam**-uh-lons), which are rounded enamel extensions on the incisal ridge from the labial or lingual views (Fig. 16.7). The mamelons are considered by some histologists to be extensions from the three labial developmental lobes (see **Chapter 6**).

The incisors are also the only permanent teeth with two **incisal angles** formed from the incisal ridge and each proximal surface (see Fig. 16.7). Incisors of both types are the only permanent teeth with an almost straight incisal ridge, which is a linear elevation on the masticatory or incisal surface of these anteriors when newly erupted, thus the reference in the name *incisors.*

The lingual surface has a cingulum that corresponds to the lingual developmental lobe, although its prominence or development differs for each type of incisor (see Fig. 16.7). These teeth also have a lingual fossa and marginal ridges on the lingual surface, again in differing developmental levels for each type of incisor. The height of contour for both labial and lingual surfaces of all incisors is at the cervical third as is the case for all anteriors.

Clinical Considerations with Permanent Incisors

Because of the anterior position of the incisors, esthetic concerns are important during restorative procedures. However, restorative replacement of any part of the incisal surfaces of these teeth after traumatic fracture may also be difficult to maintain owing to their function in biting and cutting food during mastication.

The mamelons on the incisal ridges of incisors usually undergo slight attrition, the wearing of a tooth surface caused by tooth-to-tooth contact, shortly after eruption as the teeth move into occlusion. Thus mamelons are usually most noticeable immediately after eruption, becoming less detectable as the teeth undergo some level of attrition over time.

If mamelons are still present on the incisal ridges long after eruption, it is because these teeth are not in occlusion where they usually undergo some level of attrition, such as with an anterior open bite relationship (Fig. 16.8, *A*). Many young adults do not like the appearance of mamelons and sometimes request to have them removed by minor odontoplasty; some patients even request restorative treatment to achieve straighter-appearing incisal ridges.

Part of the reason that the mamelons are so noticeable if present long after eruption is that these extensions are made of enamel with no dentin layer underneath. This factor and their thinness contribute overall to the striking translucent appearance as opposed to the rest of the clinical crown, which is usually has more opacity than the mamelons. With the addition of vital tooth whitening (or bleaching), incisal translucencies from mamelons or incisal ridges may become even more noticeable.

In addition, after eruption the incisal ridges can now appear even more flattened from the labial, lingual, or incisal views due to attrition and each

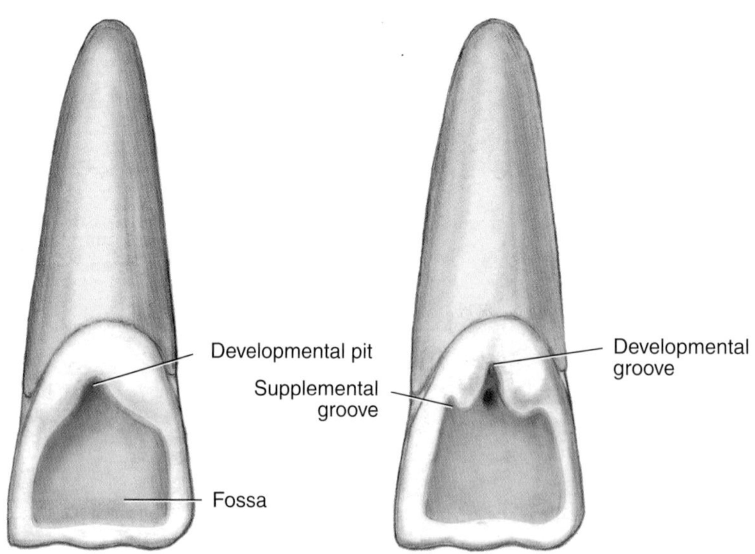

Fig. 16.6 Additional Examples of Lingual Surface Features on a Permanent Anterior Tooth.

TABLE 16.1 Permanent Incisors

	Maxillary Central Incisor	Maxillary Lateral Incisor	Mandibular Central Incisor	Mandibular Lateral Incisor
Universal number	#8 and #9	#7 and #10	#24 and #25	#23 and #26
International number	#11 and #21	#12 and #22	#31 and #41	#32 and #42
General crown features	Incisal ridge, incisal angles, cingulum, marginal ridges, lingual fossa			
Specific crown features	Widest crown mesiodistally. Greatest CEJ curve and height of contour. Pronounced distal offset cingulum and marginal ridges, with wide and deep lingual fossa	Greatest crown variation. Like smaller central. Pronounced lingual surface, with centered cingulum and prominent marginal ridges	Smallest and simplest tooth. Symmetrical. Small centered cingulum, with less pronounced marginal ridges and lingual fossa	Like larger mandibular central. Not symmetrical. Appears twisted distally. Small, distally placed cingulum, with mesial marginal ridge longer than distal marginal ridge
Height of contour	Cervical third			
Mesial contact	Incisal third			
Distal contact	Junction of incisal and middle thirds	Middle third	Incisal third	Incisal third
Distinguish right from left	Sharper mesioincisal angle and rounder distoincisal angle. More pronounced mesial CEJ curvature			
General root features	Single root			
Specific root features	Triangular on cervical cross section. Overall conical shape. No proximal root concavities. Rounded apex	Oval on cervical cross section. Same or longer than central but thinner. Overall conical shape. No proximal root concavities. Root curves distally, with sharp apex	Elliptical on cervical cross section. Root is longer than crown. Pronounced proximal root concavities can give double-rooted appearance	

CEJ, Cementoenamel junction.

becomes an **incisal edge** (see Fig. 16.8, *B*). Thus with this arrangement, the incisal edges of the maxillary and mandibular incisors are now usually parallel to one another and occlude correctly during mastication. However, with increased attrition the maxillary incisors' incisal edges can show lingual inclination and the mandibular incisors can have a labial inclination to their incisal edges as well as translucency (see Fig. 16.9, *C*).

The crown of a permanent maxillary incisor can be affected with dens in dente (see Box 6.1, *G, H*). This disturbance may leave the tooth with a deep lingual pit resulting from invagination of the enamel organ into the dental papilla. This pit may lead to pulpal exposure and pathology. Dens in dente may be hereditary and is more common within a maxillary lateral incisor.

The crowns of permanent incisors, similar to molars, can be affected in children with congenital syphilis. A pregnant woman infected with syphilis transmits the spirochete *Treponema pallidum,* a sexually transmitted microorganism, to her fetus via the placenta. This microorganism may cause localized enamel hypoplasia, which can result in **Hutchinson incisors** (**hutch**-in-suhn) occurring during tooth development (see Fig. 3.17, *A*). A Hutchinson incisor has a crown with a screwdriver shape from the labial view and is wider cervically and narrow incisally with a notched incisal ridge. Restorative treatment of these teeth may improve their oral appearance. Affected children may also have other developmental anomalies, such as blindness, deafness, and paralysis from congenital syphilis.

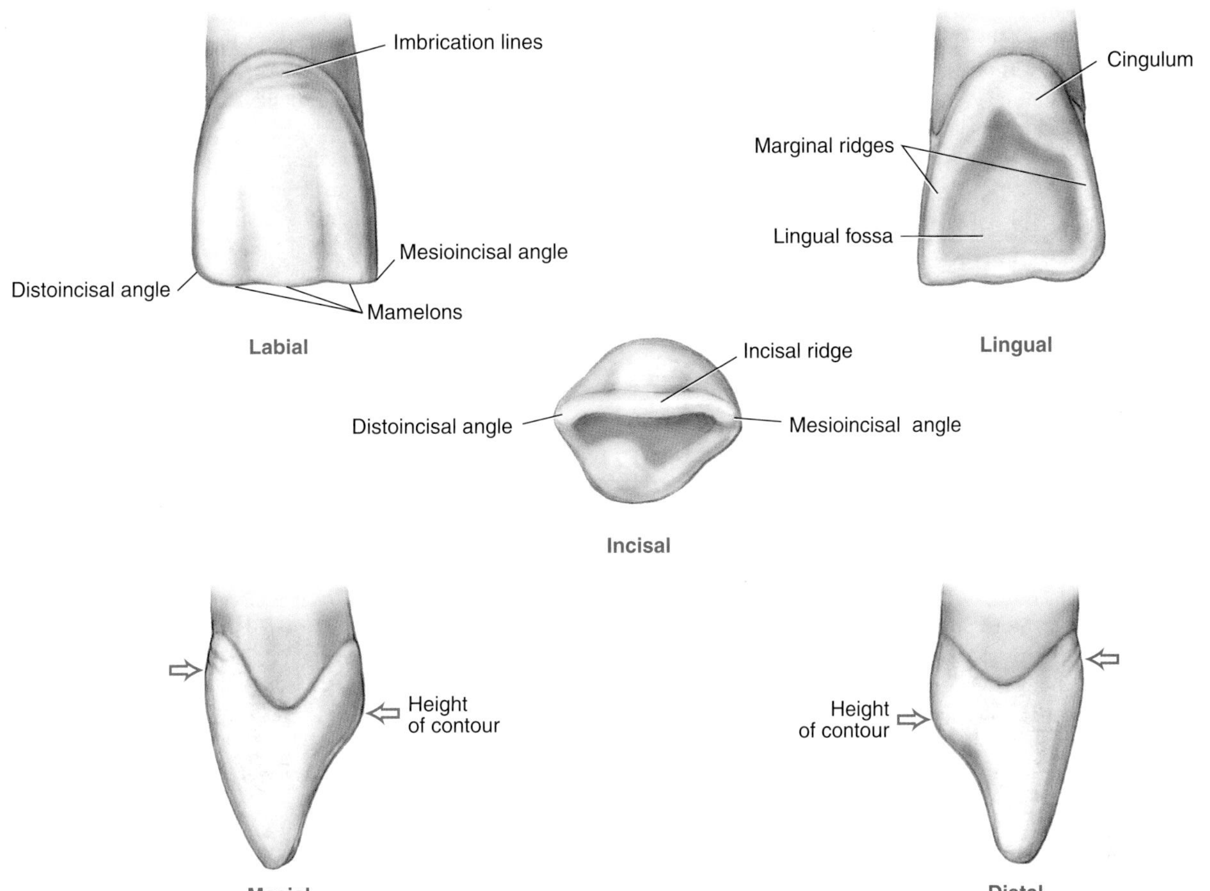

Fig. 16.7 Views of a Newly Erupted Permanent Incisor with the Features Noted.

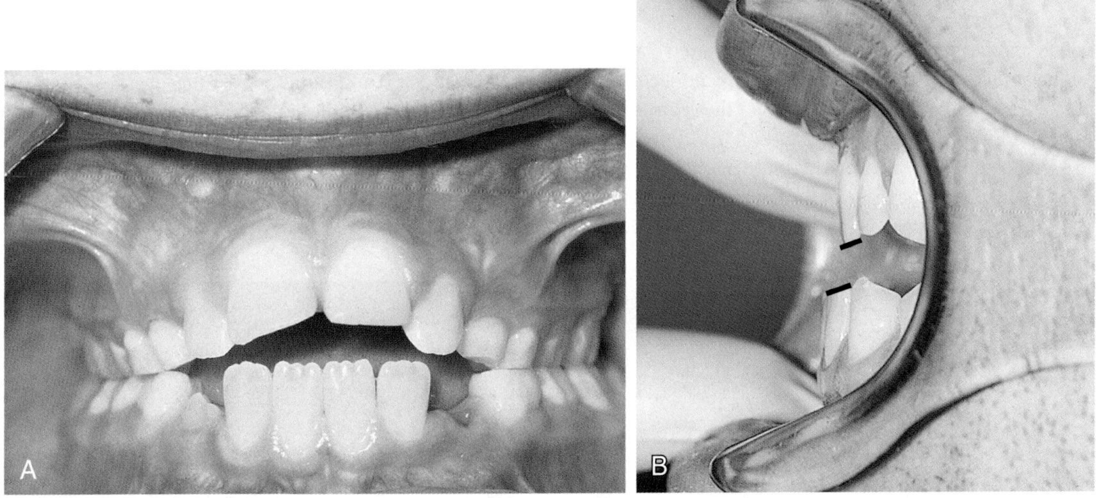

Fig. 16.8 Incisal Surface on Permanent Incisors. **A,** Mamelons present on the incisal ridges of newly erupted permanent mandibular incisors in a mixed dentition, which have been kept from attrition due to an anterior open bite. In contrast, through attrition the mamelons have been lost on the already erupted same tooth type on the maxillary arch. **B,** Lateral view of both permanent maxillary and mandibular incisors altered by higher levels of attrition on the incisal surfaces, which have transitioned from incisal ridges to incisal edges *(dark outlines)*. (Courtesy of Margaret J. Fehrenbach, RDH, MS.)

A sharp small extra cusp or **talon cusp**, which means like a claw, occasionally appears as a projection from the cingulum of incisor teeth and can happen on any tooth within both dentitions. These types of cusps can interfere with occlusion and even minor odontoplasty may be a hazardous procedure. They often contain a prominent pulp horn, which is at an increased risk of pulpal exposure during restorative procedures.

PERMANENT MAXILLARY INCISORS

General Features

Permanent maxillary incisors are the four most anteriorly placed teeth of the maxillary arch. Each has a crown that is larger in all dimensions, especially mesiodistally, compared with a mandibular incisor. In addition, the labial surfaces are rounder from the incisal aspect with the tooth tapering toward the lingual.

The central and lateral incisors of the maxillary arch both resemble each other more than they resemble the similar type of incisors of the opposing arch. Generally, a maxillary central incisor is larger than a maxillary lateral incisor but they have a similar form. Both types of maxillary incisors are wider mesiodistally than labiolingually.

All lingual surface features, including the marginal ridges, lingual fossa, and cingulum, are more prominent on the maxillary incisors than on the mandibular incisors. Finally, the incisal ridge is just labial to the long axis of the root from either proximal view.

Each root is short compared with those of other maxillary teeth and usually is without root concavities. However, the presence of bulbous and pronounced crowns may create deep mesial and distal concavities at the CEJ.

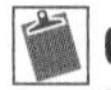

Clinical Considerations with Permanent Maxillary Incisors

If a maxillary incisor has increased prominence of the lingual marginal ridges and a deeper lingual fossa, it may be considered to have an extreme shovel-shaped form (Fig. 16.9, *A*). It presents with pronounced marginal ridges and a deeper lingual fossa. It can also have an accentuated cingulum with deepened grooves or have an incisal edge with severe attrition, giving it a lingual inclination (see Fig. 16.9, *B* and *C*, respectively). In addition, supragingival tooth deposits, such as dental biofilm and stain, can collect in the prominent lingual surface concavities of maxillary incisors (see Fig. 16.9, *D*).

The lingual pit is another lingual feature that if present on the maxillary incisors can be at increased risk of caries development due to both increased dental biofilm retention and the weakness of the enamel forming the walls of the pit (Fig. 16.10, *A* to *C*; see Fig. 12-4, *A*). If the lingual pit is deep, a developmental disturbance of dens in dente must be considered and needed changes must be made in the patient's treatment plan (discussed earlier). Also present may be a vertically placed linguogingival groove that originates in the lingual pit and extends cervically and slightly distally onto the cingulum (see Fig. 16.10, *D*). It is more common on maxillary laterals, which may result in caries with the architecture of the pit.

Clinicians need to be aware of these lingual pit and groove patterns on maxillary incisors when they examine a dentition in order to determine the patient's caries risk level. All pits and grooves must be checked for decay with an explorer and mirror. Light-induced devices that measure changes in laser fluorescence of hard tissue allow dental professionals to better diagnose early lesions in pits and grooves. Maxillary incisors with deep pit and groove patterns but without incipient decay should have enamel sealants placed as soon as they erupt. If dental caries occurs or an enamel sealant does not remain on the lingual surface, tooth-colored restorative materials can be used to achieve a more esthetic appearance and thus the past history of the lingual pit may not now be easy to discern clinically.

During instrumentation or restoration, the proximal surfaces of these teeth are more accessible from the lingual than the labial approach because of the increased tapering of the tooth to the lingual. Dental professionals must be careful to check for deposits in any mesial and distal root concavities at the CEJ if this area is exposed as a result of gingival recession.

Finally, the competency of the lips to maintain a lip seal when at a resting posture can affect the overall position of the maxillary incisors (see Fig. 20.31). Competent lips allow these tooth ridges to be inferior to the lower lip border, helping to maintain the level of inclination. Incompetent lips that fail to provide a lip seal do not control this inclination and may even allow the maxillary incisors to be anterior to the lower lip, exaggerating already buccally inclined teeth and may become lingually inclined. A tongue thrust is a complicating factor that may be associated with this occlusal challenge (see Fig. 20.28).

Permanent Maxillary Central Incisors #8 and #9 (#11 and #21)

Specific Overall Features

Permanent maxillary central incisors erupt between 7 to 8 years of age with root completion at age 10 (Fig. 16.11). Thus these teeth usually erupt after the mandibular central incisors. Many child patients want these two teeth to come in fast to fill their wide open anterior arch space when they shed their two primary maxillary central incisors as in the old song, "All I Want for Christmas Is My Two Front Teeth."

The maxillary central incisors are the most prominent teeth in the permanent dentition because of both their large size and their anterior arch position. In addition, they are the largest of all the incisors and the two usually share a mesial contact area. They have the widest crown mesiodistally of any permanent anterior tooth.

The maxillary central incisor has a single conical root, smooth and slightly straight, usually with a rounded apex. Thus the root is thick in the cervical third and narrows through the middle to the blunt apex

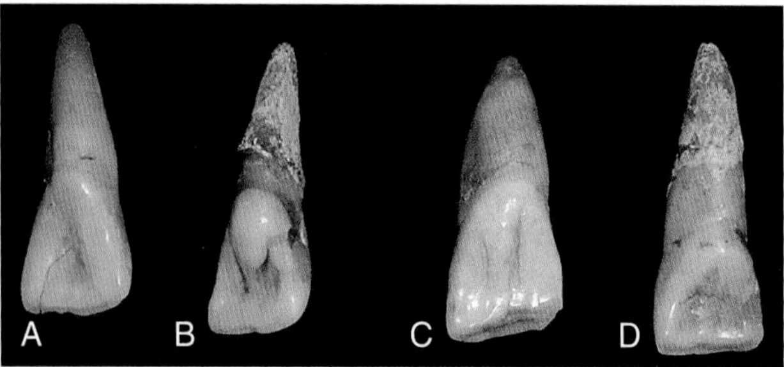

Fig. 16.9 Lingual Views of Extracted Permanent Maxillary Incisors. **A,** Extreme shovel-shape to lingual surface. **B,** Accentuated cingulum with deepened grooves. **C,** Attrition on incisal surface with formation of an incisal edge from the incisal ridge with lingual inclination. **D,** Stain in the deepened lingual fossa. (Courtesy of Margaret J. Fehrenbach, RDH, MS.)

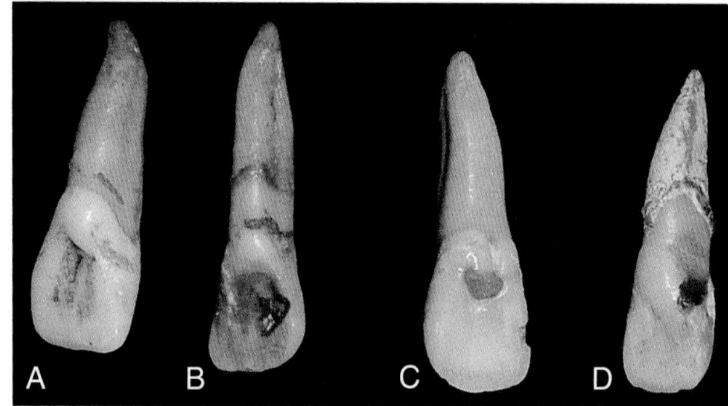

Fig. 16.10 Lingual Views of Extracted Permanent Maxillary Incisors. **A,** Lingual pit. **B,** Lingual pit with caries. **C,** Lingual pit caries repaired. **D,** Linguogingival groove with caries. (Courtesy of Margaret J. Fehrenbach, RDH, MS.)

and it is one and one-half times the length of the crown. The root is also about the same length or shorter, but wider than the lateral of the same arch. Bulbous crowns may create deep mesial and distal concavities at CEJ. The root on cervical cross section is roughly triangular, with the base at the labial aspect, being slightly wider on the labial surface and narrower at the lingual (see Fig. 15.8, *B*).

The pulp cavity mirrors the shape of the tooth; there is only one pulp canal that is quite large in form (Fig. 16.12). The pulp chamber of the maxillary central incisor has three sharp elongations: the mesial, distal, and central pulp horns. These pulp horns correspond to the three labial developmental lobes of the tooth. The central pulp horn is usually shorter than the other two and more rounded.

Labial View Features

The crown of a maxillary central incisor is narrowest at the cervical third and becomes wider toward the incisal ridge on the labial surface (see Fig. 16.11). The incisal ridge is almost straight. Two labial developmental depressions may extend the length of the crown from the cervical to the incisal, showing the division of the surface into three labial developmental lobes. The crown usually has imbrication lines or slight ridges that run mesiodistally in the cervical third and between them are the grooved perikymata (see **Chapter 12**). The CEJ on the labial surface has more curvature to the distal.

From the labial view, both incisal angles can be seen on the maxillary central incisor. The overall mesial outline is slightly rounded with a sharp mesioincisal angle. The overall distal outline is even rounder with a definite rounded distoincisal angle. The difference in sharpness of the central's mesioincisal and distoincisal angle *helps to distinguish the maxillary right central incisor from the left.*

The mesial contact with the other maxillary central is in the incisal third (see Fig. 16.7). The distal contact with the maxillary lateral is at the junction of the incisal and the middle third, located farther cervically than the mesial contact.

Lingual View Features

The lingual surface of the crown of a maxillary central incisor is narrower overall than the labial surface (see Fig. 16.11). The CEJ usually has more curvature to the distal. The single cingulum is

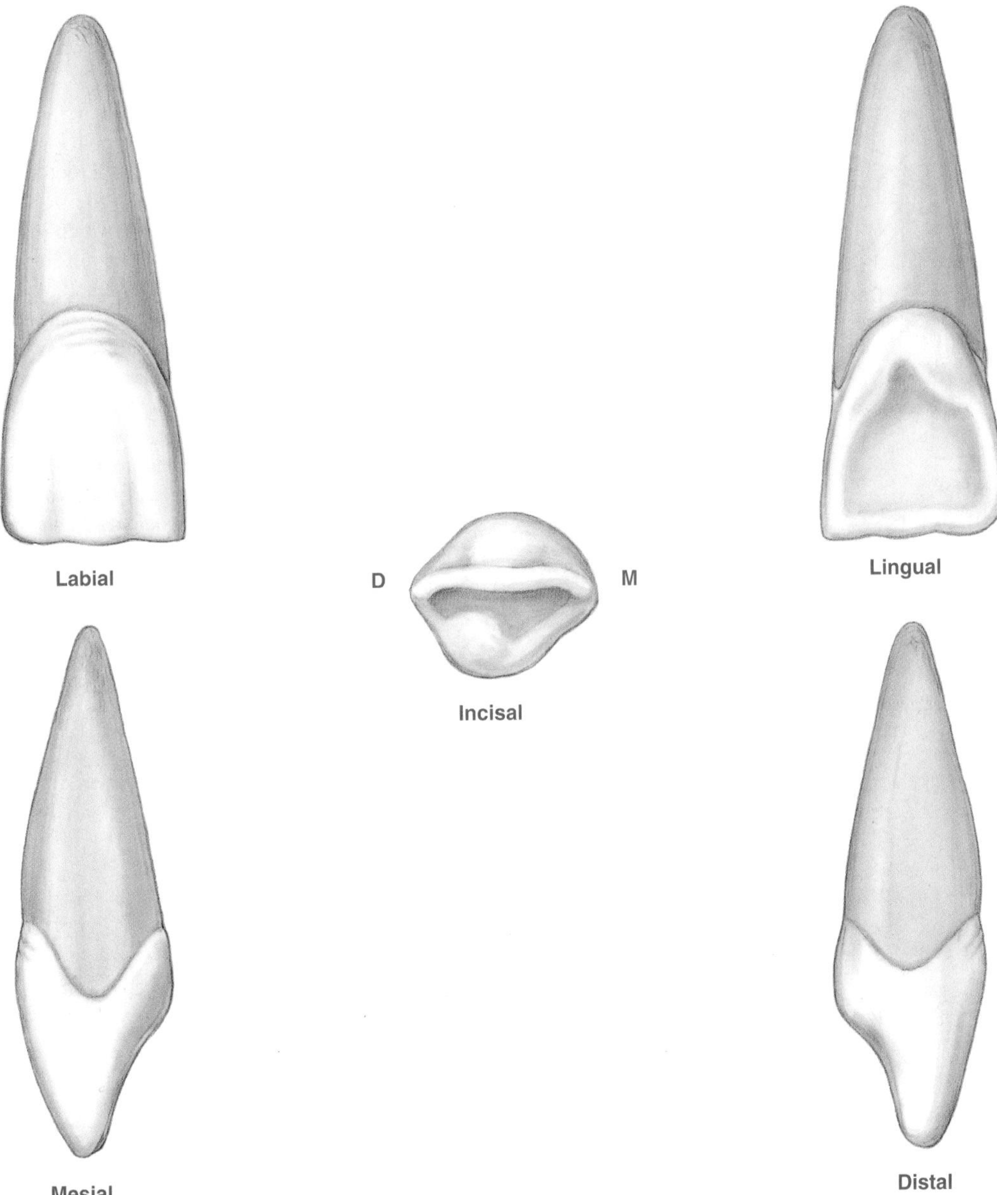

Fig. 16.11 Views of a Permanent Maxillary Right Central Incisor. *D*, Distal; *M*, mesial.

wide and well developed in size as well as being located slightly off center toward the distal.

From the lingual view, the mesial marginal ridge is longer than the distal marginal ridge. The single lingual fossa is wide yet shallow and is located immediately incisal to the cingulum. The lingual fossa varies in depth and diameter. Outlining the incisal border of the lingual fossa, the raised linguoincisal ridge is on the same level as the bordering marginal ridges.

Variations can occur on the lingual surface of the tooth (Fig. 16.13). A horizontally placed lingual groove may be present (although it is more common on maxillary laterals), separating the cingulum from the lingual fossa. The lingual groove may make the cingulum appear scalloped along its borders. A lingual pit may also be present at the incisal border of the cingulum in the lingual groove. Also present may be a vertically placed linguogingival groove (or palatogingival groove), which originates in the lingual pit and extends cervically and slightly distally onto the cingulum.

Proximal View Features

The CEJ curvature on the mesial surface is deep incisally and has the greatest depth of curvature of any tooth surface in the permanent dentition, which *helps to distinguish the maxillary right central incisor from the left* (see Fig. 16.11). The height of contour for both the labial and lingual surfaces is also greater on this tooth than on any tooth in the permanent dentition and is located at the cervical third as in all incisors.

The incisal ridge is located slightly labial to the long axis of the tooth. The incisal outline is also sloped toward the lingual from its longest and also most labial part. The distal view is similar to the mesial, although the curvature of the CEJ is less on the distal than on the mesial surface.

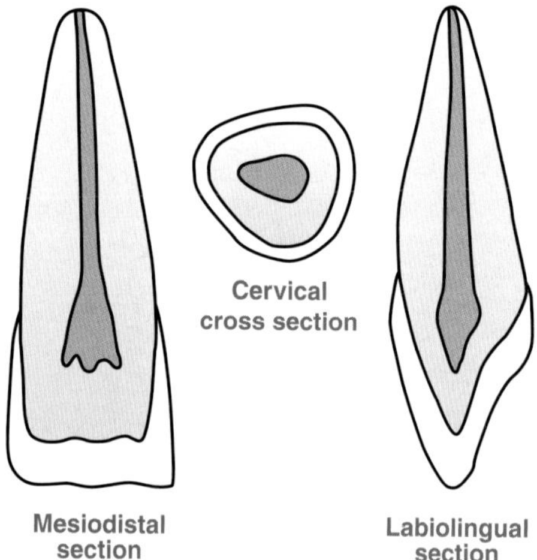

Fig. 16.12 Pulp Cavity of a Permanent Maxillary Right Central Incisor.

Incisal View Features

Overall, the shape of the crown of a maxillary central incisor from the incisal view is triangular with the labial outline broadly rounded (see Fig. 16.11). This is a useful view for observing the slight distal placement of the cingulum. On the lingual surface of the incisal view, the mesial marginal ridge again appears longer than the distal marginal ridge. Note that the incisal ridge lies just labial to the long axis of the root.

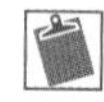 Clinical Considerations with Permanent Maxillary Central Incisors

The incisal ridge or even the entire maxillary central incisor is especially at risk for traumatic fracture or tooth displacement because of the tooth's more anterior and labial position as well as its early eruption into the oral cavity. Because of these two factors and without full root completion, the entire tooth in a child may undergo **avulsion** (uh-**vulh**-shuhn), which is complete displacement of the tooth from the tooth socket or alveolus resulting from extensive trauma to the area. Even if the tooth only undergoes fracture, pulpal pathology may occur in the tooth and result in the need for endodontic therapy or loss of tooth vitality as the pulp dies. If an avulsed permanent tooth has immature root formation with an open apex, the chances of pulpal revitalization after replantation improve considerably, especially if replantation occurs within 30 minutes after avulsion.

An open contact or **diastema** (dahy-uh-**stee**-muh) can also exist between the maxillary central incisors. It can be quite wide and to some patients it is an unattractive space. Both the cause and treatment of this type of diastema are controversial. Treatment may involve surgical release to reduce the impact of a tight maxillary labial frenum, with or without additional orthodontic therapy. Incisors may appear *winged* when looking at the patient's smile. This is not a disturbance of development but rather a case of tooth rotation, usually bilateral rotation to the mesial. This can be corrected with orthodontic therapy. Finally, in consideration of a patient's smile design, the central incisors should dominate the perspective in such a way that each adjacent tooth appears when viewed to become smaller as

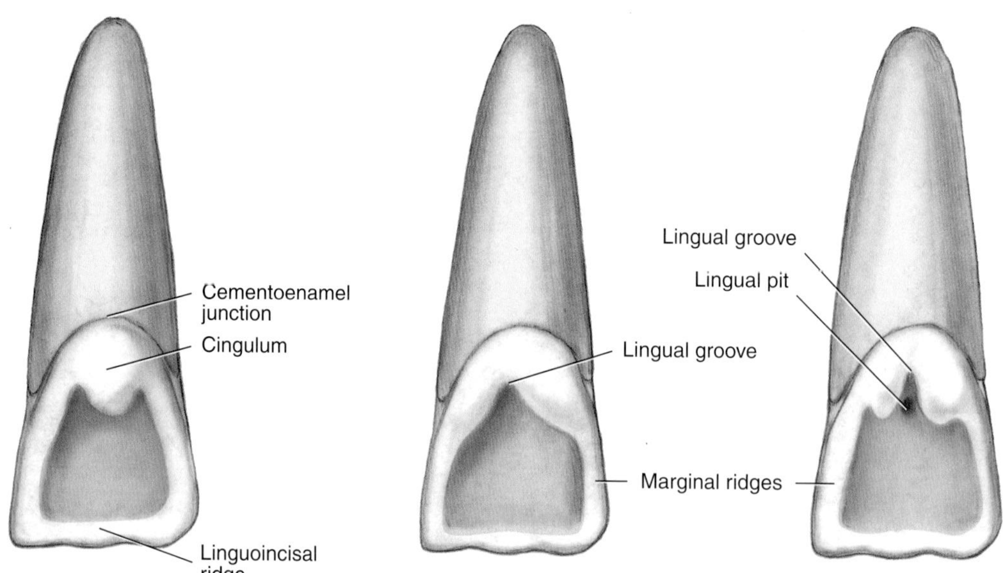

Fig. 16.13 Lingual Surface Variations of the Permanent Maxillary Right Central Incisor with the Lingual Fossae Highlighted.

one moves distally down the dental arch. There should be no deviation of midline of maxillae in its relationship to the philtrum.

One common location for a supernumerary tooth is between the two maxillary central incisors, which is considered a **mesiodens** (**me**-zee-oh-denz) (see Box 6.1, *C, D*). This developmental anomaly is due to the presence of an extra tooth germ resulting from an abnormal initiation process during tooth development, forming a supernumerary tooth. The presence of this extra tooth may affect spacing in the maxillary arch, whether it is erupted or not. The involved tooth may also have a dwarfed root, which results in a lack of periodontal support for the tooth and thus may negatively affect the prognosis of the tooth if it is involved in periodontal disease.

Permanent Maxillary Lateral Incisors #7 and #10 (#12 and #22)

Specific Overall Features

Permanent maxillary lateral incisors erupt between 8 and 9 years of age with root completion at age 11 (Fig. 16.14). Thus these teeth usually erupt after the maxillary central incisors.

The crown of a maxillary lateral incisor has the greatest degree of variation in form of any permanent tooth, except for the third molars. This tooth resembles a maxillary central incisor in all views of the tooth but is smaller and has a slightly rounder crown. This tooth when examined as an extracted tooth is frequently confused with a small permanent mandibular canine, but the root usually has no depressions on the proximal surface, which is common on a mandibular canine.

A maxillary lateral incisor has a single conical root that is almost smooth and straight but in many cases may curve slightly to the distal. Its crown is one to one and one-half times shorter than the length of the root. The root is also about the same length as or longer than the central, but it is thinner, particularly mesiodistally as well as being wider labiolingually. The shape of the root on cervical cross section is oval (as in ovoid or egg-shaped) (see Fig. 15.8, *B*). A linguogingival groove may be present on the root and may continue on the crown. The apex of the root is not rounded like the central but is sharp.

The pulp cavity of the maxillary lateral incisor is simple in form with a single pulp canal and a pulp chamber (Fig. 16.15). The pulp chamber does not have three sharp pulp horns as it does in a maxillary central incisor; instead, it usually has one rounded form or two less-sharp pulp horns: a mesial and distal pulp horn.

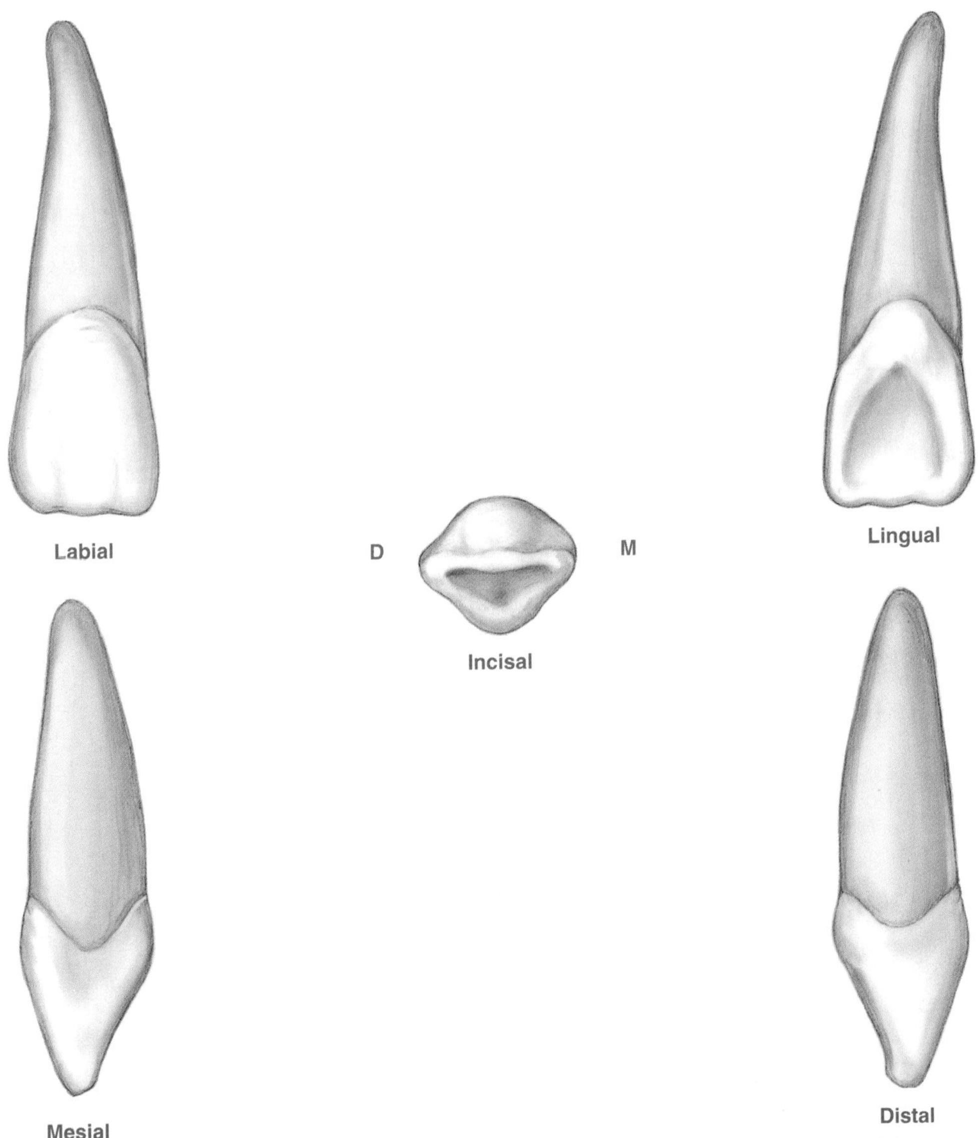

Fig. 16.14 Views of a Permanent Maxillary Right Lateral Incisor. *D*, Distal; *M*, mesial.

Labial View Features

Labial developmental depressions and imbrication lines on the labial surface are less common on a maxillary lateral than on a central incisor (see Fig. 16.14). The crown is smaller than that of a central incisor and less symmetrical.

However, it usually resembles a central in its mesial outline, with the mesial contact with the maxillary central at the incisal third. The distal outline is always rounder than the central and has a more cervical distal contact area with the maxillary canine at the middle third or at the junction of the incisal and the middle third.

From the labial view, both incisal angles are rounder on a maxillary lateral than on a central incisor. Although similar to a central incisor, a maxillary lateral has different incisal angles from the labial. The lateral's mesioincisal angle is sharper than the distoincisal angle, which *helps to distinguish the maxillary right lateral incisor from the left.*

Lingual View Features

The lingual surface of the crown of a maxillary lateral incisor is narrower than the labial surface as is the case with a central (see Fig. 16.14). It has a prominent, yet centered and narrower cingulum than does a central incisor, with a deeper lingual fossa. The marginal ridges are pronounced: The longer mesial marginal ridge is an almost straight line and the shorter distal marginal ridge is quite straight. The linguoincisal ridge is also noticeably well developed in size.

Variations can occur on the lingual surface of the tooth (Fig. 16.16). On the lingual surface, a horizontal lingual groove that separates the cingulum from the lingual fossa is more common on a maxillary lateral and better developed than on a central. A lingual pit is more common on a lateral than on a central and is located on the incisal surface of the cingulum, along the lingual groove.

Additionally present on the lingual surface may be a vertical linguogingival groove that originates in the lingual pit and extends cervically and slightly distally onto the cingulum. The linguogingival groove may extend onto the root surface. The linguogingival groove is also more common on this tooth than on a maxillary central. Rarely, the root has a deep distolingual marginal groove, a developmental groove that begins on the distal marginal ridge on the lingual surface and extends onto the root.

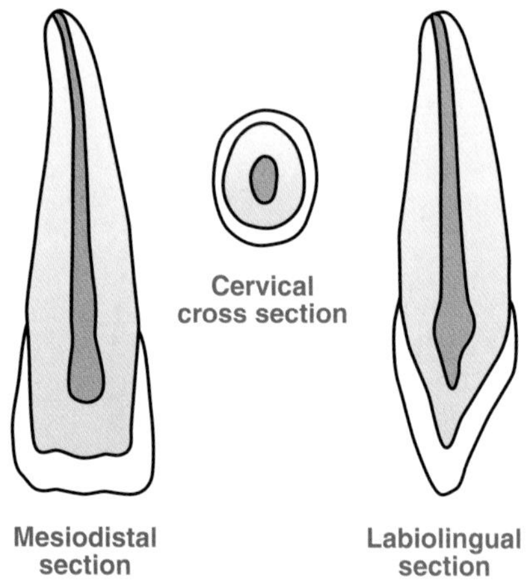
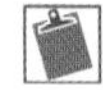

Fig. 16.15 Pulp Cavity of a Permanent Maxillary Right Lateral Incisor.

Proximal View Features

The crown of a maxillary lateral incisor is triangular on a mesial view as are all anterior teeth (see Fig. 16.14 and Table 15.4). The CEJ curvature is similar to that of a central, although it is not as deeply curved on a lateral. Also similar to a central, a lateral's CEJ is more curved on the mesial surface than the distal of this tooth, *which helps to distinguish the maxillary right lateral incisor from the left.* The incisal ridge is usually labial to the long axis of the tooth. The distal view is similar to that of the mesial, although the CEJ is not as deeply curved.

Incisal View Features

The outline of the crown of a maxillary lateral incisor is round or oval from the incisal view, not triangular as is a central (see Fig. 16.14). The crown's mesiodistal measurement is somewhat wider than the labiolingual measurement. Thus the labial surface of the lateral is rounder than that of a central.

Clinical Considerations with Permanent Maxillary Lateral Incisors

Open contacts that seem unattractive to some patients may be easily visible in this region of the dental arch due to variations in form as well as asymmetry in both tooth size and position across the maxillary arch (see

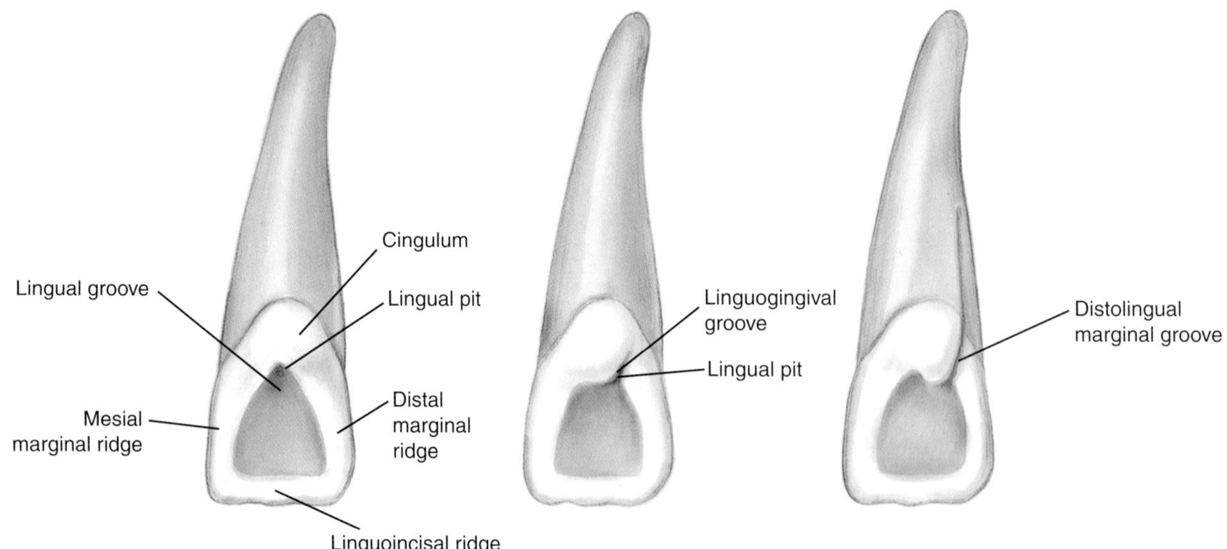

Fig. 16.16 Variations of the Lingual Surface of the Permanent Maxillary Right Lateral Incisor with the Lingual Fossae Highlighted.

Fig. 20.24 and 20.25). Because of the variations in form as well as the possibility of developmental disturbances, maxillary lateral incisors present challenges during preventive, restorative, and orthodontic procedures.

The linguogingival groove on the tooth can be considered an adverse factor because tooth deposits can accumulate in the niche-like groove. This feature then can track periodontal destruction apically following the pathway of the groove, resulting in the formation of a localized periodontal lesion, such as an abscess. A deeper mean probing pocket depth and a greater degree of severe gingivitis are usually present with this situation. Careful and repeated pocket depth probing with associated root exploration is essential to monitor these high-risk areas for periodontal complications in a patient with such a feature.

A maxillary lateral incisor is one of the most common teeth of the permanent dentition to exhibit partial microdontia (see Box 6.1, *E*). This disturbance leads to a smaller lateral incisor crown or **peg lateral** present either unilaterally or bilaterally. This disturbance occurs in the process of proliferation during tooth development. It may be hereditary or may result from other factors. To improve appearance, prosthetic treatment may be performed to increase the crown size of the tooth.

The maxillary laterals are also more commonly involved in partial anodontia and thus may be congenitally missing (see Box 6.1, *A*). This disturbance results from an absence of the appropriate individual tooth germ(s) in the area, unilaterally or bilaterally. This occurs at around 1% to 2% of the time, resulting from a failure in the initiation process during tooth development. Partial anodontia may present esthetic challenges for patients and can also result in complications with occlusion; thus these missing teeth may require a prosthetic replacement such as an implant, bridge, or partial denture.

Finally, a maxillary lateral may have one or more tubercles or accessory cusps on the cingulum. The dilaceration of the crown or root, showing angular distortion may occur, making extraction and endodontic treatment difficult.

PERMANENT MANDIBULAR INCISORS

General Features

Permanent mandibular incisors are the smallest teeth of the permanent dentition and the most symmetrical when first erupted. More uniformity in form is seen with these teeth than with any other of the permanent dentition. The lateral and central incisors of the mandibular arch resemble each other more than do the similar types of incisors of the maxillary arch.

Usually a mandibular lateral is slightly larger than a central, exactly the opposite of the situation in the maxillary arch. The incisal ridge is just lingual to the long axis of the root. Each mandibular incisor has a crown that is wider labiolingually than mesiodistally, which is also unlike the maxillary incisors. Both mandibular incisors also have less pronounced lingual surface features than the maxillary incisors, including those of the cingulum, lingual fossa, and marginal ridges.

The root is longer than the crown for both incisors (see Figs. 16.18 and 16.20). The shape of the root of a mandibular incisor is elliptical (or elongated oval) on cervical cross section (see Fig. 15.8, *B*). Thus the root is extremely narrow on the labial and lingual surfaces and wide on both proximal surfaces. Proximal root concavities are also present on both types of mandibular incisors and if deep enough give the teeth a double-rooted appearance.

Clinical Considerations with Permanent Mandibular Incisors

With attrition, the wearing of a tooth surface caused by tooth-to-tooth contact, the incisal ridge can drastically change on the mandibular incisors as it becomes an incisal edge (see **Chapter 20**). Excessive attrition can even sometimes create a bow-shaped wear pattern on the incisal edge from the incisal view, exposing the underlying dentin (Fig. 16.17). The exposed dentin is more porous and can become unattractively intrinsically stained or it can be affected by dentinal hypersensitivity (see Fig. 13.12).

Although the concavities of the lingual surfaces of all mandibular incisors are less pronounced than that of maxillary incisors, supragingival tooth deposits (such as dental biofilm, calculus, and stain) tend to collect in the concavities. This buildup of deposits is aided by the mandibular incisors' position in the oral cavity near the duct openings of both the submandibular and sublingual salivary glands in the floor of the mouth. Saliva with its mineral content is released from these glands, causing the dental biofilm to mineralize quickly into supragingival calculus, along with the addition of stain. The addition of mesial drift over time can also add to increased deposit levels on these teeth from crowding (see Fig. 20.21).

Instrumentation or restoration may be more difficult in this area because many patients have overlapping mandibular incisors owing to inadequate mandibular arch size and other occlusal factors. This crowding increases with age because of the physiologic process of mesial drift, even after orthodontic therapy, which can also complicate homecare. And if the incisors tip incisally back toward the tongue, instrumentation or restoration becomes extremely difficult; the use of a mouth mirror for indirect vision is essential.

Prolonged hand instrumentation can narrow even further the already narrow labial and lingual root surfaces of the mandibular incisors. The crowns of the teeth can thus be placed in jeopardy during mastication because of unsupported cervical enamel. Finally, the proximal surface of the roots can be difficult to explore with instruments or treat restoratively because of the limited interproximal space and the shape of the root is oval (as in ovoid or egg-shaped) on cervical cross section; the presence of proximal root concavities may also increase this difficulty.

Permanent Mandibular Central Incisors #24 and #25 (#31 and #41)

Specific Overall Features

Permanent mandibular central incisors erupt between 6 and 7 years of age with root completion at age 9 (Fig. 16.18). Thus these teeth usually erupt before the maxillary central incisors. They are the smallest and simplest teeth of the permanent dentition; and they are smaller than the lateral incisors of the same arch. Due to its smallness, the tooth has only one antagonist in the maxillary arch. This tooth and the maxillary third molar are the only teeth that have one antagonist; all others have two. Equally different is that the two mandibular centrals usually share a mesial contact area.

This tooth has a simple root, which is widest labiolingually and then mesiodistally. The root shape is a narrow oval (as in ovoid or egg-shaped) on cervical cross section (see Fig. 15.8, *B*). The root has pronounced proximal root concavities, which vary in both length and depth and a shallow depression extends longitudinally along the midportion of root. The pulp cavity of the mandibular central is quite simple because it has a single pulp canal and three pulp horns (Fig. 16.19).

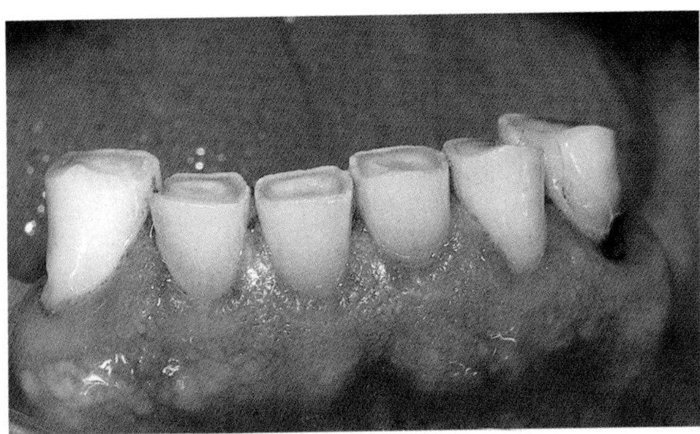

Fig. 16.17 Clinical View of Severe Attrition Noted on the Incisal Surface of the Permanent Mandibular Incisors as Well as Canines. (Courtesy of Margaret J. Fehrenbach, RDH, MS.)

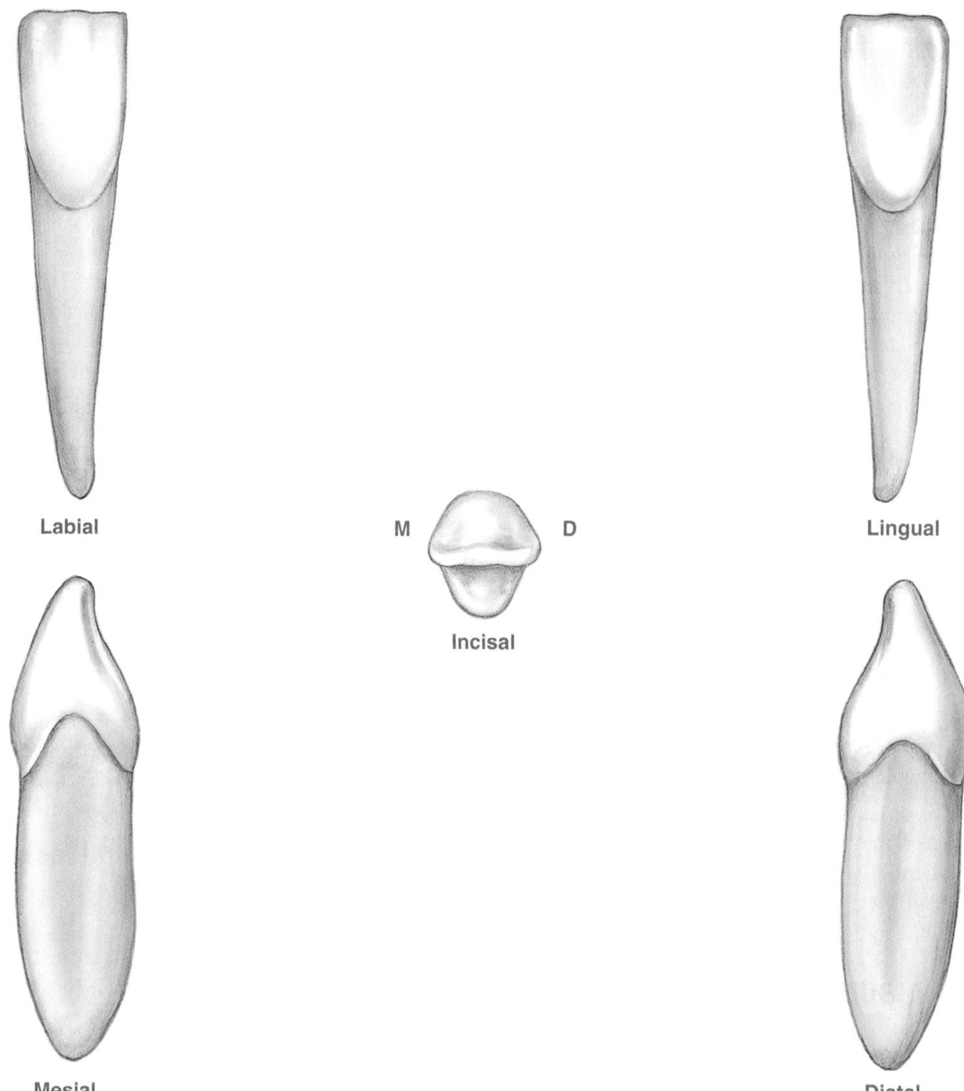

Fig. 16.18 Views of a Permanent Mandibular Right Central Incisor. *D,* Distal; *M,* mesial.

Labial View Features

The crown of a mandibular central incisor is quite symmetrical from the labial view, having a fan shape (see Fig. 16.18). The imbrication lines and developmental depressions usually are not present or are extremely faint. The mesial contact with the other mandibular central is at the incisal third. The distal contact with the lateral incisor is also at the incisal third.

From the labial view, both the incisal angles, mesioincisal angle and distoincisal angle, are sharp or only slightly rounded; the mesioincisal angle is slightly sharper than the distoincisal angle, which *helps to distinguish the mandibular right central incisor from the left.* Nevertheless, differentiating between the right and left central incisors is often difficult. The mesial and distal outlines are almost straight lines from the CEJ to the almost straight incisal ridge.

Lingual View Features

The crown outline of a mandibular central incisor is narrower on the lingual surface than the labial, which is the reverse of the labial view (see Fig. 16.18). However, its outline of the crown is the most symmetrical of all incisors, either maxillary or mandibular. Overall, the lingual surface is less pronounced and has a small centered cingulum.

On the lingual surface, the single lingual fossa is barely noticeable; therefore, the mesial marginal ridge and distal marginal ridge are barely noticeable as well. And because the cingulum is centered, the faint mesial and distal marginal ridges both have the same length.

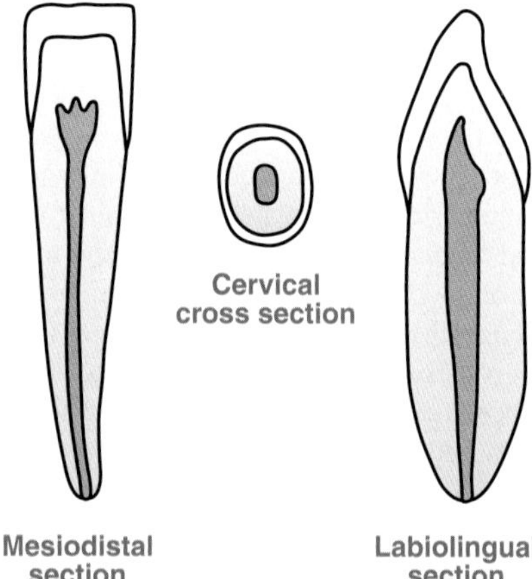

Fig. 16.19 Pulp Cavity of a Permanent Mandibular Right Central Incisor.

Proximal View Features

The CEJ curvature is higher incisally on the mesial than on the distal surface, which *helps to distinguish the mandibular right central*

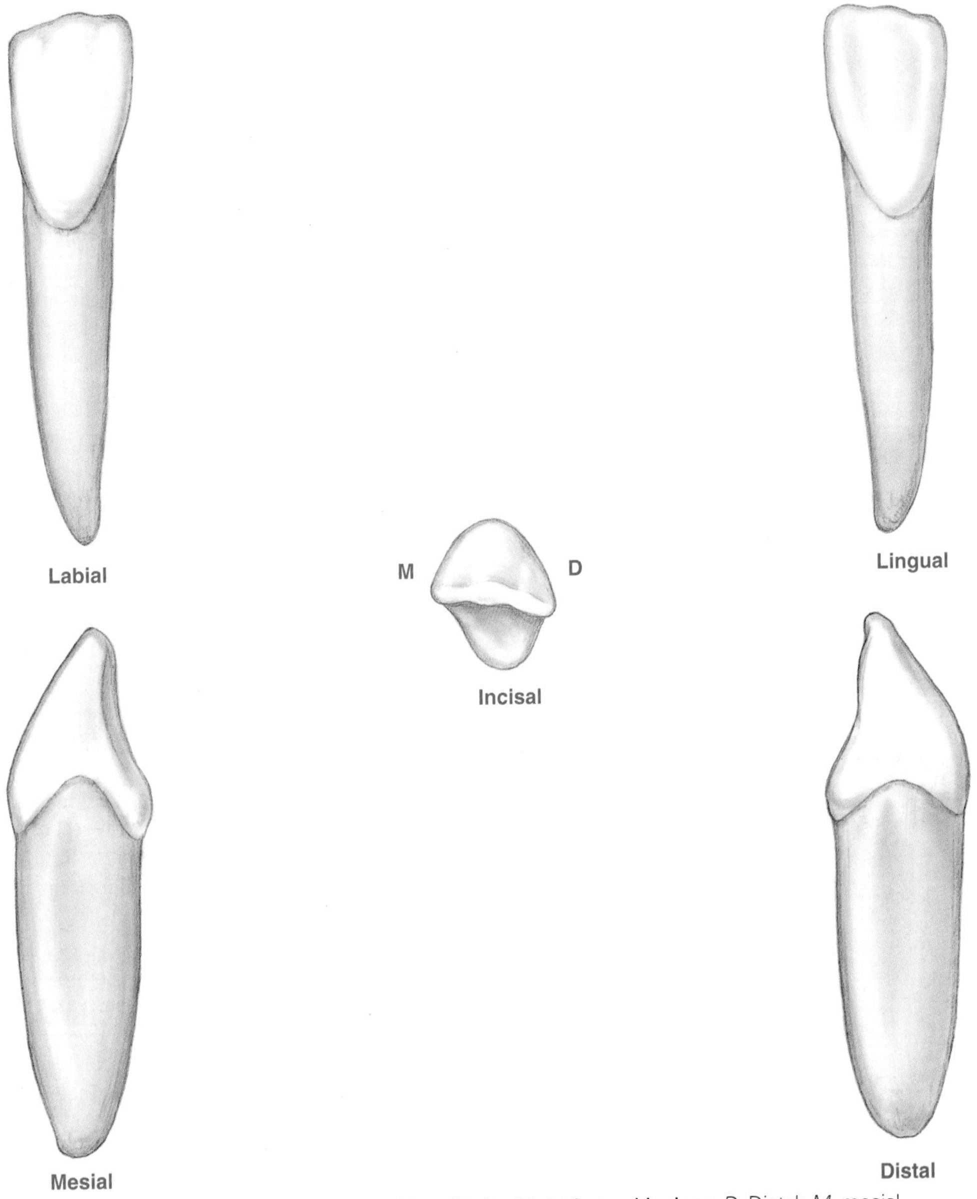

Fig. 16.20 Views of a Permanent Mandibular Right Lateral Incisor. *D*, Distal; *M*, mesial.

incisor from the left (see Fig. 16.18). The incisal ridge is usually straight but can be rounded and is lingual to the long axis of the root. The distal view is similar to the mesial view of the tooth, except that the CEJ curves less incisally on the distal than on the mesial surface.

Incisal View Features

The mandibular central incisor has an almost symmetrical crown outline (see Fig. 16.18). The incisal ridge is usually at 90° or perpendicular to the labiolingual axis of the crown of the tooth and overall it is just lingual to the long axis of the root. The labiolingual measurement is also wider than the mesiodistal measurement on incisal view. Again, on the lingual surface, the faint mesial marginal ridge and distal marginal ridge are both the same length.

 Clinical Considerations with Permanent Mandibular Central Incisors

Root proximation with the contralateral mandibular central incisor may cause access difficulty for homecare and instrumentation. Developmental disturbances are rarely noted in the mandibular central incisors. One rare exception is that the teeth may have an accessory root or bifurcated root with the two branches having labial and lingual orientations.

Permanent Mandibular Lateral Incisors #23 and #26 (#32 and #42)

Specific Overall Features

Permanent mandibular lateral incisors erupt between 7 and 8 years of age with root completion at age 10 (Fig. 16.20). Thus these teeth usually erupt after the mandibular central incisors. The tooth is slightly larger overall than a central; there is also more variation overall in form too. The crown is also slightly larger than that of a central, but it resembles a central in most other ways. From both the labial and lingual views, the crown appears tilted or twisted distally in regard to the long axis of the tooth; this gives the impression that the tooth has been bent at the CEJ.

The single root of a mandibular lateral is usually straight, slightly longer, and wider than that of a central. The root, like that of a mandibular central, has pronounced proximal root concavities, especially on the distal surface. These vary in both length and depth. The pulp cavity for this tooth is quite simple because it has a single pulp canal and three pulp horns (Fig. 16.21).

Labial View Features

The crown of a mandibular lateral incisor is not as symmetrical as that of a central and appears tilted or twisted distally on the root from the labial view (see Fig. 16.20). The tooth is not symmetrical because the distal outline is slightly rounder and shorter compared with the slightly flatter and longer mesial outline. The incisal angles are different: The mesioincisal angle of the incisal ridge is sharper than the distoincisal angle, which *helps to distinguish the mandibular right lateral incisor from the left.* The labial developmental depressions are deeper than on the central incisors of the same arch.

From the labial view, the mesial contact with a mandibular central incisor is in the incisal third. The distal contact with a mandibular canine is in the incisal third but is located more cervically than the mesial contact.

Lingual View Features

The crown of a mandibular lateral incisor lacks bilateral symmetry and again appears tilted or twisted distally on the root from the lingual view with its outline the reverse of the labial view (see Fig. 16.20). Overall, the lingual surface has more prominent features as compared to the lingual surface of a central incisor. The small single cingulum lies just distal to the long axis of the root.

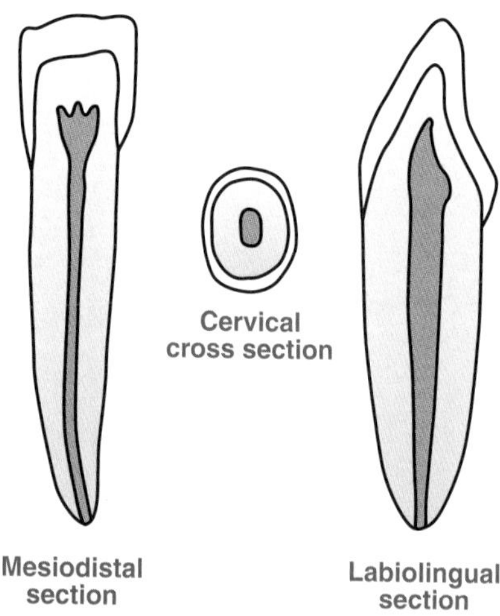

Fig. 16.21 Pulp Cavity of a Permanent Mandibular Right Lateral Incisor.

Thus on the lingual surface, both the mesial marginal ridge and the distal marginal ridge are more developed than on a central. The mesial marginal ridge is longer than the distal marginal ridge. A single lingual fossa is also present, but a lingual pit is rarely present on a lateral, although this happens more often than on a central.

Proximal View Features

The greater height of the CEJ curvature on the mesial than on the distal surface *helps to distinguish the mandibular right lateral incisor from the left* (see Fig. 16.20). Also from the mesial view, more of the lingual surface is visible because of the distal tilt or twist of the incisal ridge. The distal view is similar to the mesial view of the tooth, but the CEJ is curved less on the distal than the mesial surface.

Incisal View Features

A rounder appearance is noted both labially and lingually from the incisal view of a mandibular lateral incisor as compared with that of a central (see Fig. 16.20). The entire incisal ridge is not straight mesiodistally as it is in a central; instead the incisal ridge curves toward the lingual in its distal part. Additionally the incisal angles are noticeably different: The distoincisal angle is visibly at a distinctly lingual location compared to the mesioincisal angle, and the cingulum appears displaced toward the distal. Again on the lingual surface, the mesial marginal ridge is longer than the distal marginal ridge.

Clinical Considerations with Permanent Mandibular Lateral Incisors

Developmental disturbances are rare in a mandibular lateral incisor as is the case with the central of the same arch. One rare exception is that the tooth may have an accessory root or bifurcated root with the two root branches having labial and lingual orientation.

PERMANENT CANINES

GENERAL FEATURES OF PERMANENT CANINES

Permanent canines are the four anterior teeth located at the corners of each quadrant for each dental arch (Table 16.2). Thus it is the third

TABLE 16.2 Permanent Canines

	Maxillary Canine	Mandibular Canine
Universal number	#6 and #11	#22 and #27
International number	#13 and #23	#33 and #43
General crown features	Single cusp with tip and slopes, labial ridge, cingulum, lingual ridge, marginal ridges, lingual fossae	
Specific crown features	Longest tooth in arch	
	Prominent lingual surface. Sharp cusp tip	Less pronounced lingual surface. Less sharp cusp tip.
Height of contour	Labial: Cervical third Lingual: Middle third	
Mesial contact	Junction of incisal third and middle thirds	Incisal third
Distal contact	Middle third	Junction of incisal and middle thirds
Distinguish right from left	Shorter mesial cusp slope, with more pronounced mesial CEJ curvature. More cervical contact on distal	
	More cervical contact on distal, with shorter distal outline on labial view with depression between distal contact and CEJ	Shorter and rounder distal outline on labial view, with shorter mesial slope than distal
General root features	Long thick single root	
Specific root features	Oval on cervical cross section. Proximal root concavities. Blunt root apex	Oval on cervical cross section. Proximal root concavities, with developmental depressions on mesial and distal, giving tooth double-rooted appearance. Pointed apex

CEJ, Cementoenamel junction.

tooth from the midline in each quadrant, distal to the incisors and mesial to the posteriors. The permanent canines are succedaneous and replace the primary canines of the same type.

Patients refer to the canine as their *eyeteeth;* an older term that was also used was *cuspids* because they were the only teeth in the permanent dentition with one cusp. The more commonly used term of *canines* means dog-like because they seem to resemble dogs' teeth. Patients often complain of the slightly deeper yellow color of their permanent canines compared with their incisors, which is due to its increased thickness and thus increased opacity. This property is placed in prosthetic teeth in many cases to mimic a more natural look.

Because of their overall tapered shape and prominent cusp, the canines function to pierce or tear food during mastication (see Table 15.4). And because of their arch position, they serve as a major support of facial muscles and keep the overall vertical dimension of the face intact. Without their presence intact facial contours cannot be maintained and a loss of height occurs in the lower third of vertical dimension. Anatomists consider the canines the cornerstones of the dental arch because of their arch position, tooth form, and function.

The canines also support the incisors and premolars in their functions during mastication and speech. During occlusal movement, these teeth act as guideposts (see Fig. 20.13). In this respect, they serve as a protective functional device for a type of mandibular movement of lateral deviation (see **Chapter 20**). Finally, they can help relieve any excessive horizontal forces imposed on posteriors.

The canines are the most stable teeth in the dentition, one reason being their long root length, which offers an increased amount of periodontal tissue support. In addition, the proximal root concavities help to provide an increased periodontal anchorage for these teeth. Thus these teeth have a significantly reduced risk of loss as a result of periodontal disease or traumatic injury, usually making them the last teeth present in an overall failing dentition. The canines (or many times only the roots) often serve as the stabilizing anchors for replacements of lost teeth in prosthetic procedures, such as the placement of partial fixed or removal dentures and permanent bridges. These teeth are also important esthetically because each one holds the skin of the labial commissure in its position, reducing the appearance of any deep lip lines or wrinkles present when the skin may start to cave in this region with increasing age.

Canines are not usually involved in dental caries, which is another factor that makes them an extremely stable tooth in the dentition. This is because the crown usually has a less pronounced form that promotes self-cleansing and does not easily retain dental biofilm or other deposits.

Both the maxillary and mandibular canines resemble one another (Fig. 16.22). The crown of each is about the same size and, when viewed from the proximal, appears triangular like all anterior teeth (see Table 15.4). When viewed from the labial or lingual, however, its crown outline appears pentagonal with five sides. Canines are also wider labiolingually than the incisors, even wider than maxillary central incisors.

Similar to the other anteriors, each of the canines has an incisal ridge on its masticatory surface (see Fig. 16.22). Different from the incisors is the **cusp tip**, which is in line with the long axis of the root for both maxillary and mandibular canines when first erupted. Because of the presence of the cusp tip, the incisal ridge is divided into two **cusp slopes** or ridges rather than being straight across like the incisors.

The mesial cusp slope is usually shorter than the distal cusp slope for both the maxillary and mandibular canines when they first erupt. The mesial cusp slope of a maxillary canine occludes with the distal cusp slope of a mandibular canine. The length of these cusp slopes and position of the cusp tip can change with attrition (discussed later).

The canines are the only teeth in the permanent dentition with a centrally placed vertical **labial ridge** (see Fig. 16.22). This labial ridge is a result of greater development of the middle labial developmental lobe in comparison with the mesial and distal labial developmental lobes. Mamelons are usually not present on the incisal ridge as they are on incisors, but a small notch may be seen on either cusp slope. The height of contour on labial and lingual surfaces is in the cervical third for the canines, similar to all anteriors.

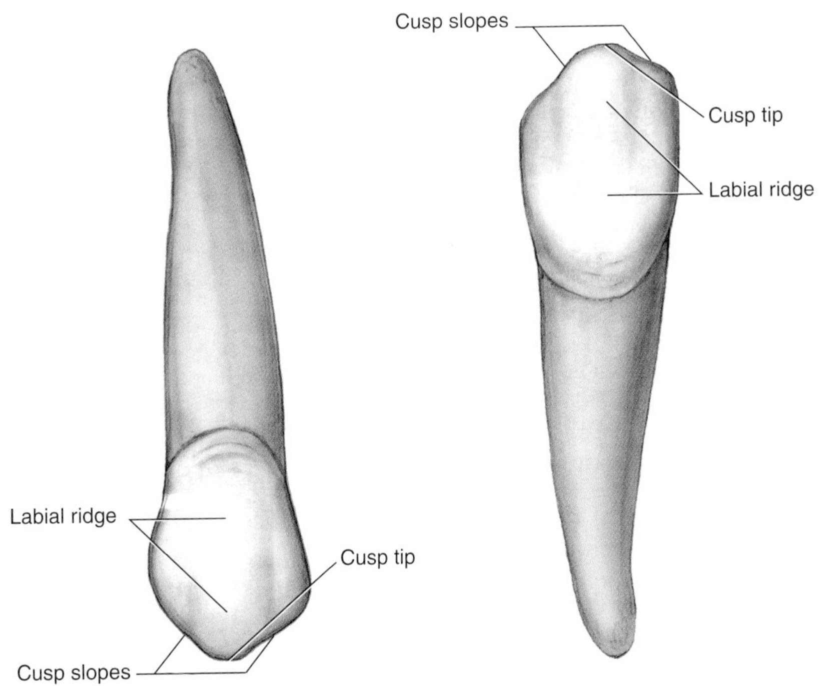

Fig. 16.22 Labial Views of Newly Erupted Permanent Canines with Features Noted; Both Teeth Resemble Each Other.

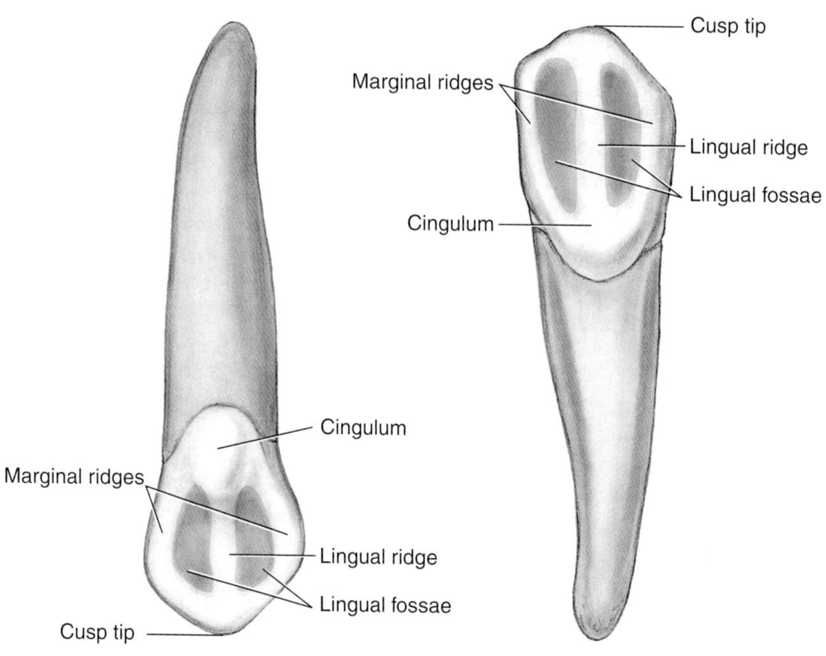

Fig. 16.23 Lingual Views of Permanent Canines and Their Features with Lingual Fossae Highlighted; Both Teeth Resemble Each Other.

Each canine also has a cingulum and marginal ridges on its lingual surface, similar to the incisors (Fig. 16.23). The cingulum corresponds to the lingual developmental lobe as in the incisors but is larger than on any incisor. As with the incisors, however, its crown is narrower on the lingual surface than on the labial surface with the crown tapering lingually.

In addition, canines have a centrally placed vertical **lingual ridge** that extends from the cusp tip to the cingulum. The lingual ridge creates two separate and shallow lingual fossae between it and the bordering marginal ridges; these lingual fossae are more pronounced on the maxillary canines than on the mandibular.

The permanent canines are the longest teeth in the dentition. Each has a particularly long, thick root, and the root is usually one and one-half times the length of the crown. The long and large root is externally manifested in the jaws by the vertically oriented and labially placed bony ridge of the alveolar process, the **canine eminence** (**em**-uh-nuhns*)*, which is especially noted on the maxillary arch. The shape of the root is oval (as in ovoid or egg-shaped) on cervical cross section (see Figs. 15.8, *B*, 16.26, 16.29). Proximal root concavities are located on both proximal root surfaces.

Clinical Considerations with Permanent Canines

Changes can occur in the length of each canine cusp slope and in the position of the usually centered cusp tip. With attrition, the lengths of the cusp slopes are often altered due to this wearing of a tooth surface caused by tooth-to-tooth contact and the overall narrower incisal ridges become wider incisal edges similar to worn incisors (Fig. 16.24). With wear, each cusp tip of the maxillary canines is placed more to the distal of center with mesial displacement of the cusp tip for the mandibular canine. This wear also lengthens the mesial cusp slope and shortens the distal slope for the maxillary canines, while it shortens the mesial cusp slope and lengthens the distal slope for the mandibular canines. The related wear pattern on a canine from the incisal view can appear either diamond-shaped or triangular.

It is also noted that proximal surfaces of the canines are more accessible from the lingual than the labial approach during instrumentation or restoration. This is because of the convergence of the proximal surfaces toward the lingual.

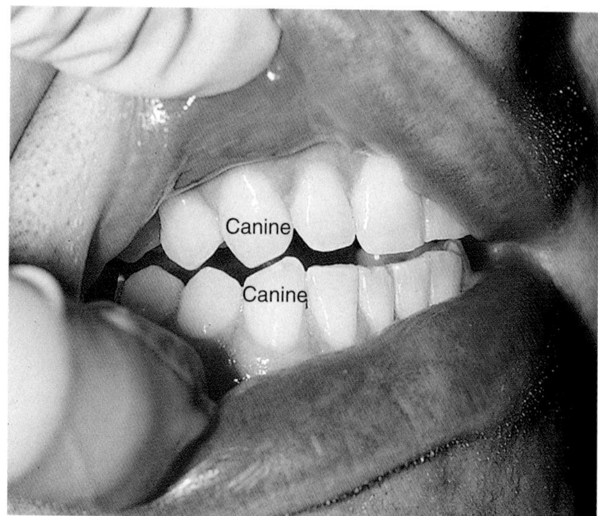

Fig. 16.24 Lateral View of Permanent Canines Altered on the Incisal Surfaces by Attrition. The cusp tip of maxillary canines is now placed more to the distal of center with mesial displacement of the cusp tip for the mandibular canine. This also lengthens the mesial cusp slope as well as shortening the distal one for the maxillary canines, while it shortens the mesial cusp slope and lengthens the distal one for the mandibular canines. (Courtesy of Margaret J. Fehrenbach, RDH, MS.)

PERMANENT MAXILLARY CANINES #6 AND #11 (#13 AND #23)

Specific Overall Features

Permanent maxillary canines erupt between 11 and 12 years of age with root completion between ages 13 and 15 (Fig. 16.25). Thus these teeth usually erupt after the mandibular canines, after the maxillary incisors and possibly also the maxillary premolars.

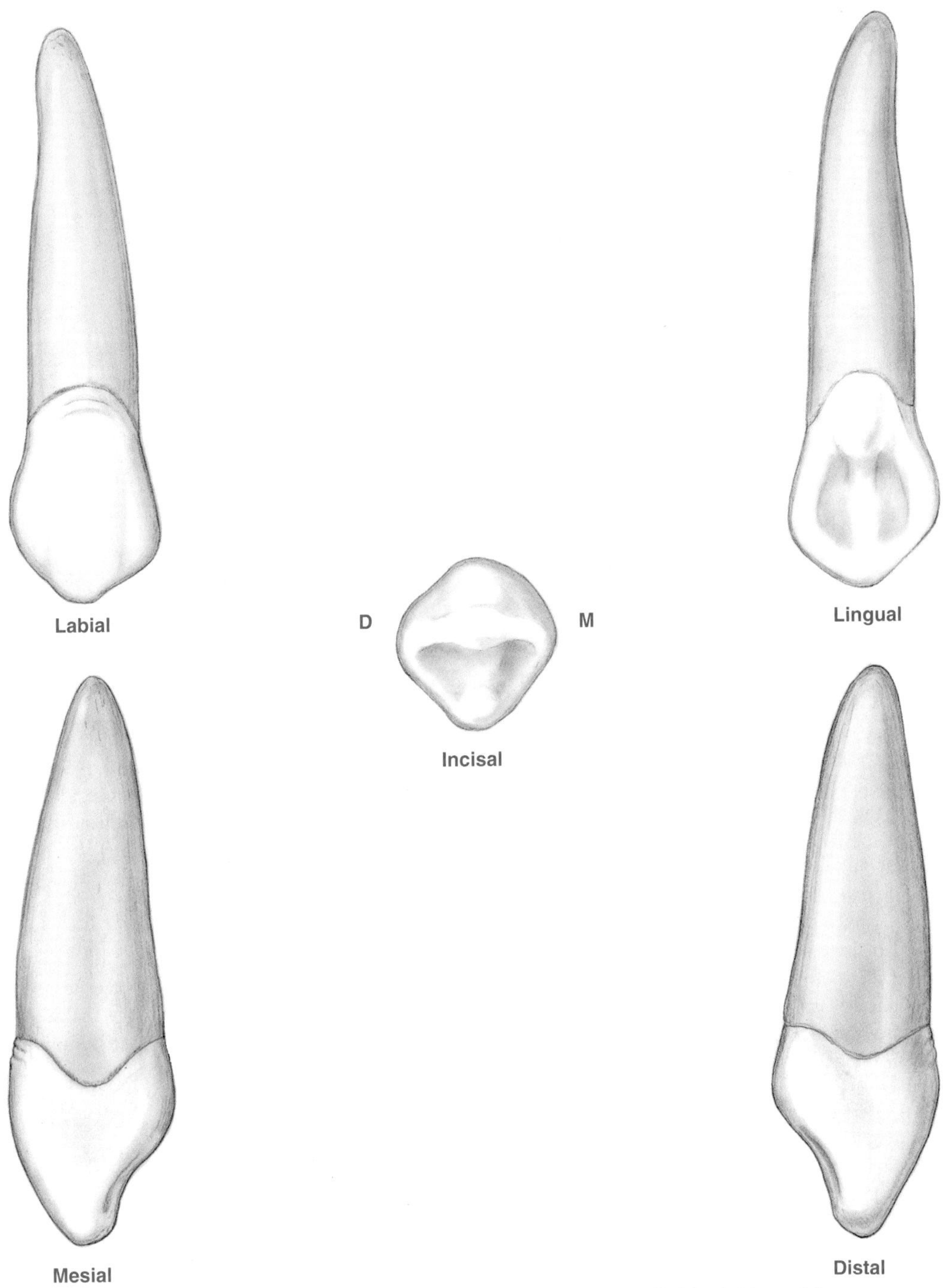

Fig. 16.25 Views of a Permanent Maxillary Right Canine. *D,* Distal; *M,* mesial.

The crown of a maxillary canine is similar in length or even shorter than that of a maxillary central incisor. Labiolingually, the crown is considerably wider than that of a central incisor, but a canine crown is noticeably narrower mesiodistally. The cingulum on the lingual surface is more developed and larger than that of a central incisor of the same arch, making the tooth stronger during mastication.

A maxillary canine does somewhat resemble a mandibular canine (see Figs. 16.22 and 16.23). However, the cusp is more developed and larger, and the cusp tip is sharper as on all maxillary teeth. In addition, the entire lingual surface features of the maxillary canine are more prominent, including the lingual ridge and marginal ridges.

Finally, an entire maxillary canine is as long as a mandibular canine, but the crown is as long as or slightly shorter than that of a mandibular canine. The long root is single and has a blunt apex; it is the longest root in the maxillary arch. Developmental depressions are evident on both proximal surfaces of the root but are especially pronounced on the distal surface owing to the distal prominence of crown at CEJ. Moderate to deep proximal concavities are also possible. The pulp cavity consists of a single pulp canal and a large pulp chamber (Fig. 16.26). The pulp chamber usually has only one pulp horn.

Labial View Features

The mesial half of the crown of a maxillary canine resembles the nearby incisor. The distal half resembles the nearby premolar, showing the transition in form from the incisors to the premolars in the maxillary arch (see Fig. 16.25). Usually both imbrication lines and perikymata

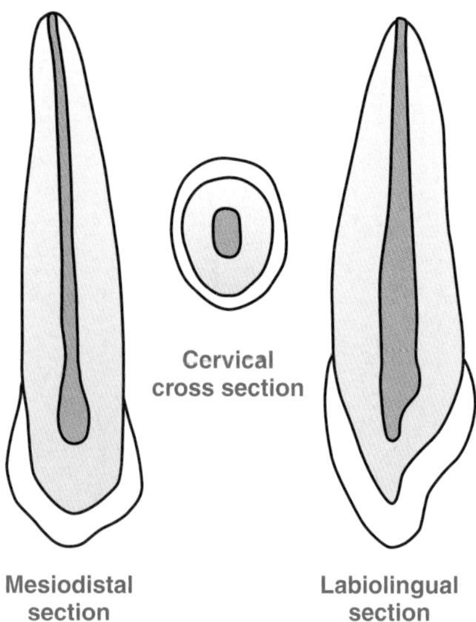

Fig. 16.26 Pulp Cavity of a Permanent Maxillary Right Canine.

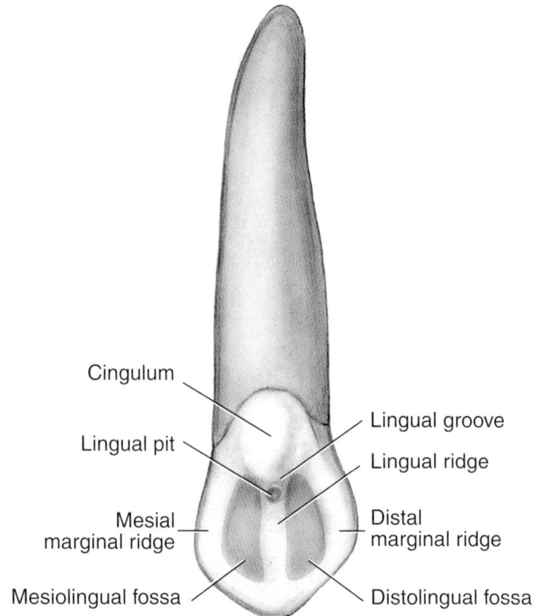

Fig. 16.27 Lingual View of a Variation of the Permanent Maxillary Right Canine and Features with Lingual Fossae Highlighted.

are present in the cervical third of the labial surface, especially in newly erupted teeth (see Fig. 12.9).

Two faint and vertical mesial and distal labial developmental depressions extend from the cervical to the incisal and separate the three labial developmental lobes. These depressions are located on either side of the centrally placed vertical labial ridge and this ridge is most noticeable in the incisal part of the labial surface.

The mesial outline of the labial surface of the maxillary canine is usually rounded from the mesial contact area to the CEJ, but overall it is straighter than the distal outline. The distal outline is shorter than the mesial outline and usually has a depression between the distal contact area and the CEJ, which *helps to distinguish the maxillary right canine from the left.* From the labial view, the mesial and distal contacts are on two different levels of the tooth, which also *helps to distinguish the maxillary right canine from the left.* The mesial contact with the lateral incisor is at the junction of the incisal and the middle third. The distal contact with the first premolar is more cervical because it is at the middle third.

As previously discussed, the single cusp is round in form and the mesial cusp slope of a maxillary canine is shorter than the distal cusp slope when first erupted, which again *helps to distinguish the maxillary right canine from the left.* The CEJ on the labial surface is evenly curved toward the root.

Lingual View Features

The mesial, distal, and incisal lingual outlines of a maxillary canine are similar to those on the labial view of the tooth. The overall dimension of the lingual surface is less than that of the labial surface, however, because the both mesial and distal surfaces converge slightly toward the lingual. The cingulum is large and usually less pronounced and is centered mesiodistally on the lingual surface.

The lingual surface also has a prominent mesial marginal ridge and distal marginal ridge. A centrally placed vertical lingual ridge is also present from the cingulum to the cusp tip, separating two lingual fossae, the shallow but visible mesiolingual fossa and distolingual fossa. Each of the major features of this tooth are "variations on a theme": the cingulum and incisal half of the lingual surface are sometimes separated by a shallow lingual groove. This groove may contain a lingual pit near its center or the pit may also be present without the lingual groove (Fig. 16.27).

Proximal View Features

The mesial and distal aspects present a triangular outline (see Fig. 16.25 and Table 15.4). They resemble the maxillary incisors but are stronger looking, especially in the cingulum region. The CEJ curves higher incisally on the mesial than on the distal surface, *which helps to distinguish the maxillary right canine from the left*. The cusp tip is toward the labial. The distal view of the tooth is similar to the mesial view, but the CEJ curvature is less on the distal than on the mesial surface.

Incisal View Features

Again the labiolingual width of a maxillary canine is large in comparison with that of any other anterior tooth, making it an extremely strong tooth during mastication (see Fig. 16.25). Additionally, the crown outline is asymmetrical; the mesial part of the crown has greater labiolingual bulk. The distal part of the crown appears thinner than the mesial and gives the impression of being stretched to in order to make contact with the first premolar.

More specifically, the mesial half of the labial outline is quite rounded in form and the distal half is frequently concave. The distal half of the lingual outline is also frequently concave because the distal fossa is deeper and thus more pronounced. The mesial marginal ridge is longer than the distal marginal ridge. The cusp slopes form an almost straight line; the tip of the cusp is displaced labially and mesial to the central long axis.

Clinical Considerations with Permanent Maxillary Canines

Because the maxillary canines erupt after the maxillary incisors and also possibly the maxillary premolars, their expected dental arch space often is partially closed. Because of this they may erupt labially or lingually to the surrounding teeth. The maxillary canines may also fail to erupt fully, remaining **impacted** (im-**pak**-ted) within the alveolar process. An impacted tooth is an unerupted or partially erupted tooth that is positioned against another tooth, bone, or even soft tissue in a way that makes complete eruption unlikely. As a result, surgical exposure and maintenance orthodontic therapy may be needed, which may in some cases be prevented by careful evaluation of mixed dentition

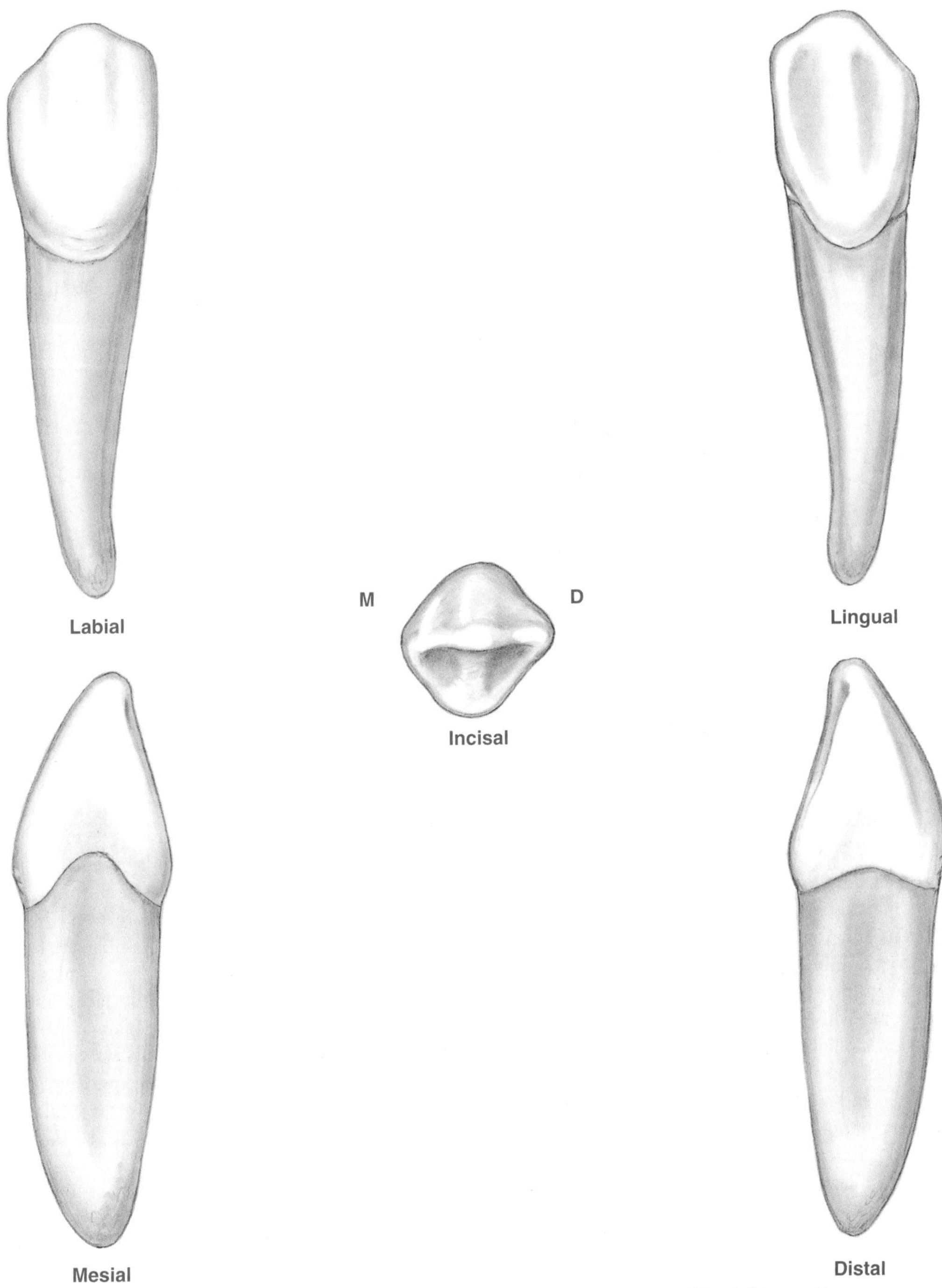

Fig. 16.28 Views of a Permanent Mandibular Right Canine. *D*, Distal; *M*, mesial.

and institution of any needed interceptive orthodontic therapy. Finally, developmental cyst formation may occur within the dental tissue of an impacted crown of a maxillary canine, resulting in a dentigerous cyst.

The cingula on the maxillary canines may exhibit tubercles or extra cusps that are located near the most incisal level of the cingulum. A lingual pit is often associated with the presence of tubercles. In addition, the distal prominence of the crown is at the CEJ, which may cause instrumentation and restoration difficulties on the distal root surface. The root of maxillary canines may also undergo distorted angulations or dilaceration and there may be several curvatures along its length. With root curvature in the apical third, the root is usually curved distally.

PERMANENT MANDIBULAR CANINES #22 AND #27 (#33 AND #43)

Specific Overall Features

Permanent mandibular canines erupt between 9 and 10 years of age with root completion between ages 12 and 14 (Fig. 16.28). Thus these teeth usually erupt before the maxillary canines and after most of the incisors have erupted.

A mandibular canine closely resembles a maxillary canine (see Figs. 16.22 and 16.23). Although the entire tooth is usually as long, a mandibular canine is narrower labiolingually and mesiodistally than a

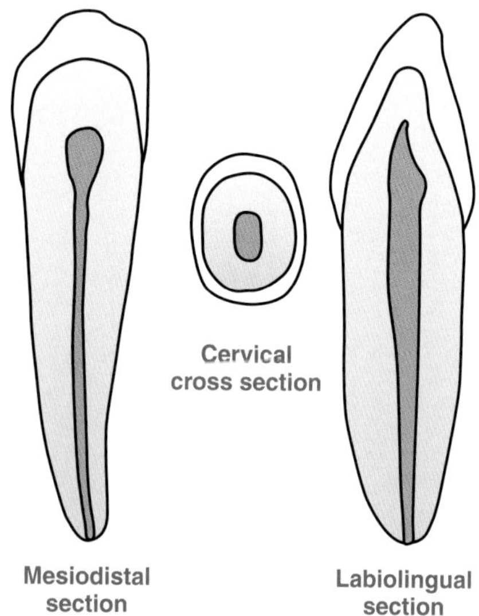

Fig. 16.29 Pulp Cavity of a Permanent Mandibular Right Canine.

maxillary canine. The crown of this tooth can be equal to in length or even longer than that of a maxillary canine.

The single cusp is not as well developed in size and the two cusp ridges are thinner labiolingually than those of a maxillary canine. The single cusp tip usually is not as sharp. In addition, the cusp tip is lined up with the long axis of the root, but it is sometimes positioned lingually, similar to the mandibular incisors.

The lingual surface of the crown of a mandibular canine is less pronounced than that of a maxillary canine, having a less developed cingulum and two marginal ridges. Thus the lingual surface of this crown more closely resembles the form of the lingual surface of the adjacent mandibular lateral incisors, despite the added feature of a lingual ridge.

The single root of a mandibular canine may be as long as that of a maxillary canine but is usually somewhat shorter, although it still has the longest mandibular root. The root has a slight mesial inclination. The mesial developmental depression on the root is more pronounced and often deeper compared with that of a maxillary canine. A distal developmental depression similar to the mesial one is also apparent. These proximal concavities may extend the full length of the root. These depressions may be extremely pronounced to the point of creating a labial and lingual component in the apical third and giving the tooth a double-rooted appearance. The root apex is also more pointed on this tooth than on a maxillary canine.

The pulp cavity of a mandibular canine resembles that of a maxillary canine in that they both usually have a single pulp canal and a large pulp chamber (Fig. 16.29). There is also only one pulp horn. The major difference is that a mandibular canine may have two separate pulp canals. If the tooth has two canals, one is placed labially and the other lingually; the canals may join at the apex or have separate apical foramina.

Labial View Features

The labial surface on a mandibular canine is not as rounded as that on a maxillary canine, especially in the incisal two-thirds of the tooth (see Fig. 16.28). In contrast, however, a mandibular canine is usually rounder than a mandibular incisor.

Imbrication lines are not usually present on the labial surface, unlike a maxillary canine. Two faint and vertically placed mesial and distal labial developmental depressions separate the three labial lobes, similar to the maxillary canine and incisors. These depressions are located on either side of the centrally placed vertical labial ridge, which is not as prominent as that of a maxillary canine.

From the labial view, the mesial outline is an almost straight line from the mesial contact to the CEJ, straighter than on a maxillary canine. The distal outline is shorter and rounder than the mesial outline, similar to that of a maxillary canine, which *helps to distinguish the mandibular right canine from the left.*

From the labial view, similar to a maxillary canine, the mesial and distal contacts are on different levels of the tooth, which also *helps to distinguish the mandibular right canine from the left.* The mesial contact with the lateral incisor is in the incisal third. The distal contact with the first premolar is at the junction of the incisal and middle thirds, at a more cervically placed location than that on the mesial side.

As discussed earlier, the cusp slopes are different: The mesial cusp slope of a mandibular canine is shorter than the distal cusp slope when first erupted from the labial view, which again *helps to distinguish the mandibular right canine from the left.* With attrition, the central cusp tip moves to the mesial, shortening the already short mesial cusp slope and further lengthening the distal cusp slope. The CEJ is evenly curved toward the root.

Lingual View Features

The lingual surface is less pronounced, except for the faintly demarcated features of a lingual ridge, mesial marginal ridge, distal marginal ridge, and two lingual fossae: the distolingual fossa and mesiolingual fossa (see Fig. 16.28). The less developed cingulum on a mandibular canine is not centered as on a maxillary canine but lies distal to the long axis of the root. In addition, the cingulum also does not extend as far incisally as it does in the maxillary canines. Rarely are there any lingual pits or lingual grooves on this surface.

Proximal View Features

A mandibular canine is again similar to a maxillary canine from a mesial view with a similar triangular shape and pointed cusp on the crown (see Fig. 16.28 and Table 15.4). However, a less developed cingulum and thinner marginal ridges are seen. The cusp tip is more lingually inclined without incisal wear, unlike the labially placed cusp tip on a maxillary canine.

The CEJ curvature on the mesial surface is more toward the incisal when compared to the same surface of a maxillary canine. Additionally the CEJ curve is more toward the incisal on the mesial surface than the distal on this same tooth, which *helps to distinguish the mandibular right canine from the left.* The distal view is similar to the mesial aspect. The one exception is that the CEJ is curved less on the distal than on the mesial surface.

Incisal View Features

A mandibular canine from this view is similar to a maxillary canine, but it is slightly more symmetrical compared with the maxillary tooth (see Fig. 16.28). Additionally the crown is wider labiolingually than mesiodistally and is offset toward the mesial. The less developed cingulum is offset toward the distal. This placement still gives the tooth only a slight asymmetrical appearance from this view, less than a maxillary canine.

The mesial marginal ridge is longer than the distal marginal ridge. The labial outline is also rounder mesiodistally than that of the mandibular incisors because of the slightly more pronounced labial ridge.

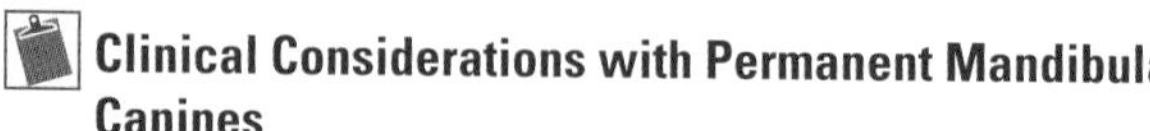

Clinical Considerations with Permanent Mandibular Canines

The dilaceration of the root can also occur with a mandibular canine, similar to a maxillary canine (see **Chapter 6**). Another developmental disturbance that may occur is an accessory root or bifurcated root in the apical third with labial and lingual root branches. This tooth is the anterior tooth most likely to have a bifurcated root, although this still is rare.

17

Permanent Posterior Teeth

Additional resources and practice exercises are provided on the companion Evolve website for this book: http://evolve.elsevier.com/Fehrenbach/illustrated.

LEARNING OBJECTIVES

1. Define and pronounce the key terms in this chapter.
2. Assign the correct names and universal or international tooth number for each permanent posterior tooth on a diagram or a skull and for a tooth model or a patient.
3. Demonstrate the correct location of each permanent posterior tooth on a diagram, a skull, and a patient.
4. Identify the permanent posterior teeth and discuss their properties and the clinical considerations concerning them, integrating it into patient care.
5. Identify the permanent premolars and their general features and discuss their clinical considerations, integrating it into patient care.
6. Describe the general and specific features of the permanent maxillary premolars and discuss the clinical considerations concerning them, integrating it into patient care.
7. Describe the general and specific features of the permanent mandibular premolars and discuss the clinical considerations concerning them, integrating it into patient care.
8. Identify the permanent molars and their general features and discuss their clinical considerations, integrating it into patient care.
9. Describe the general and specific features of the permanent maxillary molars and discuss the clinical considerations concerning them, integrating it into patient care.
10. Describe the general and specific features of the permanent mandibular molars and discuss the clinical considerations concerning them, integrating it into patient care.

PERMANENT POSTERIOR TEETH PROPERTIES

The permanent posterior teeth include the premolars and molars (Fig. 17.1; see Figs. 2.4 and 15.2). The posterior teeth are aligned with little or no curvature. These teeth appear to be in an almost straight line.

The crown of each has an occlusal surface as its masticatory surface bordered by the raised marginal ridges that are located on both the distal surface and mesial surface (Fig. 17.2). The occlusal surface also has two or more cusps. Some anatomists liken a cusp to a *gothic pyramid* with four **cusp ridges** descending from each cusp tip. Between these cusp ridges are sloping areas or four **inclined cuspal planes** (**kuhsp**-uhl). These planes are named by combining the names of the two cusp ridges that are between them. Some inclined planes are functional and thus involved in the occlusion of the teeth during mastication (see **Chapter 20**).

The occlusal surface of permanent posteriors creates an inner **occlusal table** bordered by the marginal ridges (Fig. 17.3). It is important to note that the discussion of the maxillary first premolar has extensive coverage of its occlusal table since it is the first posterior tooth discussed in this chapter; this information can then be related to the occlusal tables of other posterior teeth.

There are also **triangular ridges**, which are cusp ridges that descend from the cusp tips toward the central part of the occlusal table (Fig. 17.4). They are so named because the slopes of each side of the ridge are inclined in a way that resembles two sides of a triangle. Thus the triangular ridges are specifically named for the cusps to which they belong. Additionally present on many posteriors is a **transverse ridge** (tranz-**vurs**), a collective term given to the joining of two triangular ridges crossing the occlusal table transversely, moving from the labial to the lingual outline.

Each shallow and wide depression on the occlusal table is a fossa (plural, fossae). One type of fossa on posteriors, the **central fossa**, is located at the convergence of the cusp ridges in a central point where the grooves meet. Another type of fossa is the **triangular fossa**, which forms a triangular shape at the convergence of the cusp ridges and is associated with the termination of the triangular grooves (discussed next); the base of the triangular fossa is the marginal ridge. Located in the deepest parts of some of these fossae are **occlusal pits**; each developmental pit is a sharp pinpoint depression where two or more grooves meet.

Developmental grooves (or primary grooves) are also found on the occlusal table of posteriors, similar to those found on the lingual surface of anteriors. The developmental grooves on each different posterior tooth type are located in the same place and are thought to mark the junction between the developmental lobes. The grooves are sharp deep V-shaped linear depressions. The most prominent developmental groove on posteriors is the **central groove**, which generally travels mesiodistally and separates the occlusal table buccolingually. Lobe discussion, as was noted in **Chapter 6**, is controversial but is included for completeness when discussing in detail the various tooth types.

Other developmental grooves are **marginal grooves**, which cross the marginal ridges and serve as spillways, allowing food to escape during mastication. Finally, there are **triangular grooves** that separate a marginal ridge from the triangular ridge of a cusp and at their terminations form the triangular fossae.

In contrast, supplemental grooves (or secondary grooves) appear as shallower and more irregular linear depressions on the occlusal table of posteriors, similar to those found on the lingual surface of anteriors (Fig. 17.5). Supplemental grooves branch from the developmental grooves, but these supplemental grooves are not always present in the same pattern on the occlusal table of each different tooth type.

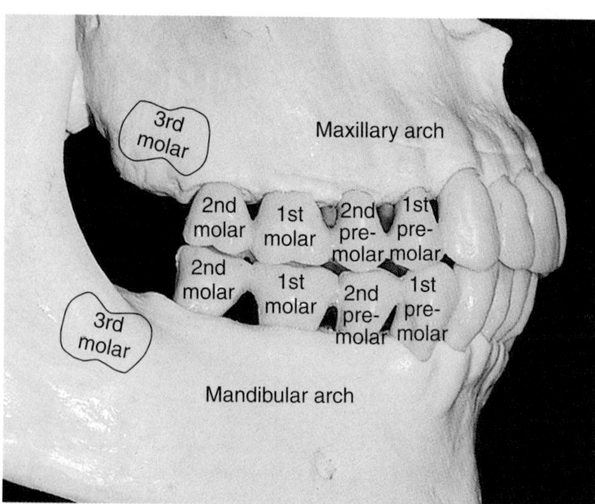

Fig. 17.1 Permanent posterior teeth identified on a skull, which include the premolars and molars. Note that the third molars have not erupted yet. (Courtesy of Margaret J. Fehrenbach, RDH, MS.)

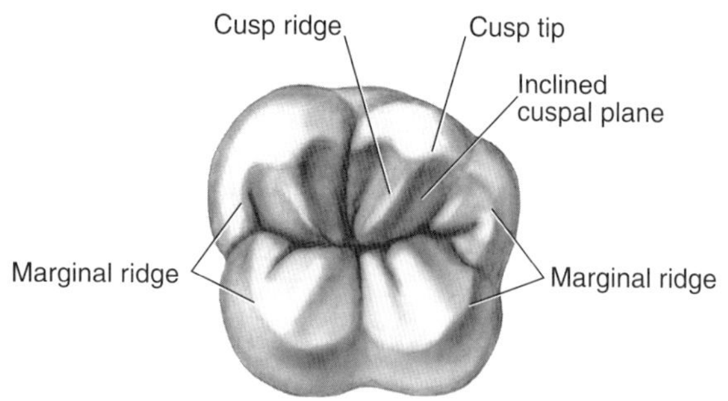

Fig. 17.2 Example of the occlusal surface on a permanent posterior tooth with its features noted.

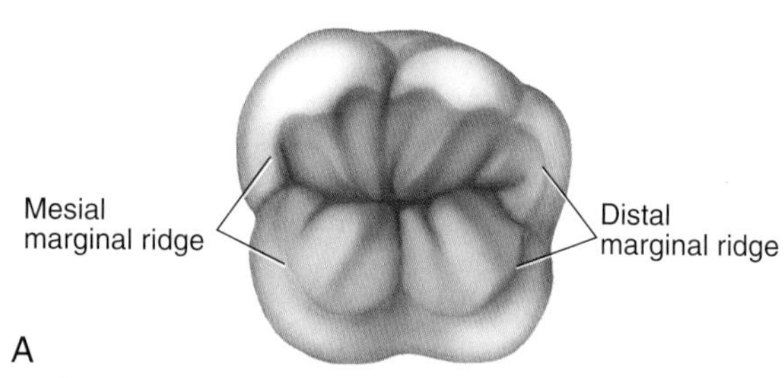

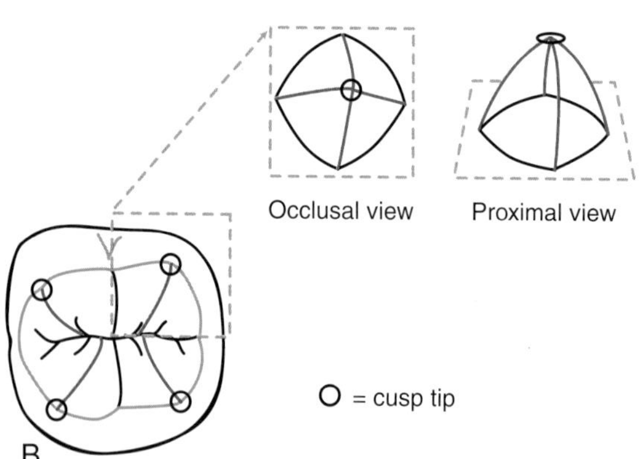

Fig. 17.3 Occlusal Views of a Permanent Posterior Tooth. A, Occlusal table highlighted. **B,** Triangular ridges highlighted with a close-up of the *gothic pyramid* shape for each of the cusps showing four cusp ridges descending from each cusp tip that many anatomists refer to when discussing these features.

In general, the more posterior a tooth is located in the dental arch, the more supplemental grooves are present, such that the occlusal table appears more wrinkled. Grooves are sometimes considered to be *fissures*.

For posteriors, the height of contour for the crown's buccal surface is in the cervical third and for the lingual surface it is in the middle third (Fig. 17.6). When compared with anteriors, most of the posteriors are wider labiolingually than mesiodistally, except for the mandibular molars.

In another comparison with anteriors, the contact areas of posteriors are wider, usually located at the buccal of center and nearer to the same level on each proximal surface (see Fig. 15.10). In addition, on each proximal surface is a cementoenamel junction (CEJ) curvature that is less pronounced on the posteriors than on the anteriors. In fact, the CEJ is often quite straight for posteriors.

Like anterior teeth, **multirooted** premolars and molars originate as a single root on the base of the crown (Fig. 17.7). This part on these posterior teeth is considered the **root trunk**. The cervical cross section of the root trunk initially follows the form of the crown (see Fig. 15.8, *B*). Unlike anteriors, the root of a posterior tooth divides from the root trunk into the correct number of root branches for its tooth type (see Fig. 6.21). This can be with either two roots, which means it

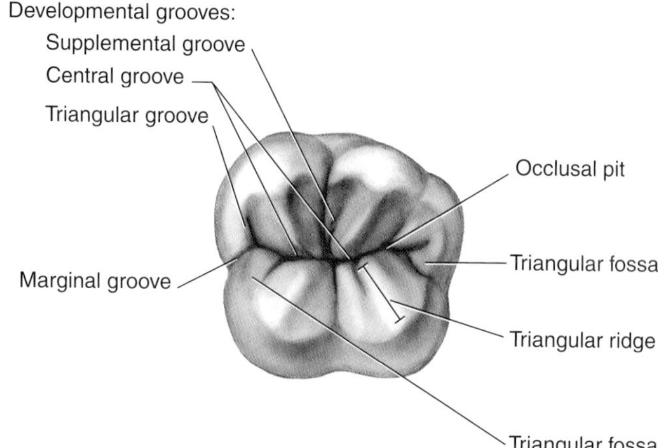

Fig. 17.4 Example of the other features of the occlusal table on a permanent posterior tooth, including the central groove with the triangular fossae highlighted.

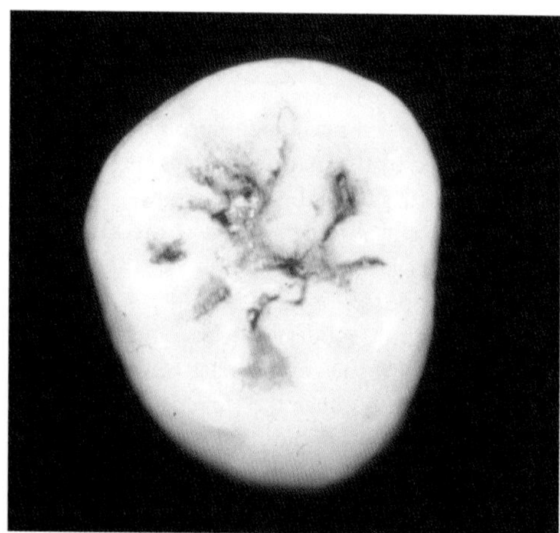

Fig. 17.5 Example of supplemental grooves on the occlusal surface of an extracted permanent posterior tooth, the maxillary third molar. The more posterior a tooth is located in the dental arch, the more supplemental grooves are present. (Courtesy of Margaret J. Fehrenbach, RDH, MS.)

is **bifurcated** (bahy-fuhr-**keyt**-tuhd) or with three roots, which means it is **trifurcated** (trahy-fuhr-**keyt**-tuhd). In some cases, a bifurcated tooth may additionally have **root fusion** with little of the remaining root trunk being truly bifurcated.

An area between two or more of these root branches before they divide from the root trunk is a **furcation** (fer-**key**-shuhn) (Table 17.1; see Fig. 17.7). The spaces between the roots at the furcation are the **furcation crotches**. Bifurcated teeth with two roots, such as the maxillary first premolar and mandibular molars, have two furcation crotches; trifurcated teeth with three roots, such as maxillary molars, have three furcation crotches. Such crotches can be located on various surfaces, depending on tooth type, each with a slightly different individual configuration. With periodontal health, these features of the root(s) are covered by the alveolar process as well as overlying gingival tissue.

Clinical Considerations for Permanent Posterior Teeth

The complex pit and groove patterns on the occlusal surface of posteriors can put them at an increased risk of caries (Fig. 17.8). This susceptibility is due to increased dental biofilm retention and the weakness of enamel forming the walls of the pits and grooves (see Fig. 12.4, *A*).

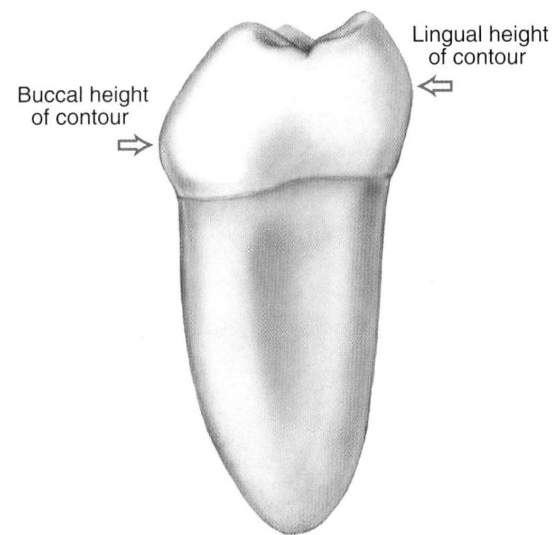

Fig. 17.6 Height of Contour on a Permanent Posterior Tooth.

Clinicians need to be aware of these pit and groove patterns on the posteriors when they examine dentitions to assess the patient's caries risk level. Thus the pits and grooves (or fissures) must be checked for decay with an explorer and mirror. In addition, using light-induced devices that measure changes in laser fluorescence of hard tissue allows dental professionals to better diagnose early lesions in pits and grooves. Posteriors with deep pit and groove patterns but without incipient decay should have enamel sealants applied as soon as possible.

PERMANENT PREMOLARS

GENERAL FEATURES OF PERMANENT PREMOLARS

Permanent premolars are the most anteriorly placed posteriors in the permanent dentition (Fig. 17.9; Table 17.2). Each dental arch has four premolars, two to each quadrant.

There are two types of premolars: first premolar and second premolar. One of each type is present in each quadrant of each dental arch. The first is closer to the midline at the fourth position from it. The second is next to the first premolar and is in the fifth position from the midline. Both types are distal to the permanent canine and mesial to the permanent first molar when full eruption of the permanent dentition has occurred. Permanent premolars are succedaneous because the first and second premolars replace the primary first and second molars, respectively.

Premolars function to assist the molars in grinding food during mastication because of the broad occlusal surface and the prominent cusps, especially the buccal cusps. Premolars are not as long as canines but they assist the canines in piercing and tearing food with those cusps. The crown outline from the buccal and lingual is pentagonal or five-sided, similar to the canines (see Table 15.4). These teeth, along with the canines, also help maintain the height of the lower third of the vertical dimension of the face, supporting the facial muscles, especially those muscles at the labial commissures. Thus the premolars are involved in both esthetics and speech, less so than the anteriors, but more so than the molars.

An older term for a premolar was *bicuspid* because of the usual presence of two cusps on the occlusal surface, which is one more cusp than in the canines. However, the mandibular second premolar frequently has three cusps. Thus the term *premolar* is more widely used since it allows for any number of cusps and also because these teeth are located anterior to the molars.

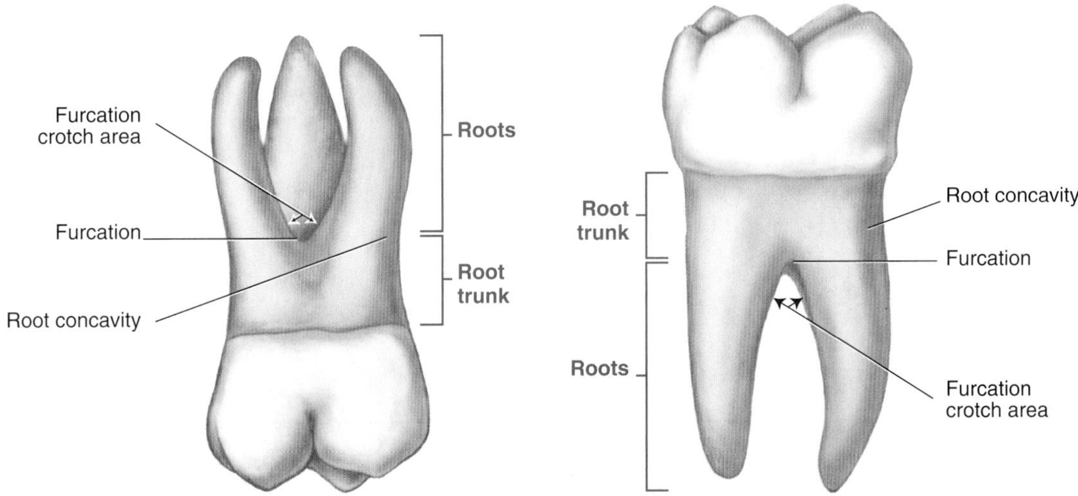

Fig. 17.7 Buccal Root Features of Both a Permanent Maxillary and a Mandibular Molar.

TABLE 17.1 Permanent Posterior Tooth Furcations and Furcation Crotches

Furcations and Furcation Crotches

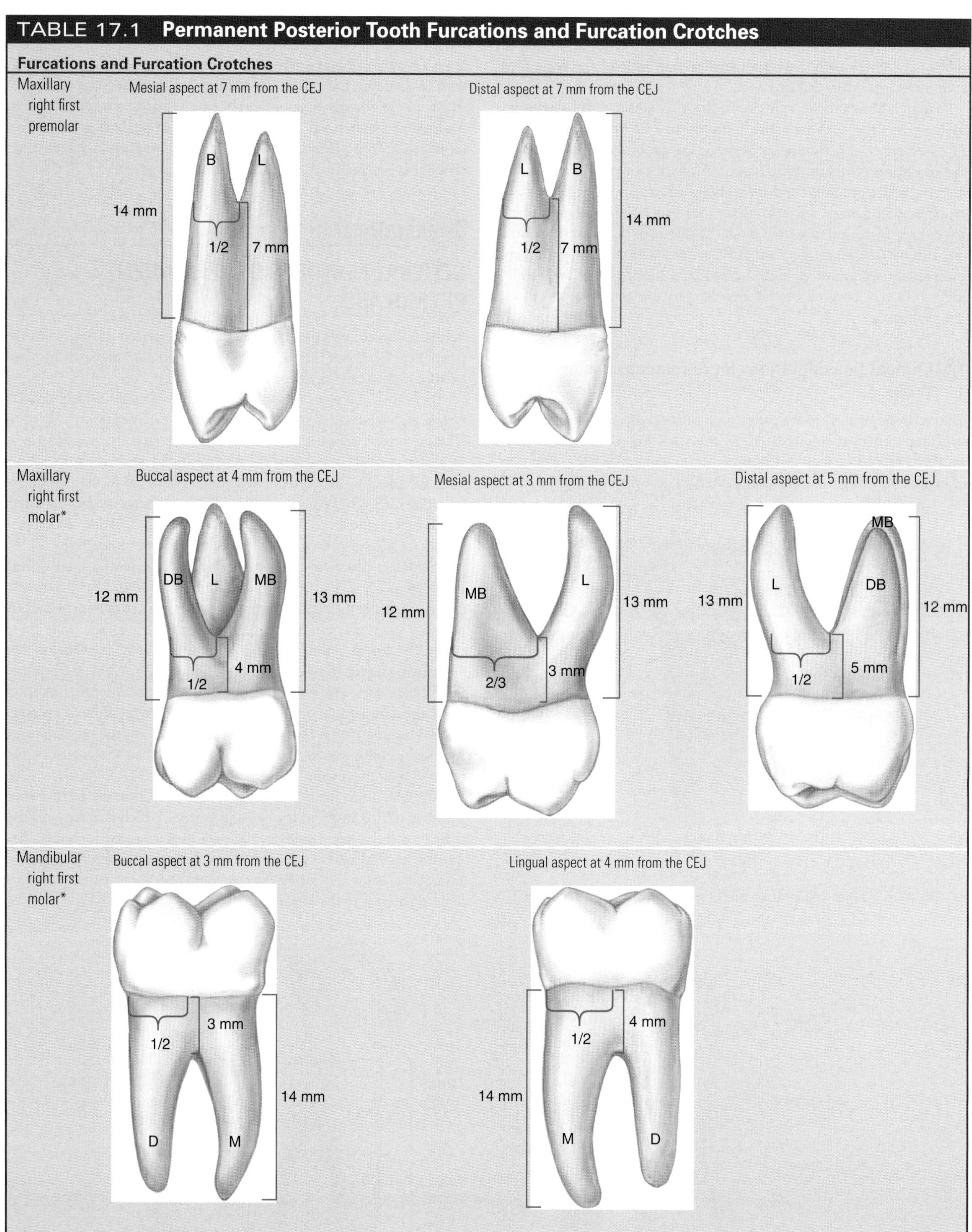

*Second and third molars for each arch are similar to first but have longer root trunks so that furcations of more posterior molars are located more apically and with roots closer together, creating tighter furcation entrances.

CEJ, Cementoenamel junction; *D*, distal; *DB*, distobuccal; *L*, lingual; *M*, mesial; *MB*, mesiobuccal.

Data from Nelson S. *Wheeler's Dental Anatomy, Physiology, and Occlusion.* 10th ed. Philadelphia: Elsevier; 2015.

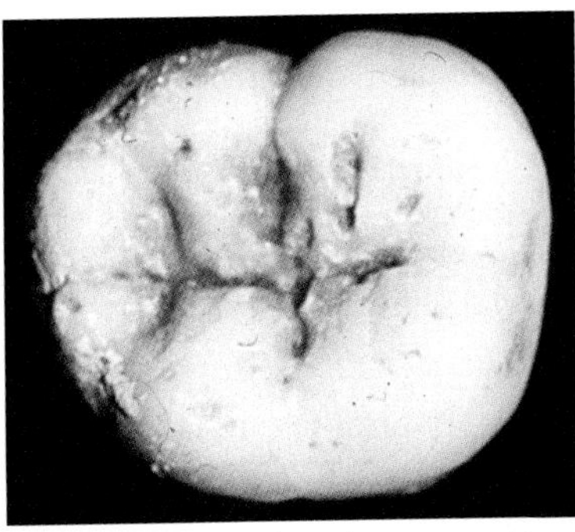

Fig. 17.8 Example of a complex pit and groove pattern on the occlusal surface of an extracted permanent posterior tooth. (Courtesy of Margaret J. Fehrenbach, RDH, MS.)

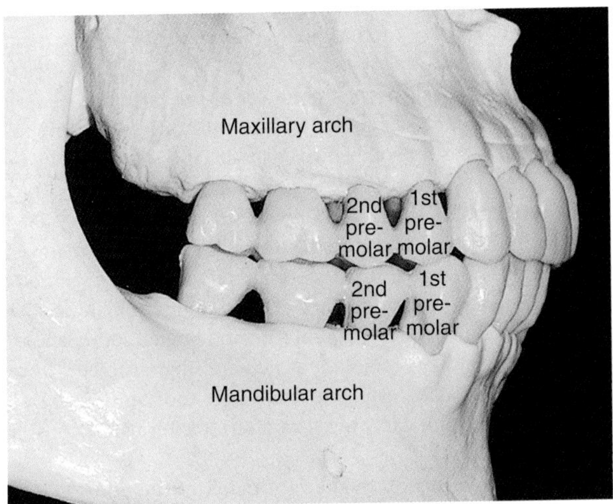

Fig. 17.9 Permanent Premolars Identified on a Skull. (Courtesy of Margaret J. Fehrenbach, RDH, MS.)

Finally, along with the cusps the occlusal surface of a premolar, similar to all posteriors, has marginal ridges, triangular ridges, developmental grooves, and occlusal pits. The boundaries of the occlusal surface created by these marginal ridges and cusp ridges form the inner occlusal table.

As posterior teeth, premolars have a shorter crown than anterior teeth. The buccal surface is rounded and has a prominent centrally located vertical **buccal ridge** (Fig. 17.10). The buccal ridge of premolars is similar to the labial ridge of the canines and may be related to the increased development of the middle buccal lobe. Two buccal developmental depressions are noted on each side of the buccal ridge. The height of contour for premolars is in the cervical third on the buccal surface, similar to all anteriors. And the height of contour on the lingual is in the middle third like all posteriors.

Most premolars usually have one root, except for the permanent maxillary first premolar, which has two roots. Whether one or two roots are present, all have proximal root concavities present.

Clinical Considerations for Permanent Premolars

In some cases, a permanent premolar can be extracted in each quadrant during orthodontic therapy to improve dental arch spacing. If a premolar has been extracted, the distinctive pit and groove patterns on the occlusal surface will help in identifying the remaining premolar when the arch space from the extraction is lost, unless the tooth has been restored. However, orthodontic therapy tends instead to now include expansion of the jaw, if needed, instead of removing premolars so as to retain a more natural rounded curved shape to the arches. If extraction is unavoidable, first premolars are usually extracted more often than second premolars. Additionally, premolars present difficulties in instrumentation of the root because they have proximal root concavities, especially on the mesial of the maxillary first premolar.

TABLE 17.2 Permanent Premolars

	Maxillary First Premolar	Maxillary Second Premolar	Mandibular First Premolar	Mandibular Second Premolar
Universal number	#5 and #12	#4 and #13	#21 and #28	#20 and #29
International number	#14 and #24	#15 and #25	#34 and #44	#35 and #45
General crown features	Occlusal table with marginal ridges and cusps with tips, ridges, inclined planes, grooves, fossae, pits			
	Buccal ridge			
Specific crown features	Larger than second. Buccal cusp longer of two cusps. Long central groove. Mesial surface features unlike second.	Smaller than first. Two cusps same length. Short central groove, with increased supplemental grooves. No mesial surface features like first.	Smaller than second. Smaller lingual cusp of two cusps. Mesial surface features.	Larger than first. Usually three cusps with: Y-shaped groove pattern or two cusps with H- or U-shaped groove pattern. Increased supplemental grooves.
Mesial and distal contact*	Just cervical to junction of occlusal and middle thirds			
Distinguish right from left	Longer mesial cusp slope than distal cusp slope, with mesial features: deeper CEJ curvature, marginal groove, developmental depression, deep mesial root concavity	Lingual cusp offset to mesial	Shorter mesial cusp slope than distal cusp slope, with mesial surface features: deeper mesial CEJ curvature and mesiolingual groove	Distal marginal ridge more cervically located, thus more occlusal surface visible from distal view
General root features	Two roots with root trunk	Single root		
Specific root features	Elliptical on cervical cross section. Proximal root concavities.		Oval or elliptical on cervical cross section. Proximal root concavities.	

*Height of contour of posteriors for the buccal is in cervical third and lingual in middle third.
CEJ, Cementoenamel junction.

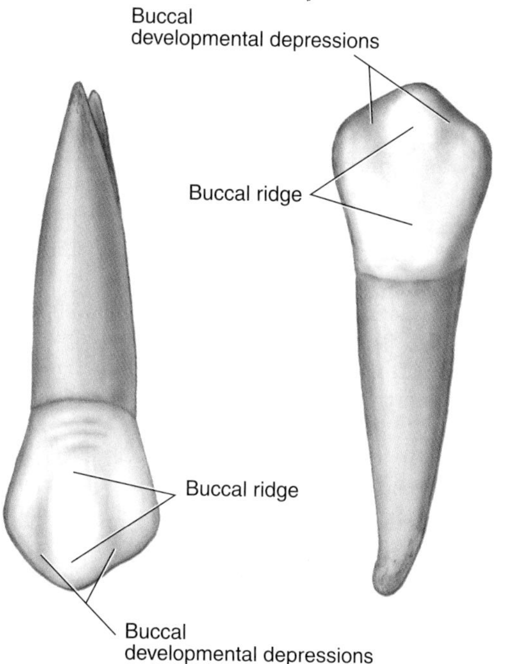

Fig. 17.10 Buccal Features of Permanent Premolars and Their Similar Features.

PERMANENT MAXILLARY PREMOLARS

General Features

Both types of maxillary premolars resemble each other more than the mandibular premolars resemble each other (see Figs. 17.11 and 17.17). However, a maxillary first premolar is larger than a maxillary second premolar. In contrast, a mandibular first premolar is smaller than a mandibular second premolar. In keeping though, both maxillary premolars erupt earlier than the mandibular premolars.

The crown of a maxillary premolar is shorter occlusocervically than that of the nearby maxillary canine but is slightly longer than that of the adjacent molars. The crown outline from each proximal aspect is trapezoidal or four-sided with only two parallel sides, similar to all maxillary posteriors (see Table 15.4). The maxillary premolars are composed of four developmental lobes: three buccal and one lingual.

The crown is also centered over the root and shows no lingual inclination, unlike the mandibular premolars, which are like other mandibular posteriors. They also have a greater buccolingual width than mesiodistal width compared with the mandibular premolars or other mandibular posterior teeth when viewed from the occlusal. The crown outline for both maxillary premolars is somewhat hexagonal from this view or six-sided; it is almost oval compared with the rounder mandibular premolars.

Both maxillary premolars have two cusps of almost equal size. In contrast, the mandibular premolars can have more than two cusps, but any lingual cusps are always smaller. Like all premolars, these cusps are centered over the long axis of the tooth from either proximal view.

The roots of the maxillary premolars are shorter than the maxillary canine's roots, but the root length is the same as that of the molars. The roots show slight lingual and distal inclination. The roots on cervical cross section are elliptical (or elongated oval), but may be slightly altered by proximal root concavities (see Fig. 15.8, *B*).

Clinical Considerations for Permanent Maxillary Premolars

The roots of maxillary premolars may penetrate the anterior part of the maxillary sinus as a result of accidental trauma or during tooth extraction because of the close relation of these roots to the sinus walls, which can occur with other maxillary posterior teeth (see Fig. 11.22). To complicate matters, the discomfort of sinusitis can be mistakenly interpreted as tooth-related from the maxillary premolar and vice versa. Thus, radiographs of the questionable tooth and maxillary sinus as well as other diagnostic tests are necessary to determine the cause of the discomfort. Cone-beam computed tomography (CBCT) images are often useful in these circumstances.

Permanent Maxillary First Premolars #5 and #12 (#14 and #24)

Specific Overall Features

Permanent maxillary first premolars erupt between 10 and 11 years of age with root completion between ages 12 and 13 (Fig. 17.11). These teeth erupt distal to the primary maxillary canines or the open arch space and thus are the succedaneous replacements for the primary maxillary first molars.

The crown of a maxillary first premolar has an angular shape with a sharply defined outline compared with a maxillary second premolar's more rounded shape. The tooth's two cusps are also sharply defined with the buccal cusp usually about 1 mm higher than the lingual cusp. The central groove on the occlusal surface is also longer on the maxillary first premolar than on the second. The tooth appears bent mesially when viewed from the occlusal compared with the second premolar of the same arch.

Most maxillary first premolars are bifurcated, having two root branches in the apical third: a buccal root and lingual (or palatal) root. This is unlike the other premolars, which are single-rooted. However, maxillary first premolars originate as a single root on the base of the crown as do other premolars as well as anteriors; this part is considered the root trunk.

A cervical cross section of the root trunk of the bifurcated tooth follows the crown form (see Fig. 15.8, *B*). The root trunk usually makes up half the length of the entire root and the root branches make up the other half. The roots are rounded overall and taper to sharp apices. The buccal root is larger but not longer than the lingual root. However, root anatomy can get even more complex with this tooth. The root trunk can also have undergone root fusion with little of the remaining root trunk being truly bifurcated.

Because the maxillary first premolar has both a buccal and a lingual root, it also has two furcations, which are located on both the mesial and distal surfaces (see Table 17.1). Both of these furcations are located midway on the root surface, with both 7 mm from the CEJ.

If a single root is present, as is the case in about 20% of the cases, it is wider buccolingually than mesiodistally. Both the buccal and lingual surfaces are rounded and the root is tapered to a blunt apex. On cervical cross section, the root becomes almost kidney-shaped. A single root also has a deep and wide mesial surface root concavity, which ranges from relatively shallow to deep enough to almost bifurcate the root. Trifurcated teeth have been occasionally found with this tooth with two buccal roots and a single lingual root.

The pulp cavity for a bifurcated tooth usually shows two pulp horns (one for each cusp) and two pulp canals (one for each root) (Fig. 17.12). Even if there is only one undivided root like the maxillary second premolar, two pulp canals are usually found, although they often combine apically to form one apical foramen.

Buccal View Features

The crown of a maxillary first premolar is the widest mesiodistally of all the premolars (Fig. 17.13). This tooth's crown is wide at the level of the contact areas, becoming narrower at the CEJ, which is similar to the adjacent maxillary canine. The mesial contact with the maxillary canine is just cervical to the junction of the occlusal and middle thirds.

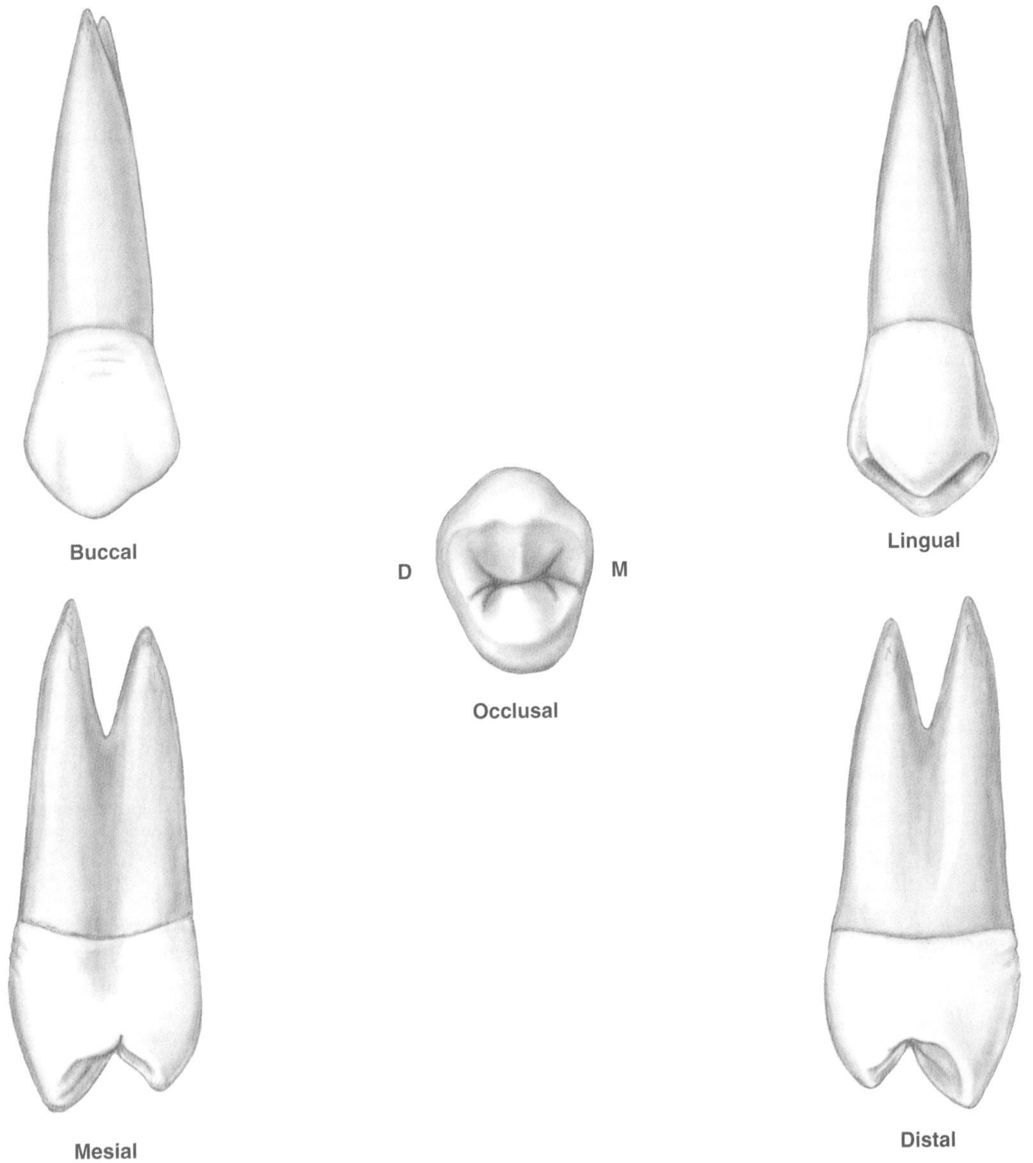

Buccal

Lingual

D

M

Occlusal

Mesial

Distal

Fig. 17.11 Views of the Permanent Maxillary Right First Premolar. *D*, Distal; *M*, mesial.

The distal contact with the maxillary second premolar is the same, just cervical to the junction of the occlusal and middle thirds.

The mesial and distal outlines of the crown of the maxillary first premolar are both almost straight from the contact areas to the CEJ, but the mesial outline is more rounded. Both of these outlines converge more toward the cervical than they do on the maxillary second premolars. Imbrication lines and perikymata are found on the buccal surface and these extend mesiodistally in the cervical third. The CEJ curvature of the tooth is evenly rounded toward the apex of the tooth and has less depth than on anterior teeth.

The buccal cusp of a maxillary first premolar is high and sharp, located slightly distal to the long axis of the tooth because the two cusp slopes of the buccal cusp are not equal in height. This tooth is the only tooth in the permanent dentition that has a buccal cusp with the mesial cusp slope longer than the distal cusp slope, which *helps to distinguish the maxillary right first premolar from the left*. This relationship of the cusp slopes usually exists upon eruption but any attrition over time may change it. A bulge may be found occasionally on the buccal cusp of this tooth.

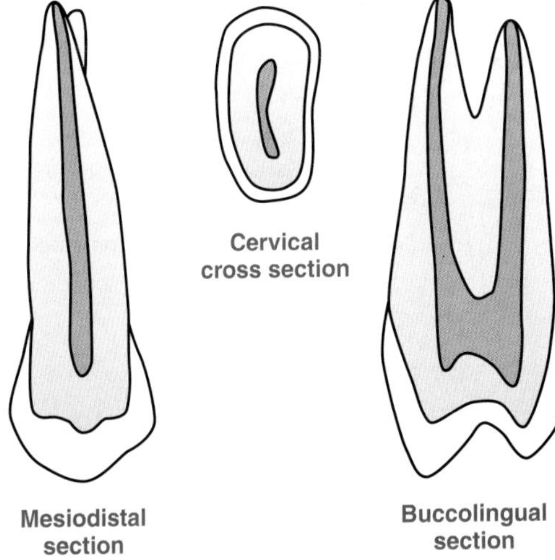

Fig. 17.12 Pulp Cavity of the Permanent Maxillary Right First Premolar.

Lingual View Features

The lingual surface of the maxillary first premolar is rounded in all directions but is smaller than the buccal surface (see Fig. 17.11). The shorter lingual cusp is sharp but not as sharp as the buccal cusp and is offset toward the mesial. Thus the cusp slopes of the lingual cusp are again not equal in length. From the lingual aspect, however, the mesial cusp slope is shorter than the distal cusp slope.

Proximal View Features

On the mesial surface of the crown of a maxillary first premolar, the mesial marginal ridge is present on the concave occlusal margin. A mesial marginal groove is also sometimes present (Fig. 17.14, *A*). This developmental groove crosses the mesial marginal ridge and extends from the occlusal to the middle third of the crown, lingual to the contact area. Also the mesial surface usually has a mesial developmental depression located cervical to the contact area, crossing the CEJ, and extending onto the root.

On the root, the mesial developmental depression joins a deep linear developmental depression, the mesial root concavity, on the root trunk, extending from the contact area to the bifurcation (see Fig. 17.14, *A*). These types of concavities increase the attachment area and produce a root shape that may be more resistant to torquing (twisting) forces. However, this concavity on the root also puts this tooth at an increased risk for periodontal disease because it allows an increased deposit level (see earlier discussion) (Fig. 17.14, *B*). The CEJ curvature is more occlusally located on the mesial than on the distal surface. All of these prominent mesial features from the proximal view *help to distinguish the maxillary right first premolar from the left.*

The distal surface is similar to the mesial, except that it does not have a depression, and more of the occlusal surface shows because the distal marginal ridge is more cervically located than is the mesial marginal ridge (see Fig. 17.11). A distal marginal groove is sometimes located across the distal marginal ridge, but this distal groove is shallower than the similar groove on the mesial surface. The distal surface of the root also has a linear concavity but it is reduced in depth, creating a less-risky convex or flat surface. Additionally, the CEJ curvature on the distal surface is not as deep cervically as the mesial.

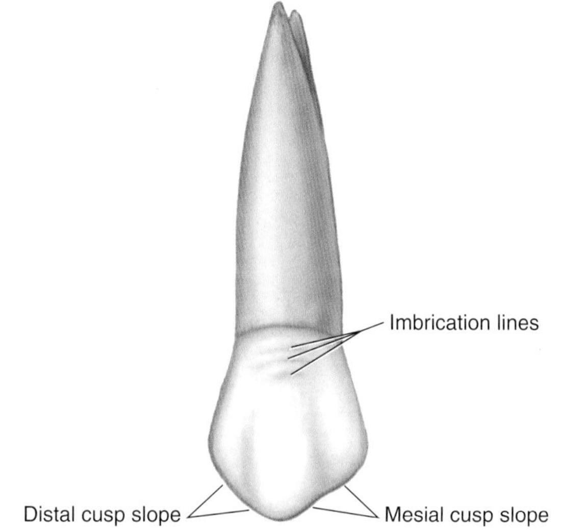

Fig. 17.13 Buccal Features of the Permanent Maxillary Right First Premolar.

Occlusal View Features

The outline of the occlusal surface of a maxillary first premolar is somewhat hexagonal or six-sided but is wider buccolingually than mesiodistally (Fig. 17.15). The buccal ridge (or buccal cusp ridge of the buccal cusp as discussed later) is prominent on the buccal margin, and the lingual margin of the occlusal outline is almost a semicircle. However, both the mesial and distal margins are straight as they converge toward the lingual. Thus the lingual part of the tooth is narrower mesiodistally than the buccal part. When the mesial marginal groove is prominent, it may create a dip in the mesial margin.

Occlusal Table Components

The buccal cusp of a maxillary first premolar is sharper and higher than the lingual cusp. The occlusal function of the buccal cusp involves only its lingual surface. Four buccal cusp ridges descend from the buccal cusp tip, each named for its location: buccal, lingual, mesial, and distal. Because this is the first occlusal table of a posterior tooth under discussion in this chapter, this text provides specific details on each of the occlusal table features; this information can then be related to the occlusal tables of other posterior teeth.

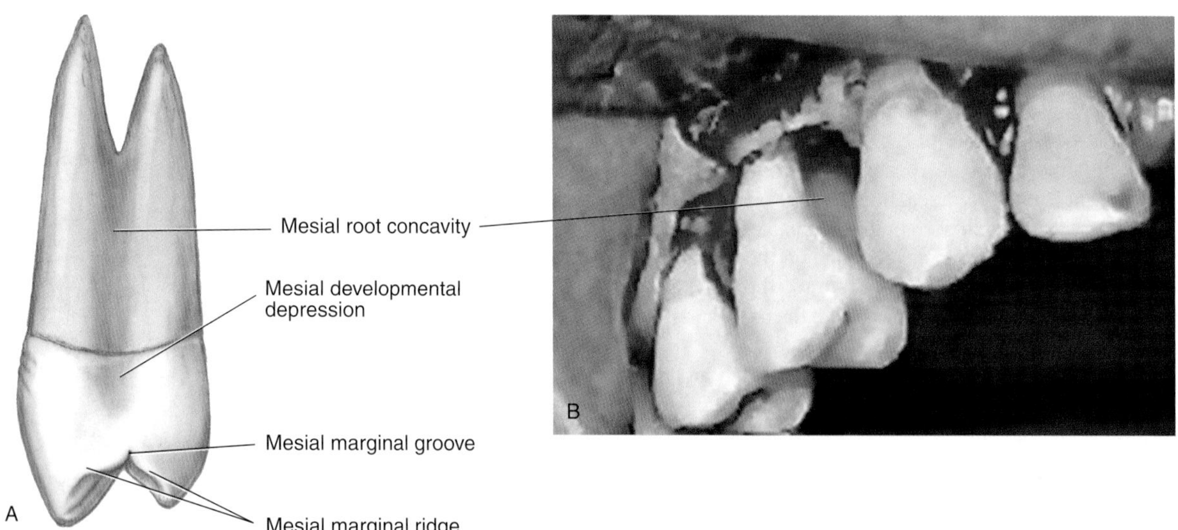

Fig. 17.14 **A**, Mesial features of the permanent maxillary right first premolar. **B**, An exposed mesial root concavity present on the root trunk from extensive periodontal disease, extending from the contact area to the bifurcation due to surgical access provided by a flap procedure (**B**, Courtesy of Margaret J. Fehrenbach, RDH, MS.).

The buccal cusp ridge of the buccal cusp extends cervically from the cusp tip on the buccal surface and corresponds to the buccal ridge. The lingual cusp ridge extends lingually from the buccal cusp tip to the central groove (or buccal triangular ridge or buccal part of the transverse ridge as discussed later). The mesial cusp ridge of the buccal cusp extends mesially from the cusp tip to the mesiobucco-occlusal point angle. The distal cusp ridge extends distally from the buccal cusp tip to the distobucco-occlusal point angle.

Between the cusp ridges are four buccal-inclined cuspal planes, named for the two cusp ridges they are between: mesiobuccal, mesiolingual, distobuccal, and distolingual. However, only the mesiolingual- and distolingual-inclined cuspal planes function during occlusion.

The lingual cusp of the maxillary first premolar is rounder, less sharp, and shorter than the buccal cusp. This cusp is also located well to the lingual and offset to the mesial. Again, there are four lingual cusp ridges and four lingual-inclined cuspal planes similar to those associated with the buccal cusp, but all the lingual-inclined cuspal planes are functional in occlusion. This is because the entire lingual cusp functions during occlusion, unlike the buccal cusp.

Extending mesiodistally across the occlusal table of the maxillary first premolar is a long central groove, evenly dividing the tooth buccolingually. The central groove is a developmental groove that is sharply defined; it is deep and V-shaped. A few supplemental grooves appear irregular in shape and shallower because they branch from the central groove. Thus the occlusal surface is relatively less pronounced compared with the adjacent maxillary second premolar.

The lingual cusp ridge, which runs from the buccal cusp tip to the central groove, is also termed the *buccal triangular ridge* (Fig. 17.16). The buccal cusp ridge of the lingual cusp is also termed the *lingual triangular ridge* because it runs from the lingual cusp tip to the central groove. Perpendicular to the central groove is a *transverse ridge,* which is the collective term given to the joining of the buccal triangular ridge and the lingual triangular ridge.

The central groove of the maxillary first premolar also crosses to the mesial marginal ridge, which is shorter than the distal marginal ridge. Extending from the central groove, another developmental groove, the mesial marginal groove, crosses the mesial marginal ridge and travels onto the mesial surface of the tooth.

Descending down the slope of the buccal cusp and just inside the distal and mesial marginal ridges are two developmental grooves: the mesiobuccal triangular groove and the distobuccal triangular groove. Across the occlusal table, the lingual cusp also has two developmental grooves: the mesiolingual triangular groove and the distolingual triangular groove.

Each of these triangular grooves ends in a triangular-shaped depression, the triangular fossa. These fossae include: the deeper mesial triangular fossa that surrounds the mesiobuccal triangular groove and the shallower distal triangular fossa that surrounds the distobuccal triangular groove. The boundaries of the mesial triangular fossa are the mesial marginal ridge, the transverse ridge, and the mesial cusp ridges of the two cusps. The distal triangular fossa has boundaries similar to those of the mesial fossa in a mirror-image fashion. Within the deepest parts of these fossae are the occlusal pits, the mesial pit, and distal pit, respectively. These developmental pits are connected by the central groove on the occlusal table.

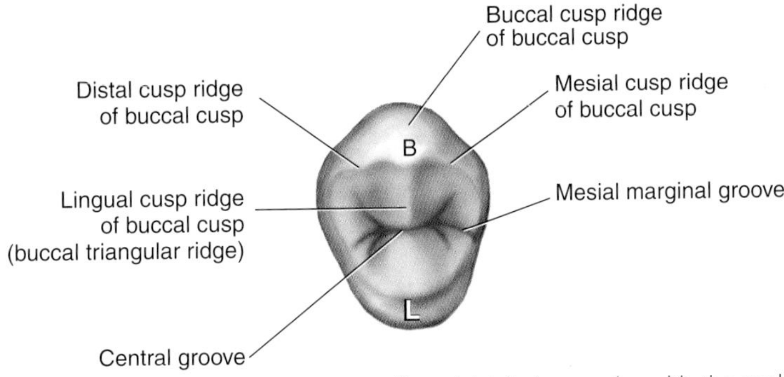

Fig. 17.15 Occlusal features of the permanent maxillary right first premolar with the occlusal table highlighted. *B*, Buccal; *L*, lingual.

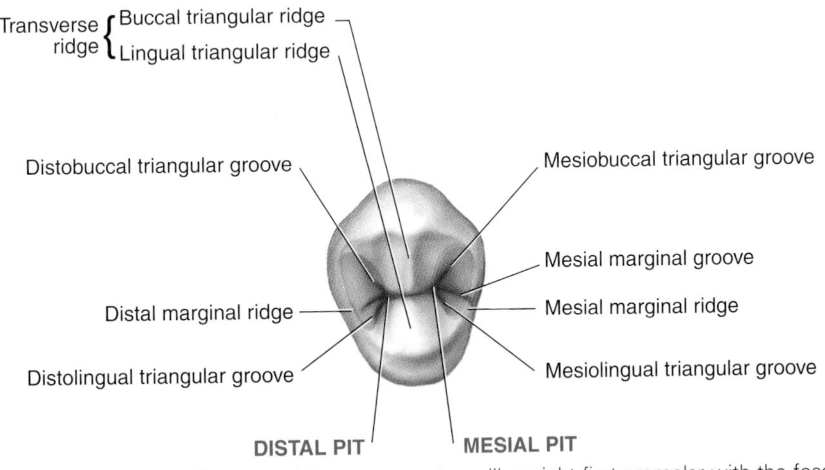

Fig. 17.16 Additional occlusal features of the permanent maxillary right first premolar with the fossae highlighted.

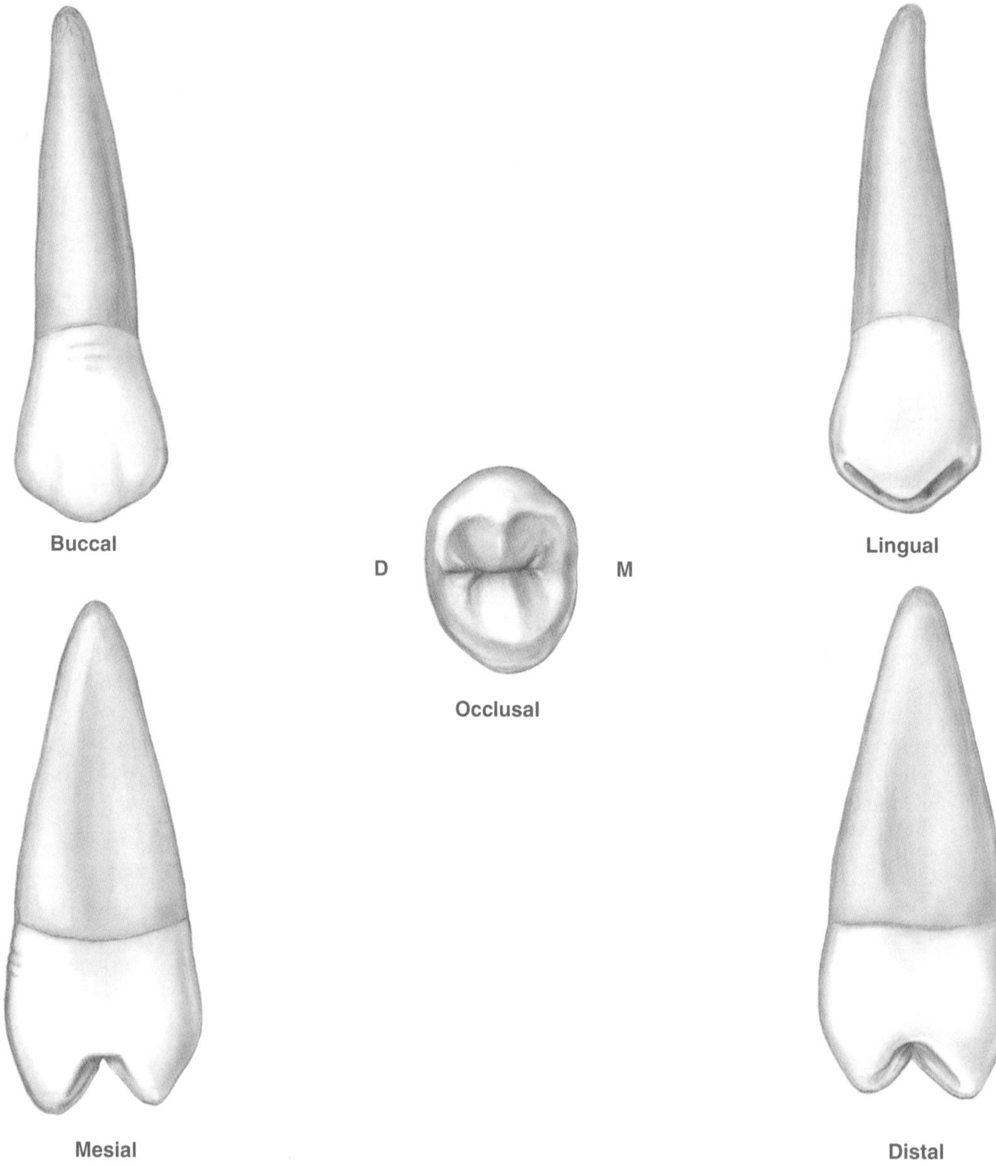

Buccal

Lingual

D

M

Occlusal

Mesial

Distal

Fig. 17.17 Views of the Permanent Maxillary Right Second Premolar. *D,* Distal; *M,* mesial.

Permanent Maxillary Second Premolars #4 and #13 (#15 and #25)

Specific Overall Features

Permanent maxillary second premolars erupt between 10 and 12 years of age with root completion between ages 12 and 14 (Fig. 17.17). These teeth erupt distal to the permanent maxillary first premolars and thus are the succedaneous replacements for the primary maxillary second molars.

A maxillary second premolar resembles a first premolar, except that its crown is less angular and more rounded. Additionally, more crown variations, especially in its occlusal surface anatomy, are noted in this tooth as compared with maxillary first premolars.

Unlike a maxillary first premolar, a maxillary second premolar usually has only a single root, but it may occasionally have two roots. The dimensions between the maxillary second and the first premolars are usually about the same overall, except for greater root length of the second. The mesial root concavity is not as pronounced as in a first premolar. The pulp cavity of this tooth has two pulp horns and one single pulp canal (Fig. 17.18).

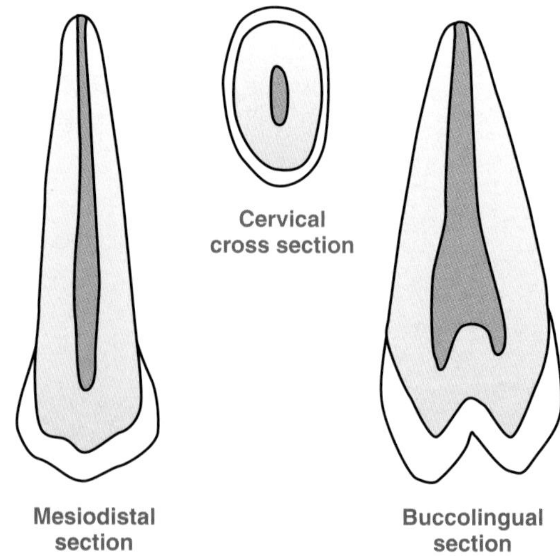

Fig. 17.18 Pulp Cavity of the Permanent Maxillary Right Second Premolar.

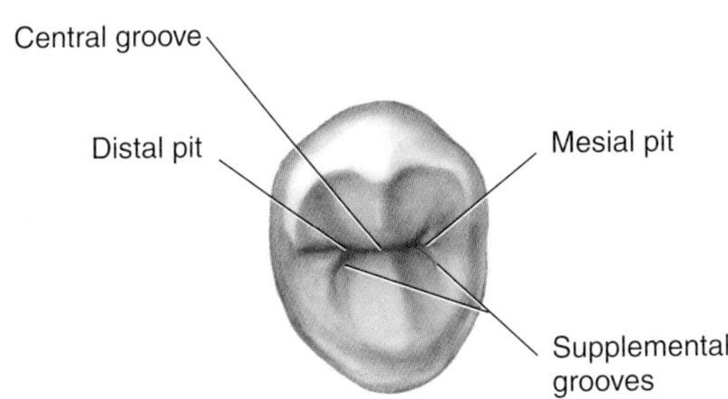

Fig. 17.19 Occlusal features of the permanent maxillary right second premolar with the occlusal table highlighted.

Buccal View Features

The buccal cusp of a maxillary second premolar is neither as long nor as sharp as that of a maxillary first premolar (see Fig. 17.17). All other features of the buccal surface of a maxillary second are similar to those of the first. Again the mesial contact with a maxillary first premolar is just cervical to the junction of the occlusal and middle thirds on the buccal surface. The distal contact with a maxillary first molar is the same, just cervical to the junction of the occlusal and middle thirds.

Lingual View Features

All lingual surface features of a maxillary second premolar are similar to those of a maxillary first premolar (see Fig. 17.17). One exception is that the lingual cusp is larger, almost the same height as the buccal cusp on a maxillary second premolar. In addition, the lingual cusp is slightly displaced to the mesial, which *helps to distinguish the maxillary right second premolar from the left*. In addition, less of the occlusal surface is seen from this view because the crown is longer on the lingual.

Proximal View Features

The mesial surface of a maxillary second premolar is similar to that of a maxillary first premolar, except that the cusps are closer to having the same size and no mesial developmental depression is present on either the crown or root. Instead, this area cervical to the contact area is rounder (see Fig. 17.17). In addition, this tooth has no mesial marginal groove. Both the contact areas and mesial marginal ridge are more cervically located than those on a maxillary first premolar. The distal surface is the same as the mesial surface without any distal marginal groove, but the contact area is larger.

Occlusal View Features

The outline of the occlusal surface of a maxillary second premolar is more rounded and larger overall than that of a maxillary first premolar from the occlusal view (see Fig. 17.17). Thus the overall hexagonal outline of the crown from the occlusal is more difficult to see.

Occlusal Table Components

The central groove is shorter on a maxillary second premolar than on a maxillary first premolar (Fig. 17.19). Thus when this groove ends in a mesial pit and distal pit at each of its ends, the pits are closer together and more to the middle on the occlusal table.

Other features and the overall anatomy of this tooth's occlusal surface are similar to those of a maxillary first premolar. An exception is that the maxillary second premolar has numerous supplemental grooves radiating from the central groove. This gives the tooth a more wrinkled appearance compared with a maxillary first premolar.

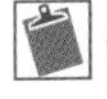 Clinical Considerations for Permanent Maxillary Second Premolars

With premature loss of a primary maxillary second molar, the developing permanent maxillary first molar inclines and drifts mesially. The developing permanent maxillary second premolar is prevented from eruption because its arch leeway space is almost closed (see **Chapter 20**). This situation can allow the maxillary second premolar to become impacted against the first molar. An impacted tooth is an unerupted or partially erupted tooth, which is positioned against another tooth, bone, or even soft tissue, making complete eruption unlikely. Additionally, the leeway space can be compromised if the permanent maxillary second molar erupts before the maxillary second premolars, the arch perimeter is now significantly shortened and occlusal disharmony is then likely to occur as with a malocclusion. These related complications may be prevented by careful evaluation of patients with a mixed dentition and the use of interceptive orthodontic therapy, such as space maintainers (see Fig. 20.4) and tooth replacement.

PERMANENT MANDIBULAR PREMOLARS

General Features

Mandibular premolars do not resemble each other as much as do the maxillary premolars (see Figs. 17.20 and 17.26). Although a maxillary first premolar is larger overall than the second premolar, a mandibular first premolar is smaller than a mandibular second premolar. Both mandibular premolars usually erupt into the oral cavity later than do the maxillary premolars.

Quite distinct from maxillary premolars, the buccal outline of the crown of all mandibular premolars shows a strong lingual inclination when viewed from the proximal, which is similar to all mandibular posterior teeth. The permanent mandibular premolars also have an equal buccolingual and mesiodistal width when viewed from the occlusal, making the outline almost round. In addition, both types of premolars have a similar buccal outline of both the crown and root.

The mesial and distal contact areas of mandibular premolars are on almost the same level. Similar CEJ curvatures are also found on both premolars. From each proximal view, both the crown outlines of mandibular premolars are rhomboidal or four-sided having the opposite sides parallel, which is like all mandibular posteriors (see Table 15.4). The crowns thus incline lingually on their root bases, bringing the cusps of these mandibular teeth into proper occlusion with their maxillary antagonists and the distribution of forces along their long axes.

Unlike the maxillary premolars, both of which have two cusps of almost equal size, the mandibular premolars can have more than two cusps; however, any lingual cusp is always smaller than the buccal cusp.

These mandibular premolars usually have a single root; the angulation of the roots of mandibular premolars may show slight distal inclination. The root on cervical cross section is either oval (as in ovoid or egg-shaped) or elliptical (or elongated oval); these shapes may be slightly altered by the presence of proximal root concavities (see Fig. 15.8, *B*). These proximal root concavities are most frequently found on the mesial surface of the root.

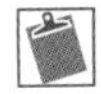 Clinical Considerations for Permanent Mandibular Premolars

Both types of mandibular premolars can present difficulties during instrumentation or restoration due to narrow lingual surfaces combined with the lingual inclination of the crown, especially with subgingival placement. In addition, patients may have difficulty performing adequate homecare because of the lingual inclination of the crown, which causes some patients to miss the cervical interface with the associated lingual gingival tissue and take care of only the occlusal surface with a toothbrush. Proximity of the nearby tongue also can make homecare procedures and instrumentation or restoration more difficult on the lingual surface.

Radiographs taken before the removal of mandibular premolars should include the mental foramen. Should a surgical flap be required

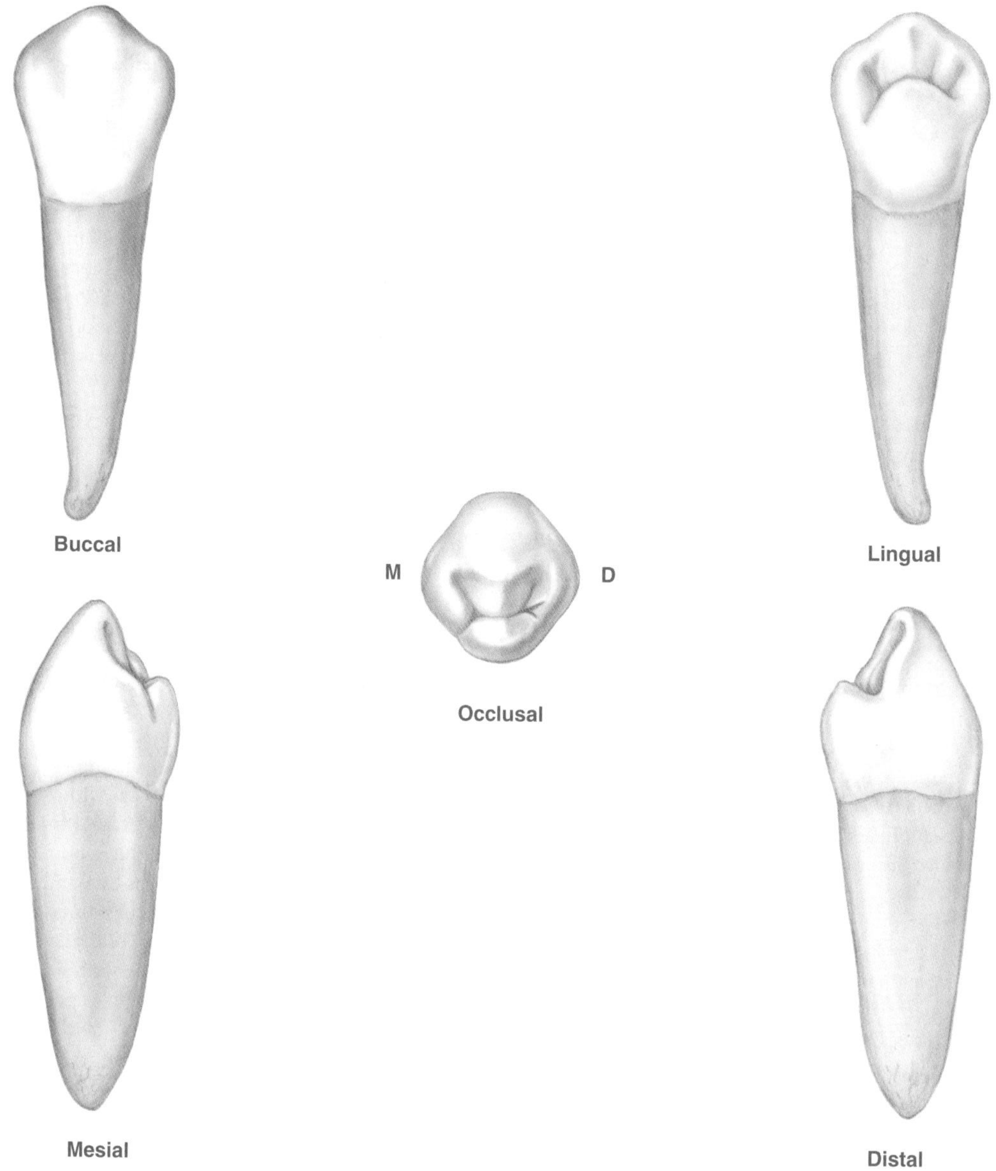

Buccal

Lingual

M

D

Occlusal

Mesial

Distal

Fig. 17.20 Views of the Permanent Mandibular Right First Premolar. *D,* Distal; *M,* mesial.

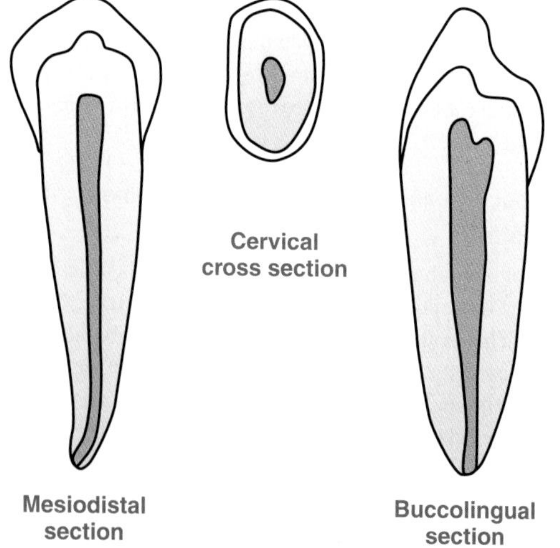

Fig. 17.21 Pulp Cavity of the Permanent Mandibular Right First Premolar.

to retrieve a premolar root, it is essential that the location of the mental foramen is known to avoid injuring the mental nerve during flap development.

Permanent Mandibular First Premolars #21 and #28 (#34 and #44)

Specific Overall Features

Permanent mandibular first premolars erupt between 10 and 12 years of age with root completion between ages 12 and 13 (Fig. 17.20). These teeth erupt distal to the permanent mandibular canines and thus are the succedaneous replacements for the primary mandibular first molars.

A mandibular first premolar resembles a mandibular canine in many more ways than it does a mandibular second premolar. This is true despite the fact that any premolar is smaller overall than a canine. However, the buccolingual width of this tooth is similar to that of a mandibular canine. Thus a mandibular first premolar shows the transition in form in the dental arch from the narrower canine to the wider molar-like second premolar.

A mandibular first premolar has a buccal cusp that is long and sharp and is the only functional cusp during occlusion, which is similar to a mandibular canine. The lingual cusp of a mandibular first premolar is usually small and nonfunctioning. The lingual cusp, then, is similar in appearance to the cingulum found on some maxillary canines but it can vary considerably. Finally, the occlusal surface of the mandibular first premolar has a similar outline and slopes sharply to the lingual and the mesiobuccal cusp ridge is shorter than the distobuccal cusp ridge; all features are similar to the mandibular canine.

A mandibular first premolar has a smaller and shorter root than a mandibular second premolar, although it is closer to the length of a second premolar than to that of a mandibular canine. The buccal aspect of the root is more conical, but the lingual aspect is tapered. A deep groove may be found on the distal root surface. The tooth occasionally has a bifurcated root with the root divided into buccal and lingual root branches.

The pulp cavity of this tooth consists of two pulp horns and a single pulp canal (Fig. 17.21). Each pulp horn is located within a cusp. The buccal pulp horn is more pronounced in form and the lingual pulp horn is smaller and less significant.

Buccal View Features

The outline of the crown of a mandibular first premolar from the buccal is almost symmetrical (see Fig. 17.20). The middle developmental lobe is visibly well developed, resulting in a prominent buccal ridge and a large pointed buccal cusp. In contrast, the buccal ridge is not as prominent as on a maxillary first premolar. Two buccal developmental depressions are often seen separating the three buccal lobes. Imbrication lines are not usually present on the buccal surface.

The buccal cusp is also located slightly to the mesial of the center of the crown, again similar to a mandibular canine. Thus the two cusp slopes of the premolar are not equal in length. The mesial cusp slope of the buccal cusp is shorter than the distal cusp slope, which *helps to distinguish the mandibular right first premolar from the left.*

The mesial outline of the mandibular first premolar is slightly concave from the mesial contact to the CEJ. The distal outline is rounder and shorter. Again the mesial contact with a mandibular canine is just cervical to the junction of the occlusal and middle thirds. The distal contact with a mandibular second premolar is the same, just cervical to the junction of the occlusal and the middle thirds.

Lingual View Features

The lingual surface is much narrower than the buccal on a mandibular first premolar, with the crown tapering to the lingual (Fig. 17.22). Most of both the mesial and distal surfaces, therefore, can be seen from the lingual. The lingual cusp is small and nonfunctional during occlusion and the lingual cusp tip is often pointed.

Because the lingual cusp is small, most of the occlusal surface can also be seen from this view. The lingual cusp tip lines up with the buccal triangular ridge. The mesial fossa and distal fossa are on each side of this ridge. A developmental groove, the mesiolingual groove, usually separates the mesial marginal ridge from the mesial cusp slope of the small lingual cusp.

Proximal View Features

From the mesial, the crown of a mandibular first premolar tilts noticeably toward the lingual at the cervix as do all mandibular posteriors (see Fig. 17.20). Thus the buccal outline is longer than the lingual outline. This lingual inclination of the crown also places the buccal cusp tip more directly over the root axis line. Thus the lingual cusp tip is usually in line vertically with the lingual surface of the cervical part of the root. The transverse ridge slopes at a 45° angle from the buccal cusp tip to the occlusal surface and then almost flattens out to the lingual cusp tip.

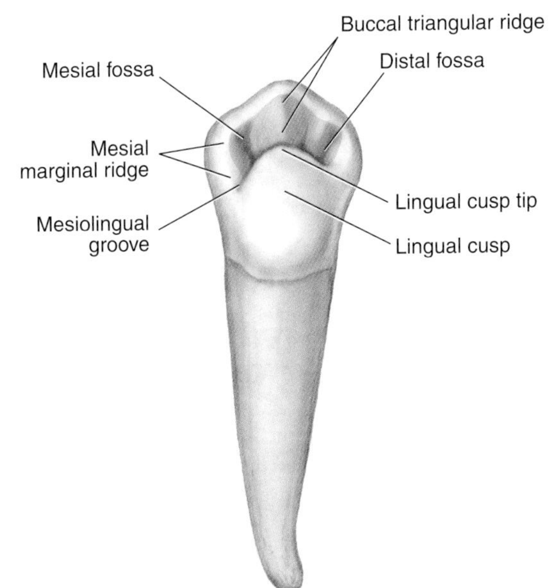

Fig. 17.22 Lingual features of the permanent mandibular right first premolar with the occlusal table highlighted.

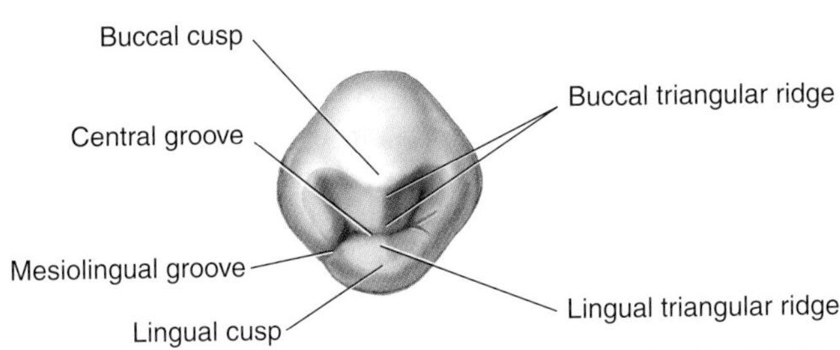

Fig. 17.23 Occlusal features of the permanent mandibular right first premolar with the occlusal table highlighted.

The mesial marginal ridge is almost parallel to the angulation of the transverse ridge at a more cervical level; the slope of the mesial marginal ridge is similar to that of anteriors. The mesiolingual groove, again, can be seen near the lingual margin. The CEJ curvature is also more occlusal on the mesial surface. Both these mesial surface features *help to distinguish the mandibular right first premolar from the left.*

The distal view of the mandibular first premolar is somewhat similar to the mesial, except for the absence of a groove near the lingual margin. And the distal marginal ridge is much more developed than that of the mesial and its continuity is unbroken by any deep developmental grooves. Additionally, the distal marginal ridge does not show quite as steep a slope toward the lingual as is present on the mesial.

Occlusal View Features

The crown outline of the mandibular first premolar is diamond-shaped from the occlusal with a notch in the mesial outline at the mesiolingual groove (Fig. 17.23). The prominent buccal ridge is located on the buccal margin. The lingual margin is much shorter than the buccal margin. The mesial margin is slightly rounded to almost straight surface, except in the area near the mesiolingual groove. The distal margin is even more rounded than the mesial margin.

Occlusal Table Components

Both the cusps and transverse ridge of the mandibular first premolar are offset to the mesial, leaving the distal part of the tooth larger than the mesial part (see Fig. 17.23). The larger and functioning buccal cusp has four buccal cusp ridges and four functioning buccal-inclined cuspal

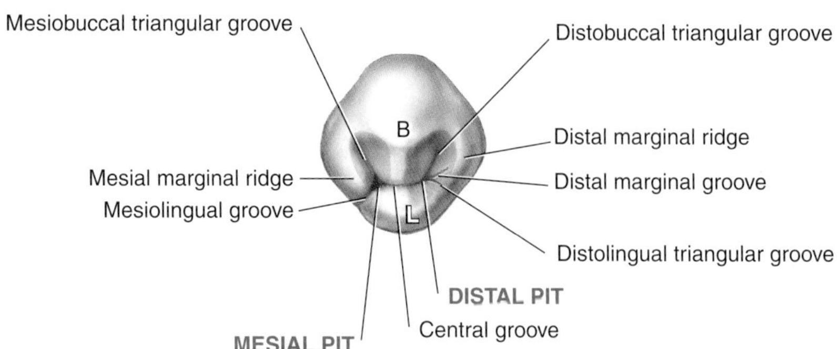

Fig. 17.24 Additional occlusal features of the permanent mandibular right first premolar with the fossae highlighted. *B*, Buccal; *L*, lingual.

planes, all of which are named for their location. The lingual cusp ridge of the buccal cusp is also considered the buccal triangular ridge.

The lingual cusp is quite small, usually no more than half the height of the buccal cusp. It also has four lingual cusp ridges and four lingual-inclined cuspal planes. The buccal cusp ridge of the buccal cusp is also considered the lingual triangular ridge.

The transverse ridge is composed of the joining of the buccal triangular ridge of the lingual cusp and the lingual triangular ridge of the buccal cusp. The buccal triangular ridge is longer than the lingual, thus making up a greater part of the transverse ridge. The transverse ridge is perpendicular to the central groove. This groove that slightly separates the two triangular ridges is sometimes rather indistinct and thus the two triangular ridges appear to be continuous.

The mesial marginal ridge closely resembles the angulation of the marginal ridges of anterior teeth, especially the canine. This is because it slopes from the buccal to the lingual at a 45° angle (Fig. 17.24). The mesial marginal ridge is less prominent and shorter than the distal marginal ridge. The distal marginal ridge also does not have quite as steep a slope toward the lingual.

The mesial fossa and distal fossa and associated deeper mesial pit and distal pit are also found on the occlusal table. The mesial fossa is shallower than the distal, and although both are circular, the mesial fossa is slightly more linear. The mesial pit is the junction of the central groove, mesiolingual groove (previously described on the lingual and mesial aspects), and mesiobuccal triangular groove (similar in location to that of the maxillary premolars). The distal pit is the junction of the central groove, distal marginal groove, distolingual triangular groove, and distobuccal triangular groove.

 Clinical Considerations for Permanent Mandibular First Premolars

When mandibular first premolars have Class I metallic (amalgam or gold) restorations that fill the both mesial and distal occlusal pits, these restorations are sometimes known as *snake eyes* because of the eye-like roundness presented (Fig. 17.25). This type of restoration can also be noted on the occlusal surface of mandibular second premolars. Tooth-colored restorative materials are now more commonly placed on the occlusal surface of these smaller posterior teeth to achieve a more esthetic appearance.

Permanent Mandibular Second Premolars #20 and #29 (#35 and #45)

Specific Overall Features

The permanent mandibular second premolars erupt between 11 and 12 years of age with root completion between ages 13 and 14 (Fig. 17.26). These teeth erupt distal to the mandibular first premolars and thus are the succedaneous replacements for the primary mandibular second molars.

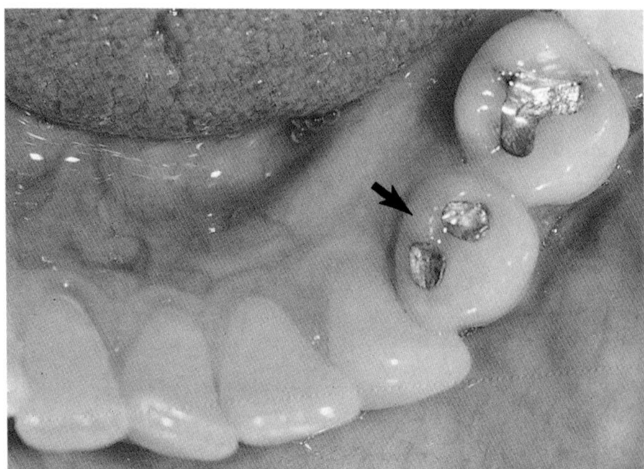

Fig. 17.25 Metallic restorations on the permanent mandibular first premolar in the oral cavity, which are considered to be like snake eyes *(arrow)*. (Courtesy of Margaret J. Fehrenbach, RDH, MS.)

There are two forms of the mandibular second premolars: three-cusp type (the tricuspidate form) and two-cusp type (the bicuspidate form; Fig. 17.27). Unlike mandibular first premolars, the more common (55% frequency) three-cusp type has three cusps: the one large buccal cusp composed of the three buccal lobes and the two smaller lingual cusps composed of the two lingual lobes (see Fig. 17.26). Thus the three-cusp type is composed of total five developmental lobes: three buccal and two lingual.

Similar to mandibular first premolars, the less common (45% frequency) two-cusp type has a larger buccal cusp and a single smaller lingual cusp (Fig. 17.28). The two-cusp type is thus composed of a total of four developmental lobes: three buccal and one lingual.

The two types of this tooth differ mostly in their occlusal features, but other surface features are similar. Both types of mandibular second premolars have more supplemental grooves than the first premolar of the same arch. The three-cusp type also appears more angular from the occlusal view and the two-cusp type appears more rounded.

Although a mandibular first premolar resembles a mandibular canine, the more common three-cusp type of mandibular second premolar resembles a small molar because its lingual cusps are well developed, which places both marginal ridges horizontal and superior on the occlusal table. A more efficient occlusion thus results with the premolars in the opposite arch, which is similar to the molars. A mandibular second premolar thus represents the transition in form from a narrow canine-like first premolar to the wider molars.

The single root of a mandibular second premolar is larger and longer than that of a first premolar but shorter than both types of maxillary premolars. Proximal root concavities are pronounced. In addition, the apex of this tooth is blunter than that of a first molar or of the maxillary premolars.

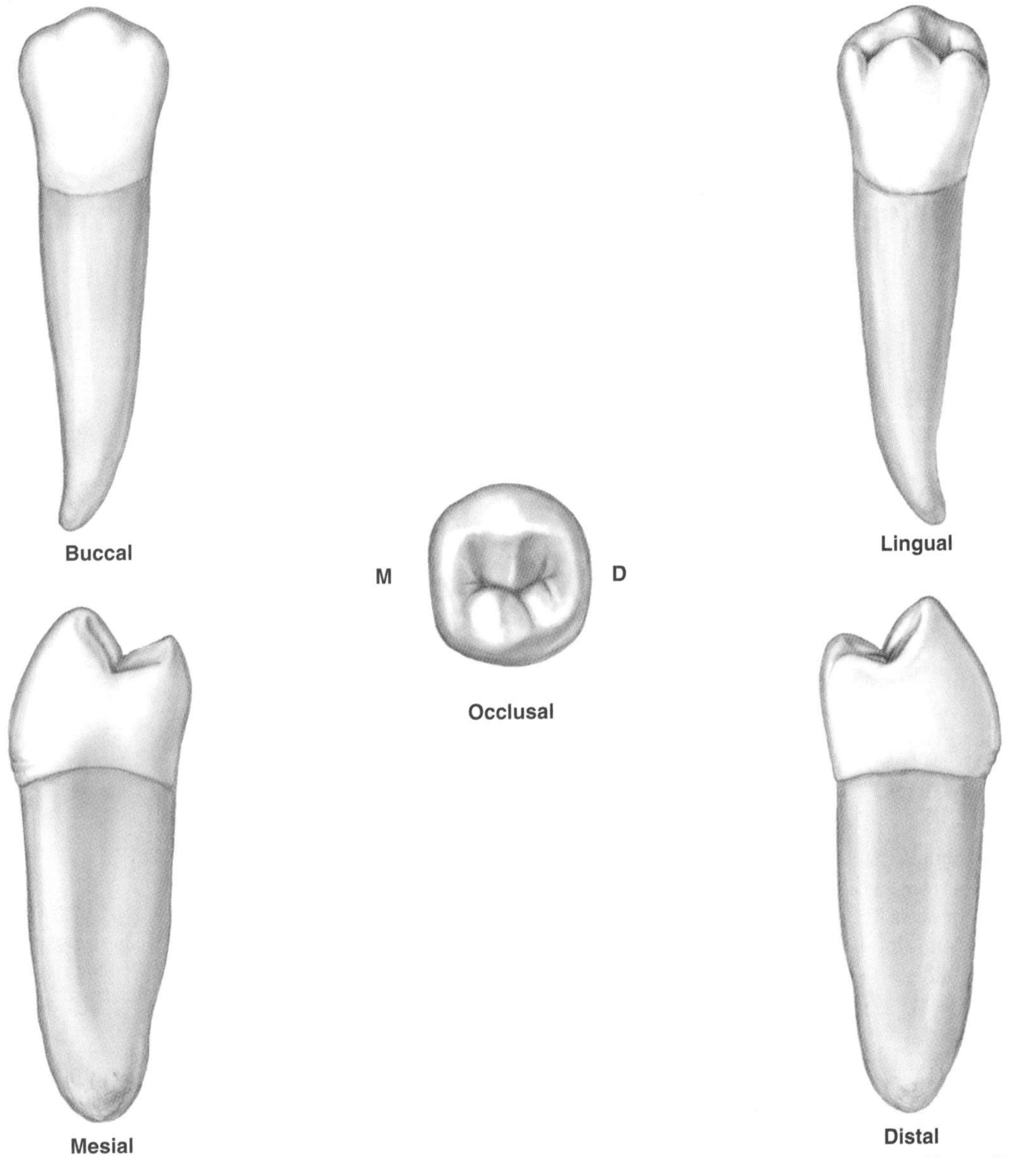

Buccal

Lingual

M

D

Occlusal

Mesial

Distal

Fig. 17.26 Views of the Permanent Mandibular Right Second Premolar of the Three-Cusp Type. *D,* Distal; *M,* mesial.

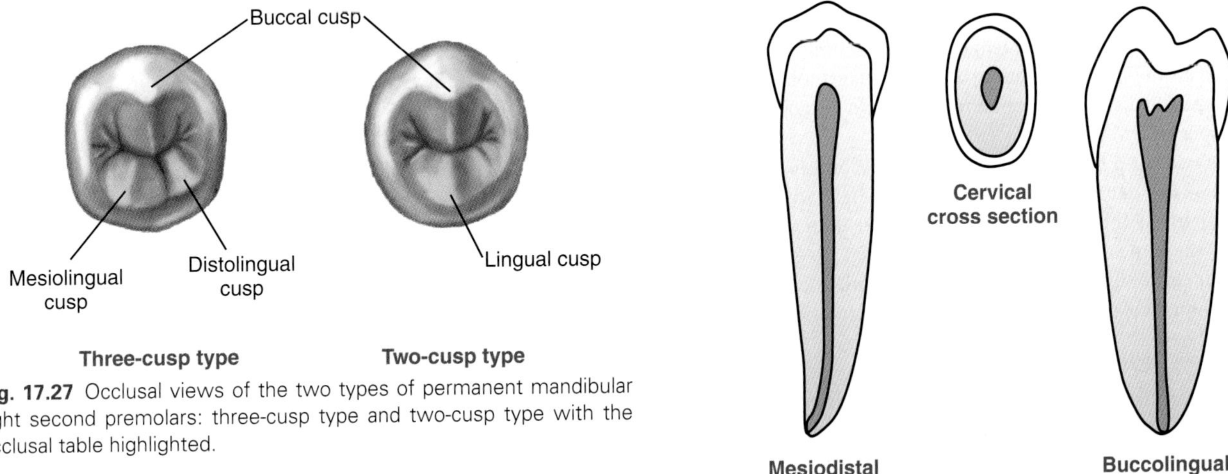

Fig. 17.27 Occlusal views of the two types of permanent mandibular right second premolars: three-cusp type and two-cusp type with the occlusal table highlighted.

Fig. 17.28 Pulp Cavity of the Permanent Mandibular Right Second Premolar of the Three-Cusp Type.

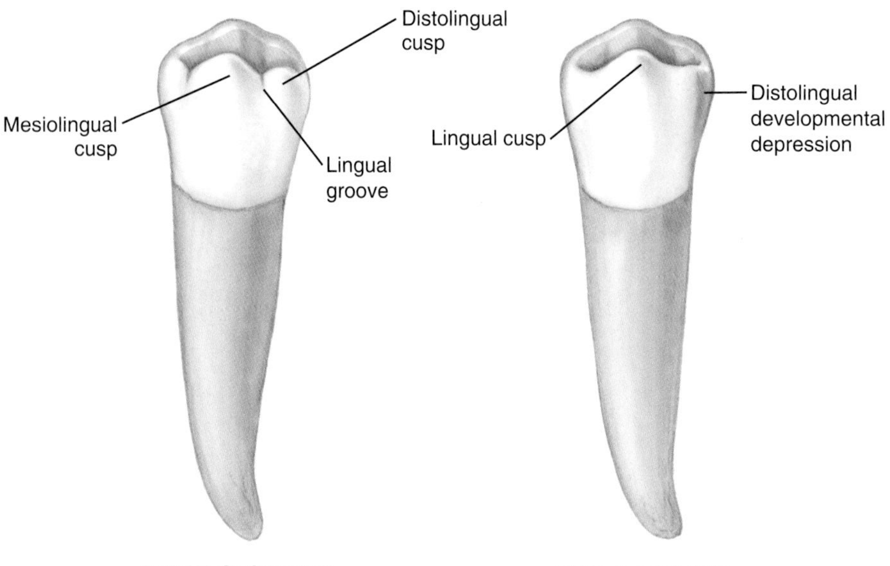

Fig. 17.29 Lingual views of both types of permanent mandibular right second premolars with the occlusal table highlighted.

The pulp cavity of the three-cusp type shows three pointed pulp horns (see Fig. 17.28). In contrasts, two pulp horns are present with the two-cusp type. No matter the number of pulp horns, all pulp horns are more pointed in the mandibular second premolar than the first.

Buccal View Features

A mandibular second premolar has a shorter buccal cusp than does a mandibular first premolar (see Fig. 17.26). The cusp slopes of the buccal cusp are also more rounded. The mesial contact and distal contact are both wide and at the same location, just cervical to the junction of the occlusal and middle thirds.

Lingual View Features

From the lingual, a mandibular second premolar shows considerable differences from a first premolar (Fig. 17.29). The lingual cusp or cusps, depending on the type, are longer. Thus less of the occlusal surface can be seen from this view. Because the lingual cusp is still smaller than the buccal cusp, however, a small part of the buccal margin of the occlusal surface may be seen.

And the differences between its two types can also be noted. In the three-cusp type, the mesiolingual cusp is wider and longer than the distolingual cusp. A developmental groove, the lingual groove, is located between the cusps, extending a short distance on the lingual surface and usually distal to the center of the crown because the mesiolingual cusp is wider.

With the two-cusp type of the mandibular second premolar, the single lingual cusp development is at an equal height with the mesiolingual cusp of the three-cusp type but is higher than that of a first premolar of the same arch. The two-cusp type has no groove noted lingually but does show a distolingual developmental depression where the lingual cusp ridge joins the distal marginal ridge.

Proximal View Features

From the mesial, a mandibular second premolar has a shorter buccal cusp and is located more to the buccal than a first premolar (see Fig. 17.26). Therefore, the distance between the cusp tips of this tooth is shorter than for the first. In addition, the crown is wider buccolingually and the lingual cusp or cusps are larger. The mesial marginal ridge is perpendicular or 90° to the long axis of the tooth. There is no mesiolingual groove.

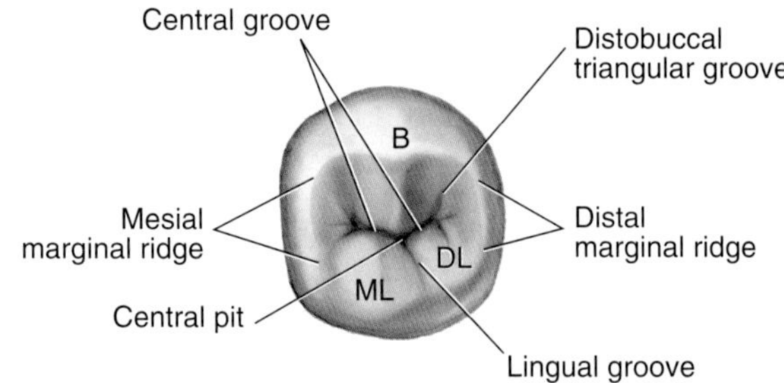

Fig. 17.30 Occlusal view of the three-cusp type of permanent mandibular right second premolar showing the Y-shaped groove pattern with the occlusal table highlighted. *B,* Buccal; *DL,* distolingual; *ML,* mesiolingual.

The distal view is similar, although more of the occlusal surface can be seen from this view because the distal marginal ridge is more cervically located than the mesial marginal ridge, which *helps to distinguish the mandibular right second premolar from the left.*

Occlusal View Features

The general shape of the crown outline of a mandibular second premolar is more nearly square, especially in the three-cusp type, than a mandibular first premolar (see Fig. 17.26). The convergence of the mesial and distal margins toward the lingual is equally severe.

Occlusal Table Components

In both the three-cusp and two-cusp types of mandibular second premolar, the buccal cusp is similar. Thus the two types are the same in that part of the occlusal table, which is buccal to the mesiobuccal and distobuccal cusp ridges. Each of the cusps has buccal ridges, triangular ridges, and cuspal inclined planes, which are each named for their location and orientation.

On the three-cusp type, the cusps are separated by two developmental grooves, a V-shaped central groove and a linear lingual groove (Fig. 17.30). The lingual groove extends lingually between the two lingual cusps and ends on the lingual surface of the crown just below the meeting of the lingual cusp ridges. These two grooves together form a distinctive Y-shaped groove pattern on the occlusal table.

On the three-cusp type, a deep central pit is located at the junction of the central groove and the lingual groove toward the lingual. The central

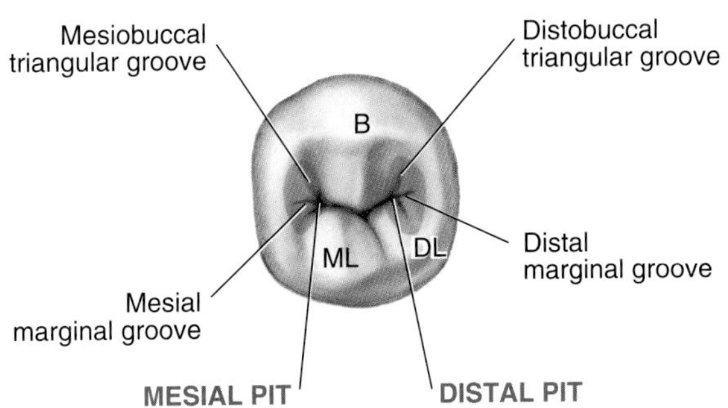

Fig. 17.31 Additional occlusal features of the three-cusp type of permanent mandibular right second premolar with the fossae highlighted. *B*, Buccal; *DL*, distolingual; *ML*, mesiolingual.

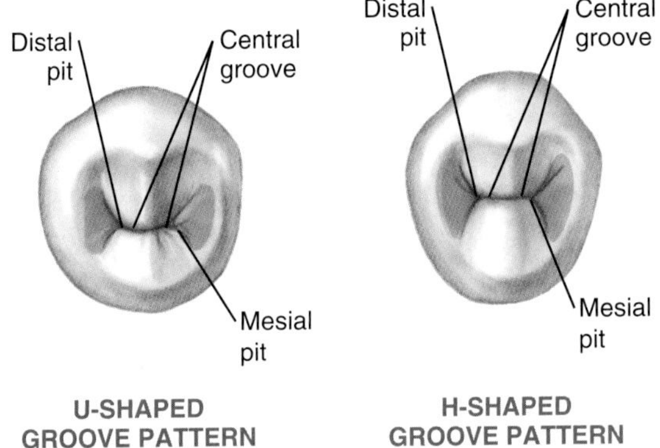

Fig. 17.32 Occlusal views of the two-cusp type of permanent mandibular right second premolar showing both the U-shaped and H-shaped groove patterns with the fossae highlighted.

pit is also more to the distal between the mesial marginal ridge and distal marginal ridge because the mesiolingual cusp is wider than the distolingual cusp. Some anatomists prefer to separate the central groove on this tooth into two grooves: a mesial groove and a distal groove.

On the three-cusp type of a second mandibular premolar, the mesial part of the central groove travels in a mesiobuccal direction and ends in a mesial pit surrounded by a mesial triangular fossa just distal to the mesial marginal ridge, which is often crossed by a mesial marginal groove (Fig. 17.31). The distal part of the central groove travels in a distobuccal direction, is slightly shorter than the mesial groove, and ends in a distal pit surrounded by a distal triangular fossa mesial to the distal marginal ridge.

These triangular fossae are shallow, irregularly shaped, but overall more linear in form than the triangular fossae of the maxillary premolars. In addition, a mesiobuccal triangular groove, which extends into the mesial pit, is on the occlusal table. The distobuccal triangular groove, distolingual triangular groove, and possibly a distal marginal groove also extend into the distal pit.

In contrast, the two-cusp type is rounder lingual to the buccal cusp ridges (Fig. 17.32). The mesial and distal margins converge slightly, making the lingual part narrower than the buccal, but never to the degree of a mandibular first premolar. The larger and longer buccal cusp is seen directly opposite the smaller and shorter lingual cusp. On the two-cusp type, a central groove on the occlusal table travels in a mesiodistal direction.

The central groove is most often cresent-shaped, forming a U-shaped groove pattern on the occlusal table. Less often, the central groove may be straight, forming an H-shaped groove pattern on the occlusal table. The lingual cusp of the type with the H-shaped groove pattern is larger and sharper than the one with the U-shaped groove pattern and is often offset to the mesial. The buccal cusp for both occlusal groove patterns of the two-cusp type has four functional inclined planes during occlusion and the lingual cusp has two.

The central groove of the two-cusp type with either groove pattern has its terminal ends centered in the mesial fossa and distal fossa, which are circular depressions having supplemental grooves radiating from them. Some two-cusp types have a mesial pit and a distal pit centered in mesial and distal fossae instead of an unbroken central groove; most have a distolingual developmental depression crossing the distolingual cusp ridge. None of the two-cusp types have a lingual groove or central pit.

Clinical Considerations for Permanent Mandibular Second Premolars

With any premature loss of a primary mandibular second molar, the developing permanent mandibular first molar inclines and drifts mesially in a mixed dentition. The developing permanent mandibular second premolar is prevented from eruption because its arch leeway space is almost closed (see Fig. 20.3). This situation can allow the mandibular second premolar to become impacted against the first molar. An impacted tooth is an unerupted or partially erupted tooth that is positioned against another tooth, bone, or even soft tissue, making complete eruption unlikely. Additionally, the leeway space can be compromised if the permanent mandibular second molars erupt before the mandibular second premolars, the arch perimeter is now significantly shortened and occlusal disharmony is likely to occur as with a malocclusion. These complications may be prevented by careful evaluation of patients with mixed dentition and use of interceptive orthodontic therapy, such as with space maintainers and tooth replacement.

Permanent mandibular second premolars are also commonly involved in partial anodontia and thus may be congenitally missing (see Box 6.1, *B*). With this disturbance, the appropriate individual tooth germ(s) in the area is absent because of failure of the initiation process during tooth development; this condition can be bilateral or unilateral. A careful patient evaluation needs to be performed when primary mandibular second molars are retained either in a mixed or permanent dentition, including radiographs. Missing permanent teeth may require prosthetic replacement (such as an implant) because they can result in complications with spacing and occlusion.

However, these retained primary molars, without the presence of the underlying succedaneous permanent teeth may not be shed for many years. Thus these primary teeth can serve as functioning stand-ins for the permanent premolar teeth and should not be extracted unless they are involved in caries, root pathology, or are uncomfortably mobile.

PERMANENT MOLARS

GENERAL FEATURES OF PERMANENT MOLARS

Permanent molars are the most posteriorly placed posterior teeth of the permanent dentition, distal to the premolars (Fig. 17.33). Molars are also the largest teeth in the dentition. Each dental arch usually has six molars with three in each quadrant, if all have erupted. Maxillary and mandibular molars differ greatly from each other in shape, size, and numbers of cusps and roots. The name *molar* means *grinder*, which is one of the functions of the molar teeth.

There are three types of molars: first molars, second molars, and third molars. The first molars and second molars are often considered the *6-year molars* and *12-year molars*, respectively, because of their eruption times.

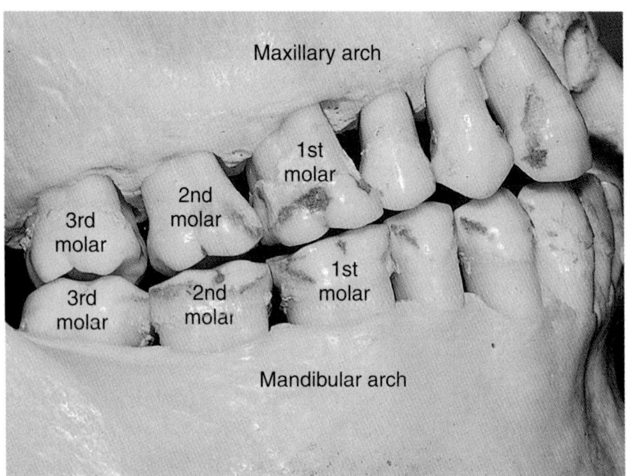

Fig. 17.33 **Permanent Molars Identified per Arch on a Skull.** (Courtesy of Margaret J. Fehrenbach, RDH, MS.)

The third molars, also known as the *wisdom teeth* by patients, are extremely variable in their eruption time as well as in their anatomic size and form. They were given this unusual reference in ancient times when it was thought that only educated men had this important type of molar. Many dental professionals jokingly argue against the wisdom sometimes shown in newly minted young adults, given that these teeth erupt between 17 and 21 years of age. Eruption of the third molars usually marks the end of the growth of the jaws.

Only the permanent dentition has three types of molars; the primary dentition only has two types. One of each type of molar is present in each quadrant of each dental arch. The first molars are closer to the midline, at the sixth position from it. And at the same time, they are distal to the permanent second premolars when full eruption of the permanent dentition has occurred. The second molars are distal to the first molars and are in the seventh position from the midline. Finally, the third molars are distal to the second molars and are in the eighth position from the midline.

All three types of molars erupt in order distal to the primary second molars, long after all the primary teeth have erupted and are functioning. Thus all the permanent molars are nonsuccedaneous because they do not replace any primary teeth. These teeth usually have enough space as they progressively erupt because of the continued elongation of the facial bones during development (except in some cases for third molars as discussed later).

Having the largest and strongest crowns of the permanent dentition, the molars, assisted by the premolars, function in grinding food during mastication. This grinding function is possible because molars have wide occlusal surfaces with prominent cusps; the molars have more cusps than do the other teeth. These teeth also support the soft tissue of the cheek, especially the facial muscles, because they maintain the height of the lower third of the vertical dimension of the face and alveolar process. Thus the molars are involved in both esthetics and speech but less so than the premolars due to their more posterior position. When viewed from the buccal or lingual, the molars' crown outline for both arches is trapezoidal or four-sided with only two parallel sides; the longer of the two parallel sides is toward the occlusal surface (see Table 15.4).

The first molar is overall the largest and the second and third are each progressively smaller. Each molar has an extremely large crown compared with the rest of the permanent dentition, but the crown is shorter occlusocervically in contrast to the teeth anterior to it. Each buccal surface of a molar has a prominent **cervical ridge** in the cervical one-third running mesiodistally.

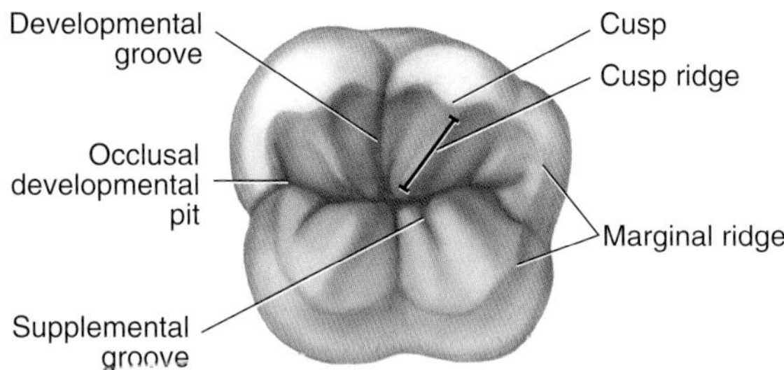

Fig. 17.34 **Occlusal View of a Permanent Molar with the Occlusal Table Highlighted.**

Like all posterior teeth, molars have an occlusal surface with usually three or more cusps of which at least two are buccal cusps (Fig. 17.34). Unlike anterior teeth and premolars, molars do not exhibit buccal developmental depressions. Evidence of developmental lobe separation is in the developmental grooves on the occlusal table.

In addition to having cusps, the occlusal table of the molar is bordered by its cusp ridges and marginal ridges. The occlusal table of molars is even more complex than that of premolars because it has more developmental grooves, supplemental grooves, and occlusal pits.

Grooves and pits are located not only on the occlusal surface of both maxillary and mandibular molars but also on the lingual surfaces of maxillary molars and buccal surfaces of mandibular molars, in some cases.

In addition, molars usually are multirooted. Maxillary molars usually have three root branches (trifurcated) and mandibular molars have two (bifurcated) (see Fig. 17.7). Molars, like other teeth, originate as a single root on the base of the crown, which is considered the root trunk. The cervical cross section of root trunk follows the form of the crown, but the root then divides from the root trunk into the number of root branches for its type (see Fig. 6.21 and see Fig. 15.8, *B*). Multiple roots give molars increased periodontal support.

As discussed earlier in this chapter, an area between two or more of these root branches before they divide from the root trunk is a furcation (see Fig. 17.7 and Table 17.1). The spaces between the roots at the furcation are the furcation crotches. Teeth with two roots (such as mandibular molars) have two furcation crotches; teeth with three roots (such as maxillary molars) have three furcation crotches. Such crotches can be located on either the buccal surfaces and the lingual surfaces or on the buccal, mesial, and distal surfaces depending on tooth type, each with a slightly different individual configuration. The furcation crotches may be close to the CEJ or far from it. Root concavities are also found on many of the root branches of molar teeth as well as on the associated furcal surfaces. In a molar, the pulp canals join the deeper pulp chamber apical to the CEJ. With periodontal health, these features of the root(s) are covered by the alveolar process as well as overlying gingival tissue.

Clinical Considerations for Permanent Molars

Even though it is a somewhat common procedure during adolescence, third molar removal remains a controversial procedure. Still it is felt that around 25% of patients need to have their third molars removed before age 25. Often patients are not aware of any difficulties associated with their third molars. More than 40% of adult patients who never had their third molars removed during adolescence may develop infection, caries, cyst formation, or associated periodontal disease by age 45, thus requiring extraction. But the risk of surgical complications in adults with removal is increased by approximately 30% compared with adolescents. However, automatically removing healthy and functioning third molars is not the norm if they are not causing any overriding complications; this can also be true of healthy impacted third molars.

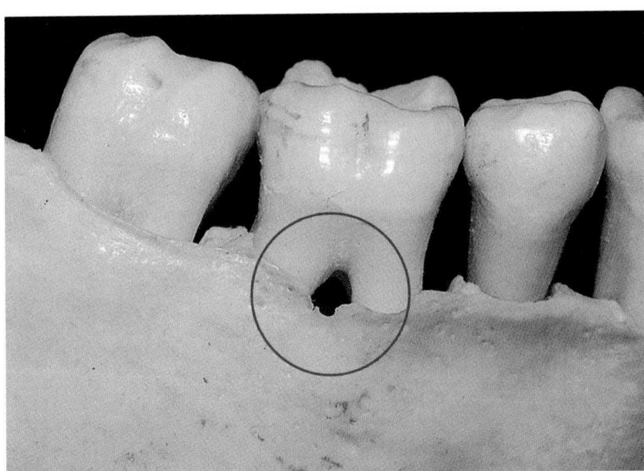

Fig. 17.35 Exposed root surface on the permanent mandibular first molar of a skull due to advanced periodontal disease, which also exposed the buccal furcation and buccal furcation crotch *(circled)*. (Courtesy of Margaret J. Fehrenbach, RDH, MS.)

Although third molars have been related with crowding, most studies do not show any relationship. Thus, an evaluation of the third molars by age 25 is usually recommended.

With periodontitis, the root features of furcations, furcation crotches, and root concavities of the molars can lose their periodontal support in varying degrees resulting in furcation involvement (Fig. 17.35; see Table 17.1). The horizontal component of a furcation invasion can be measured and classified by using a Nabors probe within a periodontal pocket because if gingival recession has occurred, they can become clinically exposed. Dental biofilm and other deposits can be retained in the exposed furcation crotches and root concavities, leading to further periodontal disease. Molars are lost to advanced periodontal disease more than single rooted teeth partially due to the presence of furcations. The cervical ridge on molars also presents challenges during instrumentation or restoration around the cervical area.

Performing periodontal debridement of roots and associated furcations involves a set instrumentation treatment plan; the best approach is to treat each root as a separate tooth when access permits, with a combination of strokes using instruments, air polisher, or ultrasonic device. The distal surface is instrumented first, followed by the buccal, lingual, and mesial surfaces. Lastly, the concavity is debrided. Furcation involvement should be suspected in the presence of a 4-mm periodontal probe reading on a multirooted tooth adjacent to a buccal or lingual furcation. In some cases, especially with mandibular molars where the bifurcation is located only 3 mm from the cervical line, invasion can occur in the early stages of periodontitis with attachment loss of only 2 to 4 mm.

Therefore, furcation crotches and root concavities on these molars present a challenge during both instrumentation and performance of homecare in the area due to lack of access. Approximately half of molar furcations are too narrow for access even by instruments or devices, decreasing the prognosis of therapy if periodontally involved. To allow better access, the furcations of a tooth may be reduced by minor odontoplasty and any occluding gingival tissue is removed during surgical intervention. In addition, when roots are extremely close to each other, access to interproximals may be even more difficult.

Finally, awareness of root trunk dimensions and their relationship to the furcations is critical to the periodontal prognosis of a molar. There is also a strong correlation between length of the root trunk and furcation invasion by advanced periodontal disease. Short root trunks are most commonly found buccally on both maxillary and mandibular molars, whereas long root trunks are more commonly found mesially in both maxillary molars. Additionally, short root length is associated with longer root trunks and these long root trunks are more commonly found on the second molars than on the first molars.

Permanent molar teeth may have one or more tubercles (or accessory cusps) on the occlusal surface. In addition, similar to incisors, the molars may be affected in children with congenital syphilis. The spirochete *Treponema pallidum*, a sexually transmitted microorganism, is passed from an infected pregnant woman to her fetus via the placenta. This microorganism may cause localized enamel hypoplasia and result in **mulberry molars** (**muhl**-ber-ee), a disturbance that occurs during tooth development (see Fig. 3.17, *B*). This tooth has a crown with an abnormally shaped occlusal surface characterized by berry-like nodules or tubercles of enamel instead of cusps. Affected children may also have other developmental anomalies, such as blindness, deafness, and paralysis caused by congenital syphilis. Treatment using full-coverage crowns may be performed to improve the appearance of these teeth.

Another developmental disturbance associated mostly with molars is the enamel pearl (see Box 6.1, *R*, *S*). Mainly found on the buccal surfaces of second molars, these deposits of enamel apical to the level on the CEJ have a tapered form and extend into root furcation areas. They are present on over 28% of maxillary and 17% of mandibular molars and on most mandibular molars with isolated furcation involvement. These teeth were also found to have deeper root concavities compared with teeth that lacked cervical enamel projections. Unlike calculus, which it somewhat resembles radiographically, the enamel pearl cannot be removed by instrumentation. Instead, it must undergo minor odontoplasty to restore the contour of the tooth.

Finally, dilaceration of the root(s) can also occur, making extraction and endodontic treatment challenging (Fig. 17.36; see **Chapter 6**). Another developmental disturbance that can be present is root fusion, which creates deep developmental grooves when the molar roots fuse. These can function as hidden niches to accumulate deposits that are not easily accessible to either periodontal therapy or homecare procedures. The highest prevalence of permanent molars with root fusion occurs in maxillary second molars, followed by mandibular second molars, maxillary first molars, and finally, mandibular first molars; women present an overall higher incidence of root fusion than men.

PERMANENT MAXILLARY MOLARS

General Features

Permanent maxillary molars erupt between 6 months and 1 year after the corresponding permanent mandibular molars (Table 17.3; see Figs. 17.39, 17.44, and 17.47). They are usually the first permanent teeth to erupt into the maxillary arch. In addition, maxillary molars are overall the largest and strongest teeth of the maxillary arch. They are usually shorter occlusocervically than are the crowns of teeth anterior to them, but they are larger still in all other measurements compared to other maxillary teeth.

All maxillary molars are wider buccolingually than mesiodistally; in contrast, the mandibular molars are wider mesiodistally. From the occlusal, the outline of the crown of maxillary molars is rhomboidal or four-sided with opposite sides parallel. Like all maxillary posteriors, the crown outline is trapezoidal from each proximal view, again four-sided but with only two parallel sides (see Table 15.4). In addition, the crown is also centered over the root and shows no lingual inclination, similar to maxillary premolars, but unlike mandibular molars.

Each maxillary molar usually has four major cusps with two cusps on the buccal part of the occlusal table and two on the lingual (Fig. 17.37). An **oblique ridge** is a unique feature present on the occlusal table of most maxillary molars except the third molar. This type of transverse ridge crosses the occlusal table obliquely, forming by the

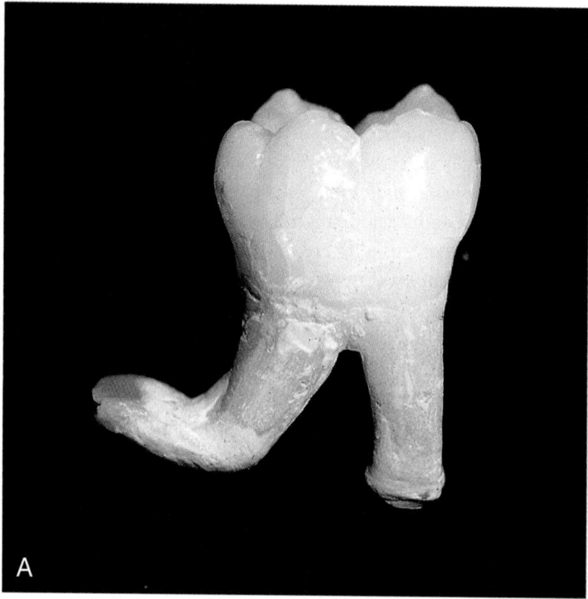

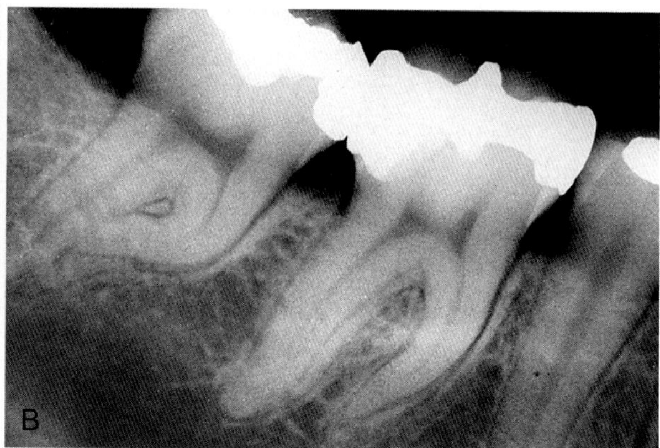

Fig. 17.36 Dilaceration of **(A)** an extracted permanent mandibular first molar and **(B)** permanent mandibular second molar on a radiograph. **(A,** Courtesy of Dr. Rudy Melfi. B, From Ibsen OAC, Phelan JA. *Oral Pathology for Dental Hygienists*. 7th ed. St. Louis: Elsevier; 2018.)

TABLE 17.3 Permanent Maxillary Molars

	Maxillary First Molar	Maxillary Second Molar	Maxillary Third Molar
Universal number	#3 and #14	#2 and #15	#1 and #16
International number	#16 and #26	#17 and #27	#18 and #28
General crown features	Occlusal table with marginal ridges and cusps with tips, inclined planes, ridges, grooves, fossae, pits		
	Buccal cervical ridge		
Specific crown features	Largest tooth in arch and largest crown in dentition. Prominent oblique ridge. Four major cusps, with buccal cusps almost equal in height. Fifth minor cusp of Carabelli associated with mesiolingual cusp	Smaller crown than first. Heart-shaped or rhomboidal crown outline, with three or four cusps. Less prominent oblique ridge. Mesiobuccal cusp longer than distobuccal cusp. Distolingual cusp smaller than on first or absent. No fifth cusp	Smaller crown than second and variable in form. Heart-shaped or rhomboidal crown outline, with three or four cusps
Mesial contact*	Junction of occlusal and middle thirds	Middle third	Middle third
Distal contact*	Middle third	Middle third	None
Distinguish right from left	Mesiolingual cusp outline longer and larger but not as sharp as distolingual cusp outline		Distobuccal cusp shorter than mesiobuccal cusp. Roots curve distally
General root features	Three roots		
Specific root features	Furcations well removed from CEJ. Root trunks and root concavities.		Usually fused roots, curving distally
	Divergent roots		Less divergent roots

*Height of contour of posteriors for the buccal is in cervical third and lingual in middle third.
CEJ, Cementoenamel junction.

union of the triangular ridge of the distobuccal cusp and distal cusp ridge of the mesiolingual cusp. In contrast, an oblique ridge is never present on mandibular molars.

Maxillary molars usually have three root branches or are trifurcated, unlike mandibular molars, which usually have only two root branches because they are bifurcated (see Fig. 17.7). These roots of the maxillary molar include: the mesiobuccal, distobuccal, and lingual (or palatal). The lingual root is usually the largest and longest for all these molars.

The farther distal a molar is in the maxillary arch, the shorter as well as more varied in size, shape, and curvature are the roots. The roots also become less divergent (or divided) on the teeth located farther distally, being less parallel with each other. Thus a first molar has longer, more divergent roots than a third molar and has more consistency in the root's size, shape, and curvature. Roots of maxillary molars show increased lingual inclination but only moderate distal inclination.

Because maxillary molars are trifurcated, there are usually three furcations, which are located on the buccal, mesial, and distal surfaces (see Fig. 17.7 and Table 17.1). All furcations on maxillary teeth usually begin near the junction of the cervical and middle thirds of the root. The buccal furcation is located midway between the mesial and distal surfaces. The mesial and distal furcations are both located more to the lingual than the buccal surface. Root concavities are found on the mesial surface of the mesiobuccal root, the lingual surface of the lingual root, and all three furcal surfaces.

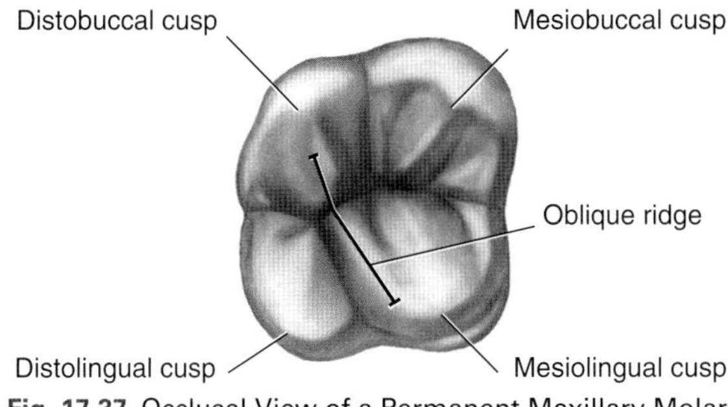

Fig. 17.37 Occlusal View of a Permanent Maxillary Molar.

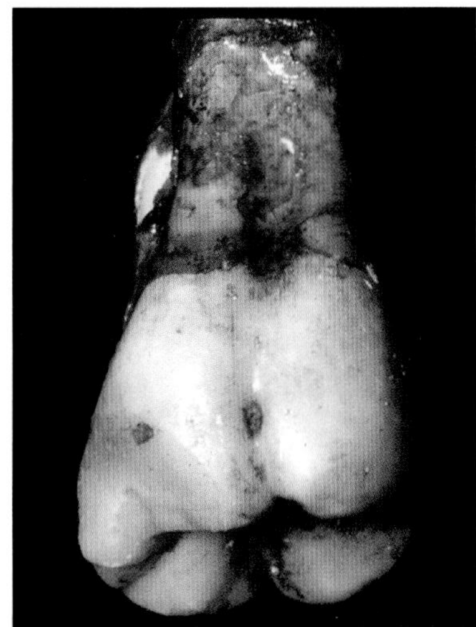

Fig. 17.38 Lingual Pit on an Extracted Permanent Maxillary First Molar. (Courtesy of Margaret J. Fehrenbach, RDH, MS.)

Clinical Considerations for Permanent Maxillary Molars

A possible lingual pit on the lingual surface of maxillary molars is at an increased risk of caries (Fig. 17.38). This is due to both increased dental biofilm retention and the thinness of enamel forming the walls of the pit (see **Chapter 12**). An enamel sealant could be placed on the lingual pit of the erupting teeth. However, because of the histology of enamel in the area, enamel sealants do not bond as easily on any lingual surface as on the occlusal surface so a full restoration procedure may be needed. A tooth-colored restorative material can be used to achieve a more esthetic appearance and provide protection or even to repair caries; thus the past presence of the lingual pit may not now be easy to discern clinically.

The roots of maxillary molars may penetrate the middle and posterior parts of the maxillary sinus as a result of accidental trauma or during tooth extraction because of the close relation of these roots to the sinus walls, as can occur with other maxillary posteriors (see Fig. 11.22). To complicate matters, the discomfort of sinusitis can be mistakenly interpreted as tooth-related from the maxillary molars and vice versa. Thus, radiographs of the questionable tooth and maxillary sinus as well as other diagnostic tests become necessary to determine the cause of the discomfort in this area. CBCT images are often useful in these circumstances.

Also due to the arch position of maxillary molars and with the natural overhang of the cheek, instrumentation, restoration, and homecare of the buccal surface may be difficult. In addition, furcation entrances of the maxillary molars can be very narrow, making access limited when desired.

Maxillary molars are some of the most common teeth of the permanent dentition to be involved in concrescence (see Box 6.1, Q). Concrescence is the union of the root structure of two or more teeth through the cementum only. The teeth involved are initially separate but join because of excessive cementum deposition surrounding one or more teeth following eruption. It occurs as a result of traumatic injury or crowding of the teeth in the area during the stages of apposition and maturation of tooth development. This disturbance may present complications during extraction and endodontic treatment; thus preoperative radiographs are important.

Permanent Maxillary First Molars #3 and #14 (#16 and #26)

Specific Overall Features

Permanent maxillary first molars erupt between 6 and 7 years of age with root completion between ages 9 and 10 (Fig. 17.39). Thus these teeth are the first permanent teeth to erupt into the maxillary arch. They erupt distal to the primary maxillary second molars and thus are nonsuccedaneous, having no primary predecessors.

The maxillary first molar is the largest tooth in the maxillary arch as well as having the largest crown in the permanent dentition. It has a much more complex crown form than the nearby maxillary premolars. However, of all the maxillary molars, the first is the least variable in form.

This tooth is composed of five developmental lobes: two buccal and three lingual. These are named in the same manner as their associated cusps: mesiobuccal, distobuccal, mesiolingual, distolingual; an additional minor cusp may be located on the lingual surface (discussed later). Evidence of lobe separation can be found in the developmental grooves on the occlusal surface.

The roots of maxillary first molars are larger and more divergent than those of the second molars as well as more complex in form than those of the maxillary premolars. The roots are also twice as long as the crown. The lingual (or palatal) root is the largest and longest, inclining lingually to extend beyond the crown outline. It has a banana-like curvature toward the buccal. A vertical depression may be present on the direct palatal surface of the root that is more pronounced at the cervical third.

The mesiobuccal root is the second largest and longest and is inclined both mesially and buccally, having its apical third curve distally. The distobuccal root is the smallest, shortest, and thus the weakest of the three. This root inclines both distally and buccally, having its apical one-third curve mesially. Both the mesiobuccal and distobuccal roots have an extreme curvature that when viewed together makes them look like the handles on a set of pliers.

The furcations of the maxillary first molar are well removed from the CEJ of the tooth (see Table 17.1). But the concavity depths are only 0.1 to 0.75 mm, limiting homecare procedures and instrumentation (see earlier discussion). The midway-placed buccal furcation on the buccal surface is about 4 mm apical to the CEJ.

The mesial furcation is located two-thirds of the way across the mesial surface from the buccal aspect or one-third of the way from the lingual aspect due to the large mesiobuccal root. Thus the mesial furcation is not centered and it is wider buccolingually than mesiodistally; its entrance is dictated by the size of mesiobuccal root. The mesial furcation is 3 mm from the CEJ; a better approach for homecare procedures and instrumentation is from the lingual aspect.

The distal furcation is 5 mm from the CEJ; it is located halfway between the buccal and lingual on the distal surface. Approach for homecare procedures and instrumentation is first from the buccal aspect and then from the lingual aspect. The distal furcation is predisposed to develop periodontal disease due to the proximity of the divergent distobuccal root to the adjacent second molar, limiting access to its already narrow furcation entrance.

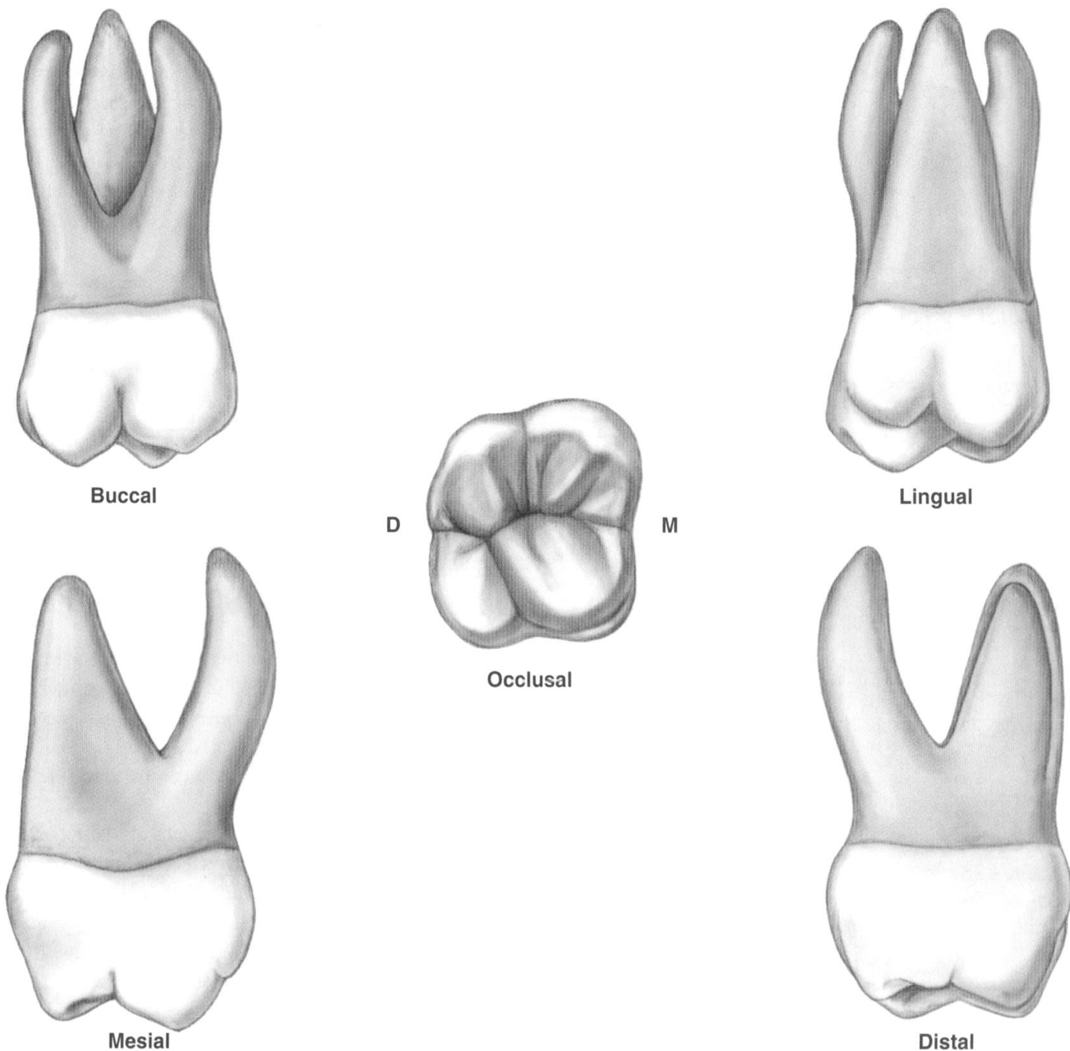

Fig. 17.39 Views of the Permanent Maxillary Right First Molar. *D,* Distal; *M,* mesial.

The pulp cavity of a maxillary first molar usually has one pulp horn for each major cusp (Fig. 17.40). Thus the four pulp horns include the mesiobuccal, distobuccal, mesiolingual, and distolingual. Three main pulp canals are usually present, one for each of the three roots. The lingual pulp canal is the largest, the distobuccal is the smallest, and the mesiobuccal is between these two in size. The tooth sometimes has four pulp canals with two pulp canals in the mesiobuccal root.

Buccal View Features

The general shape of a maxillary first molar from this view is trapezoidal, with the longer parallel side toward the occlusal (see Fig. 17.39 and Table 15.4). The entire buccal surface is larger than that of the adjacent premolar. Despite this fact, the occlusocervical measurement is slightly smaller.

Parts of all four major and functioning cusps seen from this view include: the mesiobuccal cusp, distobuccal cusp, mesiolingual cusp, and distolingual cusp. This is because the two lingual cusps are slightly offset to the distal relative to the buccal cusps. The occlusal outline of the mesiobuccal cusp is wider, but the distobuccal cusp tip is sharper. However, the two buccal cusps are almost the same height and the mesiolingual cusp tip is noted between them.

The occlusal outline of a maxillary first molar is divided symmetrically by the buccal groove. This developmental groove extends between the two buccal cusps and overall is parallel to the long axis of the tooth. It then runs apically about halfway to the CEJ, where it can fade out or end in a buccal pit or even end in two short slanting grooves, with or without a buccal pit.

The mesial outline is flat from the CEJ occlusally to the mesial contact. The mesial contact is at the junction of the occlusal and middle thirds. This mesial contact is initially with a primary maxillary second molar until that tooth is shed; later the tooth's contact is with the permanent second premolar after it erupts. As noted occlusally from the mesial contact, the mesial outline is rounded.

Instead of being flat like the mesial, the distal outline of the maxillary first molar is rounded or convex from the CEJ to the occlusal surface. The distal contact is in the middle third. However, no distal contact with a tooth occurs until the permanent maxillary second molars erupt. The CEJ is slightly but irregularly curved apically but with less curvature than that on teeth anterior to it. A sharp dip or point may be observed just occlusal to the furcation area.

Lingual View Features

The lingual surface of the maxillary first molar is almost as wide mesiodistally as the buccal surface as well as trapezoidal (see Fig. 17.39). However, the lingual surface is more rounded or convex than the buccal. Both the mesial and distal outline and CEJ curvature are about the same, except that the distal outline is shorter because the distolingual cusp is smaller than the distobuccal cusp. Being the largest cusp on the occlusal surface, the mesiolingual cusp outline is much longer and larger, but the cusp is not as sharp as the distolingual cusp, which *helps to distinguish the maxillary right first molar from the left.*

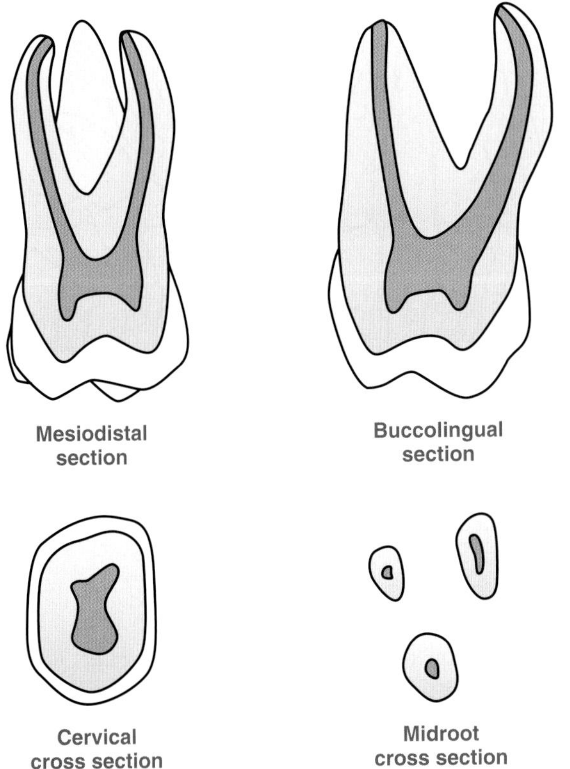

Fig. 17.40 Pulp Cavity of the Permanent Maxillary Right First Molar.

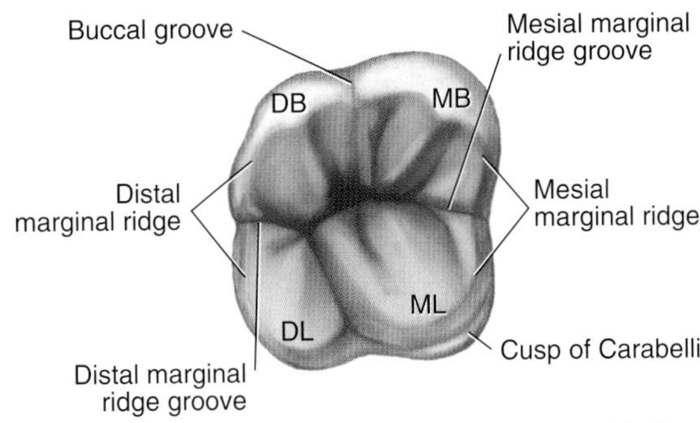

Fig. 17.41 Occlusal features of the permanent maxillary right first molar with the occlusal table highlighted. *DB*, Distobuccal; *DL*, distolingual; *MB*, mesiobuccal; *ML*, mesiolingual.

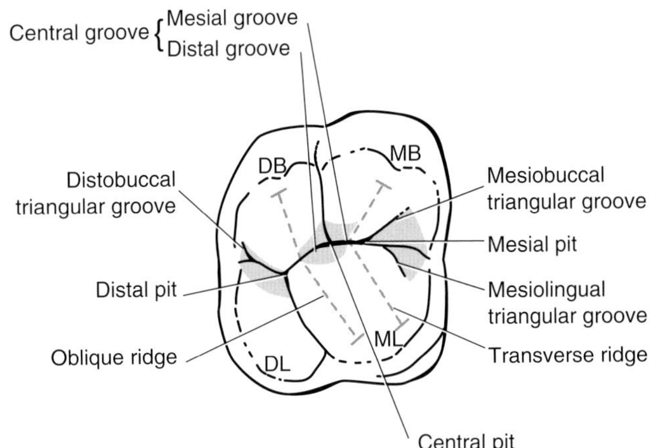

Fig. 17.42 Additional occlusal features of the permanent maxillary right first molar with the fossae highlighted. *DB*, Distobuccal; *DL*, distolingual; *MB*, mesiobuccal; *ML*, mesiolingual.

Commonly arising from the lingual surface of the mesiolingual cusp of the maxillary first molar is a fifth nonfunctioning cusp, the **cusp of Carabelli** (kare-uh-**bell**-ee), named for its discoverer (see Fig. 17.38). This minor cusp is set apart from the rest of the mesiolingual cusp by its associated **cusp of Carabelli groove**. Its presence can be variable; it is not present in all dentitions. If present, this small cusp and its equally small groove, varies in prominence from tooth to tooth.

Similar to the buccal surface, the lingual surface has a distolingual groove that divides the occlusal outline into two unequal parts. And dissimilar to the buccal surface, only the two lingual cusps can be seen from this view. The distolingual groove usually ends in a lingual pit in the middle of the lingual surface, but it also may fade out.

Proximal View Features

The only two cusps of the maxillary first molar that are seen from the mesial are the mesiobuccal cusp and mesiolingual cusp (see Fig. 17.39). A mesial marginal groove usually notches the mesial marginal ridge about midway along its length. The contact area on the mesial is situated slightly to the buccal.

The distal view is the same as the mesial, the exception being that the mesial cusp tips are seen projecting beyond the outline of the distobuccal cusp and distolingual cusp from proximal. The distal marginal ridge is less prominent and dips farther cervically than on the mesial with a distal marginal groove halfway along its length. On both proximal views, the CEJ usually curves slightly toward the occlusal and may even be a straight line on some teeth on the distal.

Occlusal View Features

The overall rhomboidal outline of the occlusal surface of a maxillary first molar is seen from the occlusal view because it is four-sided with opposite sides parallel (Fig. 17.41). The buccal outline is divided unequally into two parts by the buccal groove with the mesial part longer than the distal part. The lingual outline is also divided unequally into two parts by the distolingual groove with the mesial part longer and less rounded than the distal part.

The mesial marginal ridge is longer and more prominent than the distal marginal ridge. Both marginal ridges are crossed by a mesial marginal ridge groove and distal marginal ridge groove, respectively. Because this is the first molar discussed, an extensive coverage of the occlusal table follows; this information can be applied to the other molars, especially the maxillary molars.

Occlusal Table Components

On the maxillary first molar, the two marginal ridges and two cusp ridges of the four major cusps are found bordering the occlusal table on the buccal and lingual margins (Fig. 17.42). Each major cusp has a triangular ridge and three other cusp ridges. Also present with each major cusp are four inclined cuspal planes.

The mesiobuccal cusp has a sharp cusp tip and is the second largest cusp. It has a mesial cusp ridge that extends from the cusp tip to the mesiobuccal occlusal point angle. The mesiobuccal cusp on the first maxillary first molar is important in classifying the permanent dentition using Angle classification of malocclusion in relation to the mandibular arch (see Table 20.1).

The distal cusp ridge of the mesiobuccal cusp runs from the cusp tip to the buccal groove. The buccal cusp ridge passes from the cusp tip to the CEJ on the buccal surface. Finally, the lingual cusp ridge runs from the cusp tip to the central groove and is also considered the triangular ridge of the mesiobuccal cusp. The mesiobuccal cusp has four inclined planes with all the lingual parts functional in occlusion.

The distobuccal cusp has the sharpest cusp tip and is the third largest cusp. Its triangular ridge, cusp ridges, and inclined planes are named similarly to those of the mesiobuccal cusp.

The mesiolingual cusp is the largest cusp with a rounded cusp tip. Its cusp ridges are similar to those of the other cusps, except that the distal triangular ridge extends from the mesiolingual cusp tip in an oblique distobuccal direction. There the distal triangular ridge meets the lingual triangular ridge of the distobuccal cusp to form the defining prominent oblique ridge. The mesiolingual cusp also has four inclined planes, all of which are functional in occlusion. A typical transverse ridge is also present and is formed by the buccal triangular ridge of the mesiolingual cusp and the lingual triangular ridge of the mesiobuccal cusp.

The distolingual cusp is the smallest of the major cusps and is the most variable of this group. The triangular ridge, cusp ridges, and inclined planes are similar to those of other cusps, except that all of the inclined planes are functional in occlusion.

The smallest cusp, when present on the maxillary first molar, is the minor and nonfunctional cusp, the cusp of Carabelli with its associated cusp of Carabelli groove.

Four fossae are also present, along with associated developmental grooves and occlusal pits: central, mesial triangular, distal triangular, and distal. The central fossa is mesial to the oblique ridge and has a central pit in its most central, deepest part. The central pit divides the central groove into two parts: a mesial groove and a distal groove. Thus the central pit is at the junction of three developmental grooves: buccal, mesial, and distal.

Three triangular grooves are present: mesiobuccal triangular groove, mesiolingual triangular groove, and distobuccal triangular groove. The buccal groove extends onto the buccal surface. The mesial groove as part of the central groove extends from the central pit to the mesial pit. The mesial pit is in the mesial triangular fossa, distal to the mesial marginal ridge. Thus the mesial pit is at the junction of four developmental grooves: mesial, mesiobuccal triangular, mesiolingual triangular, and mesial marginal.

As part of the central groove, the distal groove usually extends from the central pit across the oblique ridge to the distal pit; it can also be considered the transverse groove of the oblique ridge. The distal pit is in the distal triangular fossa, mesial to the distal marginal ridge, making the distal pit located at the junction of five developmental grooves: distal, distolingual, distobuccal triangular, distal marginal, and distal lingual triangular. The last fossa noted is the distal fossa, a linear rather than circular depression that is distal and parallel to the oblique ridge and thus is within the distolingual groove. Along with the central groove and other developmental grooves, a few supplemental grooves can be present.

Clinical Considerations for Permanent Maxillary First Molars

Because of their arch position and because the permanent maxillary first molars are the first permanent teeth to erupt in the maxillary arch, they are considered important in the development of functional occlusion (see Table 20.1). The importance of their role in occlusion is demonstrated if this tooth is lost (Fig. 17.43). Loss of this tooth now commonly results from periodontal disease, whereas, in the past, it resulted mostly from caries.

Loss of the tooth is followed by mesial inclination and mesial drift of the maxillary second molar into the open arch space and the mandibular first molar, if present, also overeruption (or super-eruption) in the space (see **Chapter 14** for more discussion). Occlusion and then mastication are disabled, causing an increased risk of caries and possibly also periodontal disease around the irregularly spaced teeth. Prosthetic replacement may prevent these situations.

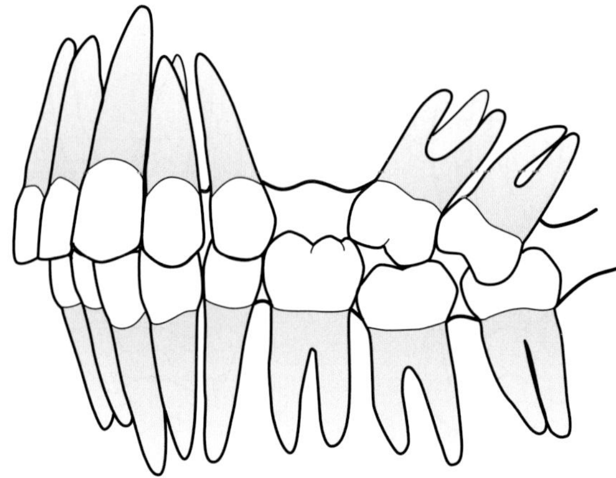

Fig. 17.43 Changes that can occur in the permanent dentition when the maxillary first molar is lost. Arch undergoes mesial inclination and drift of the maxillary second molar into the adjacent open space with overeruption (or super-eruption) of the mandibular first molar into opposing space.

The distobuccal surfaces of the permanent maxillary first molars may have increased supragingival tooth deposits. This is mostly due to the maxillary first molars' position in the oral cavity, opposite the duct openings of the parotid salivary glands on the inner cheek at the parotid papilla. Saliva, with its mineral content, is released from these glands causing the dental biofilm to mineralize quickly into supragingival calculus.

Permanent Maxillary Second Molars #2 and #15 (#17 and #27)

Specific Overall Features

Permanent maxillary second molars erupt between 12 and 13 years of age with root completion between ages 14 and 16 (Fig. 17.44). These teeth erupt distal to the permanent maxillary first molars and thus are nonsuccedaneous, having no primary predecessors.

Much variation in the form of the maxillary second molars is observed, especially in the size of the distolingual cusp. The crown usually has four cusps similar to the four major cusps of the first molar of the same arch, but it can also have three cusps. This tooth is composed of four developmental lobes, all named in the same manner as their associated cusps. Evidence of lobe separation can be found in the developmental grooves on the occlusal surface.

The three roots on maxillary second molars are smaller than the first molars. They are also less divergent as well as placed at a more parallel position than on the first molars. The lingual root is still the largest and longest, extending beyond the crown outline, but it is usually straighter and not as curved toward the buccal as the same root of the first molars.

The layout for the furcations of the maxillary second molar is similar to the first and the approach for homecare procedures and instrumentation is also the same (see Table 17.1 for general placement). Thus this tooth has three furcations: buccal, mesial, and distal. However, the furcation notches tend to be narrower in the second than those in the first molars with shallower depressions. Thus the chance of fusion, especially of the buccal roots or even of all three roots, is greater for the second than for the first molars.

The pulp cavity of a maxillary second molar consists of a pulp chamber and three main pulp canals, one for each of the three roots (Fig. 17.45). Each major cusp usually has one pulp horn, giving

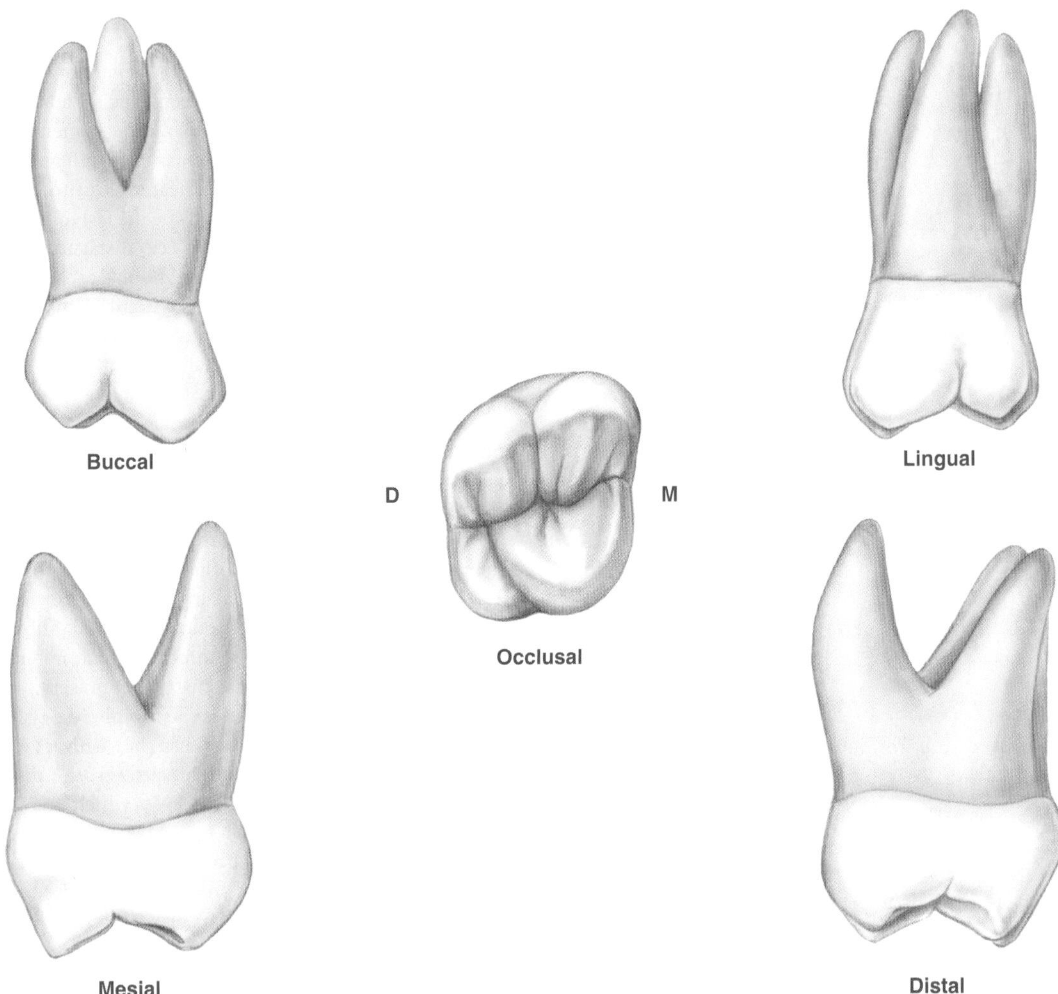

Fig. 17.44 Views of the Permanent Maxillary Right Second Molar with a Rhomboidal Crown Outline. *D,* Distal; *M,* mesial.

it four pulp horns: mesiobuccal, distobuccal, mesiolingual, and distolingual.

Buccal View Features

A maxillary second molar is shorter occlusocervically and narrower mesiodistally than a first molar (see Fig. 17.44). The buccal groove is located farther distally on the buccal surface of the second than the first. The mesiobuccal cusp is also longer and has a less sharp cusp tip than the distobuccal cusp. Both the mesial contact and distal contact are in the middle third.

Lingual View Features

The distolingual cusp of the maxillary second molar is smaller and shorter than on the first molar and is sometimes not even present (see Fig. 17.44). Thus the outline of the largest cusp of the occlusal surface, the mesiolingual cusp, is much longer and larger, but the cusp is not as sharp as the distolingual cusp, which *helps to distinguish the maxillary right second molar from the left.* In addition, a fifth cusp (or cusp of Carabelli) usually does not exist as it does in the first. From this view, the cusp tips of both the distobuccal cusp and the mesiobuccal cusp can be seen.

A lingual pit is usually present at the end of the distolingual groove, which does not extend as far mesially or cervically as the groove on the first molar. Thus the distolingual groove ends at a point that is occlusal and distal to the center of the lingual surface.

Proximal View Features

From the mesial, the mesial contact area of a maxillary second molar is larger and the cervical flattening or concavity is never as pronounced as in a first molar (see Fig. 17.44). From the distal, both the distobuccal cusp and distolingual cusp are smaller on a second than a first molar, thus showing more of the occlusal surface. Note that no distal contact area is present until the third molar possibly erupts and moves into occlusion.

Occlusal View Features

The general outline of the crown of a maxillary second molar is narrower mesiodistally than that of a maxillary first molar but is about the same width buccolingually (see Fig. 17.44). Two types of more specific crown outlines are possible on this tooth when viewed from the occlusal: rhomboidal or heart-shaped (Fig. 17.46). The more common rhomboidal type has four sides with opposite sides parallel; this type is similar to that of the first molar but with an even more accentuated outline. The heart-shaped type is the less common and is similar to the typical maxillary third molar.

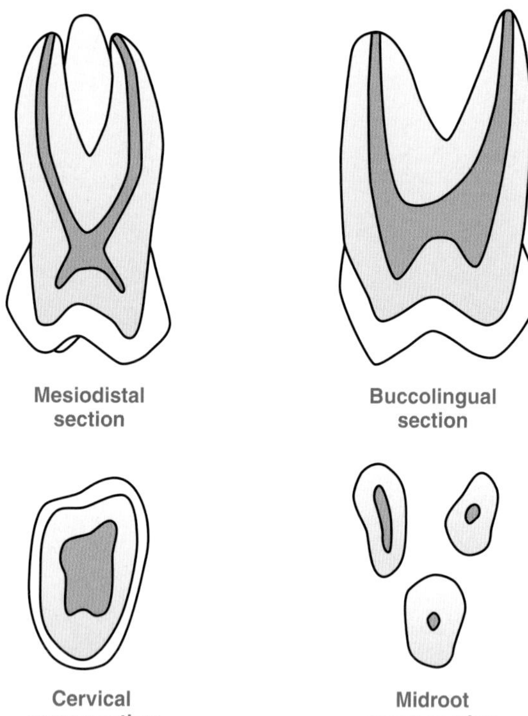

Fig. 17.45 Pulp Cavity of the Permanent Maxillary Right Second Molar with a Rhomboidal Crown.

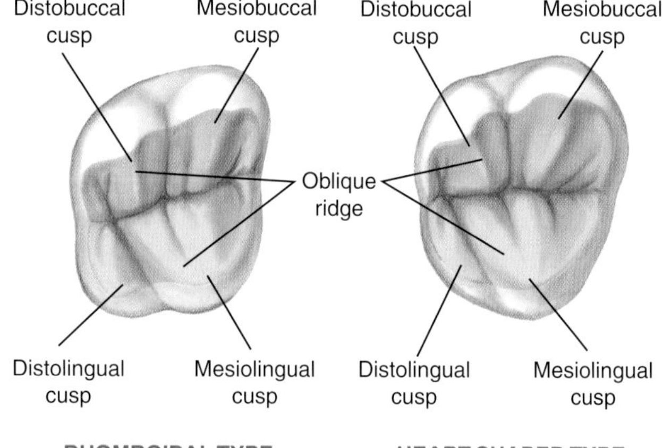

Fig. 17.46 Occlusal views of the two types of crowns of the permanent maxillary right second molars: rhomboidal and heart-shaped with the occlusal tables highlighted.

Occlusal Table Components

With the rhomboidal type on a maxillary second molar, the cusps present are similar to the major cusps of a maxillary first molar (see Fig. 17.46). With the heart-shaped type, the distolingual cusp is quite small with the other three cusps completely overshadowing by their larger size. The distolingual cusp can sometimes even be absent in the heart-shaped type with the distolingual groove confined to the occlusal table.

The cusp ridges, triangular ridges, transverse ridge, oblique ridge, developmental grooves, fossae, and occlusal pits for both types of a second molar are similar to those of the first molar of the same arch. However, the defining oblique ridge is less prominent on the second than on the first molar. Instead, an increased number of supplemental grooves are usually present on the occlusal table of the second.

Permanent Maxillary Third Molars #1 and #16 (#18 and #28)

Specific Overall Features

Permanent maxillary third molars may erupt between 17 and 21 years of age with root completion between ages 18 and 25 (Fig. 17.47). If erupted, they are located distal to the permanent maxillary second molars and thus are nonsuccedaneous, having no primary predecessors.

The tooth's mesial contact is in the middle third, but it does not have a distal tooth contact because it may be the last tooth in each maxillary quadrant. In addition, because of its very distal arch position, the tooth has only one antagonist in the mandibular arch. This tooth and the very small mandibular central incisor are the only teeth that have one antagonist in the permanent dentition; all others have two.

In addition, this tooth is the smallest molar and most variable tooth in shape in the permanent dentition. Without any standard form observed for this tooth, describing a typical maxillary third molar is therefore difficult. It is smaller generally in all dimensions than a second maxillary molar and its crown is also poorly developed when compared with the other maxillary molars. The tooth is composed of four developmental lobes.

Two types of crown outlines are possible for a maxillary third molar when viewed from the occlusal (Fig. 17.48). The most common type is heart-shaped, similar to a maxillary second molar but with more supplemental grooves present on the occlusal table. With the heart-shaped type, the tooth usually has only three cusps: mesiobuccal, distobuccal, and mesiolingual; a distolingual cusp is not present.

If a fourth cusp is present, it is the rhomboidal type, having a small and nonfunctioning distolingual cusp, but without any oblique ridge present. For both types of occlusal surfaces, the distobuccal cusp is much shorter than the mesiobuccal cusp, which *helps to distinguish the maxillary right third molar from the left.*

All roots of the third are also poorly developed like the crown and shorter than that of a second molar. And similar to other maxillary molars, the maxillary third molars are trifurcated. However, the roots are sometimes so close together that they are fused, either partially or fully, and thus may give the appearance of a single root. The distobuccal root usually is the smallest and often is found tucked under the crown. The roots are curved distally, which also *helps to distinguish the maxillary right third molar from the left.*

The pulp cavity of a maxillary third molar may have a pulp chamber and three pulp canals (Fig. 17.49). The tooth may sometimes have one large pulp canal with a fused root to as many as four pulp canals with four roots. The number of pulp horns varies and depends on the number of cusps; if there are three cusps, there are three pulp horns.

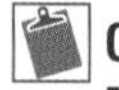

Clinical Considerations for Permanent Maxillary Third Molars

Any homecare procedures, instrumentation or restoration may be difficult when these teeth are erupted because of their extreme posterior arch position. Many times, the tooth in each quadrant has heavy deposits and an increased risk of disease, either periodontally or with caries on not only the occlusal surface but also on the cervix of the buccal surface. Having the patient open less wide, actually helps accommodate any procedures on these teeth.

However, permanent maxillary third molars may also fail to erupt and remain impacted within the alveolar process. An impacted tooth is an unerupted or partially erupted tooth that is positioned against another tooth, bone, or even soft tissue in such a way that only partial eruption is likely, if at all. This impaction usually occurs because the maxilla is underdeveloped and space or arch length is insufficient to accommodate these teeth because they are the last to erupt in the maxillary arch; thus, surgical removal may be necessary (see earlier discussion). Finally, developmental cyst formation may occur within the dental tissue of an impacted crown, resulting in a dentigerous cyst.

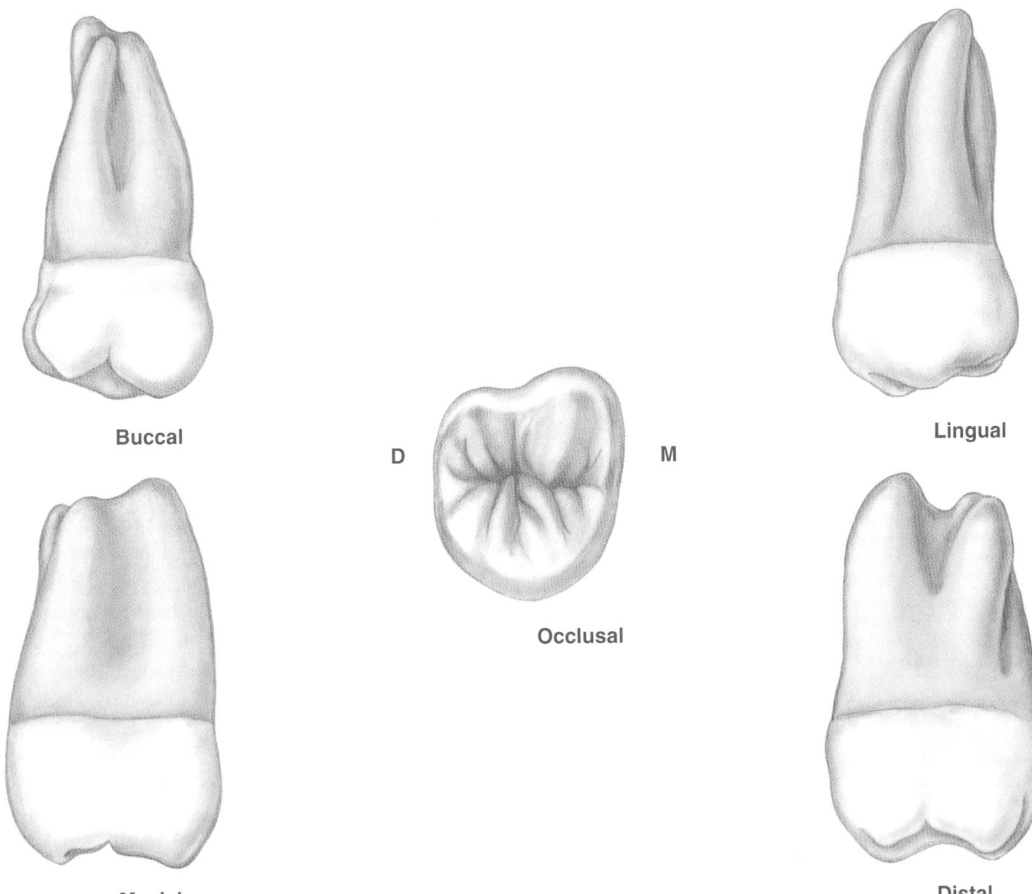

Fig. 17.47 Views of the Permanent Maxillary Right Third Molars with a Heart-Shaped Occlusal Outline. *D*, Distal; *M*, mesial.

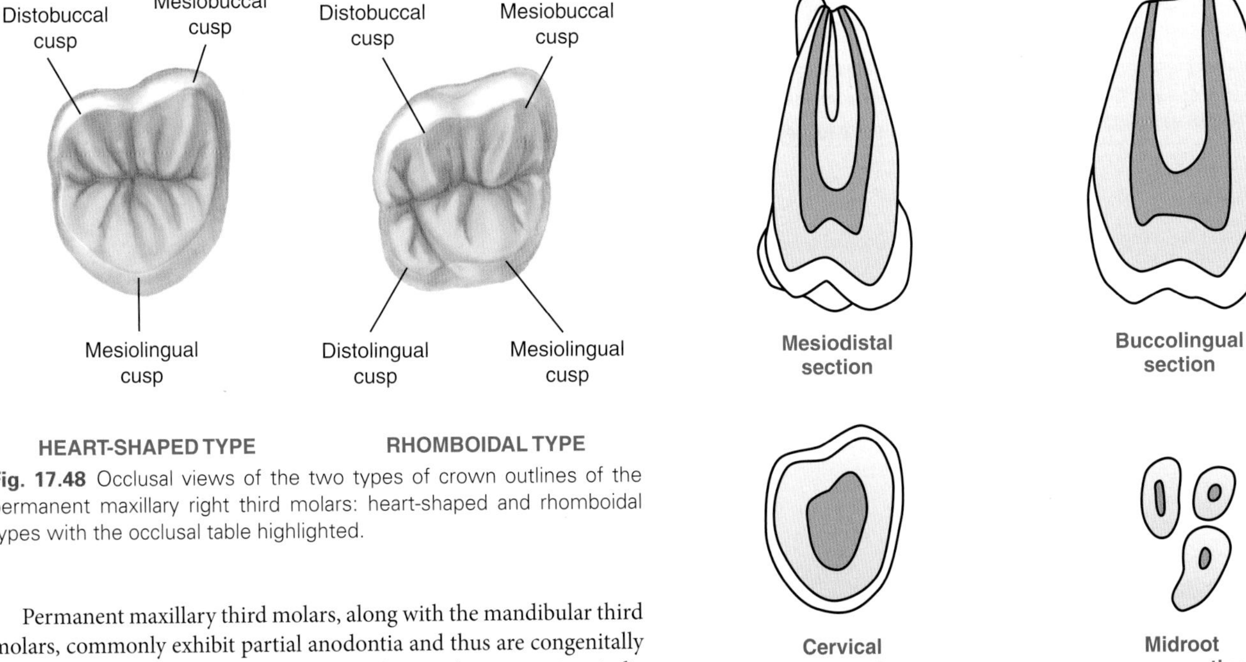

Fig. 17.48 Occlusal views of the two types of crown outlines of the permanent maxillary right third molars: heart-shaped and rhomboidal types with the occlusal table highlighted.

Fig. 17.49 Pulp Cavity of the Permanent Maxillary Right Third Molar.

Permanent maxillary third molars, along with the mandibular third molars, commonly exhibit partial anodontia and thus are congenitally missing (see **Chapter 6**). With this disturbance, the appropriate individual tooth germ(s) in the area is missing owing to failure of the initiation process during tooth development. However, the situation in this case usually has no harmful consequences.

This tooth also commonly exhibits partial microdontia, which leads to a smaller molar crown with one cusp or **peg molar**, either unilaterally or bilaterally, owing to failure in the proliferation process during tooth development (Fig. 17.50; see Box 6.1, *F*). This tooth may also have accessory roots, which can complicate extraction procedures.

PERMANENT MANDIBULAR MOLARS

General Features

Permanent mandibular molars erupt between 6 months and 1 year before the corresponding permanent maxillary molars (Table 17.4; see Figs. 17.51, 17.57, and 17.60). The crown has four or five major cusps, of which there are always two lingual cusps of about the same width. All mandibular molars are wider mesiodistally than buccolingually, which is similar to anterior teeth. In contrast, maxillary molars are wider buccolingually as are all posterior teeth. Thus from an occlusal view, the outline of the crown is also rectangular (four-sided) or pentagonal (five-sided).

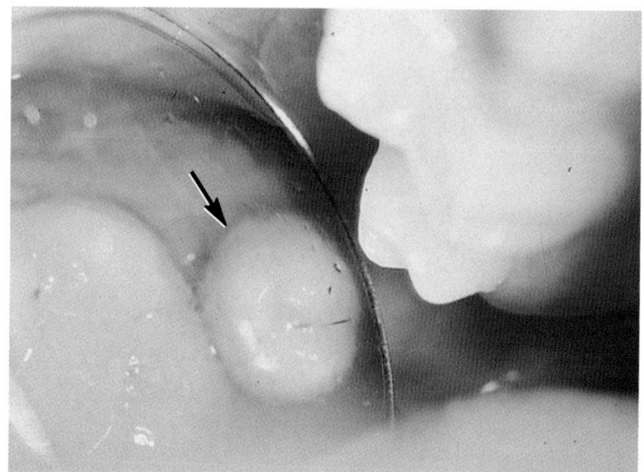

Fig. 17.50 Peg third molar of the permanent maxillary arch *(arrow)* in the oral cavity. (Courtesy of Margaret J. Fehrenbach, RDH, MS.)

Quite distinct from maxillary molars, the buccal crown outline of all mandibular molars also shows a strong lingual inclination when viewed from the proximal, like the nearby premolars. Thus from each proximal view, the crown outline is rhomboidal or four-sided with opposite sides parallel, which is like all mandibular posterior teeth (see Table 15.4). The crown is thus inclined lingually on the root base, bringing the cusps of these mandibular teeth into proper occlusion with their maxillary antagonists and distributing the forces along the long axis.

Mandibular molars are usually bifurcated, having two roots, a mesial root and distal root (see Fig. 17.7). Both of these roots show great to moderate distal root inclination. Because these teeth are bifurcated, there are two furcations located on the buccal and lingual surfaces midway between the proximal surfaces (see Table 17.1). These furcations are also at a level of one-fourth the root length from the CEJ. Root concavities are also found on the mesial surface of the mesial root and on furcal surfaces of both the mesial and distal roots. The root concavities on the mesial root are especially deep if this root also has two pulp canals.

The inferior alveolar canal may approximate the roots of mandibular molars. Although the removal of an erupted tooth rarely impinges on the inferior alveolar canal, if an impacted tooth is to be removed, it is important that the relationship between molar roots and the canal be assessed (see further discussion of impaction later in this chapter). Such an extraction may lead to injury of the canal and cause consequent damage to the inferior alveolar nerve. CBCT images are often useful in these circumstances.

Clinical Considerations for Permanent Mandibular Molars

All three types of mandibular molars can present difficulties in instrumentation or restoration because of their narrow lingual surfaces combined with the lingual inclination of the crown; therefore, instrument placement subgingivally can be even more difficult.

In addition, patients may have difficulty in performing homecare procedures because of the lingual inclination of the crown. They may miss the cervical interface with the associated lingual gingival tissue and remove deposits from only the occlusal surface with a toothbrush. And the proximity of the tongue also makes homecare procedures, instrumentation, or restoration more difficult on the lingual surface.

TABLE 17.4 Permanent Mandibular Molars

	Mandibular First Molar	Mandibular Second Molar	Mandibular Third Molar
Universal number	#19 and #30	#18 and #31	#17 and #32
International number	#36 and #46	#37 and #47	#38 and #48
General crown features	Occlusal table with marginal ridges and cusps with tips, inclined planes, ridges, grooves, fossae, pits		
	Buccal cervical ridge		
Specific crown features	First permanent tooth to erupt. Widest crown mesiodistally of dentition. Five cusps, with Y-shaped groove pattern. Buccal groove possibly ending in buccal pit.	Smaller crown than first. Four cusps with cross-shaped groove pattern.	Smaller crown than second
Mesial and distal contact*	Junction of occlusal and middle thirds	Middle third	Mesial: cervical third; Distal: none
Distinguish right from left	Distal cusp smallest with a sharp cusp	Difference in height of contour for buccal and lingual from each proximal surface and wider on the mesial than distal	Wider buccolingually on mesial than on distal
General root features	Two roots		
Specific root features	Furcations well removed from the CEJ. Root trunks and root concavities. Divergent roots.	Furcations closer to CEJ. Root trunks and root concavities. Less divergent roots.	Fused roots, irregularly curved, with sharp apices

*Height of contour of posteriors for the buccal is in cervical third and lingual in middle third.
CEJ, Cementoenamel junction.

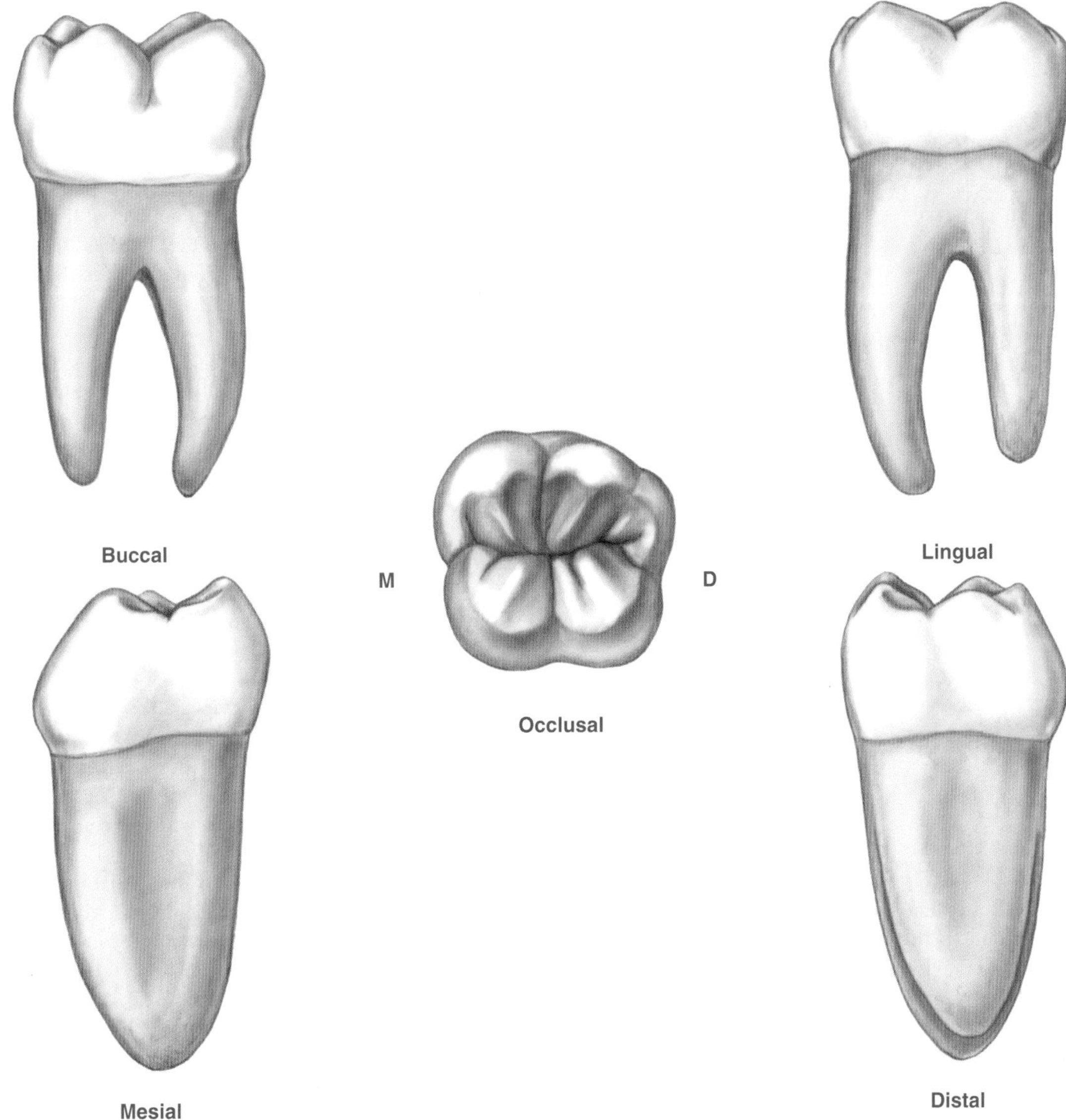

Fig. 17.51 Views of the Permanent Mandibular Right First Molar. *D,* Distal; *M,* mesial.

Permanent Mandibular First Molars #19 and #30 (#36 and #46)

Specific Overall Features

The permanent mandibular first molars erupt between 6 and 7 years of age with root completion between ages 9 and 10 (Fig. 17.51). These teeth are usually the first permanent teeth to erupt in the oral cavity. They erupt distal to the primary mandibular second molars and thus are nonsuccedaneous, having no primary predecessors.

The crown of a mandibular first molar usually has five cusps: three buccal and two lingual. Thus these teeth are usually composed of five developmental lobes, like the maxillary first molars but unlike the other mandibular molars, which have four. The lobes are named for their associated cusps. Evidence of lobe separation is found in the developmental grooves on the occlusal surface. Occasionally, the distal cusp is missing and even more rarely, the distal cusp can have an adjacent sixth cusp on larger sized ones.

The two roots, mesial and distal, of a mandibular first molar are both larger and more divergent than the second, leaving these roots widely separated buccally and no longer parallel to each other. The root trunk of the first is also shorter than that of the second. Both roots are usually the same length on the tooth, but if one is longer, it is the mesial root. The mesial root is also the wider and stronger of the two. If this molar has three roots, it is because the mesial root has developed both buccal and lingual root branches.

Fluting, an elongated developmental depression, is present on many surfaces of the root branches. This fluting especially noted on the mesial surface of the mesial root; however, it is not observed on the distal surface of the distal root.

The midway-placed furcations on both the buccal and lingual surfaces are well removed from the CEJ at 3 mm for the buccal furcation and 4 mm for the lingual furcation (see Table 17.1). But the entrance diameters for both are small at only around 1 mm or less, making access to homecare procedures and instrumentation limited. And the buccal furcation entrance tends to be smaller than that of the lingual furcation.

The pulp cavity of a mandibular first molar is more likely to have three pulp canals: distal, mesiobuccal, and mesiolingual with five pulp horns (Fig. 17.52). The distal pulp canal is much larger than the other two canals and is usually the only canal in the distal root. The mesial root usually has two pulp canals: mesiobuccal and mesiolingual. Rarely,

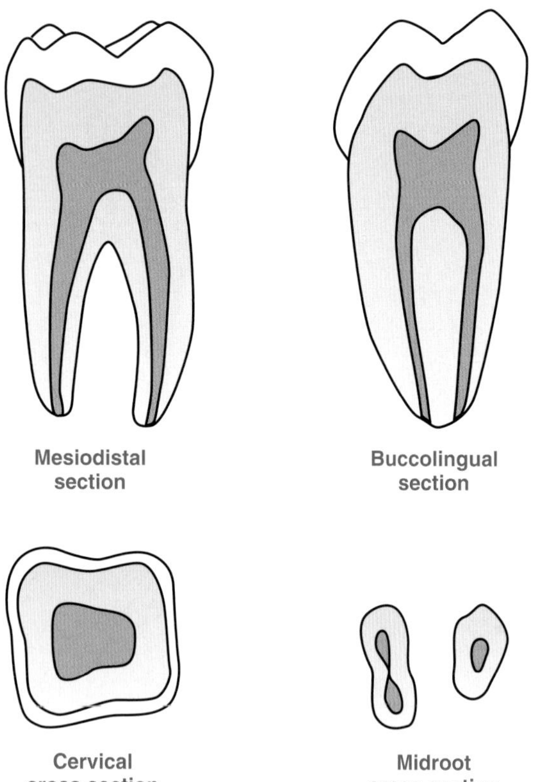

Fig. 17.52 Pulp Cavity of the Permanent Mandibular Right First Molar.

these two mesial canals are joined with one single apical foramen or only one pulp canal is found in the mesial root. Again, rarely, two canals are present in the distal root, just as in the case of the mesial root.

Buccal View Features

The crown of a mandibular first molar is larger mesiodistally than occlusocervically (see Fig. 17.51). It is also the widest tooth mesiodistally of any permanent tooth because it has a fifth major cusp. From this view, at least some part of all five cusps is visible.

The mesiobuccal cusp is the largest, widest, and highest cusp on the buccal side. The distobuccal cusp is slightly smaller, shorter, and sharper than the mesiobuccal cusp. The distal cusp, despite its name, is also considered a buccal cusp due to its position on that side; it is the lowest cusp and slightly sharper than the other two. The occlusal outline is divided into three sections by the two grooves as they pass into the buccal surface: the mesiobuccal and distobuccal grooves. These sections of the crown's buccal surface decrease in size from the distal to the mesial.

The mesiobuccal groove on a first mandibular molar is important in classifying the permanent dentition using Angle classification of malocclusion in relation to the maxillary arch (see Table 20.1). The mesiobuccal groove extends straight cervically to a point about midway occlusocervically, but slightly mesial to the center mesiodistally, and usually ends in the buccal pit. However, it may also end in two short slanting grooves or even fade out after a short distance. The distobuccal groove extends cervically, similarly to the mesiobuccal groove, but is slightly distal to the center mesiodistally, and usually ends in a distobuccal pit but sometimes just fades out.

A buccal cervical ridge, which has a mesiodistally oriented roundness in the cervical third of the buccal surface, is apparent. It is usually more prominent in its mesial part. In addition, a shallow concavity may extend mesiodistally in the middle third.

The mesial outline on a mandibular first molar is slightly concave from the contact area cervically and is rounded occlusal to the contact. The distal outline is more rounded than the mesial. Both the mesial contact and distal contact are at the junction of the occlusal and middle thirds.

Lingual View Features

The lingual surface of a mandibular first molar is smaller than the buccal surface but the mesial and distal outlines of the lingual surface are similar to the buccal surface (see Fig. 17.51). The occlusal outline is divided in this view by a lingual groove between the mesiolingual cusp and the distolingual cusp.

Proximal View Features

The crown is smaller buccolingually than mesiodistally and cervico-occlusally (see Fig. 17.51). The crown is also inclined toward the lingual as are the other mandibular posterior teeth. Additionally, the crown outline from this view is rhomboidal or four-sided with opposite sides parallel.

The buccal outline on the mesial surface is usually rounded, especially at the buccal cervical ridge. The buccal cervical ridge is in the cervical third, where the height of contour is also located. The lingual outline on the mesial is either straight or slightly rounded from the CEJ to the height of contour in the middle third. It is then rounded from the height of contour to the occlusal. The CEJ is either straight or slightly curved occlusally, but it is always located at a more occlusal level on the lingual part of the mesial surface.

The mesial marginal groove notches the mesial marginal ridge on a mandibular first molar. It has a flattened or slightly concave area centrally located in the gingival third, which is comparable to the mesial root concavity of a maxillary first premolar.

The distal surface is similar to the mesial but smaller, especially in the buccolingual dimension. The distal marginal ridge is notched by the distal marginal groove and is located more cervically than the mesial marginal ridge.

Occlusal View Features

The crown outline of the mandibular first molar is roughly pentagonal or five-sided, with the fifth side created by the distal cusp from an occlusal view (see Fig. 17.51). The distal part of the buccal outline converges toward the distal to create the fifth side of the outline. The buccal outline has rounded line angles, which is divided into three parts by the two buccal grooves, the mesiobuccal groove and the distobuccal groove. The length of each of the buccal cusps decreases distally as noted from the buccal view.

The lingual outline is divided into two parts by the lingual groove. The mesial outline is divided into two parts by the mesial marginal groove. The distal outline, the shortest of the five sides, is divided by the distal marginal groove.

Occlusal Table Components

The mandibular first molar usually has five functional cusps; listed from largest to smallest: mesiobuccal, mesiolingual, distolingual, distobuccal, and distal (Fig. 17.53). The cusps listed from highest to lowest: mesiolingual, distolingual, mesiobuccal, distobuccal, and distal cusp. Each cusp has four cusp ridges, a triangular ridge, and four inclined cuspal planes.

The mesiobuccal cusp is the bulkiest cusp, although it has a blunt tip. Except for the distal cusp, the distobuccal cusp is the smallest of the larger cusps and has a rounded tip. The mesiolingual cusp is second in size to the mesiobuccal cusp and has the sharpest tip. The tip of the distolingual cusp is also quite sharp but is slightly smaller than the mesiolingual cusp. The distal cusp is the smallest of all the cusps

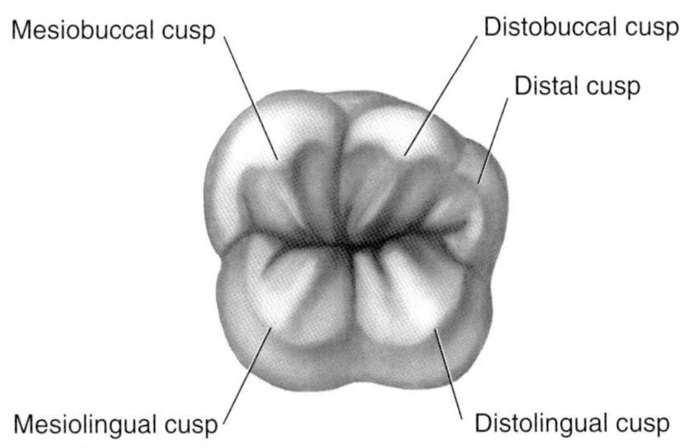

Fig. 17.53 Occlusal Features of the Permanent Mandibular Right First Molar.

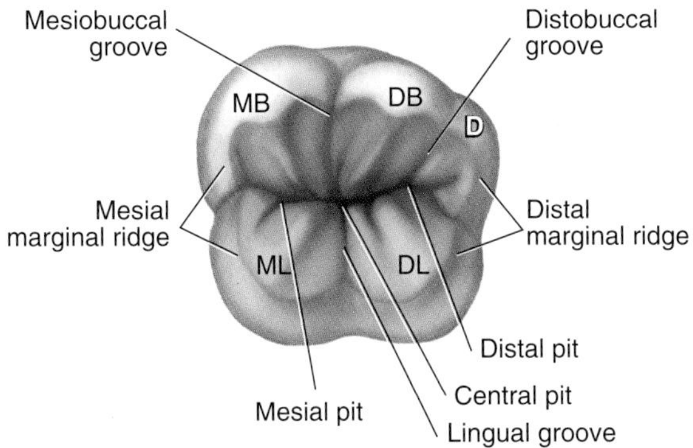

Fig. 17.54 Additional occlusal features of the permanent mandibular right first molar with the occlusal table highlighted. *D, Distal; DB,* distobuccal; *DL,* distolingual; *MB,* mesiobuccal; *ML,* mesiolingual.

and has a sharp tip, which *helps to distinguish the mandibular right first molar from the left.*

The mandibular first molar has the most complex developmental groove pattern of all the permanent mandibular molars (Fig. 17.54). A Y-shaped groove pattern is formed on the occlusal table around the cusps by the mesiobuccal groove, distobuccal groove, and lingual groove. Two marginal ridges border the occlusal table, the mesial marginal ridge and the distal marginal ridge. No transverse ridges are found on the occlusal table, unlike a maxillary first molar and a mandibular second molar.

The occlusal table also has three fossae: large central fossa, smaller mesial triangular fossa, and distal triangular fossa. Three pits are associated with the fossae: mesial pit, central pit, and distal pit. The central pit is the also the deepest pit, dividing the central groove into two grooves, the mesial groove and distal groove.

The central pit is the junction of three grooves: mesiobuccal, distobuccal, and lingual. The mesial pit is the junction of four grooves: mesial, mesiobuccal triangular, mesiolingual triangular, and mesial marginal. The distal pit is the junction of three grooves: the distal, the distolingual, and distal marginal.

Clinical Considerations for Permanent Mandibular First Molars

Buccal pits that may occur on the buccal surface of mandibular first molars are at an increased risk of caries because of both increased dental biofilm retention and the thinness of enamel forming the walls of the pit (Fig. 17.55; see **Chapter 12**). An enamel sealant could be placed on each buccal surface as the tooth begins to erupt. Sealants on the buccal surface do not bond as easily as on the occlusal surface, however, because of the histology of the area.

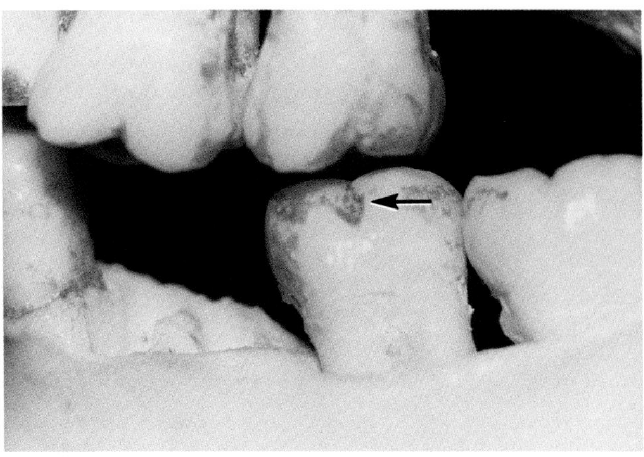

Fig. 17.55 Buccal pit *(arrow)* on the permanent mandibular first molar of a skull. (Courtesy of Margaret J. Fehrenbach, RDH, MS.)

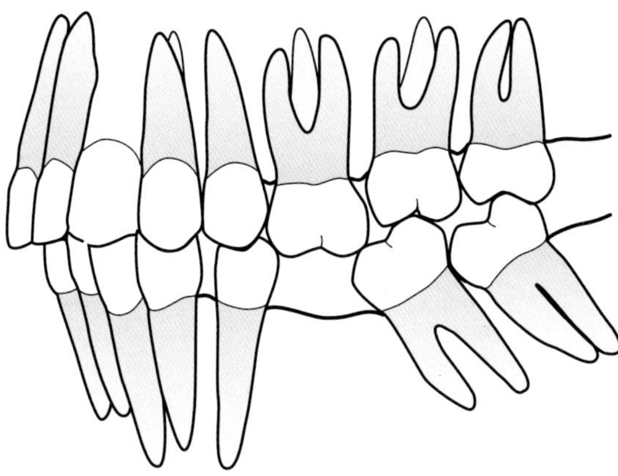

Fig. 17.56 Changes that can occur in the permanent dentition with the loss of the mandibular first molar. Teeth become inclined, then there is mesial drift of the mandibular second molar and possibly the third molar, with overeruption (or super-eruption) of the maxillary first molar into the opposing open space.

If caries occur, tooth-colored restorative materials can be used to achieve a more esthetic appearance and thus the past presence of the buccal pit or associated restoration may not be easy to discern clinically.

Because of their arch position and because the permanent mandibular first molars are the first permanent teeth to erupt in the mandibular arch, they are considered important in regard to the development of occlusion (see Table 20.1). The importance of the role of this tooth in occlusion is shown when the tooth is lost (Fig. 17.56). This loss might more easily occur because this tooth is the first permanent tooth to erupt into the oral cavity. It has a greater chance of being affected by caries because child patients are just beginning to master homecare procedures and dietary restrictions. In addition, early dental restorative intervention of the caries may be neglected with a newly present mixed dentition.

With the loss of the tooth, the mandibular second molar and possibly also the third molar start to undergo mesial incline and mesial drift into the newly opened arch space, allowing the maxillary first molar to undergo overeruption (or super-eruption) into the space (see **Chapter 14** for more discussion). Occlusion and then mastication are disabled, and the risk of caries and possibly periodontal disease around the irregularly spaced teeth is greatly increased. Interceptive orthodontic therapy as well as tooth replacement is important to prevent these situations after tooth loss.

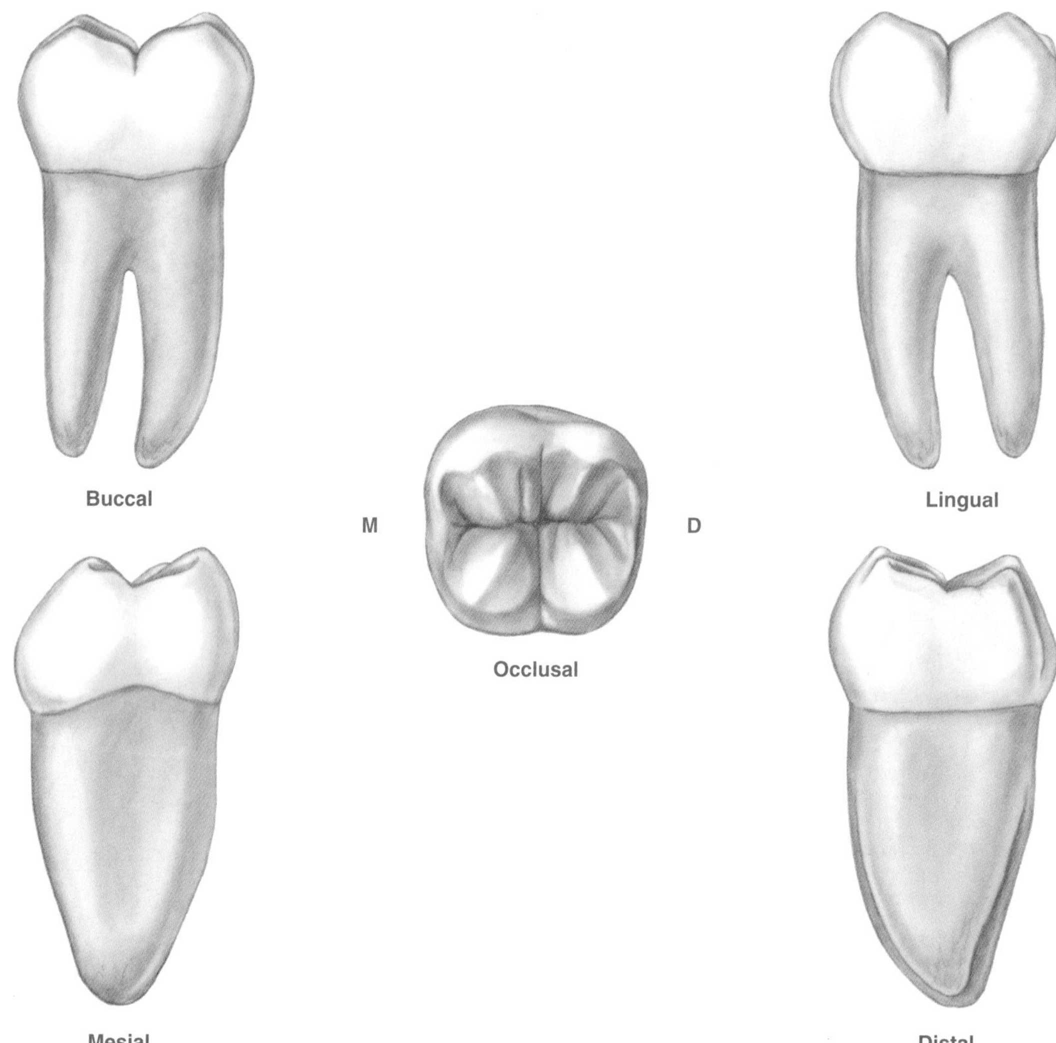

Fig. 17.57 Views of the Permanent Mandibular Right Second Molar. *D,* Distal; *M,* mesial.

Permanent Mandibular Second Molars #18 and #31 (#37 and #47)

Specific Overall Features

The permanent mandibular second molars erupt between 11 and 13 years of age with root completion between ages 14 and 15 (Fig. 17.57). These teeth erupt distal to the permanent mandibular first molars and thus are nonsuccedaneous, having no primary predecessors.

The crown measurements of a mandibular second molar are usually smaller when compared to a first molar. The four cusps of a second are almost equal in size compared with the five cusps of differing sizes of a first molar. Like the mandibular third molars, the mandibular second molars are usually composed of four developmental lobes, unlike the mandibular first molars, which are from five lobes. The lobes are named for the associated cusps and the developmental grooves on the occlusal surface show lobe division.

The two roots of a mandibular second molar are smaller, shorter, and less divergent than those of a first molar, being more parallel to each other. However, the lack of root separation makes detection and deposit removal more difficult if exposed. The root trunk of a second is also longer than that of a first. The mesial root of the second is not as broad as that of a first, but the furcation is farther from the CEJ. The rest of the general layout of the furcations for the second is similar to the first (see Table 17.1 for general placement). However, all of the root depressions are shallower. And overall, root variability is greater in the second than in the first molar.

The pulp cavity of a mandibular second molar can have two pulp canals, with one for each root. However, it is more likely to have three pulp canals, similar to a mandibular first molar: distal, mesiobuccal, and mesiolingual canals; the latter two being together in the mesial root (Fig. 17.58). The tooth usually has only four pulp horns, which correspond to the four cusps.

Buccal View Features

The buccal groove divides the same-size mesiobuccal cusp and distobuccal cusp of a mandibular second molar (see Fig. 17.57). The mesial contact is at the junction of the occlusal and middle third. The distal contact is slightly cervical, but still at the junction of the occlusal and middle third.

Lingual View Features

The mesiolingual cusp and distolingual cusp have the same size and shape as the buccal cusps, although they have sharper cusp tips (see Fig. 17.57). Because the crown converges lingually, a part of both the mesial and distal surfaces can be seen from this view.

Proximal View Features

The buccal height of contour is in the cervical third and the lingual height of contour is in the middle third for the mandibular second molar (see Fig. 17.57). The crown also tapers distally when viewed from the mesial aspect. That is because the molar is also wider buccolingually on the mesial surface

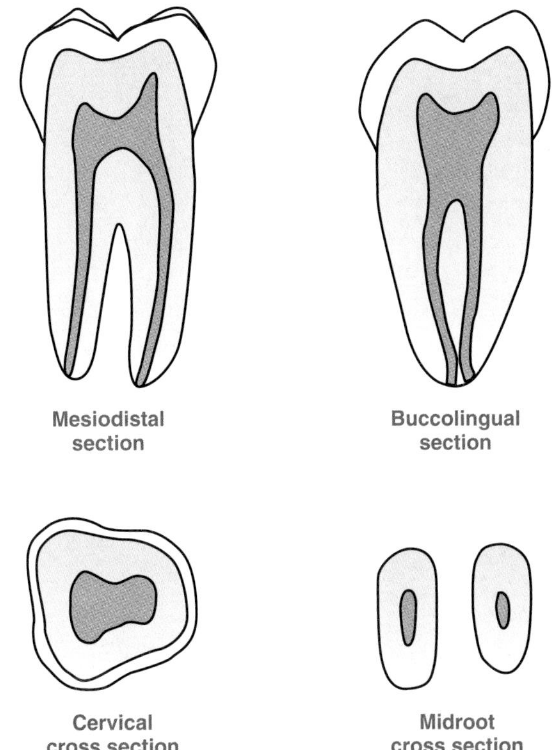

Fig. 17.58 Pulp Cavity of the Permanent Mandibular Right Second Molar.

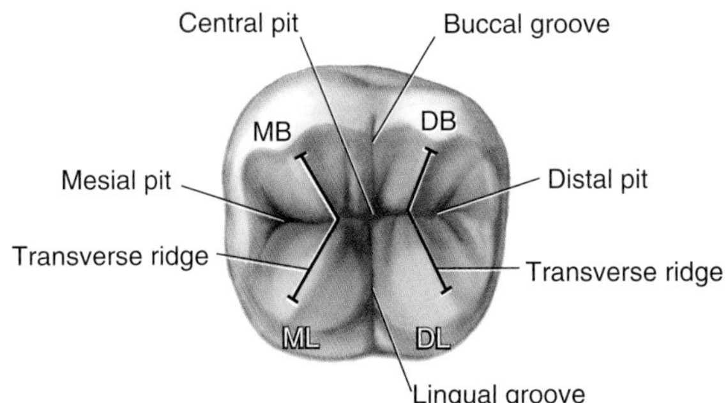

Fig. 17.59 Occlusal features of the permanent mandibular right second molar with the occlusal table highlighted. *DB*, Distobuccal; *DL*, distolingual; *MB*, mesiobuccal; *ML*, mesiolingual.

than on the distal. Both these mesial surface features *help to distinguish the mandibular right second molar from the left.* The buccal cervical ridge is less pronounced on the second molar than on the first from the proximal.

The CEJ curvature on both proximal surfaces of a second is also less pronounced than that of a first. Neither the mesial nor the distal marginal ridge is divided by a marginal groove.

Occlusal View Features

The outline of the crown of a mandibular second molar is rectangular or four-sided (Fig. 17.59). The tooth has four cusps, two buccal and two lingual cusps: mesiobuccal, distobuccal, mesiolingual, and distolingual. With this view, the occlusal surface of a second molar is considerably different from that of a first because there is no distal cusp, and all cusps are of equal size.

Occlusal Table Components

Unlike a mandibular first molar, this tooth has two transverse ridges (see Fig. 17.59). The triangular ridges of the mesiobuccal and mesiolingual cusps meet to form a transverse ridge as do the distobuccal and distolingual cusps. A cross-shaped groove pattern is formed where the well-defined central groove is crossed by the buccal groove and lingual groove, dividing the occlusal table into four parts that are almost equal like four pastry buns in a pan. Cusp slopes on a second are less smooth than on a first because second molars have an increased number of supplemental grooves. There are three occlusal pits present: central, mesial, and distal.

Permanent Mandibular Third Molars #17 and #32 (#38 and #48)

Specific Overall Features

The mandibular third molars may erupt between 17 and 21 years of age with root completion between ages 18 and 25 (Fig. 17.60). If erupted, they are located distal to the permanent mandibular second molars and thus are nonsuccedaneous, having no primary predecessors. The tooth's rounded mesial contact when fully erupted is more cervical than any other mandibular molar, meeting at the cervical third, but it does not have a distal tooth contact because it may be the last tooth present in each mandibular quadrant.

Similar to maxillary thirds, the mandibular thirds are variable in shape, having no standard form. Thus a typical mandibular third molar is difficult to describe. This molar usually is smaller in all dimensions than the second molar, and it sometimes is the same size as the first molar.

Like the mandibular second molars, the mandibular third molars are usually composed of four developmental lobes, unlike the mandibular first molars, which have five lobes. The lobes are named for the associated cusps and the developmental grooves on the occlusal surface show lobe division.

The crown of a mandibular third molar tapers distally when viewed from the mesial aspect. That is because the molar is also wider buccolingually on the mesial surface than on the distal surface, which *helps to distinguish the mandibular right third molar from the left,* like all mandibular molars. The crown is usually smaller in all dimensions than that of a second molar.

The occlusal outline of the crown is more oval than rectangular, although the crown usually resembles that of a second molar. The two mesial cusps are larger than the two distal cusps. The occlusal surface appears quite wrinkled with an irregular groove pattern, numerous supplemental grooves, and deepened occlusal pits; if an excess of these features exists, the occlusal surface is described as *crenulated.*

A mandibular third molar usually has two roots that are fused, irregularly curved, and shorter than a mandibular second molar. Additionally, the roots are usually smaller in proportion to the crown and have sharp apices. The pulp cavity is usually similar to that of the second molars with four pulp horns and two or three pulp canals (Fig. 17.61).

Clinical Considerations for Permanent Mandibular Third Molars

Permanent mandibular third molars may also fail to erupt and remain impacted within the surrounding alveolar process (Fig. 17.62), which occurs more frequently than with the maxillary counterparts. An impacted tooth is an unerupted or partially erupted tooth that is positioned against another tooth, bone, or even soft tissue, making complete eruption unlikely and may make surgical removal necessary (see earlier discussion). This impaction usually occurs because the mandible is underdeveloped and space or arch length is insufficient to accommodate these teeth, which are the last to erupt in the mandibular arch.

The mandibular third molar may also be partially erupted causing the surrounding gingival tissue to even cover a part of the occlusal surface, with this tissue now considered the *operculum.* This situation has an increased risk of periodontal infection from poor homecare, which is considered *pericoronitis.* Due to its posterior arch position, this infection can become serious with resultant Ludwig angina, cellulitis of the submandibular space, and thus impact breathing.

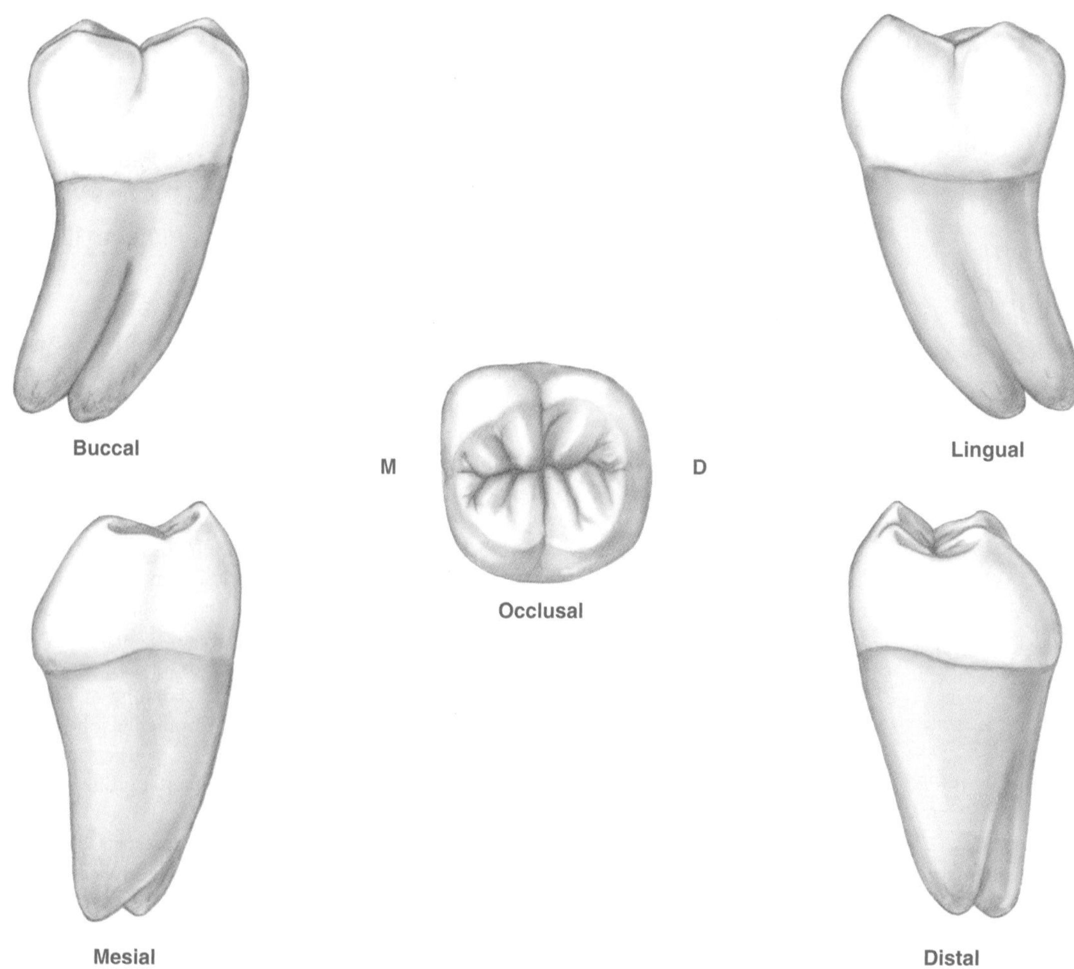

Fig. 17.60 Views of the Permanent Mandibular Right Third Molar. *D,* Distal; *M,* mesial.

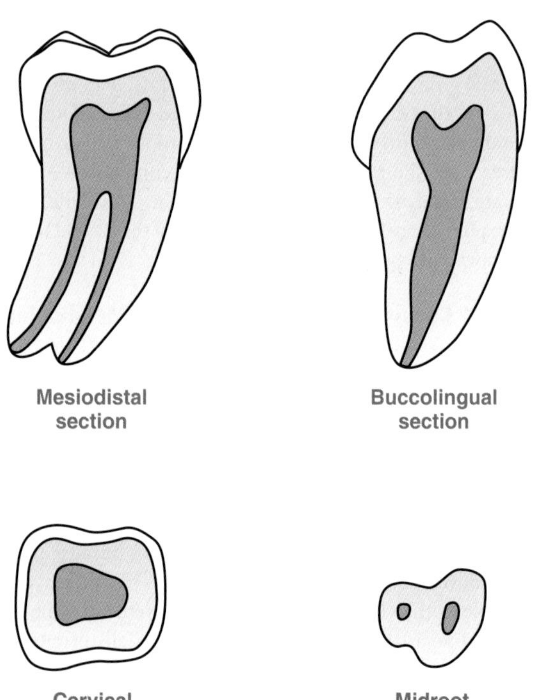

Fig. 17.61 Pulp Cavity of the Permanent Mandibular Right Third Molar.

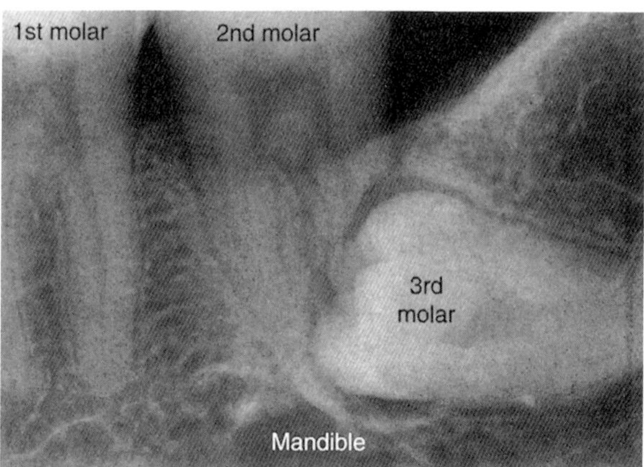

Fig. 17.62 Radiograph of an Impacted Permanent Mandibular Third Molar.

Permanent mandibular third molars, as was the case with the maxillary third molars, are permanent teeth commonly involved in partial anodontia, being congenitally missing either unilaterally or bilaterally (see **Chapter 6**). With this disturbance, the appropriate individual tooth germ(s) in the area is missing because of a failure in the initiation process during tooth development. However, this situation usually has no harmful consequences.

These teeth may also have accessory roots, which can complicate extraction procedures. Finally, developmental cyst formation may occur within the dental tissue of an impacted crown, resulting in a dentigerous cyst (see Fig. 6.30).

18

Primary Dentition

Additional resources and practice exercises are provided on the companion Evolve website for this book: http://evolve.elsevier.com/Fehrenbach/illustrated.

LEARNING OBJECTIVES

1. Define and pronounce the key terms in this chapter.
2. Assign the correct name and universal number for each primary tooth on a diagram and a patient.
3. Demonstrate the correct location of each primary tooth on a diagram and a patient.
4. Discuss primary teeth properties and the clinical considerations for primary dentition, integrating it into patient care.
5. Describe the general features of primary teeth and each primary tooth type as well as the specific features of each primary tooth.
6. Discuss the clinical considerations concerning primary molars, integrating it into patient care.

PRIMARY DENTITION PROPERTIES

The first set of teeth is the primary dentition (Fig. 18.1). The primary dentition is shed and replaced by the permanent dentition, which is why they sometimes were referred to as *deciduous*, like the type of trees that shed leaves. There are 20 total primary teeth when the primary dentition period is completed, with 10 per dental arch—as compared to 32 permanent teeth, with 16 per arch. The primary dentition includes the tooth types of incisors, canines, and molars (see Figs. 15.1 and 15.3, *A*). These are designated in the Universal Numbering System by the capital letters *A* through *T*. In the International Numbering System, the digits 5 through 8 are used for the first of two digits, numbering in a clockwise manner for the quadrants of the primary dentition. The digits 1 through 5 are used for the second digit, starting at the midline and numbering the teeth in a distal direction.

The primary molars are replaced by the permanent premolars; there are no premolars in the primary dentition like there are in the permanent dentition. The permanent molars erupt distal to the primary second molars.

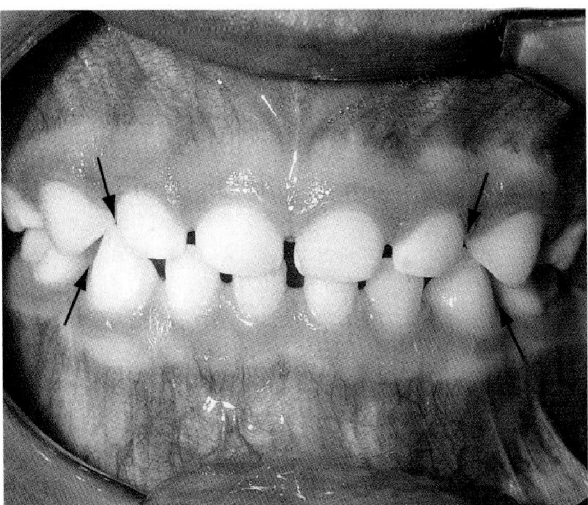

Fig. 18.1 Labial view of the primary dentition with the larger primate spaces that are usually present *(arrows)*. Note the attrition of the masticatory surfaces, which is also usually present, usually resulting in an end-to-end bite. (From Bird DL, Robinson DS. *Modern Dental Assisting.* 12th ed. St. Louis: Elsevier; 2018.)

Mineralization of the first primary teeth begin in utero at 13 to 16 weeks. By 18 to 20 weeks during prenatal development, all of the primary teeth have started to mineralize. There are usually no primary teeth visible in the oral cavity at birth. The first eruption of a primary tooth, a primary mandibular central incisor, occurs at an average age of 6 to 10 months with the further eruption of the rest of the primary dentition following (Table 18.1).

The primary dentition takes between 2 and 3 years to be completed, beginning with the initial mineralization of the primary mandibular central incisors and later being completed with root formation in the primary maxillary second molar (see Fig. 6.22, *A*). A 6-month delay or acceleration is considered usual for an individual child. However, if a child patient is unusually early or late in getting their teeth, it is important to inquire about their related dental history concerning this issue.

The actual dates are not as important as the eruption sequence because there can be a great deal of variation in the actual dates of eruption, which is noted in various texts on the subject. However, the sequence tends to be uniform (see Fig. 20.5). In addition, the specific tooth types tend to erupt in pairs so that if there is any asymmetry noted within the primary dentition, a radiograph of the area may be required. Young women tend to shed their primary teeth and have the permanent teeth slightly earlier than young men, reflecting the earlier overall physical maturation achieved.

Interproximal spaces between the primary teeth are present in most child patients because space is necessary for the proper alignment of the lager future permanent dentition. These important interproximal spaces still may concern the supervising adults and they may need reassurance. The largest spaces are considered **primate spaces**, mostly involving spaces between the primary maxillary lateral incisor and canine and also between the primary mandibular canine and first molar (see Fig. 18.1 and **Chapter 20**).

Primary teeth are smaller overall than permanent teeth. However, each primary tooth should not be considered just a "mini-me" to the permanent teeth because there are important differences that occur in the structure as well as the size of primary teeth compared with that of permanent teeth (Figs. 18.2 to 18.4).

The crown of any primary tooth is short in relation to its total length. The crowns are also more constricted or narrower at the cementoenamel junction (CEJ), making them appear bulbous in comparison

TABLE 18.1 Approximate Eruption and Shedding Ages for Primary Teeth

Type of Teeth	Mean Eruption (Range)	Mean Shedding (Range)
Maxillary Teeth		
Central incisor	10 (8–12 months)	6 7 years
Lateral incisor	11 (9–13 months)	7–8 years
Canine	19 (16–22 months)	10–12 years
First molar	16 (13–19 months for men; 14–19 months for women)	9–11 years
Second molar	29 (25–33 months)	10–12 years
Mandibular Teeth		
Central incisor	8 (6–10 months)	6–7 years
Lateral incisor	13 (10–16 months)	7–8 years
Canine	20 (17–23 months)	9–12 years
First molar	16 (14–18 months)	9–11 years
Second molar	27 (23–31 months for men; 24–30 months for women)	10–12 years

Data from Nelson S. *Wheeler's Dental Anatomy, Physiology and Occlusion.* 10th ed. St. Louis: Elsevier; 2015.

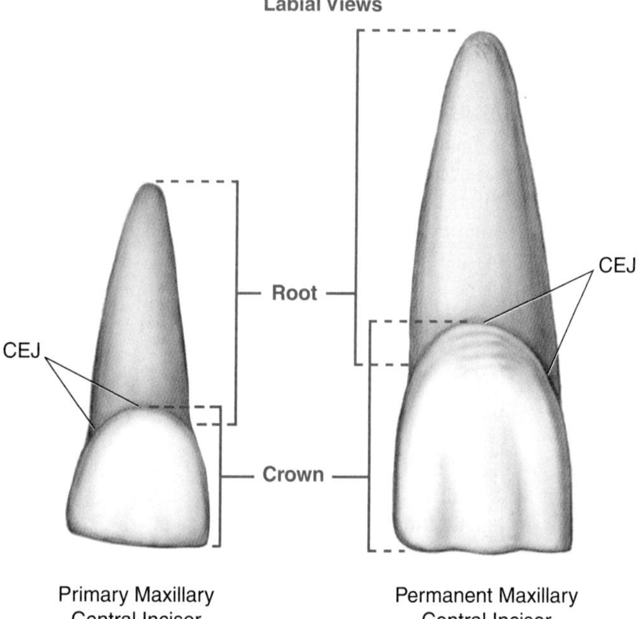

Fig. 18.2 Differences between the crowns of the primary and permanent teeth. Note the different crown-to-root ratios as well as the differences at the cementoenamel junction *(CEJ).*

to the thinner neck. The occlusal table on the primary is also narrower than on the permanent counterpart. A prominent cervical ridge is present on both the labial and lingual surfaces of anterior teeth and on buccal surfaces of the molars, more than any similar structure on the even larger permanent molars (see Fig. 18.4). The contacts are broad and flat within the primary dentition.

Roots of primary teeth are also narrower and longer than the crown length (see Figs. 18.2 to 18.4). Each crown-to-root ratio of primary teeth is smaller than those ratios of their permanent dentition counterparts. Molar roots flare more as they approach the apex. The apical foramina may be larger with the accessory canals often larger and also more numerous. Roots may also show partial resorption as the teeth begin to be shed, which can be noted radiographically (see Fig. 6.27, *A*).

The pulp cavity on primary teeth shows that both the pulp chambers and pulp horns are relatively large in proportion to those of the permanent teeth, especially the mesial pulp horns of the molars (Fig. 18.5). However, great variation in both size and location exists in this dentition, but there is usually a pulp horn under each cusp. The pulp horns are also closer to the outer surface with the pulp chambers being shallow.

Overall, the dentin of the primary dentition is thinner than that of the permanent counterparts. However, the dentin thickness between the pulp chambers and the enamel can be greater especially in the primary mandibular second molar. The enamel is also relatively thin in comparison to permanent counterparts, but it has consistent thickness overlying the dentin of the crown. Primary teeth also have whiter tone of enamel on their crowns than the permanent teeth because of the increased opacity of the enamel, which covers the underlying yellow dentin. Additionally, it needs to be noted that the enamel rods in the cervical area are directed occlusally.

Clinical Considerations for Primary Dentition

Child patients and supervising adults sometimes discount the importance of the teeth of the primary dentition because they believe they are temporary and soon replaced. It is true that a 70-year-old person will have spent 91% of his or her lifetime chewing with the permanent teeth but only 6% with the primary dentition. Thus the primary dentition generally functions in esthetics, mastication, and speech for a child for only 5 to 12 years. However, these teeth also serve the important function of holding open the eruption arch space for the succedaneous permanent teeth, which will replace the primary teeth. Individually, each primary tooth also functions in the same way as its permanent counterpart when present.

In the past, many carious primary teeth were extracted instead of repaired, resulting in crowding and potential occlusal complications in the permanent dentition as it erupted (see **Chapter 20**). Worse still many carious primary teeth were ignored, resulting in serious oral infections and discomfort for the child patient.

The value of primary teeth is now more realistically appreciated leading to more primary teeth being saved from caries because of early dental care. Still the value of these teeth must be imparted to child patients and supervising adults. Supervision of homecare procedures must begin early and at least as the first primary teeth erupt into the oral cavity to prevent premature loss of the primary teeth. Because the enamel and dentin are thinner, the risk of endodontic complications is greater for the primary dentition.

In addition, since the pulp chamber and pulp horns are also larger on primary teeth there is an increased risk of pulpal exposure during cavity preparation (see Fig. 18.5 and **Chapter 13**). If a pulpotomy (or partial removal) is performed on primary teeth, there may be perforations; a pulpectomy (or complete removal) on primary molars has increased difficulty due to the more tortuous and irregular pulp canals.

Any extraction and other surgical procedures performed during the primary dentition period must be done with extreme caution due to the presence of the deeper developing tooth germs of the permanent dentition, especially with the primary second molars with the presence of the permanent premolars located between the roots (see Figs. 6.27 and 6.28). The conical anterior roots facilitate easy surgical extraction but the flared roots of molars are more difficult to treat.

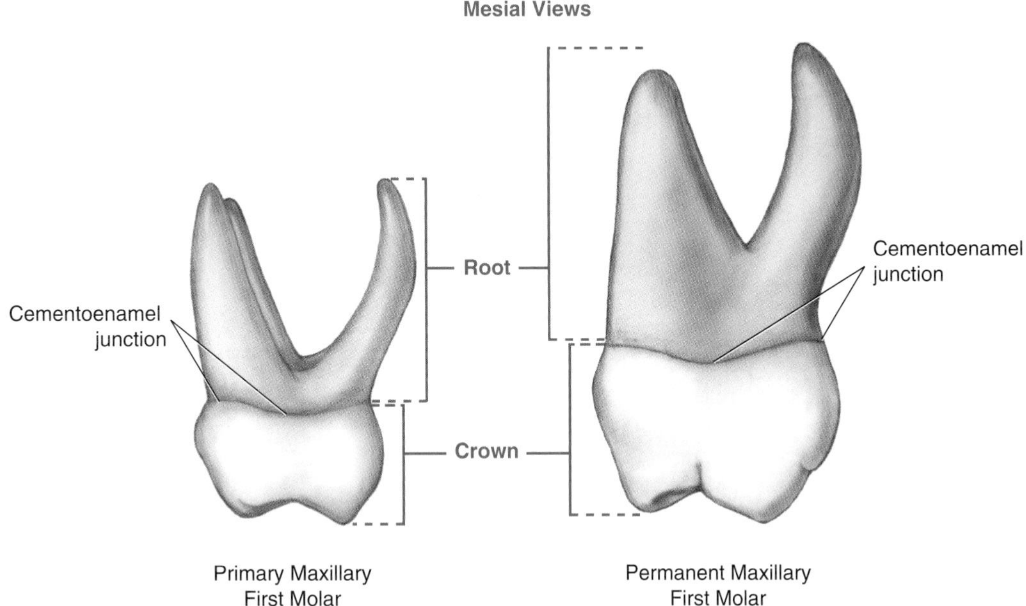

Fig. 18.3 Differences between the crowns and roots of the primary and permanent teeth, especially the differences at the cementoenamel junction.

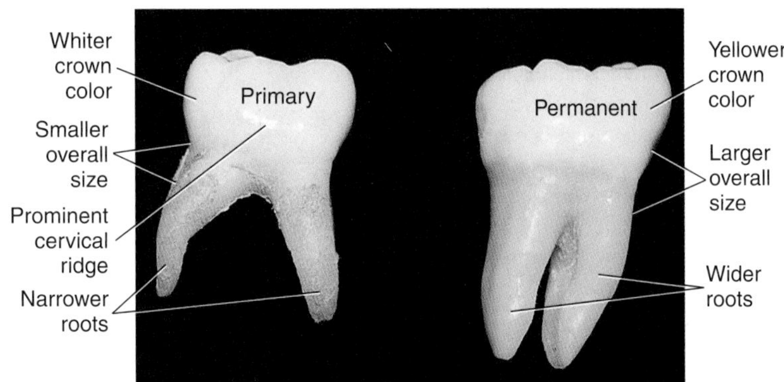

Fig. 18.4 Extracted teeth showing the differences between the primary and permanent teeth. (Courtesy of Margaret J. Fehrenbach, RDH, MS.)

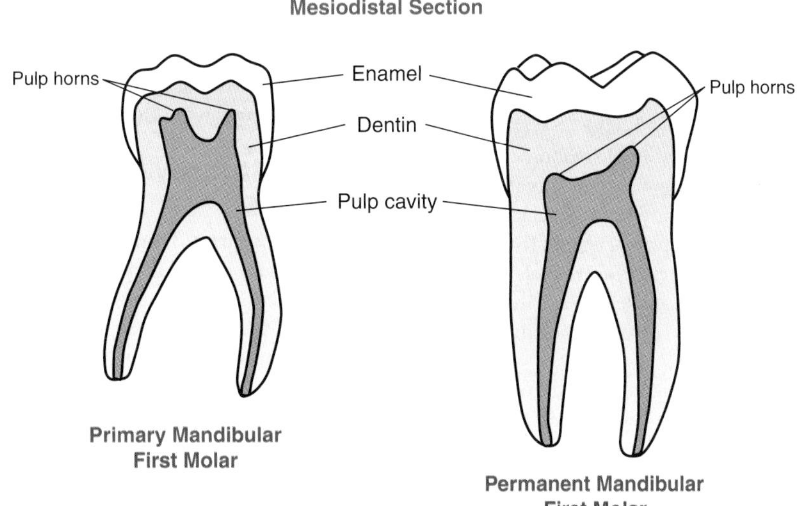

Fig. 18.5 Differences between the relatively large pulp chambers and pulp horns of the primary teeth and those of permanent teeth, which are relatively smaller.

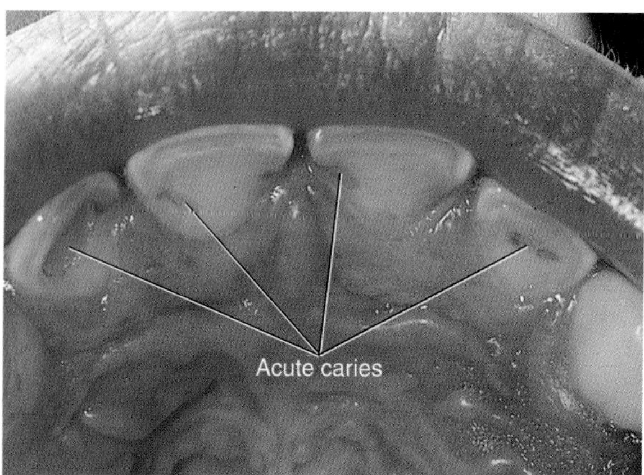

Fig. 18.6 Acute caries on the lingual surfaces of primary maxillary anterior teeth caused by early childhood caries, which is more commonly referred to as *baby bottle tooth decay.* (Courtesy of Margaret J. Fehrenbach, RDH, MS.)

Bulging of the cervical ridge of primary teeth must also be taken into account when these teeth are involved in any restorative procedure as well as restoring their broad contacts (see Fig. 18.4).

All of these complex factors are tied to the primary dentition along with the increased possibility of poor homecare in the young child patient, especially if lacking direction by supervising adults. Prolonged nighttime use of a baby bottle with a cavity-causing beverage or sugar on a pacifier must also be considered as an etiologic factor in a child patient with extensive acute caries of the primary teeth. This condition is **early childhood caries (ECC)**, which is more commonly referred to as *baby bottle tooth decay* (Fig. 18.6).

A child's first dental appointment should occur within 6 months of the eruption of the first primary tooth and no later than 12 months of age. The intent of this recommendation is to provide information to the child's supervising adults, which will help to establish positive preventive behaviors, prevent serious dental problems, and allay concerns. This early initial visit affords the dental professional the opportunity to provide basic timely information and to do this in 6-month increments.

Early dental care is important not only for keeping the primary dentition healthy but also for assessing the need for any appropriate interceptive orthodontic therapy. This may include the use of space maintainers, retainers, and removal of any extraneous bulbous proximal crown width. Also, removal of retained primary teeth (or retained roots) as needed may allow the correct eruption sequence and alignment of the permanent teeth later (see Fig. 20.4).

Extraction procedures of primary teeth should always be performed with caution and with radiographic confirmation of a permanent replacement, especially with primary second molars. If the permanent teeth are missing due to partial anodontia, which can occur with second premolars, the extraction of the primary tooth (mostly the primary molar) must be avoided because retention is preferred and may cover many years of use (see Box 6.1, *B*). Extensive extrinsic staining of the primary teeth may be attributed to Nasmyth membrane (see Fig. 6.29).

In addition, if severe periodontal inflammation and destruction in the primary and/or mixed dentition are found with evidence of little dental biofilm, either locally or within the entire dentition, aggressive periodontitis must be suspected. Early intervention with this severe yet uncommon periodontal disease can prevent further periodontal destruction. Thus a periodontal probe should always be present on the dental tray during dental examinations with child patients.

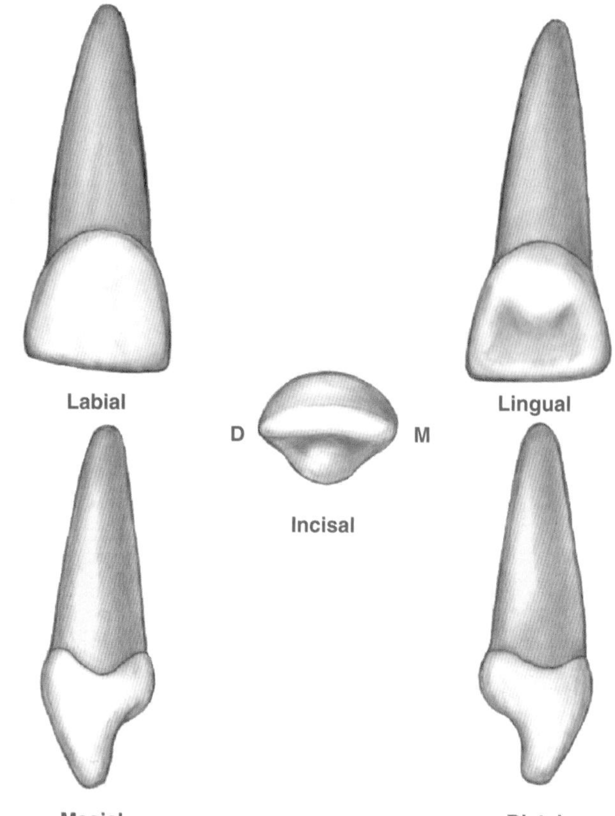

Fig. 18.7 Views of the Primary Maxillary Right Central Incisor. *D,* Distal; *M,* mesial.

PRIMARY INCISORS

General Features

Each dental arch has four primary incisors. As in the permanent dentition, each quadrant has two incisor types: central incisor and lateral incisor. Both primary incisors resemble their permanent successor with some exceptions, such as a more prominent cervical ridge present on both the labial and lingual surfaces. Also both have the same arch position, function, and general shape as the permanent counterpart, functioning as such for about 5 years.

Dental professionals sometimes note extensive wear or attrition of the incisal ridges of the primary incisors from bruxism (grinding) and the possible formation of an end-to-end bite between the arches. The significance of this finding and its possible relevance to later adult parafunctional habits are unknown (see Fig. 18.1).

Primary Maxillary Central Incisor, E and F (#51 and #61)

Specific Features. From the labial aspect, the crown of the primary maxillary central incisor (Fig. 18.7) appears wider mesiodistally than incisocervically, which is the opposite of its permanent successor. In fact, it is the only anterior tooth of either dentition with this crown dimension. Additionally, its mesial and distal outlines are more rounded than the permanent central incisor as a result of the cervical constriction. The incisal outline is relatively straight from this view, but it slopes toward the distal with attrition.

Unlike their permanent successors, the primary maxillary central incisors have no mamelons, leaving the labial surface smooth. In addition, these teeth rarely have developmental depressions or imbrication lines and no pits are evident on the lingual surface. However,

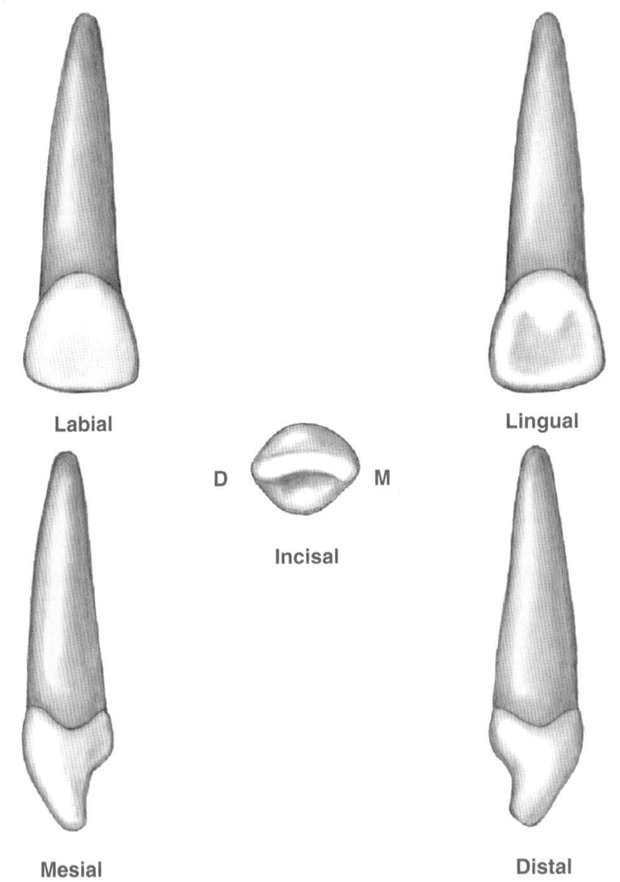

Fig. 18.8 Views of the Primary Maxillary Right Lateral Incisor. *D*, Distal; *M*, mesial.

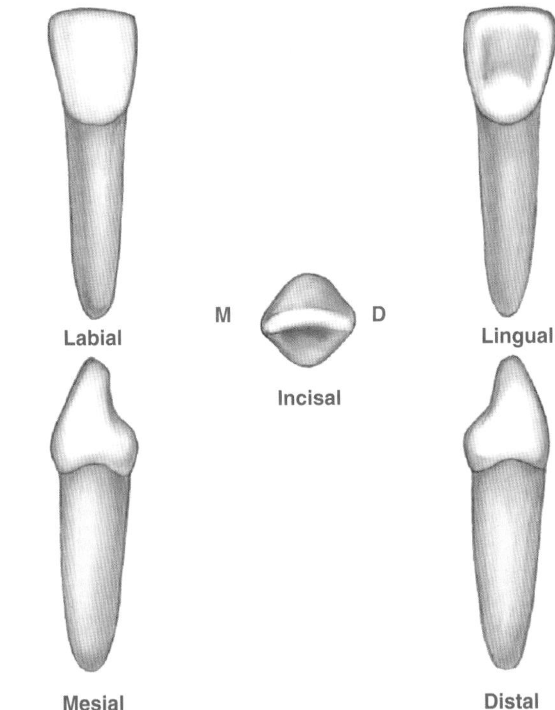

Fig. 18.9 Views of the Primary Mandibular Right Central Incisor. *D*, Distal; *M*, mesial.

the cingulum and marginal ridges on the lingual surface all are more prominent than on the permanent successor and the lingual fossa is deeper.

Both proximal surfaces of the maxillary central incisor appear similar. Because of the short crown and its wide labiolingual measurement, the crown appears thick, even at the incisal third. The CEJ curves distinctly toward the incisal but not as much as on its permanent successor. This curvature is less distal than mesial as in the permanent successor. From the incisal surface, the crown appears wider mesiodistally than labiolingually and the incisal ridge appears almost straight. The single root is generally round in shape and tapers evenly to the apex, but it is longer, relative to crown length, than the permanent central incisor.

Primary Maxillary Lateral Incisor, D and G (#52 and #62)

Specific Features. The crown of the primary maxillary lateral incisor (Fig. 18.8) is similar to the central incisor but is much smaller than the central in all dimensions. The lateral is also longer incisocervically than mesiodistally, which is exactly the opposite of the central. The incisal angles are also more rounded than the central. The root is also similar to that of the central, but the lateral's root is longer in proportion to its crown compared with the same proportions of the central and its apex is sharper.

Primary Mandibular Central Incisor, O and P (#71 and #81)

Specific Features. The crown of the primary mandibular central incisor (Fig. 18.9) looks more like the primary mandibular lateral incisor than its permanent successor or any other primary maxillary incisor. This tooth is also quite symmetrical, however, which is similar to its permanent successor. It is also not as constricted at the CEJ as the primary maxillary central incisor. From the labial aspect, the crown appears wide compared with its permanent successor. Its mesial and distal outlines from the labial aspect also show that the crown tapers evenly from the contact areas.

The lingual surface of the primary mandibular central incisor appears smooth and tapers toward the prominent cingulum. The marginal ridges are less pronounced than those of the primary maxillary incisor; the lingual fossa is also shallow. Again the CEJ curvature on the mesial surface is greater than on the distal. From the mesial aspect, this tooth is much wider labiolingually than its permanent successor.

The incisal ridge is centered over the root from both the proximal and incisal views and divides the labial and lingual into equal halves. The root is single, long, and slender. The labial and lingual surfaces of the root are both rounded, but the proximal surfaces are slightly flattened.

Primary Mandibular Lateral Incisor, N and Q (#72 and #82)

Specific Features. The crown of the primary mandibular lateral incisor (Fig. 18.10) is similar in form to the central incisor of the same arch, but the crown is wider and longer than that of the central. The cingulum is also more developed and the lingual fossa is slightly deeper than that of the central incisor.

The incisal ridge slopes distally and its distoincisal angle is more rounded as is the distal margin. From the incisal aspect, the crown is not as symmetrical as is the central because the cingulum is offset toward the distal, which has the same cingulum position as its permanent successor. The root may have a distal curvature in its apical third and it usually has a distal longitudinal groove.

PRIMARY CANINES

General Features

There are four primary canines, two in each dental arch, and one in each quadrant. These primary canines mostly resemble the outline of their permanent successors with some exceptions, such as having a more prominent cervical ridge present on both the labial and lingual surfaces.

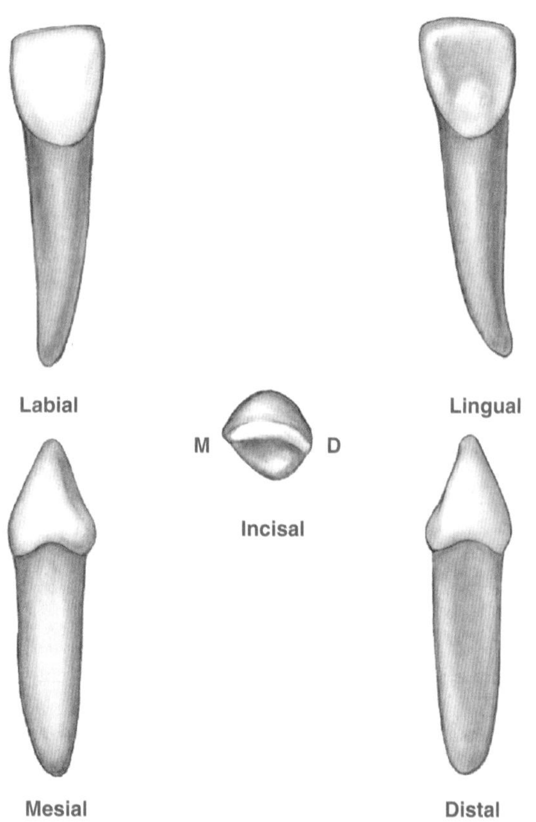

Fig. 18.10 Views of the Primary Mandibular Right Lateral Incisor. *D*, Distal; *M*, mesial.

Primary Maxillary Canine, C and H (#53 and #63)

Specific Features. The crown of the primary maxillary canine (Fig. 18.11) has a relatively longer and sharper cusp than that of its permanent successor when first erupted. The mesial and distal outlines of the primary maxillary canine are both rounder in shape, however, and greatly overhang the cervical line. The mesial cusp slope is longer than the distal cusp slope on this tooth, which is just the opposite of the primary mandibular canine and also is the opposite of its permanent counterpart.

On the lingual surface, the cingulum is well developed as are the lingual ridge and marginal ridges. The lingual ridge extends from the cingulum to the cusp tip and divides the lingual surface into a shallow mesiolingual fossa and distolingual fossa. A tubercle is often present on the cingulum, extending from the cusp tip to the cingulum.

From the incisal aspect, the crown is diamond-shaped and the cusp tip is slightly offset to the distal. The root is twice as long as the crown, more slender than that of its permanent successor, and it is inclined distally.

Primary Mandibular Canine, M and R (#73 and #83)

Specific Features. The crown of the primary mandibular canine (Fig. 18.12) resembles that of the primary maxillary canine, although some dimensions are different. This tooth is much smaller labiolingually. The distal cusp slope is much longer than the mesial cusp slope as is the case on its permanent counterpart.

The lingual surface is smoother than the primary maxillary canine and is marked by a shallow lingual fossa. The incisal ridge of the primary mandibular canine is straight and is centered over the crown labiolingually. The root is long, narrow, and almost twice the length of the crown, although it is shorter and more tapered than that of a primary maxillary canine.

PRIMARY MOLARS

General Features

There are eight primary molars with two types: a first molar and second molar. One of each type is located in each quadrant of both dental arches. Both have the similar arch position, function, and general shape as the permanent counterpart and they function as such for approximately 9 years. Primary molars are replaced by the permanent premolars when shed. However, none of the primary first molars resemble any other tooth in either dentition; instead, the crown of each

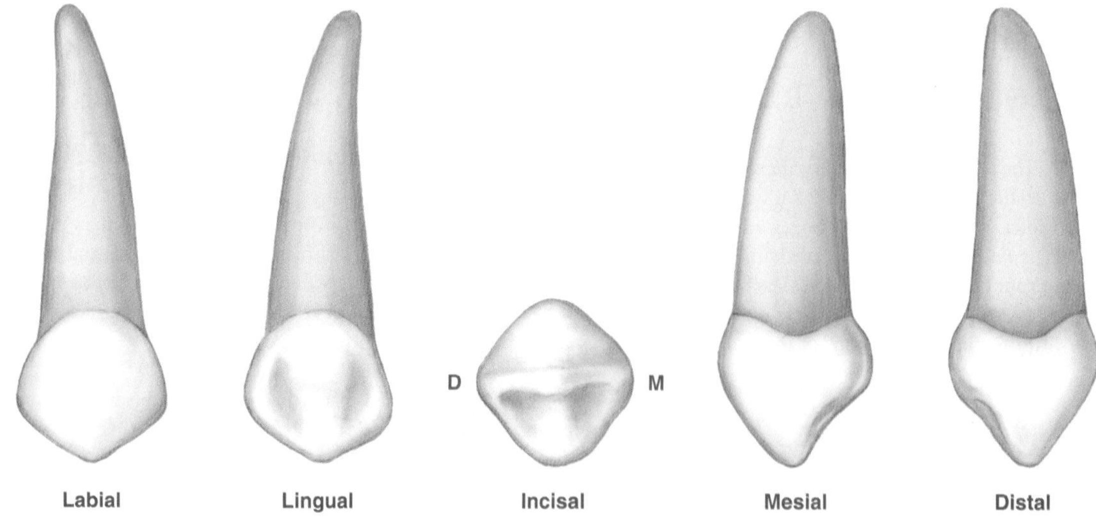

Fig. 18.11 Views of the Primary Maxillary Right Canine. *D*, Distal; *M*, mesial.

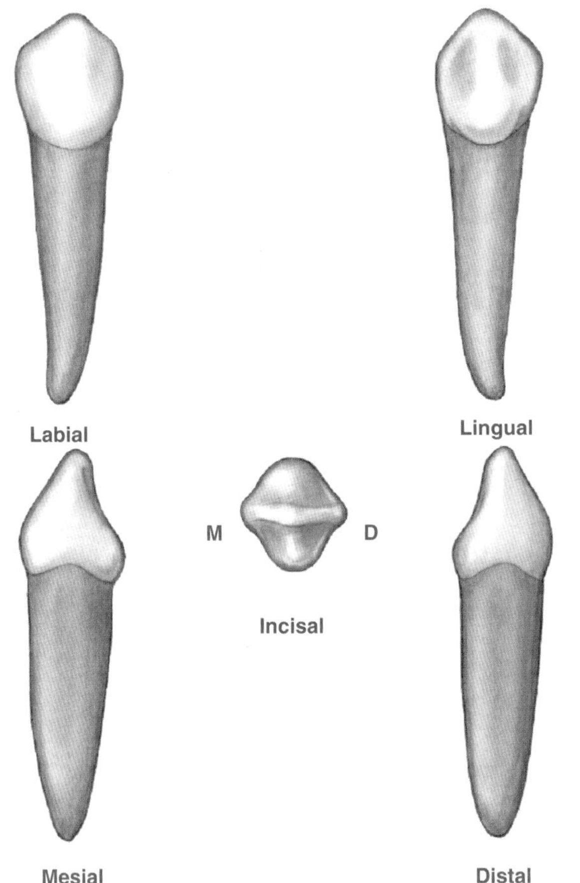

Fig. 18.12 Views of the Primary Mandibular Right Canine. *D*, Distal; *M*, mesial.

primary second molar in both arches resembles the first molars of the permanent dentition that will erupt distal to them. Each molar crown is shorter occlusocervically than mesiodistally (see Fig. 18.4). A prominent cervical ridge is present on the buccal surfaces.

The occlusal table on a primary molar is more constricted buccolingually than with a permanent molar like a rope around a corral (see Fig. 18.13 for example). This constriction is due to both the buccal and lingual surfaces of a primary molar being flatter occlusal to the CEJ curvatures, thus narrowing the occlusal table. The occlusal anatomy of the cusps is also not as pronounced as on the permanent successors.

The roots of the molars are flared beyond the crown outlines, widely separating the roots (see Fig. 18.4). Additional space is thus available between the roots for the deeper developing permanent premolar crowns. The primary molars each have a short root trunk as with permanent posterior teeth; the roots branch a short distance from the base of the crown. Thus the primary molars are wider MD than the permanent premolars, allowing for arch leeway space in each case.

Primary Maxillary First Molar, B and I (#54 and #64)

Specific Features. The crown of the primary maxillary first molar (Fig. 18.13) does not resemble any other crown of either dentition. From the buccal aspect, both the mesial and distal outlines are rounded and constricted at the CEJ. The CEJ on the mesial half of the buccal surface curves around an extremely prominent buccal cervical ridge. The height of contour on the buccal is at the cervical one-third and for the lingual at the middle one-third.

The occlusal table on the maxillary first molar can have four cusps: mesiobuccal, mesiolingual, distobuccal, and distolingual, with the two mesial cusps being the largest and the two distal cusps being quite small. It can also have only three cusps because the distolingual cusp may be absent. The occlusal table also has an extremely prominent

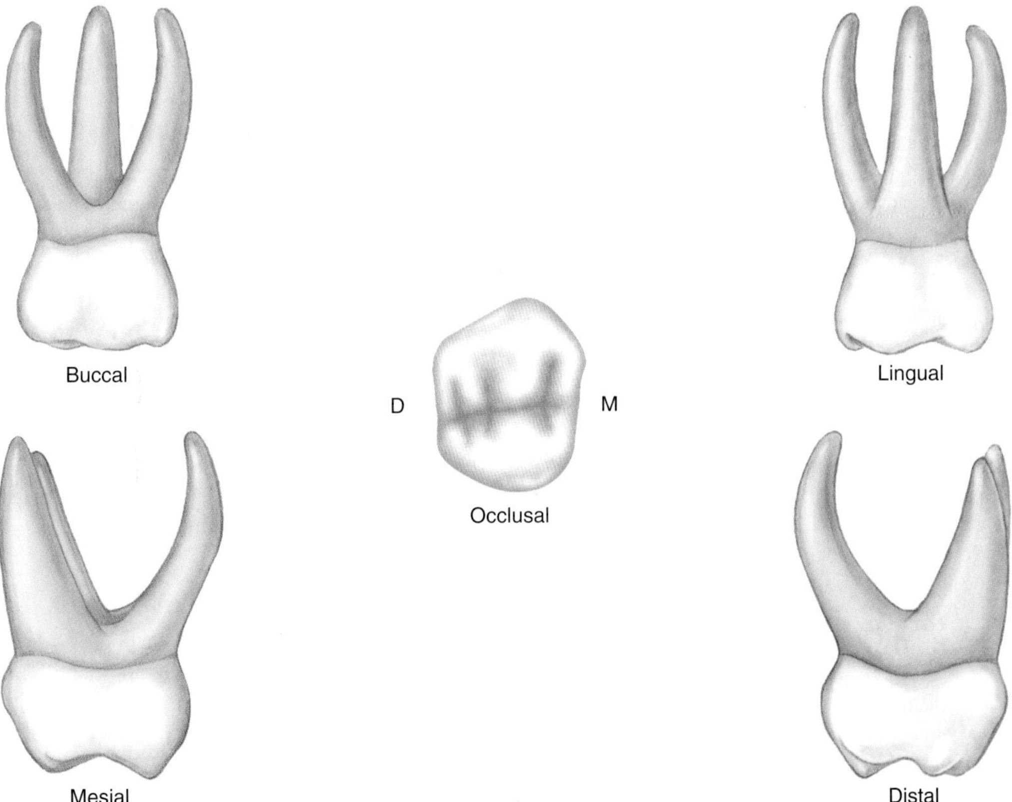

Fig. 18.13 Views of the Primary Maxillary First Right Molar. *D*, Distal; *M*, mesial.

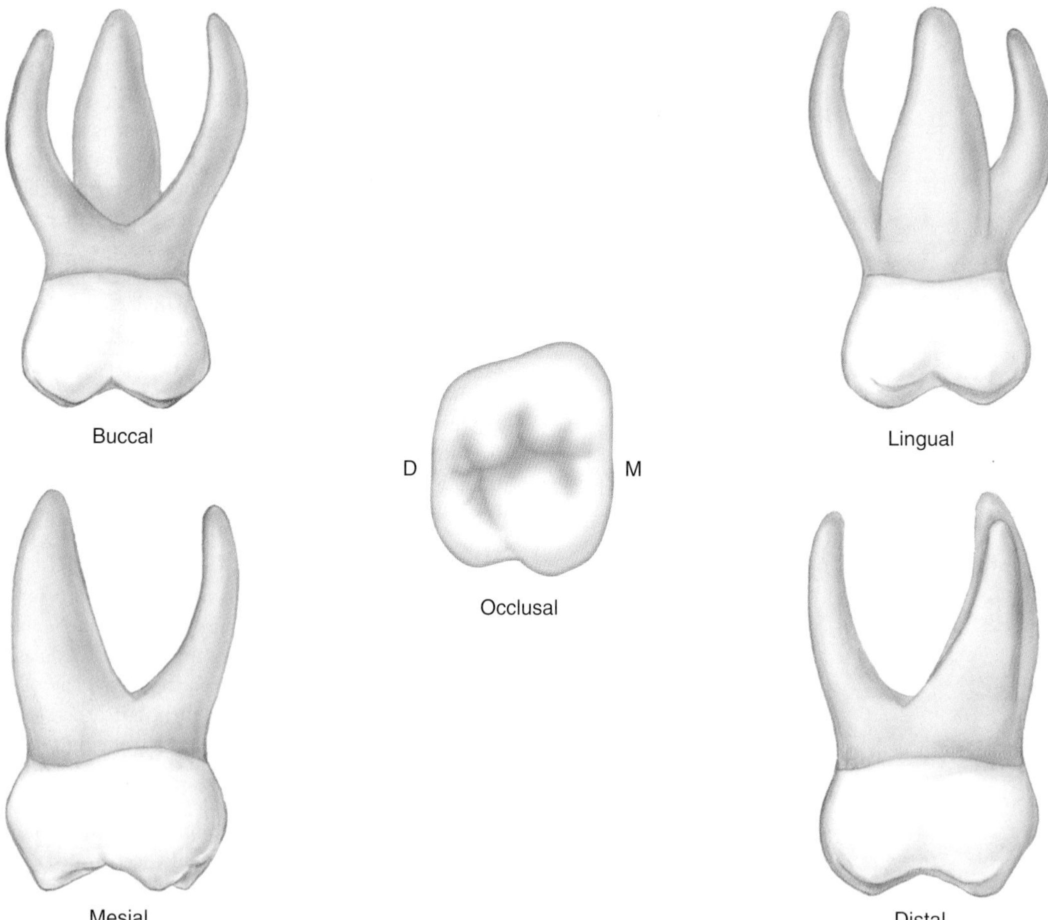

Fig. 18.14 Views of the Primary Maxillary Right Second Molar. *D,* Distal; *M,* mesial.

transverse ridge. Additionally, an oblique ridge extends between the mesiolingual cusp and the distobuccal cusp; however, it is not as prominent as the one on its permanent counterpart.

The tooth also has an H-shaped groove pattern and three fossae: central, mesial triangular, and distal triangular. The central groove connects the central pit with the mesial pit and distal pit at each end of the occlusal table.

The buccal groove originates in the central pit and extends buccally, separating the mesiobuccal and distobuccal cusps. The distal triangular fossa contains the disto-occlusal groove, which extends obliquely and is parallel to the oblique ridge just distal to it. Both the buccal and disto-occlusal grooves remain located only at the occlusal table, which is unlike its permanent counterpart.

Primary maxillary first molars do have the same number and position of the roots as the permanent maxillary molars. The three root branches are thinner and have greater flare than on the permanent molar and the root trunk is short. The mesiobuccal root is wider buccolingually than the distobuccal root and the lingual root is the longest and most divergent.

Primary Maxillary Second Molar, A and J (#55 and #65)

Specific Features. The primary maxillary second molar (Fig. 18.14) is larger than the primary maxillary first molar. This tooth most closely resembles the form of the permanent maxillary first molar but is smaller in all dimensions. Thus it usually has a cusp of Carabelli, the minor fifth cusp, as does its permanent counterpart.

Primary Mandibular First Molar, L and S (#74 and #84)

Specific Features. The primary mandibular first molar (Fig. 18.15) has a crown unlike any other tooth of either dentition. The tooth does have a prominent buccal cervical ridge, which is also on the mesial half of the buccal surface, similar to other primary molars. The height of contour on the buccal is at the cervical one-third and for the lingual is in the middle one-third. The mesiolingual line angle of the crown is rounder than any other line angles.

The tooth has four cusps with the mesial cusps larger. The mesiolingual cusp is long, pointed, and angled in on the occlusal table. A transverse ridge passes between the mesiobuccal and mesiolingual cusps. The tooth does have two roots, which are positioned similarly to those of the permanent mandibular molars.

Primary Mandibular Second Molar, K and T (#75 and #85)

Specific Features. The primary mandibular second molar (Fig. 18.16) is larger than the primary mandibular first molar. The tooth most closely resembles the form of the permanent mandibular first molar that erupts distal to it because it has five cusps. The three buccal cusps are almost equal in size, however, and the primary mandibular second molar has an overall oval occlusal shape.

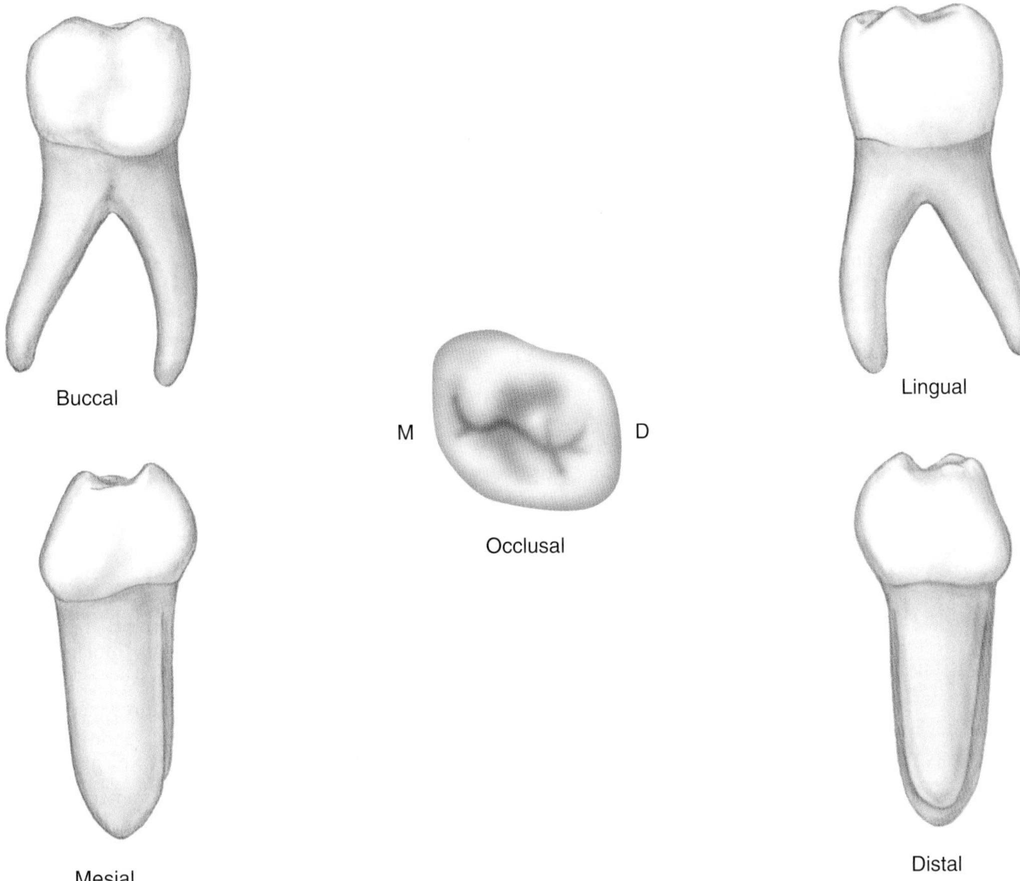

Fig. 18.15 Views of the Primary Mandibular Right First Molar. *D,* Distal; *M,* mesial.

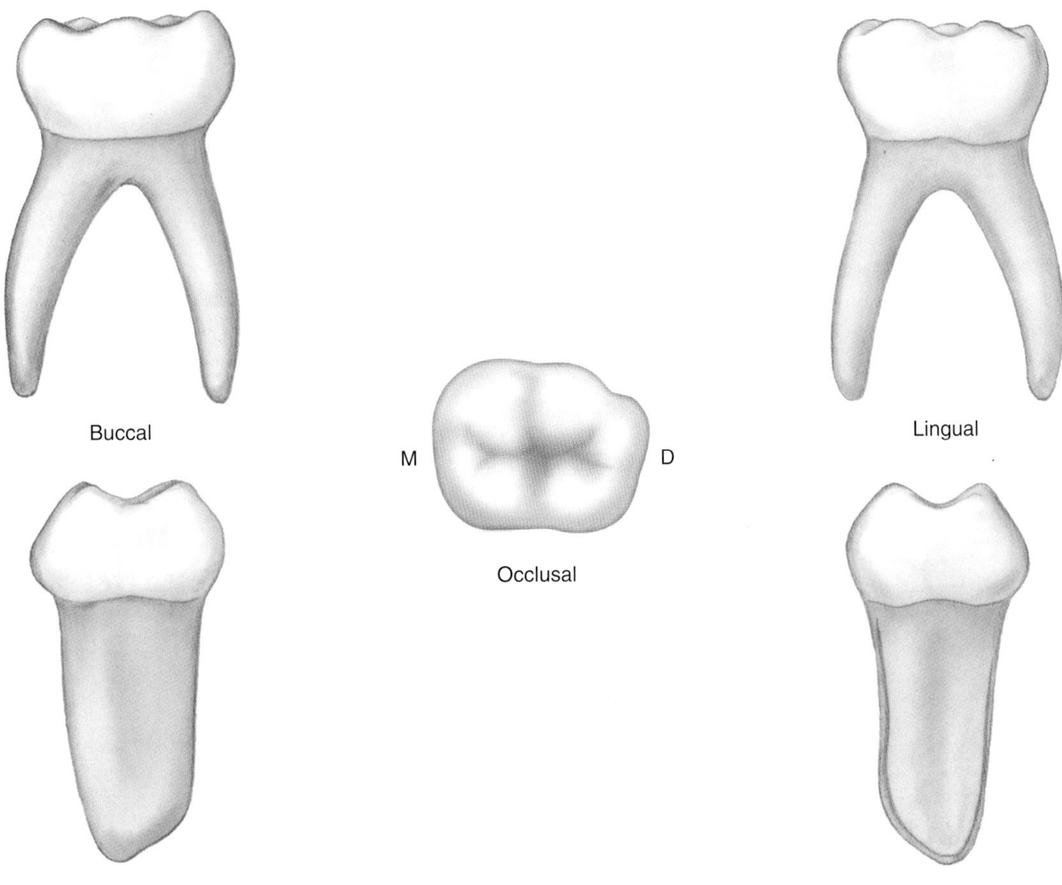

Fig. 18.16 Views of the Primary Mandibular Right Second Molar. *D,* Distal; *M,* mesial.

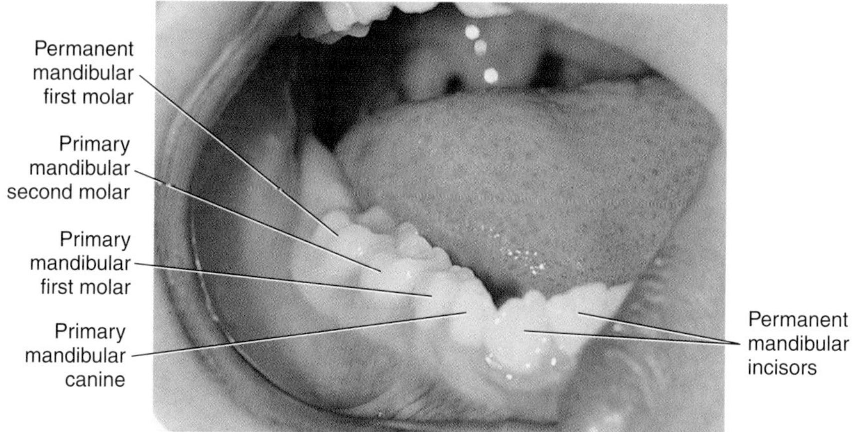

Fig. 18.17 The mixed dentition with the eruption of the permanent mandibular first molar distal to the primary mandibular second molar. Note that the newly erupted permanent first molar can be difficult to discern because it appears similar to the already erupted adjacent primary second molar. (Courtesy of Margaret J. Fehrenbach, RDH, MS.)

Clinical Considerations with Primary Molars. Child patients within the mixed dentition period and their supervising adults may not notice the presence of the newly erupted permanent first molar of either arch because when it erupts it appears similar to the larger primary second molar that is adjacent to it (Fig. 18.17). These child patients and their supervising adults must be reminded that to last a lifetime, these new posterior permanent teeth require diligent homecare and may need enamel sealants applied to the occlusal surface.

The greater root spread of primary molars, along with their narrow shape and lack of root trunk, makes primary molars susceptible to fracture during extraction procedures (see Fig. 18.4). Dental professionals should also remember that shedding of primary teeth is an intermittent process with resorption of the dental tissue being followed by apposition. A loose primary tooth may tighten and thus may not be as ready as thought for extraction, a procedure that should always be considered with caution in these young patients (see earlier discussion and **Chapter 6**).

19

Temporomandibular Joint

Additional resources and practice exercises are provided on the companion Evolve website for this book: http://evolve.elsevier.com/Fehrenbach/illustrated

LEARNING OBJECTIVES

1. Define and pronounce the key terms in this chapter.
2. Locate and identify the specific anatomic landmarks of the temporomandibular joint on a diagram, a skull, and a patient.
3. Describe the histology of each component of the temporomandibular joint and how it relates to its clinical features.
4. Outline the movements of the temporomandibular joint as well as demonstrating them on a skull, a dentition model, and a patient.
5. Discuss the clinical considerations for joint pathology and temporomandibular joint disorders, integrating it into patient care.

TEMPOROMANDIBULAR JOINT PROPERTIES

The temporomandibular joint (TMJ) is a joint located on each side of the head that allows for movement of the mandible for mastication, speech, and respiratory movements; it is the most complex set of joints in the body. The TMJ can be palpated just anterior to each ear (see Fig. 1.3).

Patients may have a disorder associated with the TMJ, which is discussed later in this chapter. Thus, dental professionals must understand the anatomy, histology, and movements of the TMJ before being able to understand any disorders associated with the joint.

The TMJ develops in the 11th to 12th week of prenatal development, during the proliferation of the associated ligaments, muscles, and bones of the joint, as well as the joint spaces and joint disc.

JOINT BONES

The TMJ is the articulation of the temporal bone and the mandible on each side of the head (Fig. 19.1). Knowing the basic anatomy of the bones is necessary for the dental professional as well as the underlying histology and actions of the TMJ.

TEMPORAL BONE

The articulating area of the TMJ on the temporal bone is located on the bone's inferior aspect (Fig. 19.2). This articulating area includes the temporal bone's articular eminence and the articular fossa. The **articular eminence** (ahr-**tik**-yuh-ler) is a smooth-surfaced rounded protuberance on the inferior aspect of the zygomatic process and is positioned anterior to the articular fossa.

The **articular fossa** (or mandibular fossa) while being posterior to the articular eminence is a depression on the inferior aspect of the temporal bone; it is also posterior and medial to the zygomatic arch (see Fig. 1.3). Posterior to the articular fossa is a sharper ridge, the **postglenoid process** (post-**glen**-oid).

The temporal bone consists of compact bone overlying cancellous bone (Fig. 19.3; see **Chapter 8**). The outermost surface of the compact bone is covered by periosteum. Like all bones, the innermost part of the bone consists of endosteum and the medullary cavity with its bone marrow. The articulating surface of the temporal bone is covered by fibrocartilage immediately overlying the periosteum.

MANDIBLE

The mandible articulates with each temporal bone at the head of each mandibular condyle, being directly on the **articulating surface of the condyle** (ahr-**tik**-yuh-late-ing), which has histology similar to the articulating surface of the temporal bone. In a mature adult, each condyle consists of compact bone overlying cancellous bone (see Figs. 19.2 and 19.3). Periosteum overlies the compact bone of the condyle, with the endosteum and bone marrow located on the innermost part of the bone. Fibrocartilage then overlies the periosteum at articulating surface of the condyle.

However, in contrast to the articulating surface of the temporal bone, a growth center is located in the head of each mandibular condyle before an individual undergoes maturity (Fig. 19.4). This growth center consists of hyaline cartilage underneath the periosteum on the articulating surface of the condyle. This is the last remaining growth center of bone in the body and is multidirectional in its growth capacity, unlike a typical long bone.

This area of cartilage within the bone grows in length by appositional growth as the individual grows to maturity. Over time the hyaline cartilage is replaced by the alveolar process, using endochondral ossification (see Fig. 8.13). This mandibular growth center in the condyle allows the increased length of the mandible needed for the larger permanent teeth as well as for the larger brain capacity of the adult. This growth of the mandible also influences the overall shape of the face; the growth pattern is charted and referred to during orthodontic therapy (see **Chapter 20**). When an individual reaches full maturity, the growth center of bone within the condyle has disappeared.

JOINT CAPSULE

A **joint capsule** completely encloses the TMJ (Fig. 19.5; see Figs. 19.1 and 19.3). To do this, the capsule wraps around the margin of the temporal bone's articular eminence and articular fossa superiorly. Inferiorly, the capsule wraps around the circumference of the mandibular condyle, at the level of the condyle's neck, but anteriorly and medially it attaches just to the margin of the articular surface of the condyle.

The joint capsule has two layers. The outer layer is a firm fibrous connective tissue supported by the surrounding ligaments associated with the joint. The inner layer is a **synovial membrane** (si-**noh**-vee-uhl), which consists of a thin connective tissue that contains nerves and blood vessels. The blood vessels in the synovial membrane produce **synovial fluid**. Synovial fluid is a thick substance that fills the joint, lubricates it, and provides nutrition to the avascular parts of the joint disc (discussed next).

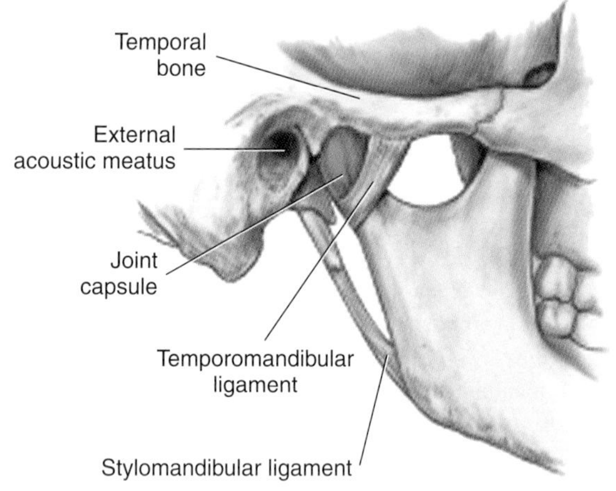

Fig. 19.1 Temporomandibular Joint and its Associated Bony Components. (From Fehrenbach MJ, Herring SW. *Illustrated Anatomy of the Head and Neck*. 5th ed. St. Louis: Elsevier; 2017.)

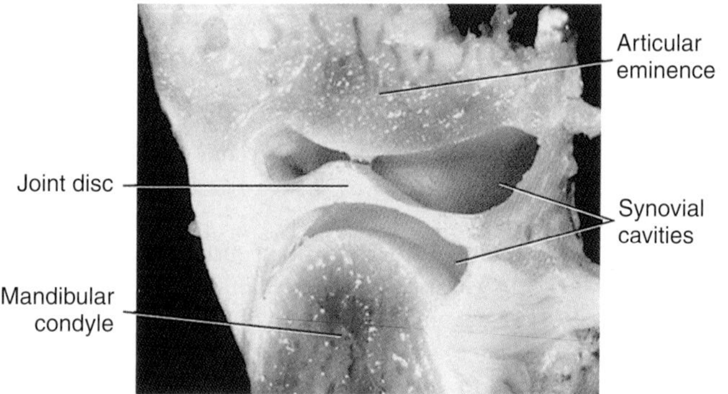

Fig. 19.2 Block Dissection of the Temporomandibular Joint. (From Nanci A. *Ten Cate's Oral Histology*. 9th ed. St. Louis: Elsevier; 2018.)

JOINT DISC

A **joint disc** is located on each side between the temporal bone and mandibular condyle (Fig. 19.6; see Figs. 19.2 and 19.3). On cross section, each disc appears caplike on the mandibular condyle, with its superior aspect concavoconvex from anterior to posterior and its inferior aspect concave. As is shown, this shape of the disc conforms to the shape of the adjacent articulating two bones of the TMJ and is related to the usual joint movements. Thus it functions as a deformable pad between the noncongruent articular surfaces of the bones of the joint.

The joint disc completely divides the TMJ into two compartments. These two compartments are considered **synovial cavities**, having both an upper and a lower synovial cavity. The synovial membrane lining the joint capsule produces the synovial fluid that fills these two cavities.

The joint disc is not free between the two bones but is attached to the lateral and medial poles of the mandibular condyle. However, the disc is not directly attached to the temporal bone anteriorly, but indirectly through the capsule. Posteriorly, the disc is divided into two areas or divisions. The upper division of the posterior part is attached to the temporal bone's postglenoid process and the lower division is attached to the neck of the mandibular condyle. The disc blends with the capsule at these two points. This posterior area of attachment of the disc to the capsule is one of the regions where nerves and blood vessels from the periosteum of the two bones enter the joint.

The joint disc itself consists of dense connective tissue (Fig. 19.7). Unlike other joint discs, it does not initially contain any cartilage. The central region of the disc is avascular (without blood vessels) and lacks innervation; in contrast, the peripheral region has both blood vessels and nerves. Few cells are present in the peripheral region and include fibroblasts and white blood cells. The central region is also thinner but of denser consistency than the peripheral region, which is thicker but has a more cushioned consistency. The synovial fluid in the synovial cavities provides the nutrition for the avascular central region of the disc. With aging, the entire disc thins and may undergo addition of cartilage in the central region, changes that may lead to impaired movement of the joint (discussed later).

JOINT MOVEMENT

Two basic types of movement of the mandible are performed by the TMJ and its associated **muscles of mastication:** a gliding movement

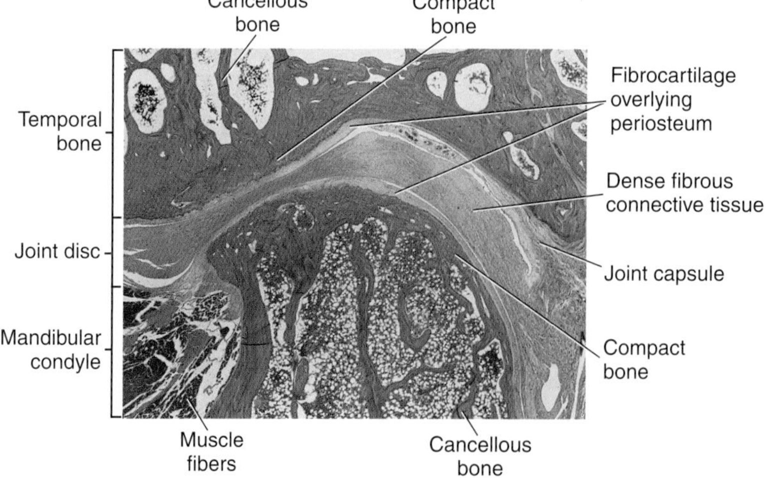

Fig. 19.3 Sagittal section of the temporomandibular joint, including the articulating area of the temporal bone, articulating surface of the condyle, joint disc, and joint capsule. (Courtesy of Major M. Ash, Jr.)

and a rotational movement (Figs. 19.8 and 19.9; Tables 19.1 and 19.2). These muscles are involved in mastication using these two movements.

The *gliding movement* of the TMJ mostly occurs between the disc and the articular eminence of the temporal bone in the upper synovial cavity, with the disc plus the mandibular condyle moving forward or backward, down and up the articular eminence. The gliding movement allows the lower jaw to move forward or backward. Bringing the lower jaw forward involves **protrusion of the mandible** (proh-**troo**-zhuhn) (see Fig. 20.15). Bringing the lower jaw backward involves **retraction of the mandible** (reh-**trak**-shuhn).

The *rotational movement* of the TMJ mostly occurs between the disc and the mandibular condyle in the lower synovial cavity. The axis of rotation of the disc plus the mandibular condyle is approximately transverse and the movements accomplished are depression or elevation of the mandible. The **depression of the mandible** is the lowering of the lower jaw. The **elevation of the mandible** (el-uh-**vey**-shuhn) is the raising of the lower jaw.

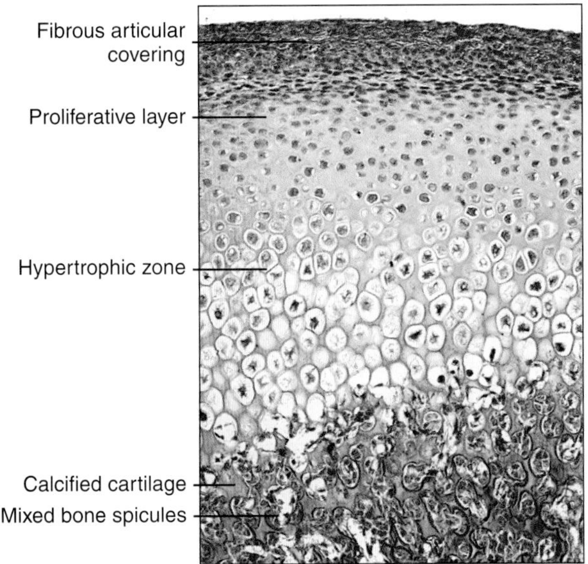

Fig. 19.4 Section taken through growth center of mandibular condyle with endochondral transformation of hyaline cartilage into the alveolar process using interstitial growth. (From Nanci A. *Ten Cate's Oral Histology*. 9th ed. St. Louis: Elsevier; 2018.)

With these two types of movements, gliding and rotation, and with the right and left TMJs working together, the finer movements of the jaws can be accomplished. These include opening and closing the jaws and shifting the lower jaw to one side.

Opening the jaws, which occurs during mastication, speech, and respiratory movements, involves both depression and protrusion of the mandible. When the jaws close, both elevation and retraction of the mandible occur. Therefore, the natural opening and closing of the jaws involve a combination of gliding and rotational movements of the TMJs in their respective joint cavities. The disc plus the condyle glides on the articular fossa in the upper synovial cavity, moving forward or backward on the articular eminence. At approximately the same time, the mandibular condyle rotates on the disc in the lower synovial cavity.

Lateral deviation of the mandible or lateral excursion involves shifting the lower jaw to one side, which occurs during mastication (see Fig. 20.13). Lateral deviation involves both gliding and rotational movements of contralateral TMJs in their respective joint cavities. During lateral deviation, the contralateral disc plus the mandibular condyle glides forward and medially on the articular eminence in the upper synovial cavity while the ipsilateral condyle and disc remain in a relatively stable position in the articular fossa, just rotating slightly in the articular fossa. This produces an orbiting of the contralateral condyle around the more stable ipsilateral condyle.

During mastication, the power stroke (when the teeth crunch the food) involves a movement from a laterally deviated position back to the midline. If the food is on the right side of the mouth, the mandible is deviated to the right. The power stroke returns the mandible to the center, and thus the movement is to the left and involves retraction of the left side; the reverse situation occurs if the food is on the left.

Clinical Considerations for Joint Pathology

Patients may have pathology associated with one or both of their TMJs or a **temporomandibular disorder (TMD)** (or dysfunction). It is the most common cause of facial pain after a toothache. Patients with TMD may experience chronic joint tenderness, swelling, and painful muscle spasms. They may also have difficulties in moving the joint, such as a limited or deviated mandibular opening. In a healthy joint, the surfaces in contact with one another (bone and cartilage) do not have any receptors to transmit the feeling of pain. The pain therefore originates from the surrounding soft tissue. When receptors from one of these areas are triggered, the pain causes a reflex to limit the mandible's movement.

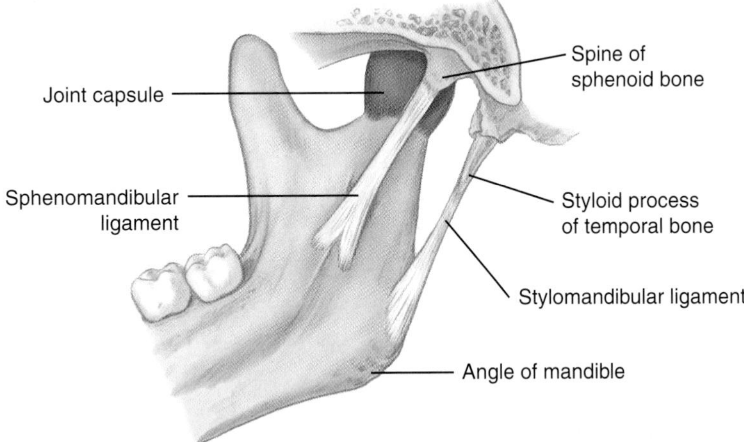

Fig. 19.5 Joint Capsule of the Temporomandibular Joint. (From Fehrenbach MJ, Herring SW. *Illustrated Anatomy of the Head and Neck*, 5th ed. St. Louis: Elsevier; 2017.)

Furthermore, inflammation of the joints can cause constant pain, even without movement of the jaw.

Recognition of TMD includes palpation of the joint as the patient performs all the movements of the joint as well as the associated muscles of mastication. The TMJ is palpated laterally at a depression inferior to each ear at the zygomatic arch and 1 to 2 cm anterior to the tragus. The posterior aspect of the joint is palpated through the external auditory canal. The joint should be palpated in both open and closed positions and also both with the mandible moving laterally and posteriorly. While palpating the clinician should feel for muscle spasm, muscle or joint tenderness, and joint sound. The muscles palpated as a part of complete TMJ examination are masseter, temporalis, medial pterygoid, lateral pterygoid, and sternocleidomastoid. See the ***Workbook for Illustrated Dental Embryology, Histology, and Anatomy*** for an exercise in the clinical identification of occlusion that includes an examination of the TMJ.

All signs and symptoms related to the TMD, such as the amount of mandibular opening and facial pain, should also be noted in the patient record as should any parafunctional habits and related systemic diseases. To aid in diagnosis a traditional skull radiograph is usually taken.

However, when conservative therapy has failed and an invasive therapy is indicated, highly sensitive diagnostic tests, such as computed tomography (CT) or magnetic resonance imaging (MRI) are selected (Fig. 19.10). CT is considered the gold standard for the assessment of bony structures and the method of choice for facial trauma, whereas MRI is similarly regarded for the study of soft tissue. The two methods often complement each other in the study of TMJ alterations, constituting important tools for muscle and joint differential diagnosis.

However, cone-beam CT (CBCT) has recently become a popular diagnostic tool mostly because of its convenience, accuracy, and reduced cost. CBCTs are office-based scanners that are capable of providing tomographic views with three-dimensional reconstructions of the mandibular condyle and articular eminence (see Fig. 19.10). For TMD, combining the CBCT scan with three-dimensional reconstruction imaging software allows the clinician to more precisely evaluate condylar changes.

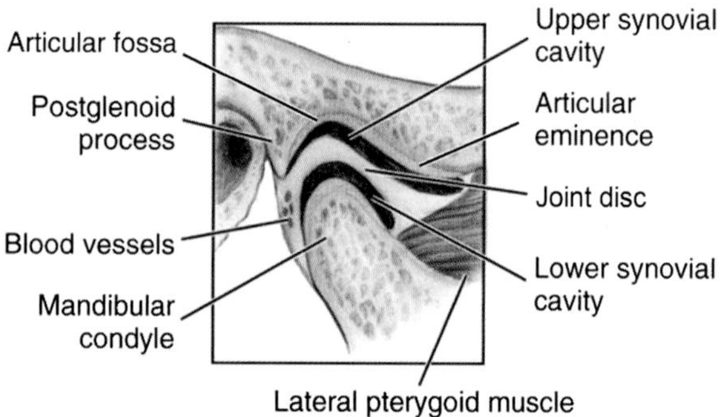

Fig. 19.6 Joint Disc of the Temporomandibular Joint and its Two Synovial Cavities. (From Fehrenbach MJ, Herring SW. *Illustrated Anatomy of the Head and Neck.* 5th ed. St. Louis: Elsevier; 2017.)

Many controversies are associated with the etiology of these disorders. TMD is a heterogeneous and complex disorder involving many factors, such as behavioral stressors and parafunctional habits (clenching and/or bruxism [grinding]) (see **Chapter 20**). Trauma to the jaw may cause TMD, with the disc having adhesions to the bony surfaces; however, this is not the most common etiologic factor as are stressors and habits. Jaw thrusting (causing unusual speech and chewing habits), excessive gum chewing or nail biting, and the size and hardness of food eaten, are other factors to be considered. Poor posture can also be an important factor in TMJ symptoms. For example, holding the head forward, while looking at a computer all day, strains the muscles of the face and neck.

Systemic diseases (such as arthritis) may involve parts of the TMJ and contribute to TMD (see Fig. 19.10). Aging of the joint disc, which causes wear and hardening, may also be a factor in TMD; however, TMD does not usually become worse with age.

Not all patients with TMD have intra-articular abnormalities in the joint disc or the joint itself; most symptoms seem to originate from the muscles. Muscle pain can sometimes be associated with muscle tissue trigger points, which is known as myofascial pain dysfunction syndrome. These trigger points can be localized by digital palpation, both intraorally and extraorally. Studies do not support the role of TMD in directly causing earaches and headaches, neck and back pain, or instability. However, cyclic episodes of TMD and other incidents of chronic body pain, are commonly encountered in the population with TMD.

Joint sounds can occur because of disc derangement as the posterior part of the disc becomes momentarily caught between the condyle head and the articular eminence. Joint sounds are not a reliable indicator of TMD because they can change over time in a patient. The clicking, grinding, and popping sounds of the joint during movement, which are commonly present with TMD, are also found in persons without TMD. In isolated cases of myofascial pain and dysfunction, joint tenderness and joint click are usually absent.

Many controversies surround the treatment of TMD and fewer than half of patients with TMD seek treatment for their disorder. Most recent studies have determined that malocclusion and occlusal discrepancies are not involved in most cases of TMD, but lack of overbite may be an additive factor. Thus, occlusal adjustment, jaw repositioning, and orthodontic therapy are not the treatments of choice for all patients with TMD, nor do these treatments seem to prevent TMD.

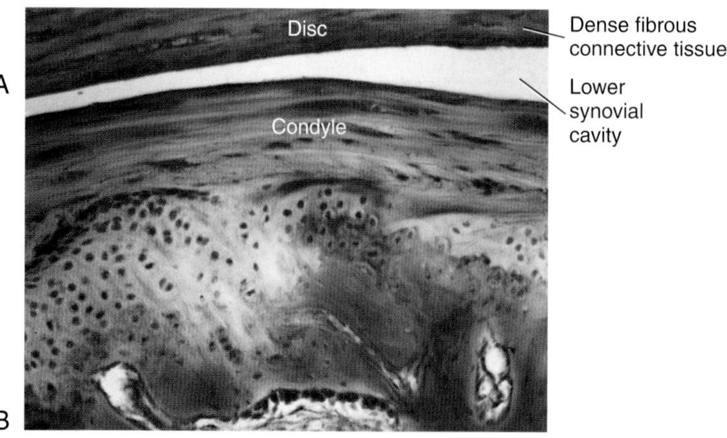

Fig. 19.7 Microscopic appearance of the temporomandibular joint from **(A)** an inferior section of the joint disc and **(B)** mandibular condyle. (Courtesy of Major M. Ash, Jr.)

Most cases of TMD improve over time with inexpensive and reversible treatments, including the adjunctive treatment with over-the-counter medications or prescriptions, such as nonsteroidal anti-inflammatory drugs (NSAIDs), including aspirin or ibuprofen to help relieve muscle pain and swelling, as well as muscle relaxants or local anesthetics with steroids in muscle trigger point injections to help relax spasming jaw muscles. The biomedical literature also supports the use of antidepressants to treat chronic pain such as TMD since it is indicated that their analgesic effects are largely independent of their antidepressant activity. In addition, heat/ice muscle applications, relaxation therapy, stress management, parafunctional habit control, moderate home-based muscular exercises with orofacial myology may be therapeutic options (see **Chapter 20**). Multiple modalities of treatment for TMD should be considered.

Many of the homecare steps to treat TMJ problems can prevent such problems in the first place, for instance, by avoiding extreme jaw movements, learning relaxation techniques to reduce overall stress and muscle tension, and maintaining good posture, especially when working at a computer. Pausing often to change position and resting hands and arms, can relieve stressed muscles. It is always important to use safety measures to reduce the risk of fractures and dislocations.

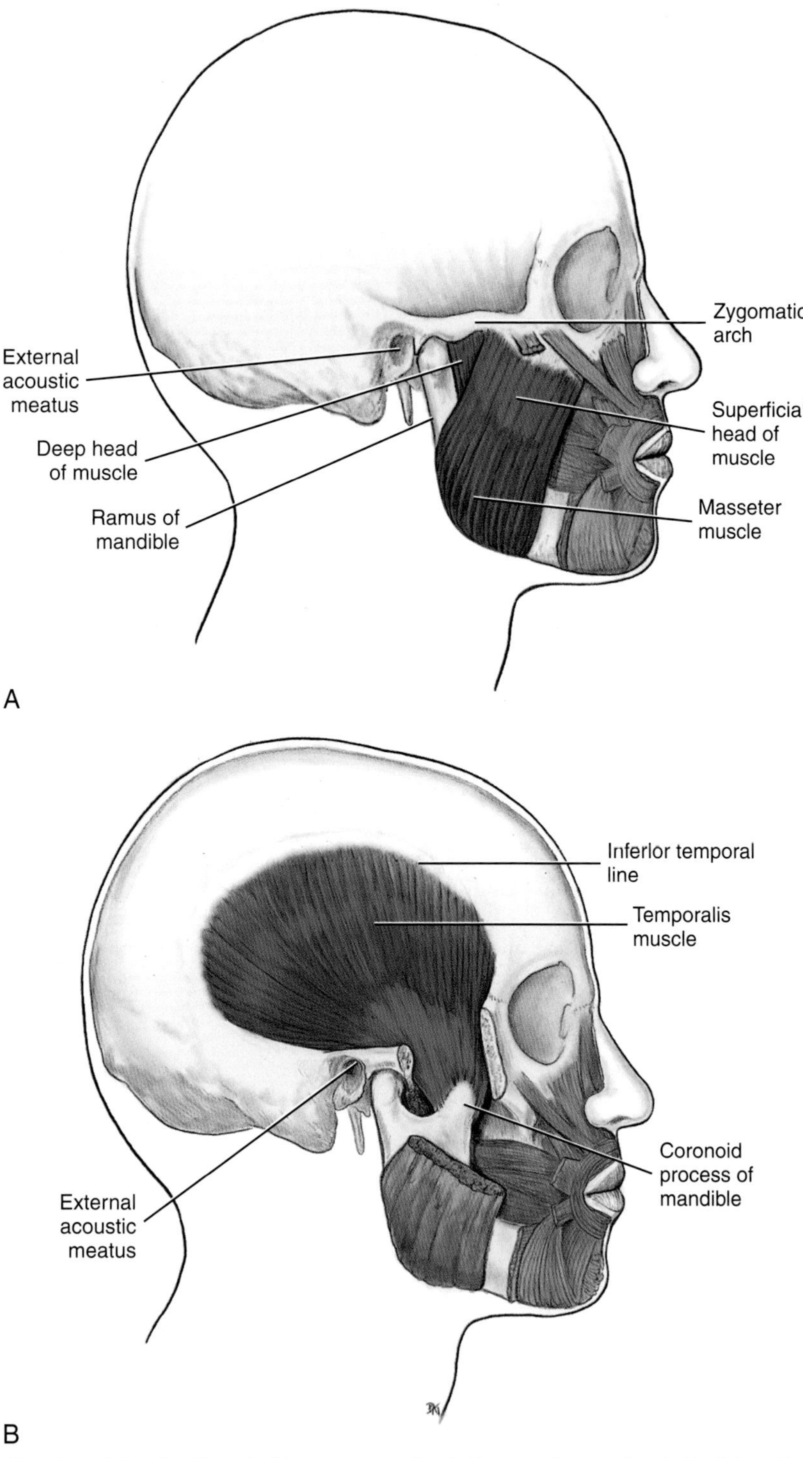

Fig. 19.8 Muscles of Mastication. A, Masseter muscle. **B,** Temporalis muscle. **C,** Medial and lateral pterygoid muscles. (**A** and **B,** From Fehrenbach MJ, Herring SW. *Illustrated Anatomy of the Head and Neck.* 5th ed. St. Louis: Elsevier; 2017.)

Continued

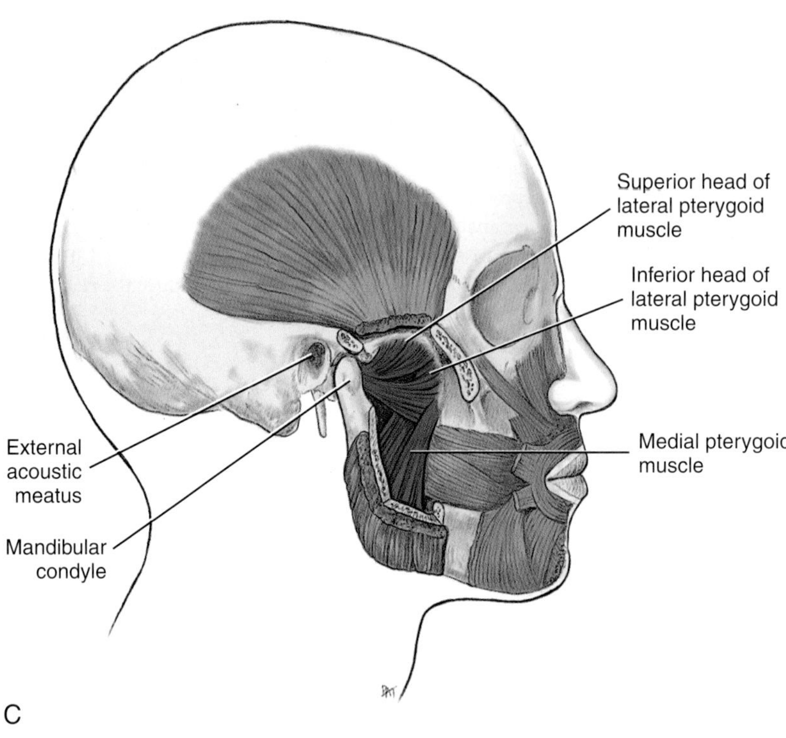

Fig. 19.8, cont'd

A flat-plane full-coverage oral appliance, for instance, a nonrepositioning stabilization splint, often is helpful to control bruxism and take stress off the TMJ, although some individuals may bite harder on it, thus worsening their condition. The anterior splint, with contact at the anterior teeth only, may then prove helpful if used short-term. Such inexpensive and reversible treatments (i.e., ones not causing permanent jaw or dentition changes) show the same success as more expensive and irreversible treatments, such as surgery. Thus, few patients with TMD require surgery or other extensive treatment. However, surgery of the TMJ can now make use of arthroscopy with an endoscope and lasers. Replacement of the jaw joint(s) or disc(s) with TMJ implants is considered as a treatment of last resort. Tissue engineering potentially offers new treatments in the future for disorders of the temporomandibular joint.

An acute episode of TMD can occur when a patient opens too wide, causing maximal depression and protrusion of the mandible as when yawning or receiving prolonged dental care. This causes **subluxation** (sub-luhk-**say**-shuhn) or partial dislocation of both joints (Fig. 19.11). Subluxation occurs when the head of each condyle moves too far anteriorly past the articular eminence. Then, when the patient tries to close and elevate the mandible, the condylar heads cannot move posteriorly because both the bony relationships serve to prevent this and the muscles have also become spastic. The patient now has **trismus (triz**-muhs) or the inability to open the mouth.

Treatment of subluxation consists of relaxation of these muscles and careful movement of the mandible downward and back. The mandibular condylar heads can then assume the usual posterior position, in relation to the articular eminence, by the muscular action of the elevating muscles of mastication. Subsequently these patients must avoid extreme depression of the mandible, such as can occur with prolonged dental work.

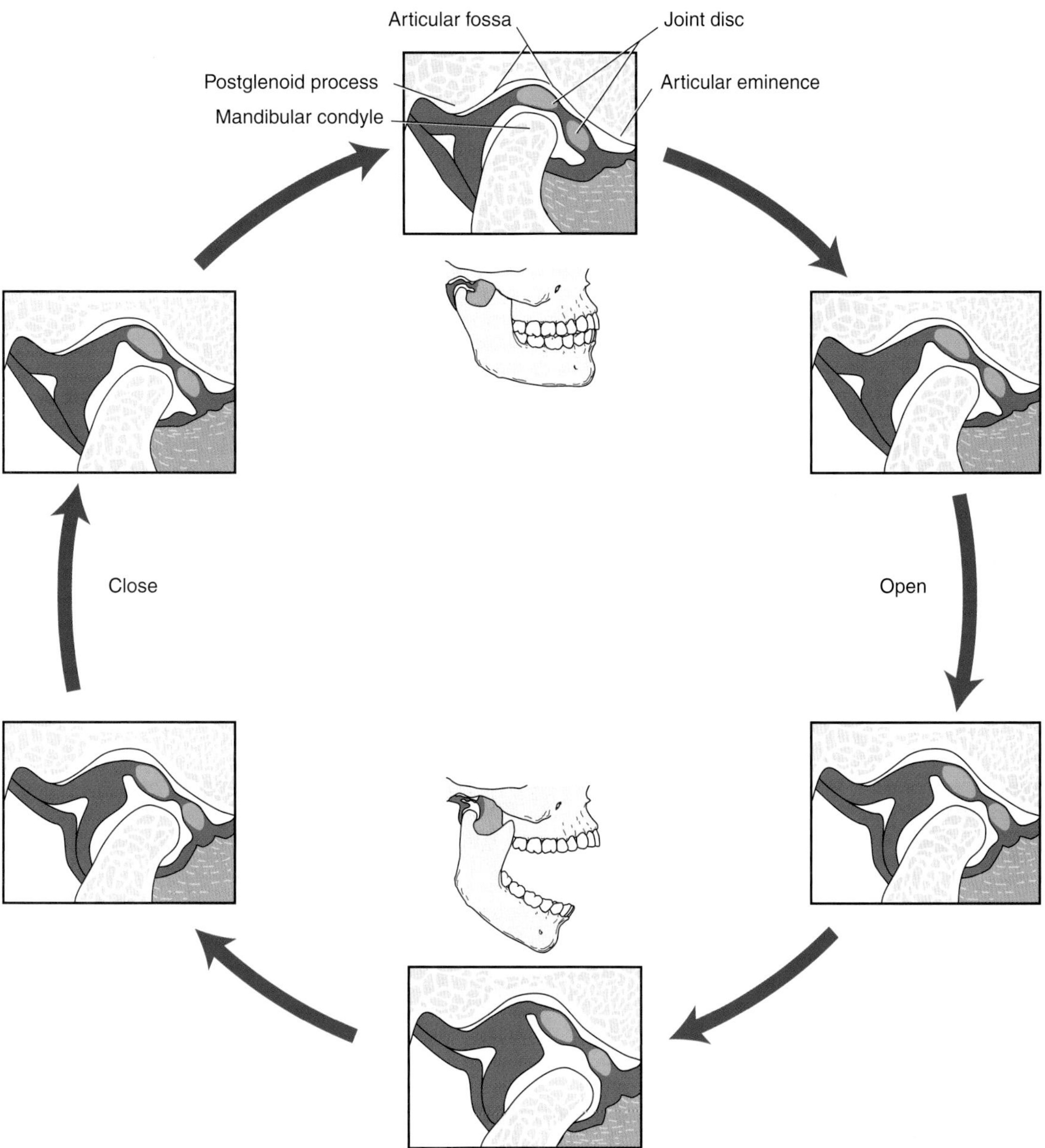

Fig. 19.9 Functional movement of the condyle and disc of the temporomandibular joint during the full range of opening and closing. Note that the disc is rotated posteriorly on the condyle as the condyle is translated out of the fossa. The closing movement is the exact opposite of the opening movement.

TABLE 19.1 Origin and Insertion of Muscles of Mastication with Associated Movements of Mandible

Muscles	Origin	Insertion	Associated Movement(s) of Mandible
Masseter	Superficial head: zygomatic process of maxilla and anterior two-thirds of inferior border of zygomatic arch Deep head: posterior one-third and medial surface of zygomatic arch	Superficial head: angle of mandible Deep head: mandibular ramus	Bilateral contraction: elevation of mandible during closing of jaws
Temporalis	Inferior temporal line superiorly and inferiorly by infratemporal crest of sphenoid bone within temporal fossa	Coronoid process of mandibular ramus	Bilateral contraction of entire muscle: elevation of mandible during closing of jaws Bilateral contraction of only posterior part: retraction of mandible, mandible backward
Medial pterygoid	Deep head: between pterygoid plates of sphenoid bone and adjoining surfaces Superficial head: pyramidal process of palatine bone and maxillary tuberosity of maxilla	Both heads: medial surface of mandibular ramus and angle of mandible	Bilateral contraction: elevation of mandible during closing of jaws
Lateral pterygoid	Superior head: infratemporal surface and infratemporal crest of greater wing of sphenoid bone Inferior head: lateral pterygoid plate of sphenoid bone	Both heads: anterior surface of neck of mandibular condyle at pterygoid fovea with superior fibers inserting on temporomandibular joint disc and capsule	Unilateral contraction: lateral deviation of mandible, shift mandible to contralateral side Bilateral contraction: mainly protrusion of mandible with mandible forward, slight depression of mandible during opening of jaws

From Fehrenbach MJ, Herring SW. *Illustrated Anatomy of the Head and Neck*. 5th ed. St Louis: Elsevier; 2017.

TABLE 19.2 Joint Movements

Mandibular Movement(s)	Temporomandibular Joint Movement(s)	Associated Muscle(s)
Protrusion of mandible moving lower jaw forward	Gliding in both upper synovial cavities	Lateral pterygoid with bilateral contraction
Retraction of mandible moving lower jaw backward	Gliding in both upper synovial cavities	Posterior part of temporalis and/or suprahyoids with bilateral contraction
Elevation and retraction of mandible closing jaws	Gliding in both upper synovial cavities with rotation in both lower synovial cavities	Masseter, temporalis, medial pterygoid with bilateral contraction
Depression and protrusion of mandible opening jaws	Gliding in both upper synovial cavities with rotation in both lower synovial cavities	Suprahyoids and lateral pterygoid with bilateral contraction
Lateral deviation of mandible to shift lower jaw to one side	Gliding in one upper synovial cavity while condyle and disc of other side spin around approximately vertical axis within upper synovial cavity	Lateral pterygoid with unilateral contraction

From Fehrenbach MJ, Herring SW. *Illustrated Anatomy of the Head and Neck*. 5th ed. St Louis: Elsevier; 2017.

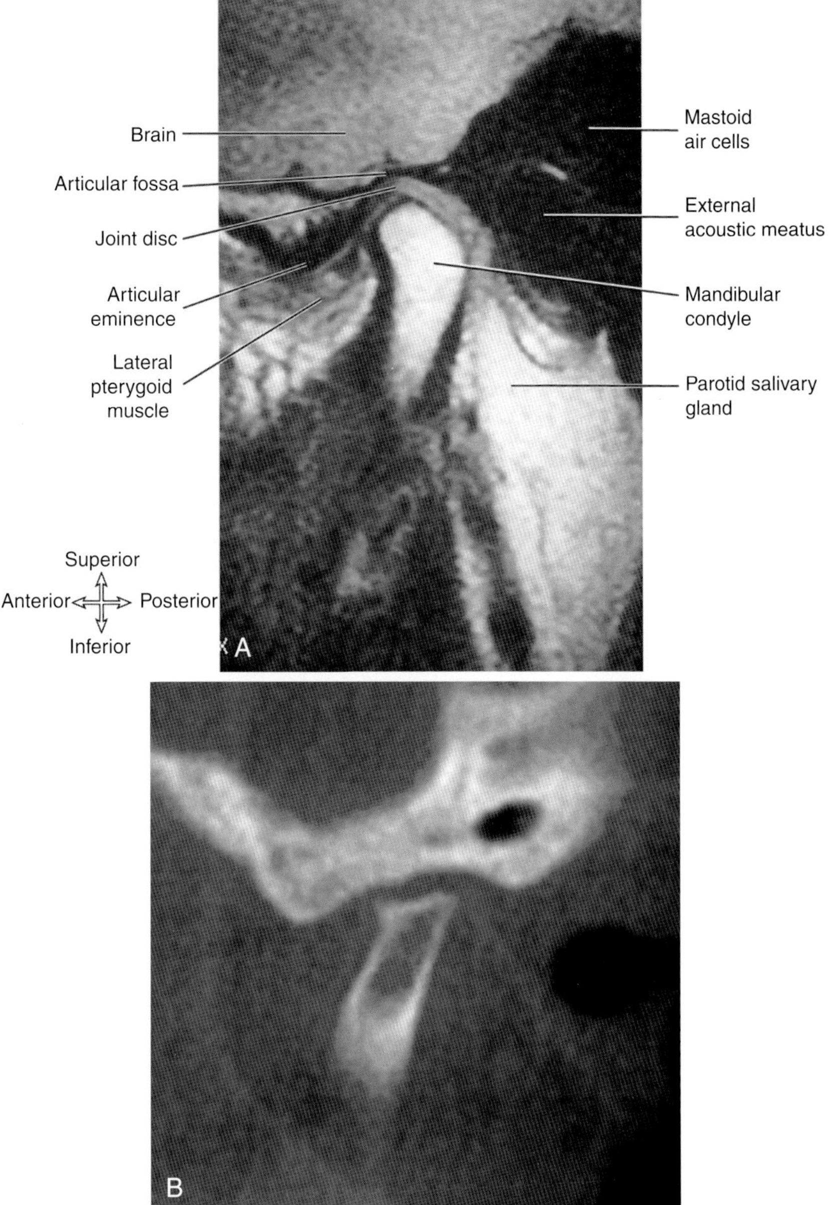

Fig. 19.10 Imaging of the Temporomandibular Joint. A, Coronal magnetic resonance imaging (MRI) that has been reconstructed as a parasagittal section of a closed temporomandibular joint in an asymptomatic individual. **B**, Cone-beam computed tomography (CBCT) of a severely deformed mandibular condyle resulting from arthritis. (**A**, From Quinn PD. *Color Atlas of Temporomandibular Joint Surgery*. St. Louis: Elsevier; 1998. **B**, From Okeson JP. *Management of Temporomandibular Disorders and Occlusion*. 7th ed. St. Louis: Elsevier; 2013.)

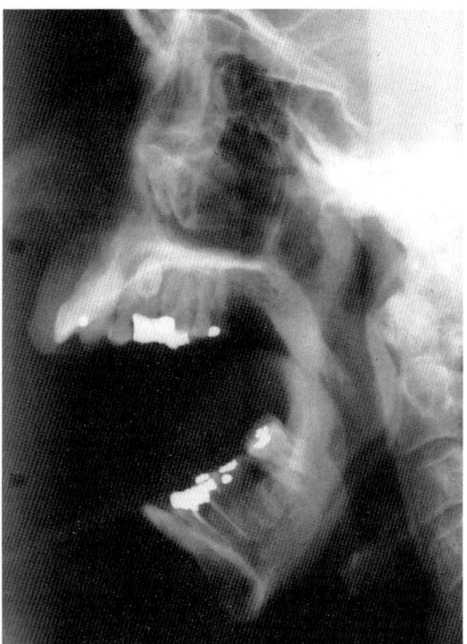

Fig. 19.11 Lateral radiographic view of an individual with a dislocation of both the joints or subluxation. (From Reynolds PA, Abrahams PH. *McMinn's Interactive Clinical Anatomy: Head and Neck.* 2nd ed. London: Mosby; 2001.)

20

Occlusion

Additional resources and practice exercises are provided on the companion Evolve website for this book: http://evolve.elsevier.com/Fehrenbach/illustrated

LEARNING OBJECTIVES

1. Define and pronounce the key terms in this chapter.
2. Discuss occlusion and centric occlusion and its relationship to functional movements and patterns of the mandible.
3. Discuss arch form and the phases of arch development.
4. Describe dental curvatures and angulations.
5. Discuss centric relation, lateral and protrusive occlusions, and the mandibular rest position and how to achieve each of them on a skull, a dentition model, and a patient.
6. Demonstrate the movements of the mandible related to occlusion.
7. Discuss primary occlusion and the clinical considerations concerning it, integrating it into patient care.
8. Identify the key concepts of occlusion on a diagram, a dentition model, and a patient.
9. Discuss malocclusion and outline Angle classification and how it relates to patient care, including clinical considerations concerning parafunctional habits.
10. Identify on dentition models each division of Angle classification of malocclusion.
11. Demonstrate an initial occlusal evaluation on a patient and record findings.

OCCLUSION PROPERTIES

Occlusion (uh-**kloo**-zhuhn) is the contact relationship between the maxillary teeth and mandibular teeth when the jaws are in a fully closed (or occluded) position as well as the relationship between the teeth in the same arch. Many patterns of tooth contact are possible; part of the reason for the variety is the substantial range of movement of the mandibular condyle within the temporomandibular joint (TMJ) (see Fig. 19.9).

Occlusion develops in a child as the primary teeth erupt. During this time, oral motor behaviors begin develop as well as the acquiring of the associated masticatory skills. The deglutition skills to accommodate the mastication process begin to develop in utero and are modified on a developmental continuum as the primary dentition erupts. Occlusion of the erupting permanent dentition is dependent on the primary teeth shedding with the exception of the permanent molars because these erupt distal to the primary dentition.

Interrelated factors, such as the associated musculature, neuromuscular patterns, TMJ functioning (see **Chapter 19**), tongue functioning and posturing, orofacial behaviors, and habit patterns are involved in the development of the occlusion. Thus occlusion is only one aspect of an entire developing orofacial masticatory and deglutition system that includes many other factors and variables. The teeth in proper alignment are relatively self-cleansing by action of the cheek and lip musculature with the neutralizing flow of saliva over the tooth surfaces.

An ideal occlusion rarely exists, but this concept provides a basis for treatment in order to improve a less than ideal occlusion. The optimum 138 occlusal contacts for the permanent dentition with the closure of 32 teeth are seldom, if ever, achieved. When occlusion is considered, the position of the dentition in centric occlusion serves as the basis for reference (discussed next). Therefore centric occlusion serves as the standard for describing an occlusion. Ideally a centric resting posture of the tongue, lips, and mandible is also present (discussed later). To prevent occlusal disharmony, all patients should have an occlusal evaluation before and after completion of their dental treatment plan with reevaluation occurring on a regular basis. See the ***Workbook for Illustrated Dental Embryology, Histology, and Anatomy*** for an exercise in the clinical identification of occlusion. Advanced digital imaging is also now available providing valuable three-dimensional views of the patient's occlusion, which can be used during orthodontic therapy as well as occlusal adjustments during periodontal therapy.

CENTRIC OCCLUSION

Centric occlusion (CO) or *habitual occlusion* is the voluntary position of the dentition that allows the maximum contact when the teeth occlude (Fig. 20.1). It is the centered contact position of the occlusal surfaces of mandibular teeth on the occlusal surface of the maxillary teeth. The position of CO is related to the functioning of the dentition. However, even when the teeth are in full closure, discrepancy between the relationships of the mandible, TMJs, and/or the maxillae may be significant (skeletal discrepancies are discussed later).

When the teeth are in the position of CO, each tooth of one arch is in occlusion with two others in the opposing arch, except for the mandibular central incisors and maxillary third molars. This structure serves to equalize the forces of impact in occlusion. Another benefit of this arrangement is that if a tooth is lost in one jaw, the alignment of the opposing jaw is not immediately disturbed or impaired. One antagonist remains until adequate restorative treatment can be performed.

If a tooth is lost for a longer period, the neighboring teeth usually tip in an effort to fill the edentulous space. The teeth become inclined, malaligned, and overeruption (or super-eruption) of the tooth opposing the space then occurs (see Figs. 17.43 and 17.56). Thus, loss of one tooth disturbs the contact relationships in that area as well as those teeth in the opposing arch, which are their antagonist(s), possibly causing changes in the occlusion of the entire dentition. Patients must understand when discussing tooth replacement that teeth are like

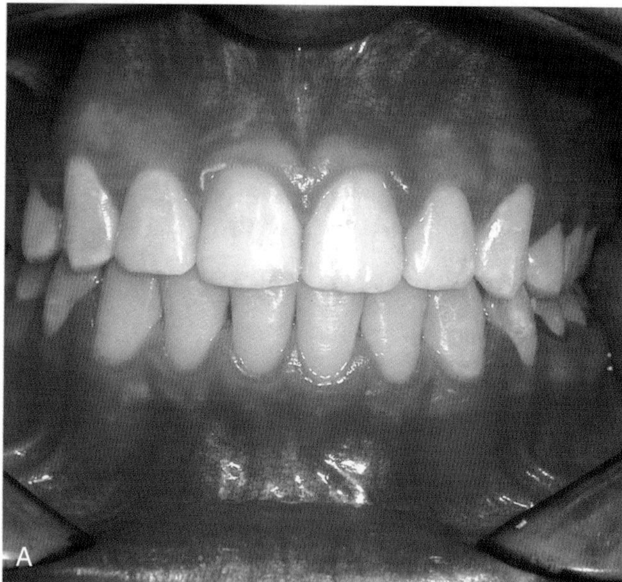

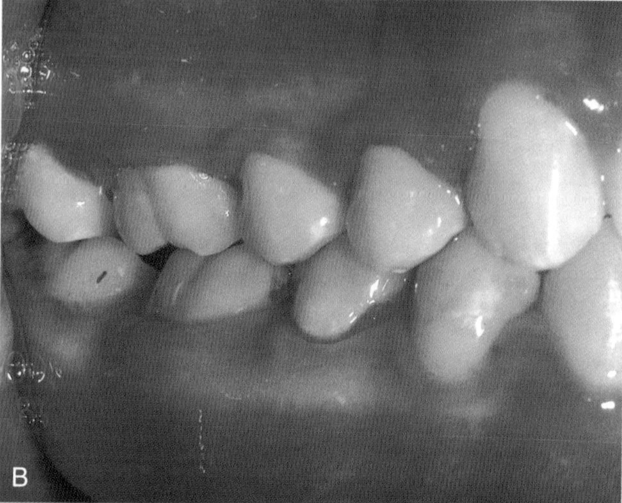

Fig. 20.1 Permanent Dentition in Centric Occlusion (CO). **A,** Facial view. **B,** Buccal view. Dentition has the usual amount of overjet present, which is the horizontal overlap between the two arches. It also has the usual amount of overbite, which is the vertical overlap between the two arches. The use of three segments can be used to describe arch form: anterior, middle, and posterior. (Courtesy of Dona M. Seely, DDS, MSD.)

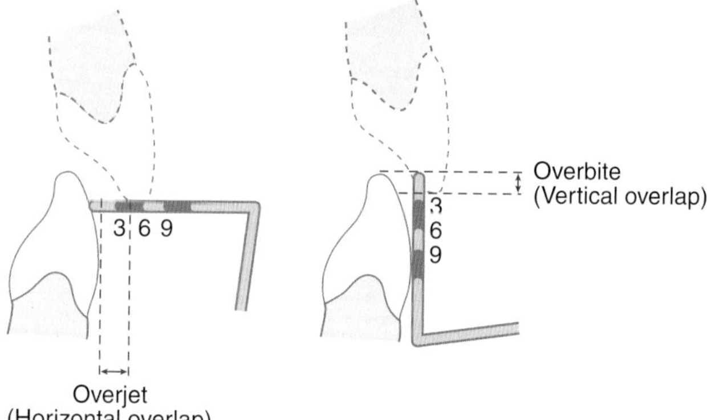

Fig. 20.2 Comparison of overjet, which is the horizontal overlap between the two arches, and overbite, which is the vertical overlap between the two arches.

building blocks: Pull one out of the overall construction and they all fall down; in the case of the dentition, tooth loss can result in occlusal disharmonies.

In addition to tooth loss, abnormal pressure or force of movement from the tongue (such as in tongue thrusting or an incorrect resting posture of the tongue) may create occlusal disharmony. An open mouth resting posture of the lips or chronic mouth breathing results in inadequate closure of the lips needed to maintain equilibrium between the lips and teeth as well as the surrounding orofacial structures. This most often leads to the teeth not being retained in the proper arch shape and thus malocclusion occurs (discussed later).

When the teeth properly occlude in CO, the maxillary arch horizontally overlaps the mandibular arch, which is referred to as **overjet** (Fig. 20.2). The amount of horizontal overlap, usually 1 to 3 mm, between the anterior segment of the two arches associated with the overjet allows extensions in the movement of the **range of motion (ROM)** of the mandible and assists in keeping the soft tissue of the oral cavity out of the way during mastication. The ROM is the maximum extent to which the parts of the TMJ can move when opening and closing as measured in degrees of a circle. The stronger posterior teeth come together first during closure.

Overjet is measured in millimeters with the tip of a periodontal probe once a patient is in CO. The probe is placed at 90° or right angle to the labial surface of a mandibular incisor at the base of the incisal ridge of a maxillary incisor. The measurement is taken from the labial surface of the mandibular incisor to the lingual surface of the maxillary incisor. Note that the labiolingual width of the maxillary incisor is not included in the measurement.

In CO, the maxillary arch also vertically overlaps the mandibular arch, which referred to as **overbite** (see Fig. 20.2). The amount of vertical overlap, usually 2 to 5 mm between the anterior sextants of the two arches allows contact between the posterior teeth during mastication. It is usually expressed as a percentage at around 20% to 30%.

Overbite is measured in millimeters with the tip of a periodontal probe after a patient is placed in CO. The probe is placed on the incisal ridge of the maxillary incisor at 90° or at right angle to the mandibular incisor. As patients open their mouths or depress their jaws, the probe is then placed vertically against the mandibular incisor to measure the distance to the incisal ridge of the mandibular incisor.

Excessive amounts of either overjet or overbite are classified as a malocclusion (discussed later). When the maxillary arch and its incisors have a more pronounced overlap with the mandibular arch and its incisors, it causes a severe overbite (or deep overbite) (see Figs. 20.24 and 20.25). When the reverse is the case and the mandibular arch and its incisors extends beyond the maxillary arch and its incisors, it is causes an **underbite** (see Fig. 20.26). Studies show that overjet measurements were equally distributed among women and men, but severe overbite was noted more often in women than men. However, neither measurement was predictably associated with any particular craniofacial pattern. Both overjet and overbite tend to diminish with age, initially because of mandibular growth and later due to incisal wear.

There is a consensus on the amount of ROM of the mandible usually present. It is measured during **maximum mouth opening (MMO)**. MMO can be expressed either as interincisal distance or as corrected interincisal distance, which is determined by adding the amount of vertical overlap between the maxillary and mandibular incisors to the incisal distance. The interincisal opening range is 40 to 50 mm. The ability to position three fingers at once (index, middle, and ring finger of nondominant hand) in the mouth usually during examination of an adult with a complete dentition is a convenient index for assessing the usual amount of MMO. Most studies show that the maximum jaw ROM and MMO is related to body size and height; thus men can usually open wider than women and taller persons more than shorter persons.

Within each dental arch, the teeth also create contact areas as they contact their same-arch neighbors at the proximal heights of contour; the exception is the last tooth in each arch of each dentition, which lacks a distal contact (see **Chapters 16 and 17**). When two teeth in the same arch come into contact, the curvatures next to the contact areas form spaces considered embrasures (see Fig. 15.11). This contact between neighboring teeth and formation of embrasures serves two purposes: It protects the interdental papillae as well as stabilizing the position of each tooth in the dental arch.

Open contacts allow areas of food impaction from opposing cusps resulting in trauma to the gingivosulcular area, now these opposing cusps are considered **plunging cusps**. Open contacts also do not allow mesiodistal stability between the teeth. Proper restorative treatment should not allow any open contacts, unless tooth position and tooth loss make this impossible to replace. Although the practice is controversial, periodontal splints are often placed in the mouth lingually with tooth-colored resins and wires to simulate this stability needed for the teeth within the dental arch. All prosthetic treatment within the mouth, including the placement of bridges, implants, and removable dentures, is an attempt to simulate this stability.

Certain topics must be considered when studying CO: arch form and its development, dental curvatures and angulations, centric stops, centric relation, lateral and protrusive occlusion, mandibular rest position, and mastication patterns.

ARCH FORM

Each dental arch of the permanent dentition is divided into three segments when describing arch form: anterior, middle, and posterior (see Fig. 20.1). The anterior segment includes the anterior teeth, the middle segment includes the premolars, and the posterior segment includes the molars. The concept of arch segments allows the arches to overlap slightly so that canines and first molars are cooperating in more than one segment. This arrangement serves to indicate that the canines and first molars function as anchor supports for both arches.

The anterior segment of each dental arch is curved and ends at the labial ridges of the canines. The middle segment is straight and extends from the distal part of the canines to the buccal cervical ridge of the mesiobuccal cusp of the first molar in each arch. The posterior segment creates a straight line starting from the buccal cusps of the first molars and remaining in contact with the buccal surfaces of the second and third molars.

Phases of Arch Development

Each dental arch goes through phases of development as the permanent teeth erupt and the primary teeth are being shed (see Fig. 6.22 for chronologic timetable). During this time, the ramus and body of the jaw develop and undergo lengthening and horizontal growth to achieve their mature form and accommodate the larger permanent teeth.

Phase one occurs when the permanent first molars erupt (see Fig. 18.17). These teeth add dramatically to chewing efficiency and jaw development during a period of rapid growth of the child. They help support the jaws while the primary anterior teeth are being shed and the other permanent teeth are erupting. The primate spaces in the primary dentition are still present to allow future space for the larger permanent dentition (see later discussion in this chapter and **Chapter 18**).

Phase two occurs with eruption of the permanent anterior teeth near the midline of the oral cavity. First the permanent centrals and then the laterals generally erupt lingually to the primary anterior roots.

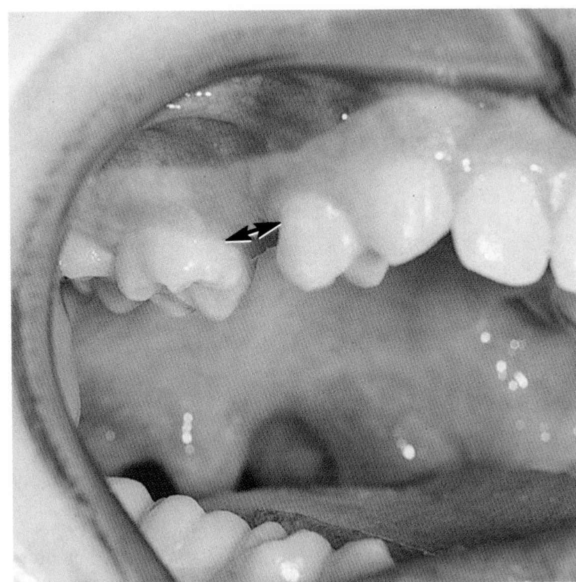

Fig. 20.3 Leeway space in the maxillary arch *(arrow)* during the mixed dentition period and phase three of the dental arch development. This space is due to the difference in size, mesiodistally, between primary molars and permanent premolars. (Courtesy of Margaret J. Fehrenbach, RDH, MS.)

However, shedding of the primary teeth and jaw growth finally place them labial to the position of the primary teeth they replaced (see Figs. 6.26 and 18.17).

In addition, the permanent location of the permanent anterior teeth is not established until the development of the arch form is complete. Some degree of transient anterior crowding may occur between 8 and 9 years of age and persist until the emergence of the permanent canines when the arch space for the teeth is adequate again. However, permanent incisor crowding that persists into a permanent dentition is considered a type of malocclusion (discussed later).

Phase three in the development of the form of the dental arches begins when the permanent premolars erupt anterior to the permanent molars (see Figs. 6.27 and 6.28). Developmentally this is quite significant because the premolars are so much smaller than the primary molars that they replace. This difference in size, mesiodistally between the two types of teeth, is referred to as the **leeway space** (Fig. 20.3). The contour of the alveolar process covering the narrower roots of the premolars, in addition to the state of flux of the bone formation in this area, furnishes adjustment for dental arch measurements, making the middle segment of the arches important architecturally. Thus this arch space allows the future forward movement of the permanent molars, which is discussed later with regard to the occlusion of the primary teeth.

However, if there is early loss of the primary second molars and impaction of the second premolar, the necessary leeway space can become compromised. Also if permanent second molars erupt before the premolars, the arch perimeter is significantly shortened and occlusal disharmony is likely to occur as is a case of malocclusion (discussed later) because the second premolar is also unable to erupt. A fixed or removable space maintainer may be used to save this leeway space from the shed primary molars for the permanent premolars (Fig. 20.4).

Phase four begins when the permanent canines erupt and wedge themselves between the lateral incisors and the first premolars. Contact relations between the teeth are established and the arch is complete from the permanent first molar forward. Simultaneously the

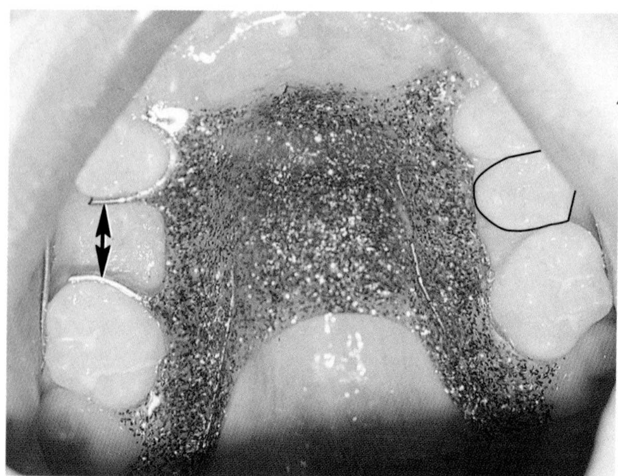

Fig. 20.4 Removable maxillary space maintainer (wonderful sparkle variety) to hold the necessary leeway space present from the shed primary second molar *(arrow)* to allow future eruption of the permanent second premolar. The permanent second molars have already erupted and may narrow the existing space in the premolar segment. Note that the permanent second premolar on the contralateral side is already fully erupted *(outlined)*, so leeway space does not need to be maintained any longer in this region. (Courtesy of Margaret J. Fehrenbach, RDH, MS.)

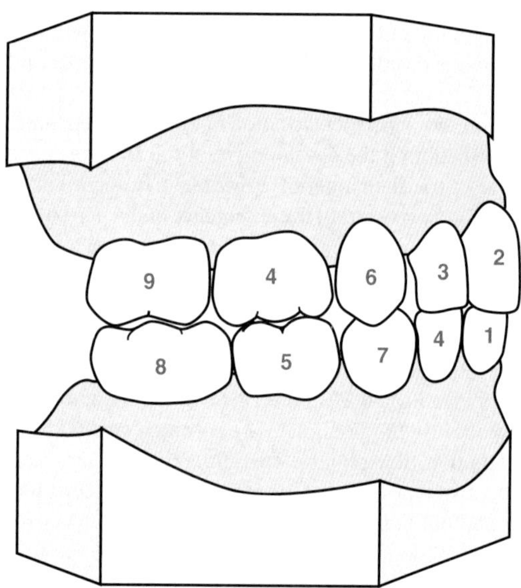

Fig. 20.5 Favorable Sequence of Eruption per Dental Arch of the Primary Dentition.

permanent second molars are due to emerge distally to the permanent first molars and support them during the wedging activity of the canines.

Phase five is the final phase of the development of the final dental arch form and consists of eruption of the third molars. Often the jaw length is not sufficient for eruption of these last teeth and dental treatment plan changes need to be considered (see **Chapter 17**).

Therefore, the usual sequence for eruption of both the primary and permanent dentition is favorable to the development of the arches (Figs. 20.5 and 20.6). Keeping this sequence in mind for each dentition is part of the interceptive considerations to prevent occlusal disruption in patients during the mixed dentition period. Disruption of this sequence, with overlong retention or too-early loss of primary teeth, may allow complications to occur with the eruption of the permanent dentition. Proper treatment of these cases of

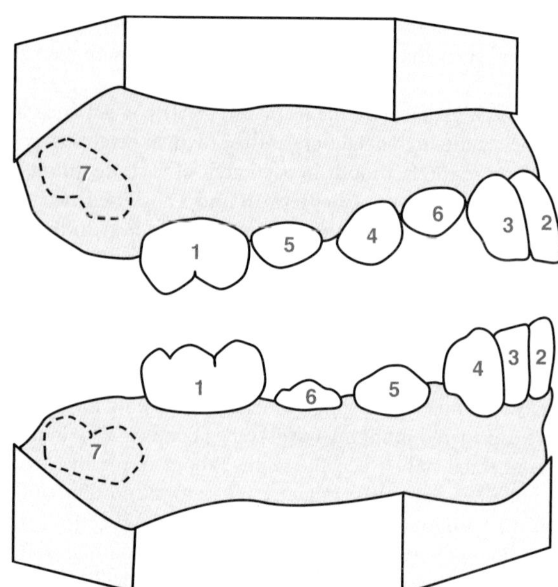

Fig. 20.6 Favorable Sequence of Eruption per Dental Arch of the Permanent Dentition.

disruption in the eruption sequence and possibly early orthodontic interceptive therapy increase the chances for a more ideal occlusion. A series of panoramic radiographs of the mixed dentition is important in order to monitor tooth eruption sequence and arch development (see Fig. 6.27, *A*).

It is important to note that attrition of the proximal surfaces also reduces the mesial-distal dimensions of the teeth and significantly reduces arch length over a lifetime, which causes crowding or spacing challenges after age 40.

DENTAL CURVATURES AND ANGULATIONS

A common mistake is to assume that the forces of occlusion act on squared and flat teeth in straight lines or planes and that the axes of the teeth are at 90° or right angle to their masticatory surfaces. Many dental curvatures and angulations must be considered when studying occlusion.

If imaginary planes are placed on the masticatory surfaces of each dental arch, the arches do not conform to these flat planes; the maxillary arch is convex occlusally and the mandibular arch is concave (Fig. 20.7, *A*). Thus when the maxillary and mandibular teeth come into CO, they align along anteroposterior and lateral curves. This anteroposterior curvature is called the **curve of Spee**, which is produced by the curved alignment of all the teeth and is especially evident when viewing the posterior teeth from the buccal view.

Another curve of the dentition is the **curve of Wilson** (see Fig. 20.7, *B*). This lateral curve results when a frontal section is visually compared to each set of maxillary and mandibular molars—the firsts, seconds, and then thirds. These imaginary dental curvatures are interesting, but it is important to note that modern dentistry does not directly use these curves often in practice because they have only a remote association with functional relationships. Both of these curves also tend to be lost with age as a result of attrition (Fig. 20.8).

The composite of these curves created by the contact of the maxillary and mandibular teeth forms a line called the **occlusal plane**, which can be noted in some cases as the linea alba (see Fig. 2.3, *B*). This plane is an imaginary curved plane formed by the incisal edges of the anteriors and the occlusal surfaces of the posteriors. It follows the natural

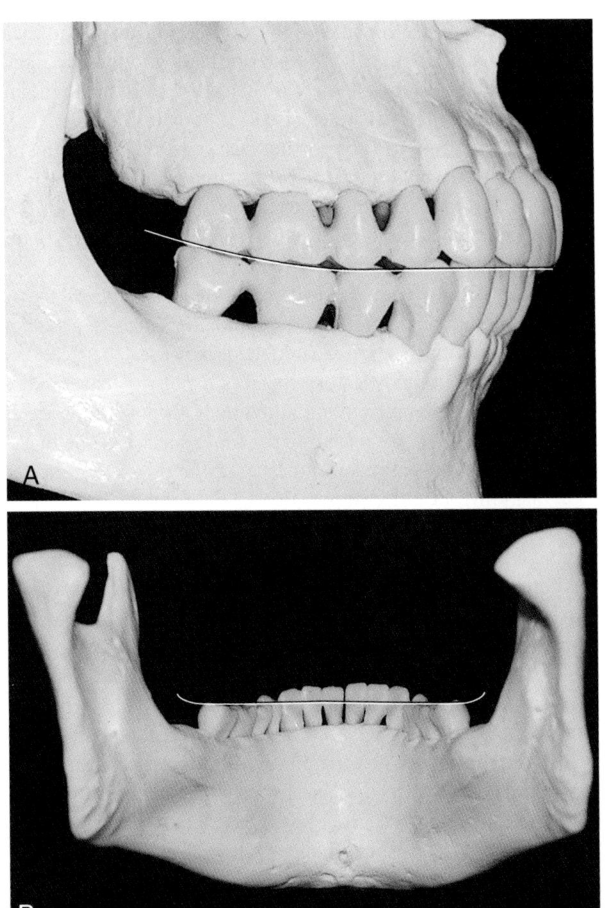

Fig. 20.7 Curves of the Teeth Noted Within the Permanent Dental Arches. **A,** Curve of Spee with the maxillary arch convex and the mandibular arch concave. **B,** Curve of Wilson is a concave curve that occurs when a frontal section is taken through each set of molars (only one is shown). (**A** and **B,** Courtesy of Margaret J. Fehrenbach, RDH, MS.)

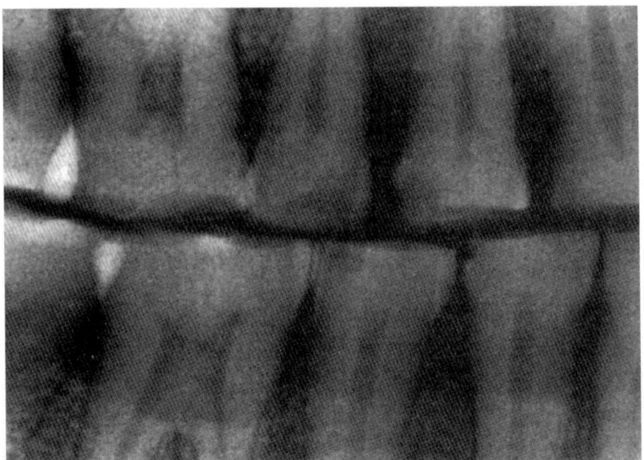

Fig. 20.8 Attrition or mechanical wear of the masticatory surfaces of the permanent teeth in this case is noted on a radiograph. The result is a loss of the curvatures of the teeth within the dental arches. (Courtesy of Margaret J. Fehrenbach, RDH, MS.)

curvature of the teeth, curving higher in back following the curve of Spee, and curving higher as it extends outward, following the curve of Wilson.

Individual teeth also exhibit some forms of curvature. Curves are found in the basic form of each tooth type. Every third of a tooth represents a curved surface, except where a tooth is worn or fractured. These curvatures of the teeth should be noted when studying the

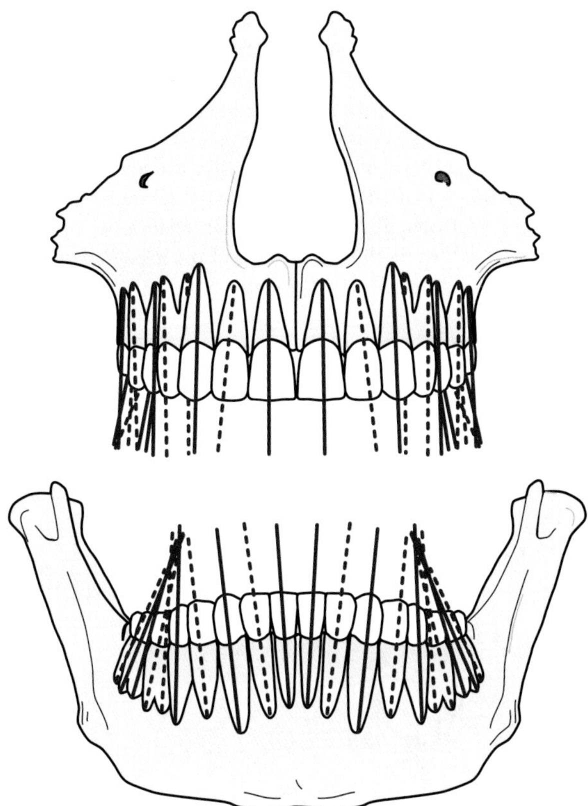

Fig. 20.9 Each tooth of both arches of the permanent dentition is bisected by its root axis line, showing the angulations of the root within the alveolar process of each dental arch.

dentitions and especially when drawing them hoping to achieve lifelike drawings of each tooth. These curves also must be noted when restoring the teeth for proper function and esthetics.

When a tooth is bisected by its root axis line (RAL), the angulations related to each tooth's root(s) within the alveolar process are noted (Fig. 20.9 and discussed per tooth type in **Chapters 16 and 17**). This angled arrangement of the teeth allows proper spacing between the roots for blood and nerve supply and for securing anchorage of the roots in the jaws.

Each tooth is placed at the angle that best withstands the lines of forces brought against it while functioning during occlusion. The angle at which it is placed depends on the function that the tooth must perform. If the tooth is placed at a disadvantage because of misalignment in the dental arch or continued incorrect pressures against it from the tongue, lips, or cheeks, its functional efficiency is limited and the permanence of its position is endangered. The anterior teeth seem to be placed at a disadvantage because they are more vertically situated in the alveolar process, but their function is only the momentary biting and cutting of food and not the full force of mastication that occurs in the posterior teeth, which usually have more angulation (see Table 15.4).

The masticatory surfaces of teeth do not have any flat planes, unless some are created over time by wear, traumatic accident, or orofacial myofunctional disorders (discussed later). Therefore, during occlusion, the curved surface of one tooth always comes into contact with the curved surfaces of another tooth. As the teeth come together in occlusion, the escapement spaces for the masticated food are provided for by each individual tooth's cusps, ridges, sulci, developmental grooves, and embrasures (see Fig. 15.11). Thus these escapement spaces are necessary for efficient occlusion during mastication.

However, the location and form of the escapement spaces change when the occlusal relation is changed as with attrition, inappropriate functional patterning of the mandible, tongue thrusting, or even with restorative treatment. These changes can be related to loss of function of the teeth, tongue, lip, and mandibular function and the masticatory system. These changes can add up to an adverse functioning of the dentition and must be noted on the patient's chart. Additionally, knowing the angulation of the roots within the alveolar process is essential for the proper adaptation during the taking of radiographs and when performing instrumentation or restorative procedures. This measurement of tooth angulation is also considered when evaluating a patient's smile.

CENTRIC STOPS

When the teeth are in CO, they should have maximal interdigitation with the locking of the two arch positions. The three areas of centric contacts or **centric stops** between the two arches are height of cusp contour, marginal ridges, and central fossae (Fig. 20.10). Those cusps that function during CO are considered the **supporting cusps** and include the lingual cusps of the maxillary posterior teeth and the buccal cusps of the mandibular posterior teeth. The incisal ridges of the mandibular anterior teeth are usually included also as supporting cusps.

These centric stops and supporting cusps are checked using articulating paper when restorative or prosthetic treatment is performed (Fig. 20.11). An occlusal adjustment involving the removal of restorative, prosthetic, or natural tooth material may be necessary, depending on the results of the occlusal evaluation.

A dental manikin with unworn plastic teeth can show the ideal location of these centric stops and supporting cusps if articulating paper is used and mastication is simulated. However, the relationship of centric stops to the masticatory surfaces is not rigidly set and may in reality vary considerably among individuals. Centric stops are often in the central fossa and are related to the inner surface of the marginal ridges rather than the embrasure surfaces of the ridges as indicated in an ideal mapping of centric stops.

These contact relationships change with wear of the dentition. With advancing attrition, the supporting cusps are seated closer and closer to the bottoms of the opposing fossae. This process continues until there is development of numerous flat surface contacts, of which each are considered a **wear facet**. When active tooth grinding occurs, the enamel rods are fractured and become highly reflective to light. The angle of the wear facet on the tooth surface is potentially significant to the periodontium. Horizontal facets tend to direct forces on the vertical axis of the tooth to which the periodontium can adapt most effectively. Angular facets direct occlusal forces laterally and increase the risk of periodontal damage.

These contact relationships change with wear of the dentition. With advancing attrition, the supporting cusps are seated closer and closer to the bottoms of the opposing fossae. This process can result in the loss of a definite locking of the two jaws in CO, in addition to creating an unstable occlusal environment. In addition, early noting of wear facets throughout the dentition may mean the patient has a parafunctional habit as the teeth undergo attrition from additional functioning (discussed later).

The position of the centric stops helps determine the height of the lower one-third of the vertical dimension of the face when the teeth are in CO. This dimension cannot be exactly measured in patients with teeth, and thus its loss requires clinical judgment and is based on the

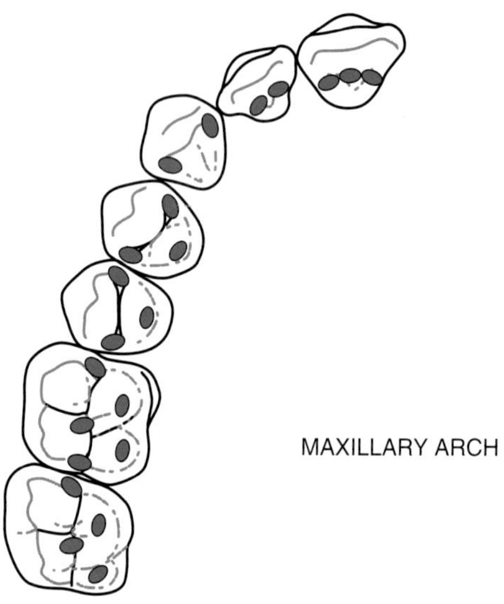

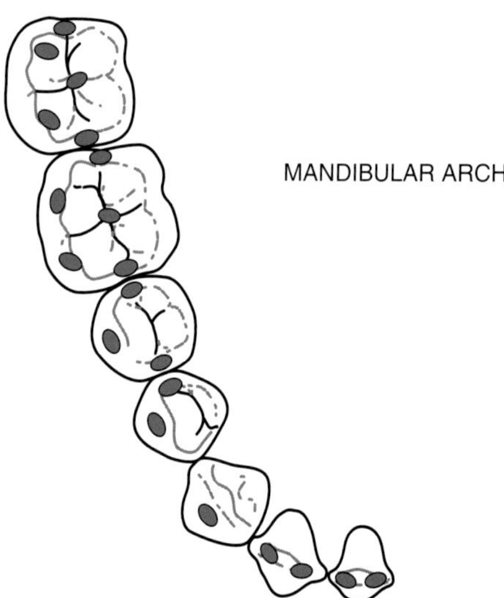

Fig. 20.10 Ideal centric stops showing articulation between the two arches of the permanent dentition are highlighted. Note that the stops include the height of cusps, incisal ridges, marginal ridges, or cingula, as well as any central fossae of the teeth.

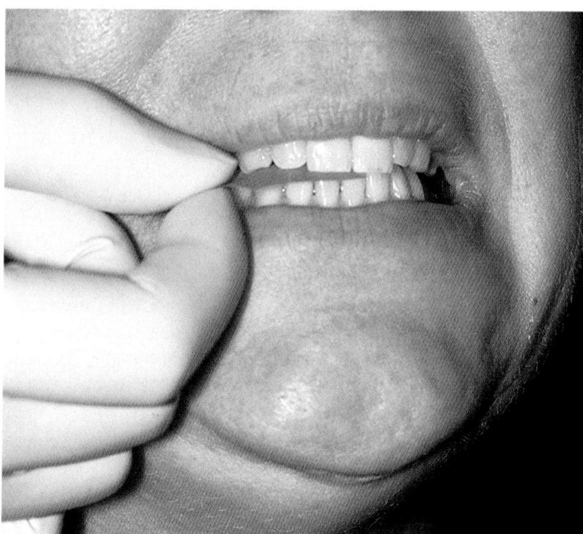

Fig. 20.11 Articulating paper is used to check the centric stops during an occlusal evaluation or after restorative treatment. (Courtesy of Margaret J. Fehrenbach, RDH, MS.)

Golden Proportion as it relates to the face. This dimension is involved in the proper functioning of the teeth and jaws and the esthetic appearance of a patient. Loss of this part of the vertical dimension is based on the resorption of the alveolar process and the attrition of the dentition (see Fig. 14.22).

CENTRIC RELATION

Centric relation (CR) is the end point of closure of the mandible; the mandible is in the most retruded position to which it can be carried by the musculature and ligaments (see **Chapter 19**). Even though a patient is rarely in CR, except sometimes when swallowing, CR is a baseline measurement from which to evaluate a patient's occlusion because it can be easily repeated.

To attain CR, the mandible must undergo complete retraction (Fig. 20.12). The position of CR must be determined by the clinician and without a patient's muscle participation. To do this, the clinician must gently establish the hinge movement of the mandible on the patient by gently arcing the mandible with the fingers in a closing and opening manner several times before attempting placement of the loosened jaw into CR. Researchers are currently exploring various ways of clinically relaxing patients' jaws to determine this position of the mandible more precisely in addition to promoting this during myofascial release and orofacial myofunctional therapy (discussed later).

Ideally, when the mandible is in CR, the dentition should be in CO (thus centric relation equals centric occlusion or CR = CO). The centric resting position also remains in a neutral pattern with an adequate freeway space maintained. Therefore, no major shift of the dentition from CR occlusion to CO should occur. However, the average distance of shift or slide from a patient's occlusion in CR to CO is approximately 1 mm or less.

The position of CO can be attained by having a patient who is in CR clench the teeth together after achieving CR. The amount and direction of the shift in the dentition can then be recorded during the occlusal evaluation. One can easily simulate this procedure with their own dentition by putting the head back (now in CR) and then clench the teeth while bringing the head forward (now in CO).

However, if disorders such as those related to function are present (for instance, orofacial myofunctional disorders, discussed later), striving to achieve CR in this manner may exacerbate the disorder. Clinicians should seat the patient in an upright position, inform the patient where the correct tongue placement is on the palate and having them bite the molars together (now in CO), followed by relaxing the mandible and allowing the maxillary and mandibular teeth to gently come apart until the masseter muscle is relaxed (note that CR is also the same as centric rest).

A slide or shift in the position of the dentition from CR to CO (centric relation does not equal centric occlusion or CR ≠ CO) should be noted. It is most often caused by **premature contacts** where one tooth or two teeth initially contact before the other teeth, an orofacial myofunctional disorder (discussed later), an incorrect habit pattern of the tongue and/or mandible, or deviation in the ROM patterning of the TMJ. The premature tooth contact, orofacial myofunctional disorder, and ROM deviation may contribute to occlusal disharmony. Additional slide between the teeth in CR to CO is also associated with tooth malalignment, improper intercuspation of the teeth, improper restorative treatment, and inherited arbitrary arch lengths and relationships.

LATERAL AND PROTRUSIVE OCCLUSION

Masticatory movement entails not only the mandible going through elevation and depression but also deviations or excursions from side-to-side and forward during lateral and protrusion occlusion (see Fig. 19.9). Therefore, other movements besides CO and its relationship to the teeth must be evaluated.

Evaluation of **lateral occlusion** is made by undergoing lateral deviation of the mandible or excursion by moving the mandible either to the right or to the left until the opposing canines on that side are in an edge-to-edge relationship (Fig. 20.13).

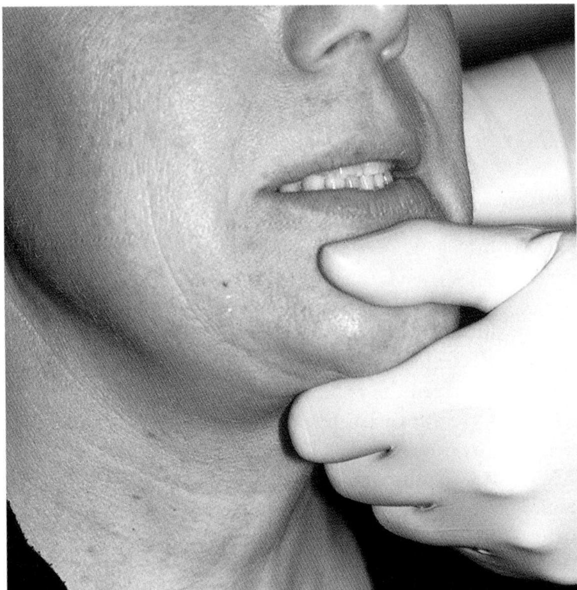

Fig. 20.12 Attaining centric relation by establishing the hinge movement of the mandible. This is achieved by gently arching the mandible with the fingers in a closing and opening manner, several times. This is performed before attempting placement of the loosened jaw into centric relation—the end point of mandible closure in which the mandible is in the most retruded position. (Courtesy of Margaret J. Fehrenbach, RDH, MS.)

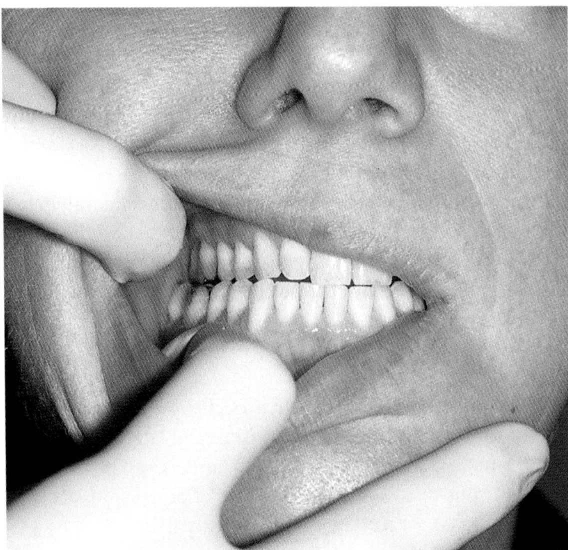

Fig. 20.13 Undergoing lateral deviation or excursion while checking the lateral occlusion on the working side (side to which the mandible has been moved) and balancing side (contralateral side of the arch from working side). Note that the mandible is being moved until the opposing canines are edge-to-edge during canine rise. (Courtesy of Margaret J. Fehrenbach, RDH, MS.)

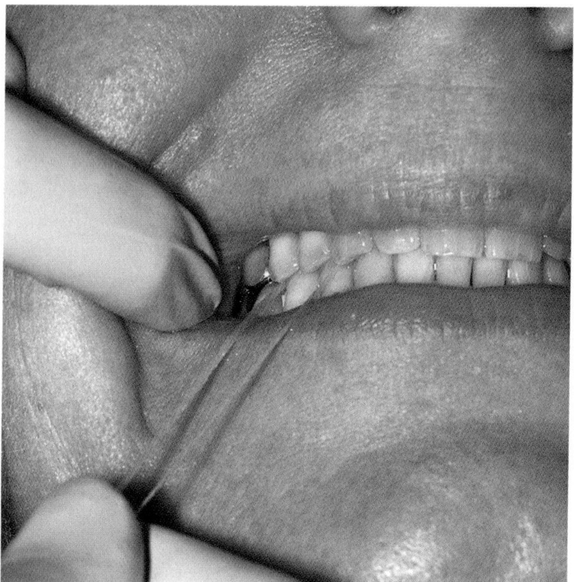

Fig. 20.14 Using floss to confirm balancing interferences where teeth contact on the balancing side during lateral occlusion. (Courtesy of Margaret J. Fehrenbach, RDH, MS.)

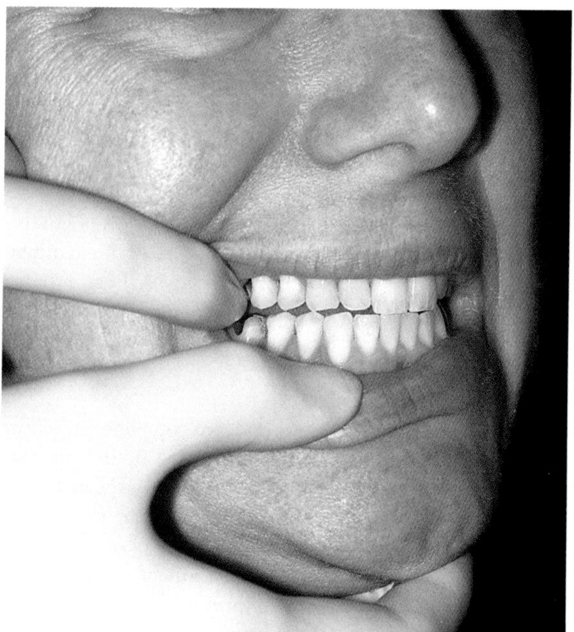

Fig. 20.15 Undergoing Protrusion to Evaluate Protrusive Occlusion. (Courtesy of Margaret J. Fehrenbach, RDH, MS.)

Before the canines contact on each side, no other individual teeth should be contacting during lateral occlusion. The side to which the mandible has been moved is called the **working side**. Two working sides are noted in an occlusal evaluation: right lateral and left lateral. The side of the arch contralateral to the working side during lateral occlusion is referred to as the **balancing side** or *nonworking side*.

During occlusion, the canine should be the only tooth in function during lateral occlusion; this is **canine rise** (or cuspid rise). Thus, the mandible is moved to the working side when checking lateral occlusion, until the opposing canines are edge-to-edge. If other teeth are involved in function during lateral occlusion, they must be noted; for example, the first molars if in function may present complications for the dentition.

If the canine rise does not exist on the working side because of cusp wear caused by parafunctional habits or tooth malalignment, it is acceptable that most of the entire posterior quadrant of each arch functions during lateral occlusion. This is considered **group function** because all opposing posterior teeth are sharing the occlusal stress during function.

No teeth should make contact on the contralateral balancing side during lateral occlusion. If teeth are in contact on the balancing side, this is considered a **balancing interference**. Balancing interference can be involved in occlusal disharmonies. For further confirmation of any balancing interferences during lateral deviation, floss can be placed over the occlusal surfaces on the appropriate side (Fig. 20.14).

With the mandible in **protrusive occlusion** (proh-**troo**-siv), all eight of the most anterior teeth, the centrals and laterals of both arches are usually in contact as the mandible undergoes protrusion (Fig. 20.15). If only one or two assume the stress of protrusion, occlusal disharmony may occur.

MANDIBULAR REST POSITION

The physiologic rest position the mandible is achieved when the mandible is being held in a relaxed state and is not being used in mastication, speech, or respiratory movements (Fig. 20.16). With this rest position, an average space of 2 to 3 mm is noted between the masticatory surfaces of the maxillary and mandibular teeth. This space or gap between the arches when the mandible is at rest is the **interocclusal clearance** (in-ter-uh-**kloo**-zhul) or more commonly referred to as *freeway space*.

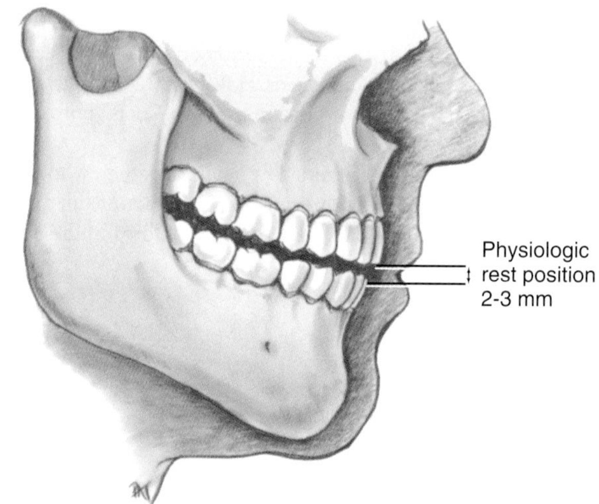

Fig. 20.16 Physiologic rest position of the mandible or interocclusal clearance of about 2 to 3 mm as shown in the permanent dentition.

This position of the mandible at rest is considered fairly stable, although it can be influenced by posture, fatigue, and tension. Thus, failure to assume this position when the jaws are not at work may mean that the patient is temporarily tense or has parafunctional habits, such as clenching or grinding (bruxism) that may be involved in occlusal difficulties (discussed later).

Overall, **resting posture** is the physiologic position of the tongue, lips, and mandible when not functioning during mastication swallowing, or speech (see earlier discussions). Correct resting posture is achieved when the tongue is resting on the palate, the teeth are not in occlusion, and the lips are gently closed without any signs of facial

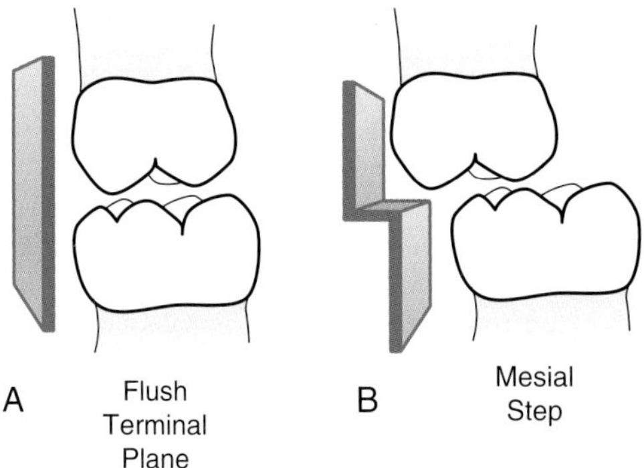

Fig. 20.17 Evaluation of the primary dentition from buccal view of right side. **A,** Flush terminal plane in which the primary maxillary and mandibular second molars are in an end-to-end relationship. This allows the proper molar relationship to occur in the permanent dentition. **B,** Mesial step in which the mandibular second molar is mesial to the maxillary molar. This will most likely allow the proper permanent molar relationship to occur in the permanent dentition when the permanent molars erupt and the primary teeth are shed.

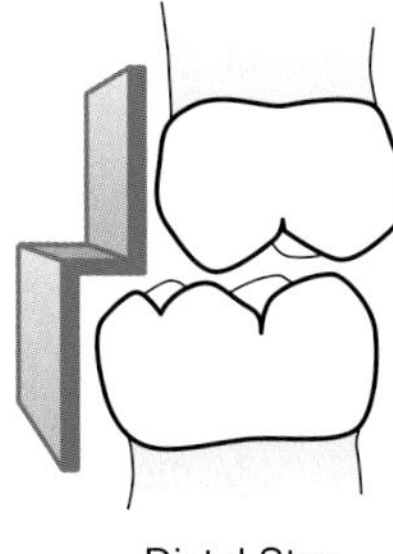

Fig. 20.18 Primary dentition from buccal view of right side in which distal step relationship exists with the primary mandibular second molar distal to the maxillary second molar. This is not a beneficial molar relationship because it will not usually result in the proper molar relationship in the permanent dentition when the permanent molars erupt and the primary teeth are shed.

grimacing. In addition, an **interlabial gap** (in-ter-**ley**-bee-uhl) is the distance between the inferior border of the upper lip and the superior border of the lower lip when the mandible is in a physiologic resting position. Patients being apprised of resting posture are more likely to assume it when early parafunctional habits are just starting to make themselves known within the oral cavity.

PRIMARY OCCLUSION

Similar to the permanent dentition, the primary dentition also has an ideal form (Fig. 20.17). The canine relationship between the arches in primary teeth is the same as that of the permanent dentition. The ideal molar relationship within the primary dentition when in CO is referred to as the **terminal plane**. The terminal plane relationship then determines the anteroposterior position of the permanent first molars at the time of their eruption. This can involve either a **flush terminal plane** in which the primary maxillary and mandibular second molars are in an end-to-end relationship or a **mesial step** in which the primary mandibular second molar is mesial to the maxillary second molar.

With the presence of a mesial step, an ideal permanent molar relationship usually occurs after the eruption of the permanent dentition. In about 80% of those individuals with mesial step less than 2 mm, Angle Class I molar relationship will result. However, if the mesial step is more than 2 mm, Angle Class III molar relationship will result in 20% of those individuals. The flush terminal plane will result in either Angle Class I (with 56% of individuals) or Angle Class II (with 44% of individuals) molar relationship, depending on the amount of mandibular anterior growth and forward drift of the mandibular primary molars in relationship to the maxillary ones.

A **distal step** relationship in which the primary mandibular second molar is distal to the maxillary second molar is not an ideal molar relationship in the primary dentition; thus it is not a type of terminal plane relationship (Fig. 20.18). Distal step of the primary second molars almost invariably results in an Angle Class II molar relationship in the permanent dentition. Thus, an ideal molar relationship in the permanent dentition may still occur with a flush terminal plane, but rarely with the presence of a distal step relationship.

Within a primary dentition, primate spaces may be present between the primary teeth; a larger space can be noted between the maxillary lateral incisor and the canine and between the mandibular first molar and canine (see Fig. 18.1). If primate spacing exists in the primary mandibular arch after the eruption of the permanent first molar, the permanent first molar puts pressure on the primary second and first molars causing forward movement of the primary mandibular canine and first molar (discussed earlier with regard to arch development). Thus this primate space actually allows for this movement, which then facilitates the development of an ideal permanent molar relationship along with the presence of a mesial step relationship. If there are no primate spaces or even crowding in the primary dentition, crowding is inevitable in the permanent dentition.

When the child patient enters the mixed dentition period, analysis of arch space is performed so as to allow for early interceptive orthodontic therapy (see Fig. 15.4 and 18.17). This analysis can range from a general examination to a specific arch length analysis by radiographs, size of erupted permanent mandibular incisors, and prediction scheme by orthodontists. This analysis is performed during this period because there is no appreciable growth of the jaws anterior to the permanent first molars after age 7 or 8 without intervention.

 CLINICAL CONSIDERATIONS WITH OCCLUSION

When the teeth in the dentition are not aligned properly or there are orofacial myofunctional imbalances and/or parafunctional habit patterns present, they lose the ability to self-cleanse. More importantly, when teeth of either dentition are not occluding properly, the teeth and periodontium may not be able to perform the functions for which they were designed. Unnatural occlusal stress is then placed on the dentition, which often results in occlusal disharmony. Occlusal disharmony may then lead to occlusal trauma (see previous discussion in Chapter 14).

The dentition and the periodontium are usually able to withstand many of these daily stresses; however, these stresses can become excessive, such as with incorrect tongue, lip, and/or mandibular resting posture patterns and/or parafunctional habits (discussed later). Structural changes within the periodontium can occur with occlusal trauma (see Figs. 14.33 and 14.34).

Dental professionals must remember that occlusal trauma does not directly cause pathogen-based periodontal disease, but it may create an overriding adverse force factor in initiating or contributing to an already weakened and diseased periodontium. It also may be associated on an acute basis with the production of a cracked tooth from masticatory impact on a hard object and fracture of the restoration margin may also occur. Occlusal trauma can usually be halted if the etiologic factors are eliminated or if the involved teeth are protected from these stresses.

Unfortunately, the effects of occlusal trauma are often irreversible if not intercepted early enough. These occlusal disharmonies, orofacial myofunctional patterns, and parafunctional habits should be controlled or eliminated during dental treatment and preventive maintenance therapy before initiating occlusal therapy (see later discussion). Signs or symptoms indicating abnormal patterns and habits must be addressed to eliminate the harmful occlusal disharmonies on a long-term basis. The effects on a patient's occlusion must also be kept in mind during all phases of dental treatment, especially during restorative treatment or when treating a temporomandibular disorder (TMD) (see **Chapter 19**).

MALOCCLUSION CONSIDERATIONS

Malocclusion (mal-uh-**kloo**-zhuhn) is related to lack of an overall ideal form in the dentition while in CO. However, it is rare that malocclusion is directly associated with severe occlusal trauma. Malocclusion or "bad bite" by patients may affect them by having a negative impact on their appearance and increasing their difficulty with homecare procedures. Poor care favors dental biofilm retention and increases the possibility that periodontal disease or caries will affect the dentition with a malocclusion. Many malocclusions stem from hereditary factors.

An orthodontist working with other specialists, such as an orofacial myologist or speech therapist, can correct many malocclusions related to the teeth and possibly the rest of the masticatory system (see Fig. 14.20). Therefore when correcting a malocclusion to achieve a more ideal form for the dentition, the occlusal functioning of the dentition also must be considered. Early intervention in the primary and mixed dentitions can prevent many malocclusions from occurring.

Approximately 80% of children and teenagers show some degree of malocclusion. The most common occlusal difficulties are crowding, which is a type of malocclusion that affects 40% of children and 80% of teenagers. The second most common type of malocclusion is excessive overjet of the maxillary incisors, which affects approximately 15% of children and teenagers.

Other factors are also involved in the consideration of smile design, such as gender, symmetry of color or shape, and position of teeth in relationship to the midline. Any negative spaces (dark areas) are also a consideration within an ideal smile and highlight the rest of the smile. The back of the mouth is considered a desired negative space because no light enters when standing. An example of an undesirable negative space is anterior or posterior crowding of teeth creating shadows, a noticeable diastema, or even a loss of a prominent tooth that stands out from the overall curve of whiteness of the rest of the teeth.

MALOCCLUSION CLASSIFICATION

For a long time clinicians have used the **Angle classification of malocclusion** because it has not been adequately replaced by another system (Table 20.1). Although the Angle system has many inadequacies, it does serve to initially and simply address malocclusion. However, many malocclusions do not fit neatly into the Angle system, but this classification system of malocclusion does give clinicians a starting point in describing a particular case.

The Angle classification of malocclusion does *not* describe the occlusion usually present or even ideal occlusion, only malocclusion of the molars and canines. The basis of the Angle classification system was the simple hypothesis that the permanent maxillary first molar was the key to occlusion. Later, the relationship of the opposing canines was also evaluated. Therefore, the Angle system does not describe lateral or protrusive discrepancies, only those that are mesiodistally placed as related to the molars or canines.

The Angle system also assumes that a patient is occluding in a position of CO; thus it does not address the potential functional discrepancies between CR and CO. Additional information is needed to more fully evaluate a patient's occlusion than just a basic classification system. It was also assumed that patients in malocclusion had all their permanent teeth. Thus, this classification system does not describe primary or mixed dentition malocclusions, although there are specific ways to classify the relationships of canines and molars in a primary dentition (discussed earlier).

In the Angle classification, most cases of malocclusion are grouped into three main classes, according to the position of the permanent maxillary first molar to the mandibular first molar. This classification system is based on the relationship of the teeth and *not* the skeletal considerations that are due to the disproportionate size or position of the jaws (discussed later). These three main classes are designated by Roman numerals (I to III), and they assume that both sides of the dentition are affected equally, unless specifically noted. Separate defining classifications can be made, depending on which side is affected. Placement into the Angle system is only an initial baseline classification and *not* a complete diagnosis of a complex occlusal situation that may be present.

Class I Malocclusion

All cases in a **Class I malocclusion** (or neutroclusion) within a permanent dentition are characterized by an ideal mesiodistal relationship of the jaws and dental arches (Fig. 20.19). Thus in these cases, the mesiobuccal cusp of the maxillary first molar occludes with the mesiobuccal groove of the mandibular first molar. In relation to the opposing canines, the maxillary canine occludes with the distal half of the mandibular canine and the mesial half of the mandibular first premolar.

Class I malocclusion is due to dental malalignments, such as crowding (patients refer to these as "crooked teeth") or irregular spacing within the jaws. These patients usually have a facial profile as described by many clinicians with the older term **mesognathic** (mez-uhg-**nath**-ik). This facial profile in CO has slightly protruded jaws, giving the facial outline a relatively flat appearance or straight profile (Fig. 20.20); see the discussion of later cases for the differing facial profiles. Each type of facial profile present can be measured by the **gnathic index** (**nath**-ick) (or alveolar index), which is the ratio of the distance from the middle of the nasion to the basion. This measurement gives the degree of prominence of the maxillae as opposed to the mandible.

Complications from crowding, in which the teeth are out of line within the dental arch, occur because of a disproportion between the size of the teeth and arch size. Spacing challenges occur within an arch where the teeth are small relative to the size of the arch or where teeth are missing. Included in this class of malocclusion is crowding that occurs because of mesial drift as the dentition ages (Fig. 20.21; see also **Chapter 14**). Mesial drift or physiologic drift is the movement phenomenon in which all the teeth move slightly toward the midline of the oral cavity over time. This can cause crowding of a once-perfect dentition late in life. It occurs slowly depending mostly on the degree of wear of the contact points between adjacent teeth and on the number of missing teeth. Overall, drift distances usually total no more than 1 cm over a lifetime. However, even this small amount may eventually lead to poor homecare and esthetics in the area of crowding.

TABLE 20.1 Angle Classification of Malocclusion*

Class	Model	Arch Relationships	Features
Class I		Molar: MB cusp of maxillary first occluding with MB groove of mandibular first molar Canines: Maxillary occluding with distal half of mandibular canine and mesial half of mandibular first premolar	Dental malalignment(s) present (see text), such as crowding or irregular spacing; mesognathic profile
Class II	Division I	Molar: MB cusp of maxillary first occluding (by more than width of premolar) mesial to MB groove of mandibular first molar	Division I: Maxillary incisors protruding facially from mandibular incisors with severe overbite; retrognathic profile
	Division II	Canines: Distal surface of mandibular canine distal to mesial surface of maxillary canine (by at least width of premolar)	Division II: Maxillary central incisors either upright or retruded and maxillary lateral incisors either tipped labially or overlapping central incisors with severe overbite; mesognathic profile
Class III		Molar: MB cusp of maxillary first occluding (by more than width of premolar) distal to MB groove of mandibular first molar Canines: Distal surface of mandibular mesial to mesial surface of maxillary (by at least width of premolar)	Mandibular incisors protruding facially from maxillary incisors with underbite and are in complete crossbite; prognathic profile

MB, Mesiobuccal.
*Note that this system deals only with classification of permanent dentition.

Class I cases frequently have some protrusive or retrusive discrepancies in the anterior teeth, but other classes can also have these discrepancies (Fig. 20.22). Within this grouping, overbites may be slight, moderate, or severe. Certain Class I cases have an **open bite** in which the anterior teeth do not occlude (see Figs. 16.8, *A* and 14.3). In addition, Class I cases may have an **end-to-end bite** (or edge-to-edge bite) in which the teeth occlude without the maxillary teeth overlapping the mandibular teeth. With this type of occlusion, the anterior teeth of both jaws meet along their incisal ridges when the teeth are in CO. An end-to-end bite can occur both anteriorly and posteriorly, unilaterally or bilaterally.

Class I cases can also include a **crossbite**, which occurs when a mandibular tooth or teeth are placed facially to a maxillary tooth or teeth, which is the reverse situation within a proper occlusion (see Fig. 14.3) (for other class crossbite involvement, see Fig. 20.26, *A* and *B*). A crossbite can occur either anteriorly or posteriorly, unilaterally or bilaterally. Individual teeth may be slightly deviated labially or lingually relative to the adjoining teeth in the same arch; they may be in labioversion or linguoversion.

Class II Malocclusion

All cases in **Class II malocclusion** (or distoclusion) within a permanent dentition are characterized by the mesiobuccal cusp of the maxillary first molar occluding (by more than the width of a premolar) mesial to the mesiobuccal groove of the mandibular first molar (Fig. 20.23). The distal surface of the mandibular canine is distal to the mesial surface of the maxillary canine (by at least the width of a premolar). A tendency to this type of malocclusion (less than the width of a premolar) can be noted. The major group of Class II malocclusion has two subgroups, a division I and a division II, based on the position of the anterior teeth, shape of the palate, and resulting facial profile.

In **Class II malocclusion, division I**, within a permanent dentition, the maxillary incisors protrude facially from the mandibular incisors causing a severe overbite (or deep bite) (Fig. 20.24). The palate is often narrow and V-shaped. The facial profile shows a protruding upper lip and recessive mandible, resulting in a convex profile. The older term for describing the facial profile in Class II, division I, is **retrognathic** (reh-troh-**nath**-ik) (see Fig. 20.20).

In **Class II malocclusion, division II**, within a permanent dentition, the molars are in the same position as division I, but rather than having protrusive maxillary incisors, the maxillary central incisors are either upright or retruded (Fig. 20.25). The maxillary lateral incisors are either tipped labially or overlap the maxillary central incisors. Overbite is still severe (or with deep overbite), yet the palate is the proper width

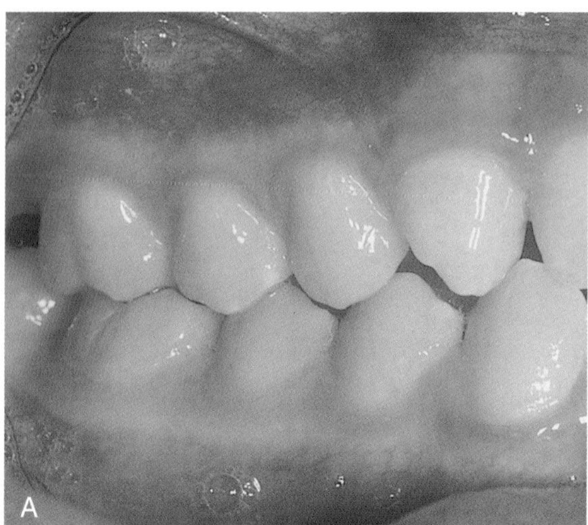

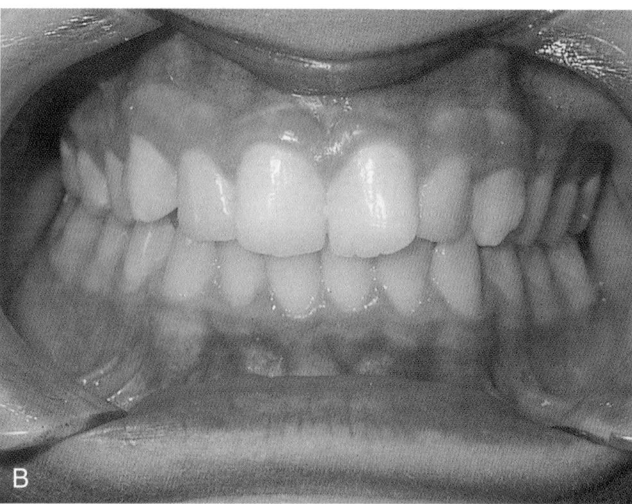

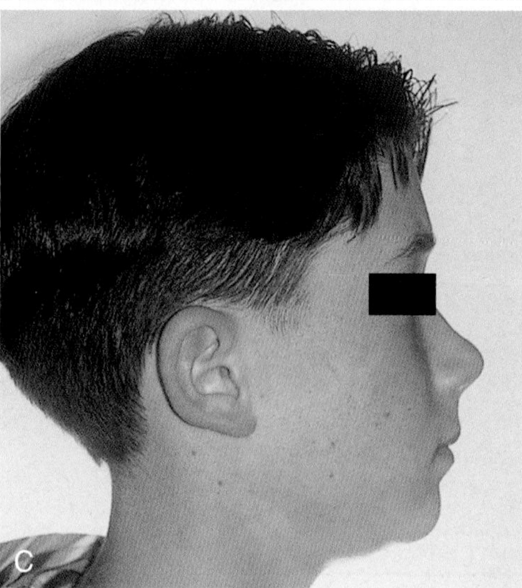

Fig. 20.19 Class I Malocclusion in a Permanent Dentition. **A,** Buccal view. **B,** Facial view. **C,** Facial profile. Mesiobuccal cusp of the maxillary first molar occludes with the mesiobuccal groove of the mandibular first molar, and the maxillary canine occludes with the distal half of the mandibular canine and the mesial half of the mandibular first premolar. Malocclusion in this specific case is due to dental malalignments, such as anterior crowding, and with a mesognathic profile (see completed orthodontic therapy case in Fig. 20.1). (Courtesy of Dona M. Seely, DDS, MSD.)

or wider compared with division I. The facial profile for Class II, division II, is usually a mesognathic profile, often with a prominent mandible (see Fig. 20.20).

Class III Malocclusion

All cases of a **Class III malocclusion** (or mesioclusion) within a permanent dentition are characterized by the mesiobuccal cusp of the maxillary first molar occluding (by more than the width of a premolar) distal to the mesiobuccal groove of the mandibular first molar (Fig. 20.26). The distal surface of the mandibular canine is mesial to the mesial surface of the maxillary canine (by at least the width of a premolar).

In comparison with Class II, division I, in which the maxillary incisors are protruding facially, the mandibular incisors extend facially from the maxillary incisors and are usually in complete crossbite. In most cases, the mandibular incisors are also inclined lingually despite the crossbite. The facial profile usually shows a prominent mandible and may also have a retrusive maxillae, thus resulting in a concave profile. The older term that describes the facial profile with a Class III malocclusion is **prognathic** (prog-**nath**-ik) (see Fig. 20.20). A tendency to this type of malocclusion (less than the width of a premolar) can be noted.

Malocclusion Subdivisions

As was noted, the Angle system of malocclusion does recognize that a case of malocclusion may occasionally have differing classifications on each side of the dentition. These asymmetrical cases are noted as *subdivisions* and usually demonstrate the main characteristics of the main class and division.

Thus the Angle classification of malocclusion allows for a Class II malocclusion, division I subdivision in which the patient has both a Class II and Class I malocclusion, showing a division I anterior pattern. Another situation that may present is a Class II malocclusion, division II subdivision, in which a patient has both a Class II and Class I, showing a division II anterior pattern. Finally, yet another situation that may present is a Class III malocclusion subdivision, in which a patient has both a Class III and Class I malocclusion on each side of the dentition.

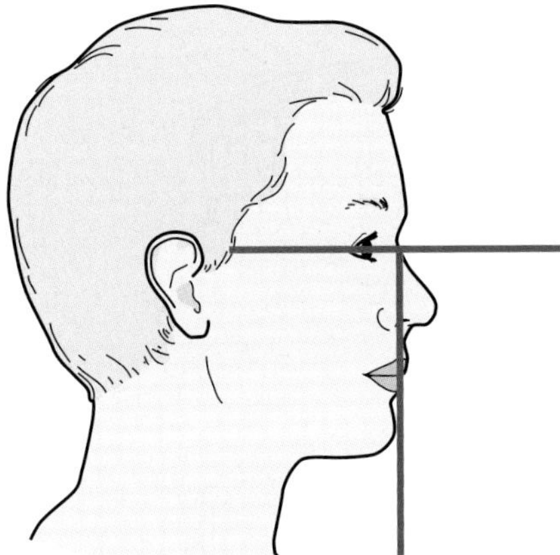
Mesognathic

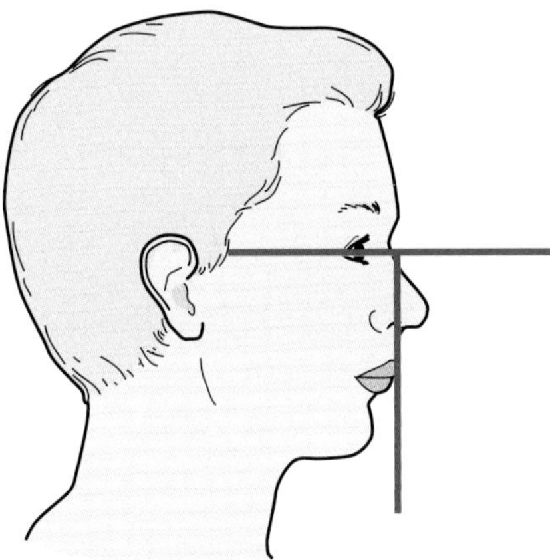
Retrognathic

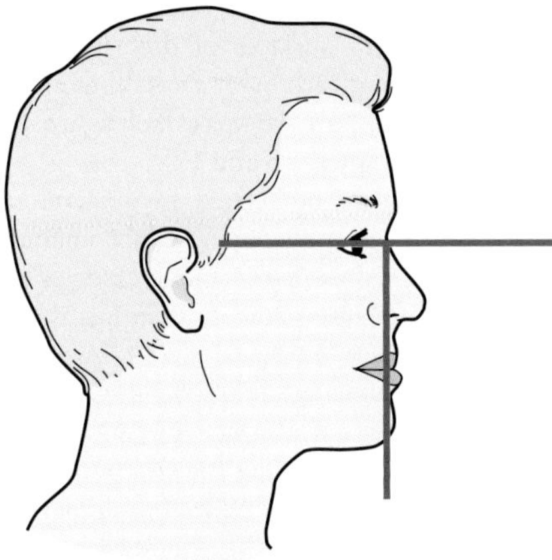
Prognathic

Fig. 20.20 Three facial profiles: mesognathic, retrognathic, and prognathic; all of which can be measured by the gnathic index (or alveolar index), that is, the ratio of the distance from the middle of the nasion (intersection of frontal bone and two nasal bones) to the basion (midpoint on anterior margin of the foramen magnum on the occipital bone). This measurement gives the degree of prominence of the maxillae as opposed to the mandible. Note that an index below 98 is retrognathic, from 98 to 103 is mesognathic, and above 103 is prognathic.

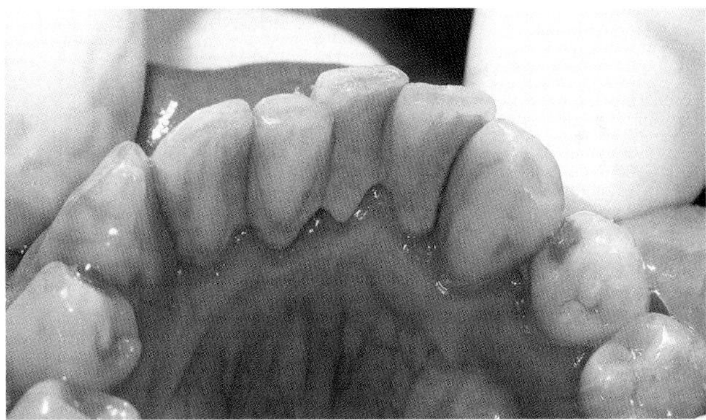

Fig. 20.21 Mesial drift is the movement phenomenon in the permanent dentition in which all the teeth move slightly toward the midline of the oral cavity over time. It can cause crowding late in life of a once-perfect dentition and may lead to poor homecare in the area of crowding, as the presence of calculus in this region demonstrates. (Courtesy of Margaret J. Fehrenbach, RDH, MS.)

Clinical Considerations with Skeletal Discrepancies

Many malocclusions are linked not only to the teeth, such as in the Angle classification of malocclusion, but also to discrepancies between the maxillae and mandible, which then can affect the occlusion of the teeth. An oral and maxillofacial surgeon when working along with an orthodontist can correct skeletal discrepancies of the jaws; orthodontic therapy with tooth movement alone is not effective.

However, in many cases, timely orthodontic intervention in young children using certain orthodontic appliances can direct bone growth of the jaws by arch expansion and by increasing arch length and level of the dentition. These interventions may prevent the need for surgical intervention. In contrast, adults and those patients whose jaw bone growth is complete, orthognathic surgery may be the only remedy for jaw discrepancies because orthodontic appliances do not in themselves produce ideal results at this point in time.

Generally orthodontic patients requiring orthognathic surgical intervention undergo an initial period of orthodontic therapy before surgery so that the teeth occlude properly after surgery. Any orthodontic appliances used to align the teeth before surgery are left in place during the surgical procedure to stabilize the teeth and jaws. After surgery, a period of follow-up orthodontic therapy helps achieve the final alignment of the teeth.

In addition to aligning the jaws, the most commonly corrected difficulties using surgical intervention include a protruding or retruding mandible, an unsightly display of gingiva superior to the maxillary anterior teeth (or "gummy smile"), an inability to achieve resting lip closure (also considered lip incompetence), and an overall elongation of the face. Associated TMDs may also be minimized with surgery in severe cases (see **Chapter 19**).

Three basic spatial planes are involved in the classification of skeletal malocclusions: horizontal, vertical, and transverse. Horizontal malocclusions are further classified as either Class II or Class III malocclusions, similar to the Angle classification of malocclusion system. Vertical malocclusions include open bites and severe overbites. Transverse malocclusions include crossbites. Most patients undergoing orthognathic surgery have a combination of these types of skeletal malocclusions.

The use of computerized treatment planning can now minimize treatment times, recovery periods, and the overall surgical efficacy, as well as use of titanium plates and miniature screws that provide stability,

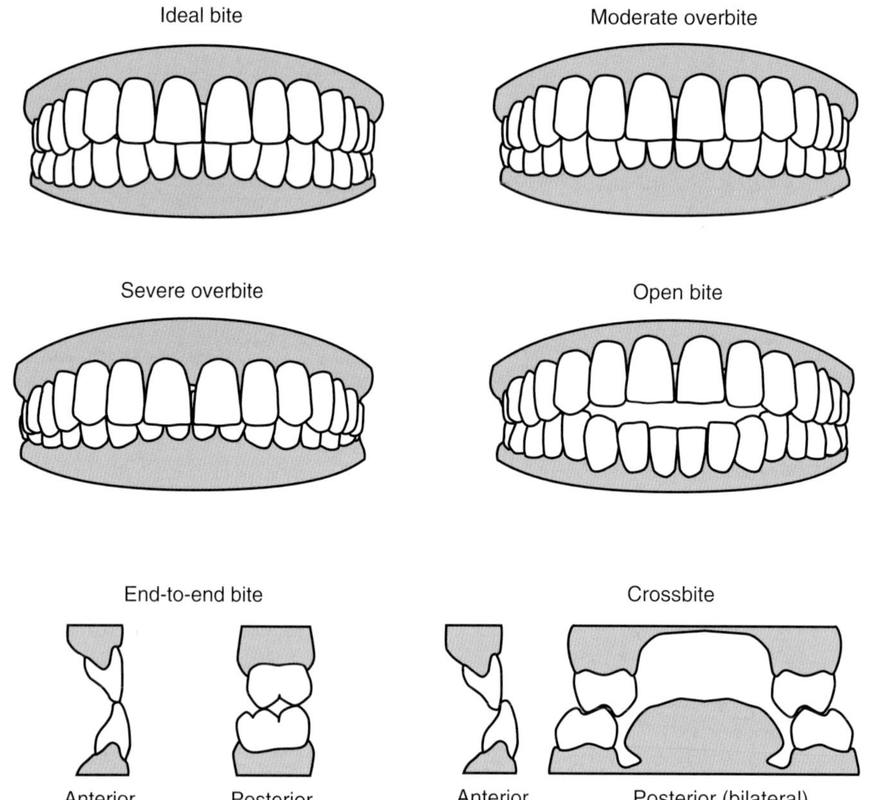

Fig. 20.22 Moderate and severe overbites contrasting with the ideal bite; open bite, end-to-end bites, and crossbites noted within the permanent dentition.

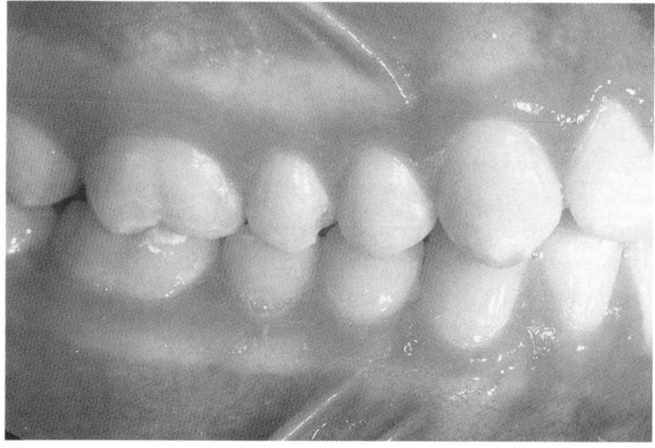

Fig. 20.23 Class II malocclusion within a permanent dentition from buccal view. Mesiobuccal cusp of the maxillary first molar is occluding (by more than the width of a premolar) mesial to the mesiobuccal groove of the mandibular first molar, and the distal surface of the mandibular canine is distal to the mesial surface of the maxillary canine (by at least the width of a premolar). (Courtesy of Dona M. Seely, DDS, MSD.)

strength and predictability to the treatment. These advances in technology, procedures, and equipment reduce postsurgical recovery time, thus allowing patients to return to their usual routines soon after the surgery.

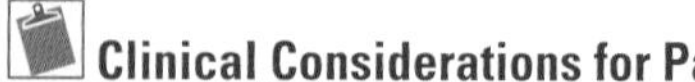

Clinical Considerations for Parafunctional Habits

Parafunctional habits (pahr-uh-**fuhngk**-shun-uhl) are those movements of the mandible that are *not* within the usual ROM associated with mastication, speech, or respiratory movements. Thus these movement habits occur more commonly and in longer duration than motions usually associated with functioning.

Parafunctional habits include **clenching** the teeth in CO or a pattern deviation for long periods, without breaking into a mandibular rest position or interocclusal clearance. Grinding the teeth or **bruxism** (**bruhk**-iz-uhm) is also a parafunctional habit. Grinding the teeth involves forceful meshing of the teeth, often causing audible noises. Attrition of the masticatory surfaces of differing levels is evident in cases of grinding, causing early wear facets that are not related to aging, especially on the canines' cusp tips as well as any contacting restorations (see Fig. 20.8; **Chapters 16 and 17**).

Parafunctional habits can be related to gingival recession and abfraction including a shearing or flaking of the enamel surface (see **Chapter 10** and Fig. 12.1, *B*). Also in many cases of parafunctional habits, a larger area of the buccal mucosa than just the linea alba can become hyperkeratinized (see Fig. 9.7).

These parafunctional habits are often subconscious and occur when a person is sleeping or concentrating deeply, such as when driving, reading, watching television, or using the computer. Usually around 20 to 30 pounds per square inch are exerted on molars during mastication, but grinders, especially at night without restraint, can exert as much as 200 pounds per square inch on the teeth. A person with these habits may have overdeveloped masseter muscles and facial and masticatory tension is considered the norm for them (Fig. 20.27). Stress may be a factor in the etiology of these habits, although it is not always present. Parafunctional habits may be linked to the individual ways one can process neurologic impulses; about 10% to 15% of adults grind their teeth moderately to severely.

Patients who grind their teeth can wear a professionally made flat-plane nonrepositioning oral splint or mouthguard during waking hours or when sleeping. This oral splint consists of a removable hard plastic, acrylic or silicone appliance(s) that covers the dental arch (or arches). These types of devices can protect the teeth from further damage, such as attrition or recession from abfraction and can reduce the occlusal

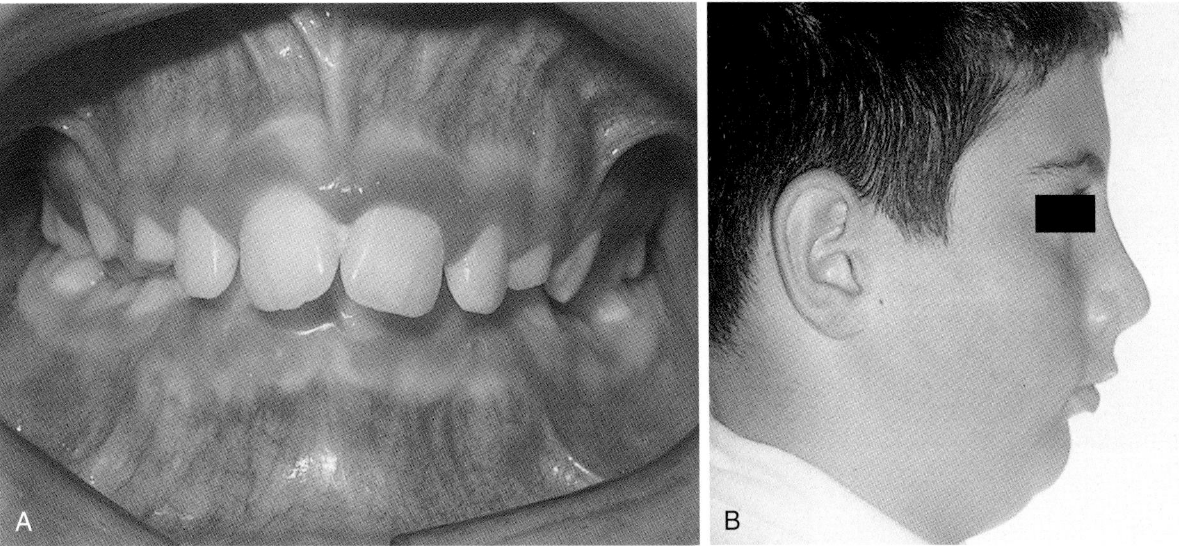

Fig. 20.24 Class II Malocclusion, Division I, Within a Permanent Dentition. **A,** Facial view. **B,** Facial profile. Maxillary incisors protrude facially from the mandibular incisors, with a severe overbite and the resulting facial profile is convex or retrognathic. (Courtesy of Dona M. Seely, DDS, MSD.)

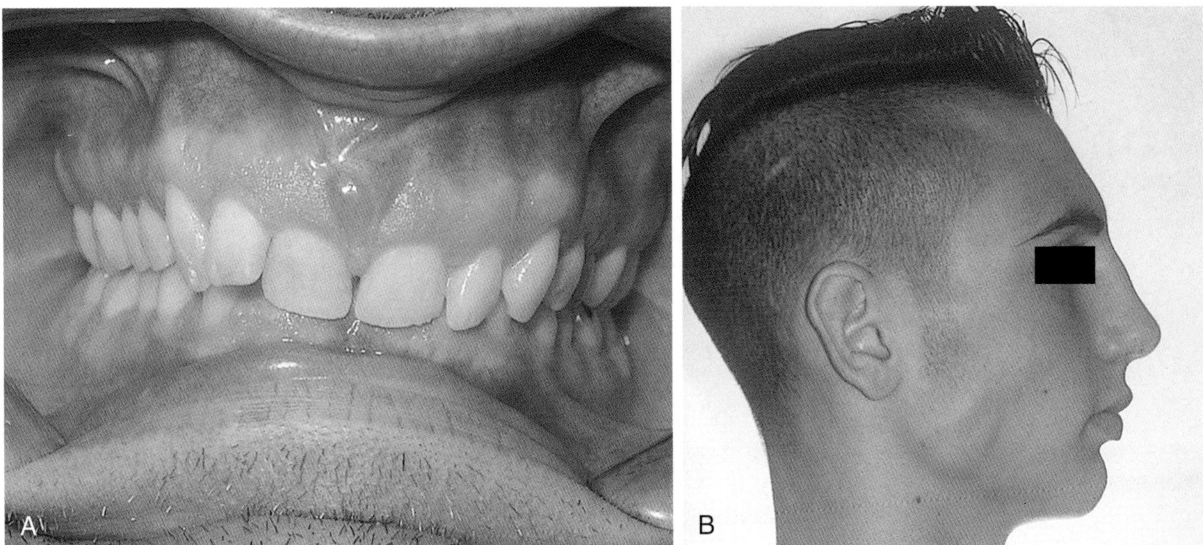

Fig. 20.25 Class II Malocclusion, Division II, Within a Permanent Dentition. **A,** Facial view. **B,** Facial profile. Maxillary central incisors in this specific case are in a retruded position and the maxillary lateral incisors are tipped labially with a severe overbite, but the resulting facial profile is mesognathic unlike division I. (Courtesy of Dona M. Seely, DDS, MSD.)

stress of the habit throughout the dentition. In contrast, individuals who clench need a mouthguard made of a softer material in order to provide a cushion to the teeth. An oromotor chewing appliance also can be used to cushion and protect the buccal, lingual, and occlusal surfaces of the teeth.

Another consideration when discussing parafunctional habits and occlusion is **orofacial myology (OM)** (ohr-oh-**fehy**-shuhl mahy-**ol**-uh-jee), a specialized professional discipline that evaluates and treats a variety of orofacial muscle postural and functional disorders as well as habit patterns that may contribute to the disruption of dental development and be involved in orofacial esthetic challenges. Each of these disorders is considered an **orofacial myofunctional disorder (OMD)** (mahy-oh-**fuhngk**-shuh-nl). OMDs involve behaviors and patterns created by inappropriate muscle function and incorrect habits involving tongue, lips, and jaws, as well as the face. Functional difficulties in speech may be associated with OMDs. Importantly studies have found a prevalence of OMDs of around 38% in the general population to 81% in children exhibiting speech difficulties.

Treatment for an OMD is through the use of **orofacial myofunctional therapy (OMT)**, a program used to retrain the patterning of the oral and facial muscles that is established by a certified orofacial myologist (COM). Individuals practicing in this specialty area may also be licensed in a dental discipline or speech pathology. Orofacial myologists work in a collaborative and team approach with other dental professionals, especially orthodontists, periodontists, and oral and maxillofacial surgeons as well as other healthcare professionals, such as speech pathologists, physical therapists, and occupational therapists.

With OMT, a variety of facial and tongue exercises and behavior modification techniques are included that work with functional head and neck postures, basing it all on individual evaluation and treatment protocols. The treatment goals for OMT include the improvement of muscle tonicity and establishing correct functional activities of the

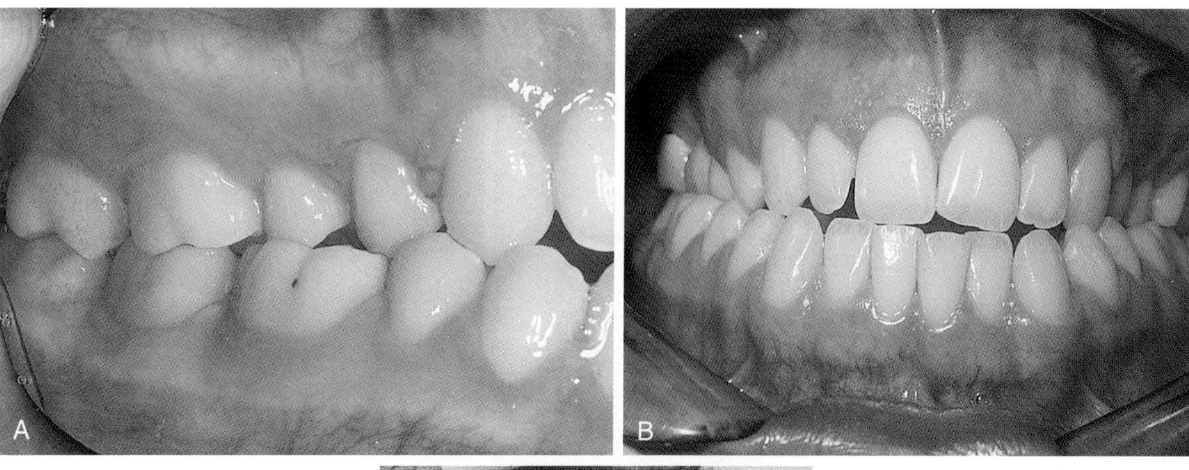

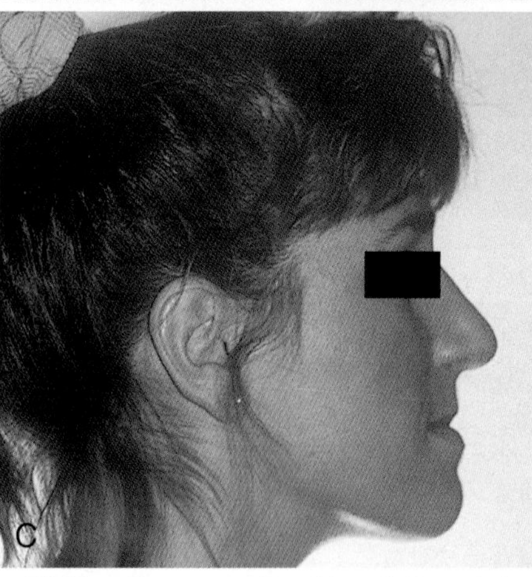

Fig. 20.26 Class III Malocclusion Within a Permanent Dentition. **A,** Buccal view. **B,** Facial view. **C,** Facial profile. Mesiobuccal cusp of the maxillary first molar is occluding (by more than the width of a premolar) distal to the mesiobuccal groove of the mandibular first molar, and the distal surface of the mandibular canine is mesial to the mesial surface of the maxillary canine (by at least the width of a premolar). Mandibular incisors protrude facially from the maxillary incisors with an underbite and are also in complete crossbite as are other teeth in this specific case and the resulting facial profile is concave or prognathic. (Courtesy of Dona M. Seely, DDS, MSD.)

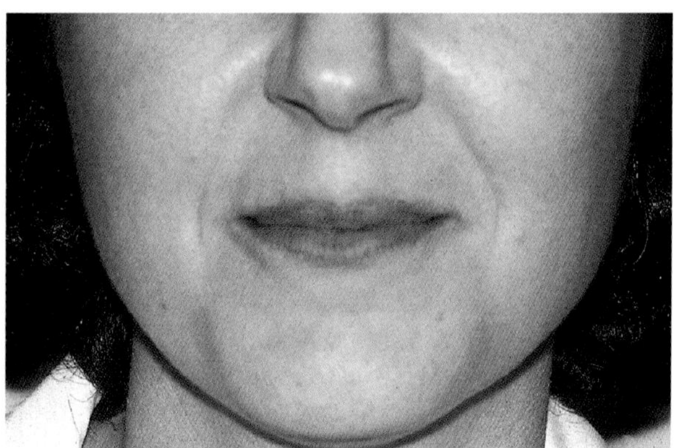

Fig. 20.27 Overdevelopment of the masseter muscles with bilateral enlargement. Patient has a history of the parafunctional habit of bruxism (grinding). (From Fehrenbach MJ, Herring SW. *Illustrated Anatomy of the Head and Neck*. 5th ed. St. Louis: Elsevier; 2017.)

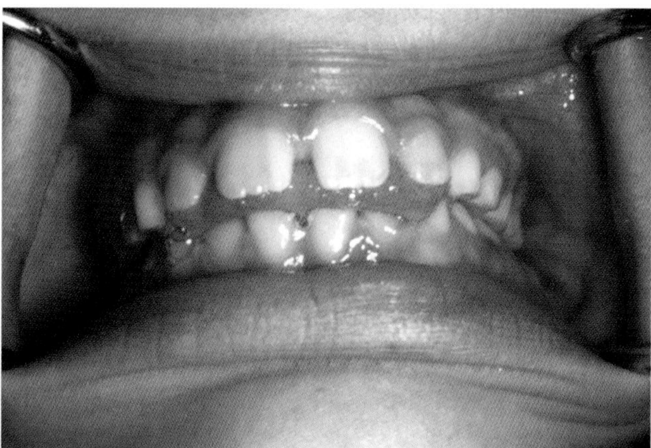

Fig. 20.28 Anterior open bite resulting from a tongue thrust swallowing pattern. (From Dean JA, McDonald RE, Avery DR. *McDonald and Avery's Dentistry for the Child and Adolescent*. 10th ed. St. Louis: Elsevier; 2016.)

tongue, lips, and mandible so that growth and development can take place or progress in a stable homeostatic oral environment. Studies have shown that OMT can be 80% to 90% effective in correcting swallowing and rest posture function and that these corrections are retained years after completing therapy. The most recent studies show that OMT with orthodontic therapy was effective in closing and maintaining closure of open bites in Angle Class I and Class II malocclusions and it reduced the relapse of open bites in patients with improper tongue movement and position.

Thus the most common OMD cited by many orofacial mycologists relative to occlusion is incorrect patterning during tongue function, which is commonly referred to as a **tongue thrust** (Fig. 20.28).

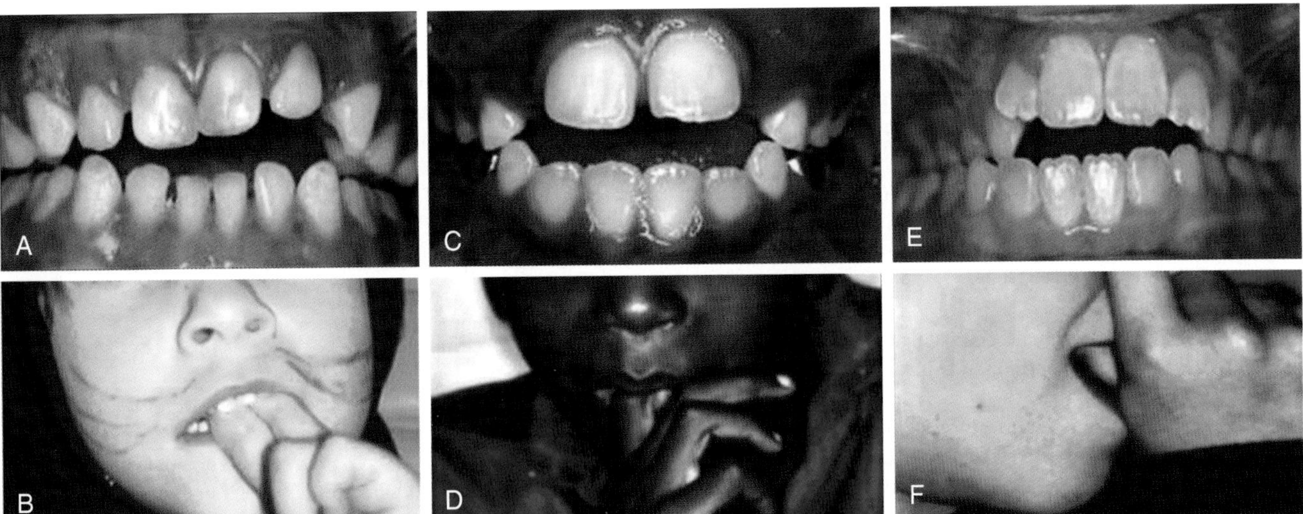

Fig. 20.29 A to **F,** Occlusion of three children with differing patterns of a retained (digit) sucking habit and the open bites that can result from this orofacial myofunctional disorder. (From Dean JA, McDonald RE, Avery DR. *McDonald and Avery's Dentistry for the Child and Adolescent,* 10th ed. St. Louis: Elsevier; 2016.)

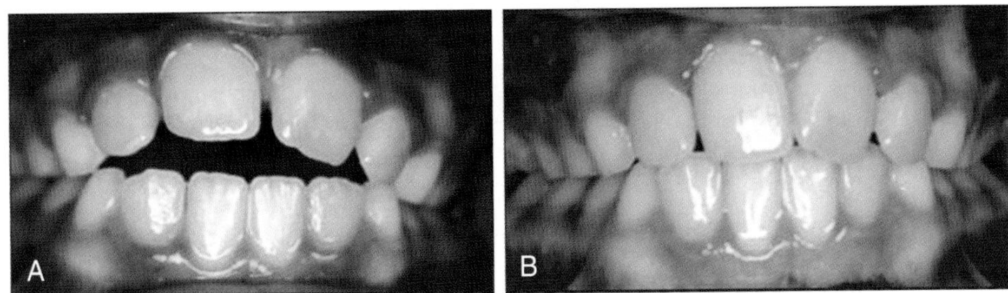

Fig. 20.30 A, Open bite in the mixed dentition of an 8-year-old child associated with the orofacial myofunctional disorder of a retained (digit) sucking habit. **B,** Bite improved after orofacial myofunctional therapy 1 year later at age 9. (From Dean JA, McDonald RE, Avery DR. *McDonald and Avery's Dentistry for the Child and Adolescent.* 10th ed. St. Louis: Elsevier; 2016.)

During the act of swallowing, and/or during the rest posture, an incorrect positioning of the tongue may contribute to improper orofacial development and maintenance of the misalignment of the teeth from this parafunctional habit. The tongue should naturally rest against the palate during swallowing as well as during the rest posture. The current view in OM is that a tongue thrust and forward interdental resting posture of the tongue serve as clues that there is likely a retained sucking habit or unresolved airway issue. Such patients are also in need of referral to pediatricians, family physicians, allergists, or specialists of the ear, nose, and throat (ENT) for definitive evaluation of the airway as appropriate.

A prime example of an OMD familiar to all pediatricians and dental professionals is a **retained sucking habit** past age 4 or 5, through digit sucking as well as excessive use of a pacifier or "sippy" cup (Fig. 20.29). While it is tempting to ignore such habits because some children do outgrow them, many children do not spontaneously discontinue noxious habits (such as digit sucking) and will need help in eliminating the habits. A range of malocclusion in a developing dentition is associated with a retained sucking habit, such as overbite and open bite, as well as a posterior crossbite. The behavioral approaches of the orofacial myologists may be effective in eliminating thumb and finger and other associated digit sucking habits (Fig. 20.30).

Another OMD cited by many orofacial myologists is an open mouth with lips apart at the resting posture. This is often referred to as **lip incompetence** (Fig. 20.31). The patient's lips should be in repose during the examination to obtain a clear indication of this OMD; patients

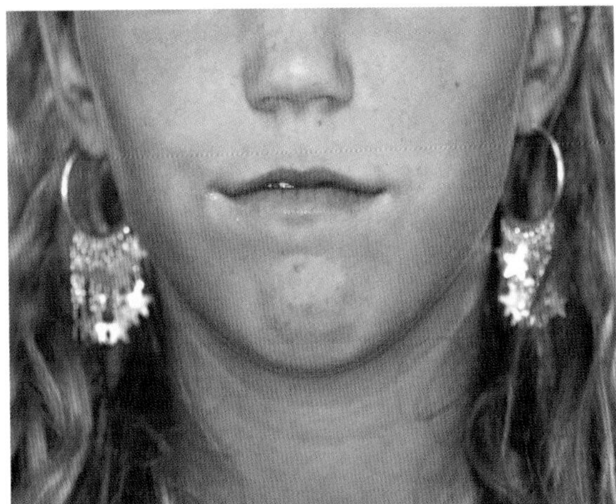

Fig. 20.31 Young patient has lip incompetence. She also has a hyperactive mentalis muscle, which is commonly associated with this orofacial myofunctional disorder as shown here during forced lip closure. (From Dean JA, McDonald RE, Avery DR. *McDonald and Avery's Dentistry for the Child and Adolescent.* 10th ed. St. Louis: Elsevier, 2016.)

frequently mask lip incompetence by forcing their lips together. This open mouth habit can distract from an esthetic facial appearance as well as compromising the beneficial influence that closed lips (considered a lip seal) have on the development and maintenance of correct dental arch form (see earlier discussion). A chronic open mouth rest posture may contribute to an increased vertical height of the face, a retrognathic profile with a downward and backward growth of the lower one-third of the face (rather than downward and forward), and hypotonic (or flaccid) lips.

Less than optimal nasal breathing may be associated with lip incompetence, so referral again may be necessary because nasal breathing must at all times be facilitated. At birth, infants instinctively are all nasal breathers with many benefits, such as filtering and warming air, increasing the ability to absorb oxygen, reducing pulse rate, and aiding in correcting tongue thrust habit as well as reducing snoring by helping maintain airflow. Instead, there may be mouth breathing associated with open lip posture, which may be associated with nasal airway obstruction, such as enlarged palatal tonsils and adenoids, a deviated nasal septum, and persistent allergies as well as a restricted labial frenum.

Mouth breathers may have a low forward tongue posture with the tongue no longer providing support for the upper jaw, thus affecting the palatal vault as well as other bones of the skull. Dry mouth (or xerostomia) and lack of air filtering are also noted. Mouth breathers often carry the head forward in order to open their airway.

In many instances, therapy to achieve a resting lip seal can avoid the need for any further tongue therapy and can also lead to a functioning freeway space dimension. Thus the concept of the freeway space is an important component associated with OMDs. This importance of the freeway space with the development of OMDs distinguishes the focus of orofacial myologists from orthodontists and other forms of dental treatment that mostly deal with a closed mouth and the role of occlusion. A primary goal of orofacial myologists is to recapture or establish a more functional level of freeway space.

Another issue for occlusal harmony can be the length of the lingual frenulum. If the lingual frenum is restricted as with ankyloglossia, it limits the possibility of creating appropriate pressure against the maxillary arch for usual level of expansion, where it may cause low and forward tongue resting posture (see Fig. 5.10). Thus it may be associated with an anterior open bite (see Fig. 16.8). It may also contribute to the developing shape of the palate. This is because the tongue cannot move up to rest properly on the palate and a crossbite often develops. It also increases the risk factors of having incorrect functional speech patterns and articulation difficulties as well as challenges with feeding by the infant. Surgery is now considered after OMT, which in many cases can help lengthen the shorter lingual frenum.

Early identification and treatment of an OMD by an orofacial myologist within an OMT program has its advantages, as does early intervention orthodontic therapy, but individuals at any age can benefit from either therapy. However, the general rule in dentistry and affirmed in pediatric medicine is that orofacial parafunctional habits should be addressed and eliminated prior to the eruption of the permanent incisors or by age 6. Individuals with special needs and syndromes also may benefit significantly from including an OMT program into their medical treatment plan. Thus, an initial OM examination and parafunctional habit pattern assessment should be incorporated into the examination procedure by dental professionals and speech pathologists as well as medical personnel to allow the patient to benefit from this area of specialized treatment.

BIBLIOGRAPHY

JOURNAL ARTICLES

Acri TM, Shin K, Seol D, et al. Tissue engineering for the temporomandibular joint. *Adv Healthc Mater.* 2019;8(2):e1801236.

Arzate H, Zeichner-David M, Mercado-Celis G. Cementum proteins: role in cementogenesis, biomineralization, periodontium formation and regeneration. *Periodontol 2000.* 2015;67(1):211–233.

Bosshardt DD. The periodontal pocket: pathogenesis, histopathology and consequences. *Periodontol 2000.* 2018;76(1):43–50.

Caton JG, Armitage G, Berglundh T, et al. A new classification scheme for periodontal and periimplant diseases and conditions - introduction and key changes from the 1999 classification. *J Clin Periodontol.* 2018;45(suppl 20):S1–S8.

Dym H, Bowler D, Zeidan J. Pharmacologic treatment for temporomandibular disorders. *Dent Clin North Am.* 2016;60(2):367–379.

Ebersole JL, Dawson DA 3rd, Emecen Huja P, et al. Age and periodontal health—immunological view. *Curr Oral Health Rep.* 2018;5(4):229–241.

Fehrenbach MJ. *Hyposalivation with Xerostomia Screening Tool,* Access (ADHA). 2010.

Ferreira LA, Grossmann E, Januzzi E, de Paula MV, Carvalho AC. Diagnosis of temporomandibular joint disorders: indication of imaging exams. *Braz J Otorhinolaryngol.* 2016;82(3):341–352.

Iafisco M, Degli Esposti L, Ramírez-Rodríguez GB, et al. Fluoride-doped amorphous calcium phosphate nanoparticles as a promising biomimetic material for dental remineralization. *Sci Rep.* 2018;8(1):17016.

Jang JK, Kwak SW, Ha JH, Kim HC. Anatomical relationship of maxillary posterior teeth with the sinus floor and buccal cortex. *Oral Rehabil.* 2017;44(8):617–625.

Lacruz RS, Habelitz S, Wright JT, Paine ML. Dental enamel formation and implications for oral health and disease. *Physiol Rev.* 2017;97(3):939–993.

Neves VC, Babb R, Chandrasekaran D, Sharpe PT. Promotion of natural tooth repair by small molecule GSK3 antagonists. *Sci Rep.* 2017;7:39654.

Noguchi S, Ukai T, Kuramoto A, et al. The histopathological comparison on the destruction of the periodontal tissue between normal junctional epithelium and long junctional epithelium. *J Periodontal Res.* 2017;52(1):74–82.

Potdar PD, Jethmalani YD. Human dental pulp stem cells: applications in future regenerative medicine. *World J Stem Cells.* 2015;7(5):839–851.

Priyadarsini S, Mukherjee S, Mishra M. Nanoparticles used in dentistry: a review. *J Oral Biol Craniofac Res.* 2018;8(1):58–67.

Silva BSE, Fagundes NCF, Nogueira BCL, et al. Epithelial rests of Malassez: from latent cells to active participation in orthodontic movement. *Dental Press J Orthod.* 2017;22(3):119–125.

Vilhena KFB, Nogueira BCL, Fagundes NCF, et al. Dental enamel bleached for a prolonged and excessive time: morphological changes. *PLoS One.* 2019;14(4):e0214948.

Yang B. Application of stem cells in oral disease therapy: progresses and perspectives. *Front Physiol.* 2017;8:197.

Yang Z. Role of the epithelial cell rests of Malassez in periodontal homeostasis and regeneration - a review. *Curr Stem Cell Res Ther.* 2015;10:398–404.

TEXTBOOKS

Dean JA. *McDonald and Avery's Dentistry for the Child and Adolescent.* 10th ed. St. Louis: Elsevier; 2016.

Fehrenbach MJ, ed. *Dental Anatomy Coloring Book.* 3rd ed. St. Louis: Elsevier; 2019.

Fehrenbach MJ. Extraoral and intraoral patient assessment. In Bowen DM and Pieren JA, eds. *Darby And Walsh Dental Hygiene Theory And Practice.* 5th ed. Philadelphia: Elsevier; 2020.

Fehrenbach MJ. Inflammation and repair; immunity. In: Ibsen AC, Phelan JA, eds. *Oral Pathology for the Dental Hygienist.* 7th ed. St Louis: Elsevier; 2018.

Fehrenbach MJ, ed. *Mosby's Dental Dictionary.* 4th ed. St. Louis: Elsevier; 2019.

Fehrenbach MJ, Herring SW. *Illustrated Anatomy of the Head and Neck.* 5th ed. St. Louis: Elsevier; 2017.

Gartner L. *Textbook of Histology.* 4th ed. St. Louis: Elsevier; 2017.

Hupp JR, Ellie III E, Tucker MR, eds. *Contemporary Oral and Maxillofacial Surgery.* 7th ed. St. Louis: Elsevier; 2019.

Moore KL, Persaud TVN, Torchia MG. *The Developing Human: Clinically Oriented Embryology.* 10th ed. Philadelphia: Elsevier; 2016.

Nanci A. *Ten Cate's Oral Histology.* 9th ed. St. Louis: Elsevier; 2018.

Nelson SJ. *Wheeler's Dental Anatomy, Physiology, and Occlusions.* 10th ed. Philadelphia: Elsevier; 2015.

Newman MG, Takei H, Klokkevold PR, Carranza FA, eds. *Newman and Carranza's Clinical Periodontology.* 13th ed. St. Louis: Elsevier; 2019.

Odell E. *Cawson's Essentials of Oral Pathology and Oral Medicine.* 9th ed. London: Elsevier; 2017.

Okeson JP. *Management of Temporomandibular Disorders and Occlusion.* 7th ed. St. Louis: Elsevier; 2013.

Perry DA, Beemsterboer PL, Essex G. *Periodontology for the Dental Hygienist.* 4th ed. St. Louis: Elsevier; 2014.

Proffit W, et al. *Contemporary Orthodontics.* 6th. St Louis: Elsevier; 2019.

Stevens A, Lowe J. *Human Histology.* 4th ed. St. Louis: Elsevier; 2015.

Young B, O'Dowd G, Woodford P. *Wheater's Functional Histology: A Text and Colour Atlas.* 5th ed. London: Elsevier; 2014.

GLOSSARY

A

Abfraction (ab-**frak**-shuhn) Hard tooth tissue loss from tensile and compressive forces during tooth flexure.

Abrasion (uh-**brey**-zhuhn) Hard tooth tissue loss caused by friction from toothbrushing and/or toothpaste.

Accessory canals Extra openings located on lateral parts of roots.

Accessory root Extra root on tooth.

Acellular cementum (si-**men**-tuhm) First layers of cementum deposited without embedded cementocytes.

Acinus (plural, **acini**) (**as**-uh-nuhs, **as**-uh-nahy) Group(s) of secretory cells of salivary gland.

Active eruption Vertical tooth movement through oral tissue.

Adipose connective tissue (**ad**-uh-pohs) Specialized connective tissue composed of fat, little matrix, adipocytes.

Afferent nerve (**af**-er-uhnt) Sensory nerve carrying information or relaying impulses from periphery of the body to brain (or spinal cord).

Afferent vessels Lymphatic vessels that allow flow of lymph into lymph node.

Ala (plural, **alae**) (**ey**-luh, **ey**-lee) Winglike cartilaginous structure(s) bounding nares laterally.

Alveolar bone proper (**ABP**) (al-**vee**-uh-ler) Bone lining alveolus.

Alveolar crest Most cervical rim of alveolar bone proper.

Alveolar crest group Alveodental ligament subgroup originating in alveolar crest to insert into cervical cementum.

Alveolar mucosa (myoo-**koh**-suh) Oral mucosa immediately apical to mucogingival junction.

Alveolar process Dental arch or tooth-bearing part of each jaw that contains alveoli.

Alveolodental ligament (al-**vee**-uh-loh-**dent**-uhl) Main principal fiber group with subgroups that include alveolar crest, horizontal, oblique, apical, interradicular.

Alveolus (plural, **alveoli**) (al-**vee**-uh-luhs, al-**vee**-uh-lahy) Socket(s) of tooth.

Ameloblasts (**am**-uh-loh-blastz) Cells that differentiate from preameloblasts to form enamel during amelogenesis.

Amelogenesis (am-uh-loh-**jen**-uh-sis) Apposition of enamel matrix by ameloblasts.

Amelogenesis imperfecta (im-per-**fek**-tuh) Hereditary enamel dysplasia with absent or thin enamel.

Amelogenins (am-uh-loh-**jen**-inz) Principal extracellular matrix protein component involved in process of mineralizing enamel.

Amniocentesis (am-nee-oh-sen-**tee**-sis) Prenatal diagnostic procedure sampling amniotic fluid.

Amniotic cavity (am-nee-**ot**-ik) Fluid-filled cavity facing epiblast layer.

Anaphase (**an**-uh-feyz) Third phase of mitosis with separation of two chromatids of each chromosome and migration.

Anatomic crown Part of crown covered by enamel.

Anatomic root Part of root covered by cementum.

Anchoring collagen fibers (**kol**-uh-juhn) Fibers from connective tissue involved in basement membrane.

Angle classification of malocclusion (mal-uh-**kloo**-zhuhn) System used to initially classify malocclusion.

Angle of the mandible (**man**-duh-buhl) Thickened area on posterior-inferior border of mandibular ramus.

Ankyloglossia (ang-kuh-lo-**glaw**-see-uh) Lingual frenum with abnormally short attachment.

Anodontia (an-uh-**don**-shee-uh) Absence of single tooth or multiple teeth owing to lack of initiation.

Anterior faucial pillar (**faw**-shuhl) Anterior lateral folds of tissue in pharynx created by underlying muscle forming structure of fauces.

Anterior teeth Incisors and canines at front of oral cavity.

Antibody (**an**-ti-bod-ee) Another term for immunoglobulin.

Antigen (**an**-ti-juhn) Another term for immunogen.

Apex of the nose (**ey**-peks) Tip of nose.

Apex of the tongue Tip of tongue.

Apical foramen (**ey**-pi-kuhl fuh-**rey**-muhn) Opening from pulp near apex of tooth.

Apical group Alveolodental ligament subgroup radiating apically from cementum to insert into alveolar bone proper.

Apposition (ap-uh-**zish**-uhn) Deposition of successive layers upon those already present.

Appositional growth (ap-uh-**zish**-uhn-uhl) Growth by addition of layers to outside of tissue mass such as that occurs to firm or hard tissue such as cartilage, bone, enamel, dentin, cementum.

Arrest lines Smooth, stained microscopic lines caused by appositional growth in cartilage, bone, cementum.

Articular eminence (ahr-**tik**-youh-ler **em**-uh-nuhns) Rounded protuberance on inferior aspect of zygomatic process for articulation of temporomandibular joint.

Articular fossa (**fos**-uh) Depression on inferior aspect of temporal bone for articulation of temporomandibular joint.

Articulating surface of the condyle (ahr-**tik**-yuh-late-ing) (**kon**-dyahl) Head of mandibular condyle within temporomandibular joint.

Attached gingiva (jin-**jahy**-vuh) Gingiva that tightly adheres to alveolar process around roots of teeth.

Attrition (uh-**trish**-uhn) Hard tooth tissue loss caused by tooth-to-tooth contact during mastication or parafunctional habits.

Avulsion (uh-**vulh**-shuhn) Complete tooth displacement from socket due to extensive trauma.

Axon (**ak**-son) Process that conducts impulses away from cell body.

B

B cell Lymphocyte that matures in lymph nodes and works during humoral immune response.

Balancing interference Teeth in contact on balancing side during lateral occlusion.

Balancing side Other side of arch from working side during lateral occlusion.

Basal bone (**bey**-suhl) Part of jaws that forms body of the maxilla or mandible.

Basal lamina (**lam**-uh-nuh) Superficial part of basement membrane within the dentogingival junction that has both an external and internal basal lamina surrounding junctional epithelium.

Basal layer Single layer of cuboidal epithelial cells overlying basement membrane.

Base of the tongue Most posterior part of tongue.

Basement membrane Extracellular material consisting of basal and reticular lamina produced by either epithelium or connective tissue.

Basophil (**bey**-suh-fil) White blood cell containing granules of histamine.

Bell stage Fourth stage of odontogenesis with enamel organ assuming bell shape.

Bifurcated (bahy-fuhr-**keyt**-tuhd) Tooth having two root branches.

Bilaminar embryonic disc (bahy-**lam**-uh-nuhr em-bree-**on**-ik) Circular plate of bilayered cells developed from blastocyst.

Bilateral symmetry (**sim**-uh-tree) Each half of embryo mirrors other half.

Biologic width Combined heights of suprabony soft tissue around tooth.

Black hairy tongue Tongue lesion marked by dead cells and keratin buildup that becomes extrinsically stained.

Blastocyst (**blas**-toh-sist) Structure formed during prenatal development consisting of trophoblast cells and inner mass of cells that develop into embryo.

Blood Fluid connective tissue containing cells and plasma.

Body of the mandible (**man**-duh-buhl) Horizontal part of lower jaw inferior to teeth.

Body of the maxilla (mak-**sil**-uh) Horizontal part of upper jaw superior to teeth.

Body of the tongue Anterior part of tongue.

Bone Rigid connective tissue.

Bone marrow (**mar**-oh) Innermost part of bone in medullary cavity.

Branchial (or pharyngeal) apparatus (**brang**-kee-uhl/fuh-**rin**-jee-uhl ap-uh-**rat**-uhs) Group that includes branchial or pharyngeal arches, grooves and membranes, with pharyngeal pouches.

Branchial (or pharyngeal) arches Six stacked bilateral swellings of tissue that appear inferior to stomodeum, including mandibular arch.

Branchial cleft cyst Developmental cervical cyst due to obliteration failure of second branchial or pharyngeal groove.

Branchial (or pharyngeal) grooves Grooves between neighboring branchial or pharyngeal arches on each side of embryo.
Bruxism (**bruhk**-iz-uhm) Parafunctional habit of tooth grinding.
Buccal (**buhk**-uhl) Structures or facial surface of tooth close to inner cheek.
Buccal fat pad Pad of underlying adipose connective tissue in vestibules.
Buccal mucosa (myoo-**koh**-suh) Mucosa that lines inner cheek.
Buccal region Region of face composed of soft tissue of cheek.
Bud stage Second stage of tooth development marked by growth of dental lamina into buds.

C

Calcium hydroxyapatite (**kal**-see-uhm hahy-drok-see-**ap**-uh-tahyt) Main inorganic crystal with chemical formula of $Ca_{10}(PO_4)_6(OH)_2$ in enamel, alveolar bone, dentin, cementum.
Canaliculi (kan-l-**ik**-yuh-lahy) Tubular canals in both bone and cementum.
Cancellous (kan-**suh**-luhs) **bone** Spongy bone within compact bone with trabeculae instead of Haversian system.
Canine eminence (**kahy**-nahy **em**-uh-nuhns) Vertically oriented and labially placed bony ridge of alveolar process.
Canine rise Contralateral canine should be only tooth in function during lateral occlusion.
Canines (**kahy**-nahyz) Anterior teeth that are third from midline in each quadrant.
Cap stage Third stage of tooth development with dental lamina growing into cap shape.
Capillary plexus (**kap**-uh-ler-ee **plek**-suhs) Capillaries located between papillary layer and deeper layers of lamina propria.
Capsule (**kap**-suhl) Connective tissue that surrounds outer part of entire gland or lesion.
Cartilage (**kahr**-ti-lij) Firm non mineralized connective tissue.
Caudal end (**kawd**-l) Tail end of structure.
Cell Smallest unit of organization in body.
Cell membrane Membrane that completely surrounds cell.
Cellular cementum (si-**men**-tuhm) Outer layers of cementum that contain embedded cementocytes.
Cemental caries (si-**men**-tuhl) Shallow carious lesion of cementum.
Cemental spurs Symmetrical spheres of cementum attached to root surface.
Cementicles (si-**men**-tih-kuhlz) Mineralized bodies of cementum either attached to root or free in periodontal ligament.
Cementoblasts (si-**men**-tuh-blastz) Cells that form cementoid and are differentiated from dental sac.
Cementocytes (si-**men**-toh-sahytz) Cementoblasts entrapped by cementum they produce.
Cementoenamel junction (**CEJ**) (si-**men**-toh-ih-**nam**-uhl) Tooth anatomy where crown enamel and root cementum are close.
Cementogenesis (si-**men**-toh-**jen**-i-sis) Appositional growth of cementum in root area.
Cementoid (si-**men**-toid) Cementum matrix laid down by cementoblasts.
Cementum (si-**men**-tuhm) Outermost layer of root of tooth.
Central cells of the dental papilla (puh-**pil**-uh) Primordium of pulp.
Central fossa (**fos**-uh) Fossa located at convergence of cusp ridges in central point on occlusal surface of posteriors.
Central groove Most prominent developmental groove on posteriors traveling mesiodistally to separate occlusal table buccolingually.
Centric occlusion (**CO**) (uh-**kloo**-zhuhn) Voluntary position of dentition that allows maximal contact when teeth occlude.
Centric relation (**CR**) End point of closure of mandible in which mandible is in most retruded position.
Centric stops Centric contacts between two arches that includes height of cusp contour, marginal ridges, central fossae.
Centrioles (**sen**-tree-ohlz) Pair of cylindrical structures in centrosome.
Centromere (**sen**-truh-meer) Clear constricted area where two chromatids of chromosome are joined.
Centrosome (**sen**-truh-sohm) Organelle associated with centrioles.
Cephalic end (suh-**fal**-ik) Head end of structure.
Cervical loop (**ser**-vih-kal) Most cervical part of enamel organ responsible for root development.
Cervical ridge Ridge running mesiodistally in cervical one-third of buccal crown surface on primary dentition and permanent molars.
Chondroblasts (**kon**-droh-blastz) Cells that produce cartilage tissue.
Chondrocytes (**kon**-droh-sahytz) Mature chondroblasts.
Chromatids (**kroh**-muh-tids) Two filamentous daughter chromosomes joined at centromere during cell division.
Chromatin (**kroh**-muh-tin) Chief nucleoprotein in nondividing nucleoplasm.
Chromosomes (**kroh**-muh-sohms) Separate concentrations of chromatin in dividing nucleus of cell.
Cilia (**sil**-ee-uh) Projections on the cell surface that are more numerous and shorter than flagella.
Cingulum (**sing**-gyuh-luhm) Raised and rounded area on cervical third of lingual surface on anteriors.
Circumpulpal dentin (sur-kuhm-**pul**-puhl) Layer of dentin around outer pulpal wall.
Circumvallate lingual papillae (sur-kuhm-**val**-yet **ling**-gwuhl puh-**pil**-ee) Larger mushroom-shaped lingual papillae that line up along anterior side of sulcus terminalis on tongue.
Class I malocclusion (mal-uh-**kloo**-zhuhn) Malocclusion characterized by ideal mesiodistal relationship of jaws and dental arches with minor dental malalignments.
Class II malocclusion Malocclusion with mesiobuccal cusp of maxillary first molar occluding by more than width of premolar mesial to mesiobuccal groove of mandibular first molar.
Class II malocclusion, division I Class II malocclusion with permanent maxillary anteriors protruding facially.
Class II malocclusion, division II Class II malocclusion with maxillary central incisors either upright or retruded.
Class III malocclusion Malocclusion with mesiobuccal cusp of maxillary first molar occluding by more than width of premolar distal to mesiobuccal groove of mandibular first molar.
Cleavage (**klee**-vij) Process during prenatal development when mitosis converts zygote to blastocyst.
Cleft lip (**kleft**) Developmental disturbance of upper lip from failure of fusion of maxillary processes with medial nasal process.
Cleft palate (**pal**-it) Developmental disturbance from failure of fusion of palatal shelves with primary palate or with each other.
Cleft uvula (**yoo**-vyuh-luh) Mildest form of cleft palate.
Clenching Parafunctional habit with teeth held in centric occlusion for long periods without interocclusal clearance.
Clinical attachment level (**CAL**) Measurement of position of gingiva in relation to cementoenamel junction.
Clinical attachment loss True attachment loss based on histology related to clinical attachment level.
Clinical crown Part of anatomic crown visible in oral cavity and not covered by gingival tissue.
Clinical root Part of anatomic root visible in oral cavity and not covered by gingival tissue.
Cloacal membrane (kloh-**ay**-kuhl) Membrane at caudal end of embryo that is location of future anus.
Col (**kohl**) Interdental gingiva apical to contact area assumes nonvisible concave form between facial and lingual gingival surfaces.
Collagen fibers (**kol**-uh-juhn) Main protein fiber.
Collagenous connective tissue (**kuh**-laj-uh-nuhs) Tissue with large amount of collagen fibers.
Colloid (**kol**-oid) Material in follicles of thyroid reserved for production of thyroxine.
Compact bone (**kuhm**-pakt) Bone deep to periosteum with Haversian system of bone with lamellae.
Concrescence (kon-**kres**-uhns) Union of root structure of two or more teeth through cementum only.
Congenital malformations (kuhn-**jen**-i-tuhl mal-fawr-**mey**-shuhns) Birth defects or developmental problems evident at birth.
Connective tissue Basic tissue mainly composed of cells and matrix.
Connective tissue papillae (puh-**pil**-ee) Interdigitation of loose connective tissue with epithelium.
Connective tissue proper Two adjacent layers consisting of loose and dense connective tissue.
Contact area Tooth anatomy where adjacent tooth crowns in same arch touch on each proximal surface.
Contour lines of Owen Adjoining imbrication lines in dentin that demonstrate disturbance in body metabolism.

Copula (**kop**-yuh-luh) Posterior swelling formed from third and fourth branchial or pharyngeal arches that overgrows second arches to form tongue base.

Core bundles Fascicles found in innermost part of nerve.

Coronal pulp (**kuh**-rohn-nl) Pulp located in tooth crown.

Coronoid notch (**kawr**-uh-noid) Main part of anterior border of mandibular ramus.

Coronoid process Bony projection at anterior border of mandibular ramus.

Cortical bone (**kawr**-ti-kuhl) Plates of compact bone on facial and lingual surfaces of alveolar process.

Crossbite Malocclusion in which mandibular tooth or teeth are placed facially to maxillary tooth or teeth.

Crown Part of tooth composed of dentin and pulp covered by enamel.

Curve of Spee Anteroposterior curvature produced by planes placed on masticatory surfaces of each dental arch.

Curve of Wilson Concave curve produced when frontal section is taken through maxillary and mandibular molars.

Cusp (**kusp**) One or more major elevations on masticatory surface of canine and posteriors.

Cusp of Carabelli (kare-uh-**bell**-ee) Small cusp on permanent maxillary first and second molar in some cases.

Cusp of Carabelli groove Groove associated with cusp of Carabelli.

Cusp ridge Ridge that descends from each cusp tip on posteriors.

Cusp slope Two ridges on incisal edge of canines divided by cusp tip.

Cusp tip Tip of cusp on incisal surface of canines and occlusal table of posteriors.

Cytodifferentiation (sy-toh-dif-uh-ren-she-**ay**-shuhn) Development of different cell types.

Cytoplasm (**sahy**-tuh-plaz-uhm) Fluid part contained within cell membrane.

Cytoskeleton (**CSK**) (sahy-tuh-**skel**-i-tn) Three-dimensional system of support within cell.

D

D-A-Q-T System System to designate teeth with *D* for dentition, *A* for arch, *Q* for quadrant, *T* for tooth type.

Dendrite (**den**-drahyt) Process of neuron that conducts impulses toward cell body.

Dens in dente (**denz in den**-tehy) Developmental disturbance caused by invagination of enamel organ into dental papilla.

Dense connective tissue Deepest layers of dermis or lamina propria.

Dense layer Dense connective tissue in dermis and lamina propria.

Dental anatomy Area of dental sciences dealing with tooth morphology.

Dental arch Alveolar process or tooth-bearing part of each jaw in either maxillary or mandibular arch.

Dental fluorosis (floo-**roh**-sis) Hypomineralization occurs due to excess systemic fluoride level.

Dental lamina (**lam**-uh-nuh) Growth from oral epithelium giving rise to tooth buds.

Dental papilla (puh-**pil**-uh) Inner mass of ectomesenchyme of tooth germ that produces dentin and pulp.

Dental placodes (**plak**-ohdz) Plate-like thickened epithelium and underlying neural crest derived mesenchyme or neuroectoderm in specific areas.

Dental pulp stem cells (**DPSCs**) Undifferentiated mesenchyme type of stem cells in pulp tissue.

Dental sac Tooth germ part consisting of ectomesenchyme surrounding outside of enamel organ.

Dentigerous cyst (den-**tij**-er-uhs) Odontogenic cyst that forms from reduced enamel epithelium.

Dentin (**den**-tin) Hard inner layer of tooth crown overlying pulp.

Dentin dysplasia (dis-**pley**-zhuh) Faulty development of dentin.

Dentinal caries (**den**-tin-uhl) Carious lesion gone beyond dentinoenamel junction from enamel invasion.

Dentinal fluid Fluid within dentinal tubule in dentin.

Dentinal hypersensitivity (hahy-per-sen-si-**tiv**-i-tee) Exposed dentin sensitive to various stimuli.

Dentinal tubules Long tubes in dentin.

Dentinocemental junction (**DCJ**) (den-tin-oh-si-**ment**-uhl) Junction between dentin and cementum formed during root development.

Dentinoenamel junction (**DEJ**) (den-tih-noh-ih-**nam**-uhl) Junction between dentin and enamel formed by mineralization of disintegrating basement membrane.

Dentinogenesis (den-tin-noh-**jen**-uh-sis) Appositional growth of predentin by odontoblasts.

Dentinogenesis imperfecta (im-per-**fek**-tuh) Dentin dysplasia with hereditary basis and blue-gray or brown teeth with opalescent sheen.

Dentition (den-**tish**-uhn) Natural teeth in jaws of either primary and permanent or mixed grouping of teeth.

Dentition periods Three periods that occur throughout lifetime, primary, mixed, permanent.

Dentogingival junction (den-toh-jin-**juh**-vuhl) Junction between tooth surface and gingival tissue.

Dentogingival junctional tissue (**juhngk**-shuhn-uhl) Tissue that includes sulcular epithelium and junctional epithelium.

Depression of the mandible Lowering of lower jaw.

Dermis (**dur**-mis) Connective tissue proper in skin.

Desmosome (**dez**-moh-sohm) Intercellular junction between cells.

Developmental depression Depression usually evident in specific tooth area.

Developmental groove Primary groove that marks junction among developmental lobes on lingual surface of anteriors or occlusal table of posteriors.

Developmental pits Pits on lingual surface of anteriors or on occlusal table and buccal, lingual surface of posteriors.

Diastema (dahy-uh-**stee**-muh) Open contact that can exist between permanent maxillary central incisors.

Differentiation (dif-uh-ren-shee-**ay**-shuhn) Change in embryonic cells to become quite distinct structurally and functionally.

Dilaceration (dih-las-uh-**rey**-shuhn) Crown or root(s) showing angular distortion.

Distal (**dis**-tl) Surface of tooth farthest away from midline.

Distal step No terminal plane relationship exists because primary mandibular second molar is distal to maxillary second molar.

Dorsal surface of the tongue (**dawr**-suhl) Top surface of tongue.

Down syndrome (**sin**-drohm) Developmental disturbance that involves trisomy of chromosome number 21.

Duct Passageway that allows glandular secretion to be directly emptied.

Duct(s) of Rivinus (**reh**-vee-nuhs) Smaller ducts of sublingual gland.

E

Early childhood caries (**ECC**) Extensive acute caries of primary teeth.

Ectoderm (**ek**-tuh-durm) Layer in trilaminar embryonic disc derived from epiblast layer and lining stomodeum.

Ectodermal dysplasia (ek-tuh-**durm**-uhl dis-**pley**-zhuh) Syndrome involving abnormal development of one or more ectodermal structures including anodontia.

Ectomesenchyme (ek-toh-**mes**-eng-kahym) Mesenchyme from ectoderm influenced by neural crest cells.

Ectopic pregnancy (ek-**top**-ik) Implantation occurring outside uterus.

Edentulous (ee-**den**-chuh-luhs) Dentition with either partial or complete loss of teeth.

Efferent nerve (**ef**-er-uhnt) Motor nerve carrying information away from brain to periphery of body.

Efferent vessel Lymphatic vessel in which lymph flows out of lymph node.

Elastic cartilage (e-**las**-tik **kahr**-ti-lij) Cartilage found in ear and epiglottis.

Elastic connective tissue Specialized connective tissue with mostly elastic fibers.

Elastic fiber Protein fiber in connective tissue composed of microfilaments.

Elevation of the mandible (el-uh-**vey**-shuhn) Raising of lower jaw.

Embrasures (em-**bray**-zhuhrs) Spaces from curvatures where two teeth in same arch contact.

Embryo (**em**-bree-oh) Structure derived from implanted blastocyst.

Embryoblast layer (**em**-bree-oh-blast) Small inner mass of embryonic cells in blastocyst.

Embryology (em-bree-**ol**-uh-jee) Study of prenatal development.

Embryonic cell layers (em-bree-**on**-ik) Germ layers derived from increased number of embryonic cells.

Embryonic folding Embryonic folding of embryo placing tissue in proper position.
Embryonic period Prenatal developmental time period for embryo from second to eighth week.
Enamel (ih-**nam**-uhl) Hard outer layer of tooth crown.
Enamel caries Carious lesion invaded through enamel either by pits and grooves or through smooth surface.
Enamel dysplasia (dis-**pley**-zhuh) Faulty development of enamel.
Enamel hypocalcification (hahy-puh-kal-sey-fih-**kay**-shuhn) Dysplasia from reduction in quality of enamel maturation.
Enamel hypoplasia (hahy-puh-**pley**-zhuh) Dysplasia from reduction in quantity of enamel matrix.
Enamel knot Region noted in molars' enamel organ involved in crown form.
Enamel lamellae (luh-**mel**-ee) Partially mineralized vertical sheets of enamel matrix.
Enamel matrix (**mey**-triks) Matrix of enamel formed during amelogenesis by ameloblasts.
Enamel organ Cap or bell-shaped part of tooth germ that produces enamel.
Enamel pearl Small spherical enamel projections on tooth surface.
Enamel rod Crystalline structural unit of enamel.
Enamel spindles Microscopic feature present in mature enamel as short dentinal tubules near dentinoenamel junction.
Enamel tufts Microscopic feature in mature enamel of small dark brushes near dentinoenamel junction.
Endochondral ossification (en-doh-**kon**-druhl os-uh-fi-**key**-shuhn) Formation of osteoid within cartilage model.
Endocrine gland (**en**-duh-krin) Ductless gland that secretes directly into blood.
Endocytosis (en-doh-sahy-**toh**-sis) Uptake of materials from extracellular environment into cell.
Endoderm (**en**-doh-durm) Layer in trilaminar embryonic disc derived from hypoblast layer.
Endoplasmic reticulum (**ER**) (**en**-duh-**plaz**-mik ri-**tik**-yuh-luhm) Membrane-bound organelle with channels that is either rough or smooth.
Endosteum (en-**dos**-tee-uhm) Lining of medullary cavity of bone.
Endothelium (en-doh-**thee**-lee-uhm) Unstratified squamous epithelium lining vessels and serous cavities.
End-to-end bite Teeth that occlude without maxillary teeth overlapping mandibular teeth.
Eosinophil (ee-uh-**sin**-uh-fil) White blood cell involved in parasitic diseases because primary function is phagocytosis of immune complexes.
Epiblast layer (**ep**-uh-blast) Superior layer in bilaminar disc.
Epidermis (ep-i-**dur**-mis) Superficial layers of skin.
Epiglottic swelling (ep-i-**glot**-ik) Posterior swelling that develops from fourth branchial or pharyngeal arches marking development of future epiglottis.
Epithelial attachment (**EA**) (ep-uh-**thee**-lee-uhl) Device that attaches junctional epithelium to tooth surface.
Epithelial pearls Persistent discrete clusters of epithelial cells that usually degenerate from dental lamina.
Epithelial rests of Malassez (**ERM**) (mal-uh-**say**) Epithelial cell groups in periodontal ligament after disintegration of Hertwig epithelial root sheath.
Epithelium (plural, **epithelia**) (ep-uh-**thee**-lee-um, ep-uh-**thee**-lee-uh) Basic tissue that covers and lines external and internal body surfaces.
Erectile tissue (ih-**rek**-tl) Thin-walled vessels in nasal cavity capable of considerable engorgement.
Erosion (ih-**roh**-zhuhn) Hard tooth tissue loss through chemical means not involving bacteria.
Erythrocyte (ih-**rith**-ruh-sahyt) Another term used for red blood cell.
Excretory duct (**ex**-sri-tawr-ee) Duct of salivary gland through which saliva exits into oral cavity.
Exocrine gland (**ek**-suh-krin) Gland having ducts associated with it.
Exocytosis (ek-soh-sahy-**toh**-sis) Active transport of material from vesicle out into extracellular environment.
Exostoses (ek-os-**stoh**-seez) Small localized bone growths noted usually on facial surface of alveolar process of maxilla.
External basal lamina (**bey**-suhl **lam**-uh-nah) Basal lamina between the junctional epithelium and the lamina propria.
External nose Surface of the nose in the nasal region.

F

Facial Structure or tooth surface closest to outer face.
Fascicles (**fas**-i-kuhlz) Numerous muscle bundles that compose muscle.
Fauces (**faw**-seez) Opening posteriorly from the oral cavity proper into pharynx.
Fertilization (fur-tl-uh-**zey**-shuhn) Process by which sperm penetrates ovum during preimplantation period.
Fetal alcohol syndrome (**FAS**) (**feet**-l) (**sin**-drohm) Syndrome in infant during embryonic period resulting from ethanol ingested by pregnant woman.
Fetal period Prenatal development period for fetus from third to ninth month.
Fetus (**fee**-tuhs) Structure of fetal period of prenatal development derived from enlarged embryo.
Fibrils (**fahy**-bruhlz) Smaller subunits of collagen fibers.
Fibroblast (**fahy**-bruh-blast) Cell that synthesizes protein fibers and intercellular substance.
Fibrocartilage (fahy-broh-**kahr**-ti-lij) Cartilage of parallel and thick compact collagenous bundles.
Fibroclasts (**fahy**-bruh-klastz) Cells that destroy remaining connecting collagen fibers holding primary tooth.
Fifth branchial (**or pharyngeal**) **arch**(**es**) (**brang**-kee-uhl/fuh-**rin**-jee-uhl) Rudimentary embryonic branchial or pharyngeal arch(es) that is absent or included with fourth branchial or pharyngeal arch(es).
Filiform lingual papillae (**fil**-uh-fawrm **ling**-gwuhl puh-**pil**-ee) Slender threadlike lingual papillae giving dorsal surface of tongue its velvety texture.
First branchial (**or pharyngeal**) **arch**(**es**) (**brang**-kee-uhl/fuh-**rin**-jee-uhl) Mandibular arch(es) in embryo.
Flagella (fluh-**jel**-uh) Projections on the cell surface that are fewer and longer than cilia.
Floor of the mouth Area of oral cavity proper underneath ventral surface of the tongue and bordered by mandibular arch.
Flush terminal plane Terminal plane relationship where primary maxillary and mandibular second molars are in end-to-end relationship.
Fluting Elongated developmental depression on surface root branches.
Foliate lingual papillae (**foh**-lee-it **ling**-gwuhl puh-**pil**-ee) Vertical ridges of lingual papillae on lateral tongue surface.
Follicles (**fol**-i-kuhls) Masses embedded in meshwork of reticular fibers within lobules of thyroid.
Foramen cecum (fuh-**rey**-muhn **see**-kuhm) Small pitlike depression located where sulcus terminalis points backward toward pharynx.
Fordyce spots (**for**-dice) Small yellowish elevations of sebaceous glands on oral mucosa.
Foregut (**fawr**-guht) Anterior part of future digestive tract or primitive pharynx that forms oropharynx.
Fossa (plural, **fossae**) (**fos**-uh, **fos**-ee) Shallow wide depression(s) on lingual surface of anteriors or occlusal table of posteriors.
Fourth branchial (**or pharyngeal**) **arch**(**es**) (**brang**-kee-uhl/fuh-**rin**-jee-uhl) Branchial or pharyngeal arch(es) in embryo that participates in formation of laryngeal cartilages.
Free gingival crest (jin-**juh**-vuhl) Most coronal part of marginal gingiva.
Free gingival groove Groove that separates attached gingiva from marginal gingiva.
Frontal region (**fruhn**-tl) Region of face that includes forehead and area above eyes.
Frontonasal process (fruhn-toh-**ney**-zuhl) Prominence in upper facial area at cephalic end of embryo.
Fungiform lingual papillae (**fuhn**-juh-fawrm **ling**-gwuhl puh-**pil**-ee) Smaller mushroom-shaped lingual papillae on dorsal surface of the tongue.
Furcation (fer-**key**-shuhn) Area between two or more root branches before division from root trunk.
Furcation crotches Spaces between roots at furcation.
Fusion (**fyoo**-zhunh) Joining of embryonic tissue of two separate surfaces, elimination of furrow between two adjacent swellings or developmental disturbance in which adjacent tooth germs unite to form large tooth.

G

Ganglion (plural, **ganglia**) (**gang**-glee-uhn, **gang**-glee-uh) Aggregation of neuron cell bodies outside central nervous system.
Gemination (jem-uh-**ney**-shuhn) Developmental disturbance with single tooth germ trying to divide forming large single-rooted tooth.
Generalized resorption (ri-**sawrp**-shuhn) Resorption of hard tissue or entire skeleton

of bone in varying amounts resulting from endocrine activity.

Geographic tongue Lesion that appears as red and then paler pink to white patches on the tongue body.

Germinal center (jur-muh-nl) Center region of lymphatic nodule of lymph node where lymphocytes mature.

Gingiva (plural, **gingivae**) (jin-**jahy**-vuh, jin-**juh**-vee) Gingival tissue composed of mucosa surrounding maxillary and mandibular teeth while covering alveolar processes.

Gingival apex of the contour (jin-**juh**-vuhl) Cervical peak of individual gingival contour.

Gingival biotype (bahy-uh-tahyp) Thickness of gingiva in faciolingual dimension.

Gingival crevicular fluid (GCF) (krey-**vik**-yoo-ler) Fluid in gingival sulcus.

Gingival fiber group Fiber groups within gingiva that have no bony attachments.

Gingival hyperplasia (hahy-per-**pley**-zhuh) Overgrowth of mainly interproximal gingiva.

Gingival recession (ri-**sesh**-uhn) Inferiorly placed margin of free gingival crest.

Gingival sulcus (suhl-kuhs) Space facing sulcular gingiva.

Gingivitis (jin-juh-**vahy**-tis) Periodontal disease of gingival tissue.

Gland Structure that produces secretion necessary for body functioning.

Globular dentin (glob-yuh-ler) Dentin with both primary and secondary mineralization.

Gnathic index (nath-ick) Measurement that gives degree of maxillary arch prominence.

Goblet cells (gob-lit) Cells in respiratory mucosa that produce mucus for moisture.

Goiter (goi-ter) Enlarged thyroid.

Golden Proportions Principle that provides guide for esthetically pleasing proportion.

Golgi complex (gawl-jee) Organelle of cell involved in protein segregation, packaging, transport.

Granular layer Layer superficial to prickle layer in some forms of keratinized epithelium.

Granulation tissue (gran-yuh-**ley**-shuhn) Immature connective tissue formed during initial repair.

Group function Entire posterior quadrant functions during lateral occlusion.

Gubernacular canal (GC) (goo-ber-**nak**-yuh-lahr) Tunnel with fibrous cord connected to dental sac containing remnants of dental lamina.

Guided tissue regeneration (GTR) (ri-jen-uh-**rey**-shuhn) Surgical procedures that utilize barrier membranes to direct growth of new bone and soft tissue at sites.

H

Hard palate (pal-it) Anterior part of palate.

Haversian canal (huh-**vur**-zuhn) Vascular tissue space in osteon.

Haversian system Organized arrangement of lamellae and canals in compact bone.

Height of contour Crest of curvature that is greatest elevation of tooth crown either incisocervically or occlusocervically.

Hemidesmosome (hem-eye-**dez**-moh-sohm) Forms intercellular junction involving attachment of cell to nearby noncellular surface.

Hertwig epithelial root sheath (HERS) (**hurt**-wig) Part of cervical loop that functions to shape the root(s) and induce root dentin formation.

Hilus (hih-luhs) Depression on one side of lymph node.

Hindgut (haynd-guht) Posterior part of future digestive tract.

Histodifferentiation (his-toh-dif-er-en-shee-**ay**-shuhn) Development of different tissue types.

Histology (hi-**stol**-uh-jee) Study of microscopic structure and function of tissue.

Horizontal group Alveodental ligament subgroup originating in alveolar bone proper to insert horizontally into cementum.

Howship lacuna (how-ship luh-**kyoo**-nuh) Large shallow pit in bone created by osteoclast.

Hunter-Schreger bands (HSB) (**hun**-ter-**shray**-ger) Alternating light to dark lines noted in certain sections of enamel using reflected rather than transmitted light.

Hutchinson incisors (huhch-in-suhn in-**sahy**-zers) Developmental disturbance in permanent incisors with screwdriver-shaped crowns caused by congenital syphilis.

Hyaline cartilage (hahy-uh-lin **kahr**-ti-lij) Cartilage that contains no nerves or blood vessels and serves as growth center in temporomandibular joint.

Hyoid arch(es) (**hahy**-oid) Second branchial or pharyngeal arch(es) that lies inferiorly to mandibular arch(es) in embryo.

Hyoid bone Bone suspended in anterior midline of neck that has many muscle attachments.

Hypercementosis (hahy-per-si-mehn-**toh**-sis) Excessive production of cellular cementum.

Hyperkeratinization (hahy-per-ker-uh-tn-ah-**zey**-shuhn) Excessive production of keratin.

Hypoblast layer (hahy-puh-blast) Inferior layer in bilaminar disc.

Hypodermis (hahy-puh-**dur**-mis) Deeper to dermis.

Hyposalivation (hahy-puh-sal-uh-**vey**-shuhn) Decreased production of saliva.

I

Imbrication lines (im-bri-**key**-shuhn) Slight ridges that extend mesiodistally in cervical third associated with lines of Retzius in enamel.

Imbrication lines of von Ebner (von eb-ner) Incremental lines in mature dentin.

Immunogen (ih-**myoo**-nuh-juhn) Antigen treated as foreign capable of triggering immune response.

Immunoglobulin (Ig) (im-yuh-noh-**glob**-yuh-lin) Blood protein or antibody produced by plasma cells during immune response.

Impacted (im-**pak**-ted) Unerupted or partially erupted tooth positioned against another tooth, bone, soft tissue preventing eruption.

Implantation (im-plan-**tey**-shuhn) Embedding of blastocyst in endometrium.

Incisal angles (in-**sahy**-zuhl) Two angles on permanent incisors formed from incisal ridge or edge and each proximal surface.

Incisal edge Flattened incisal ridge on permanent incisors due to attrition after eruption.

Incisal ridge Linear elevation on incisal or masticatory surface of incisors when newly erupted.

Incisal surface Masticatory surface for anteriors.

Incisive papilla (in-**sahy**-ziv puh-**pil**-uh) Small bulge of tissue at anterior hard palate.

Incisors (in-**sahy**-zuhrz) First and second anteriors from midline, centrals and laterals.

Inclined cuspal planes (kuhsp-uhl) Sloping planes located between cusp ridges on posteriors.

Inclusions (in-**kloo**-zhuhz) Metabolically inert substances or transient structures within cell.

Induction (in-**dunk**-shuhn) Action of one group of cells on another leading to developmental pathway in responding tissue.

Infraorbital region (in-fruh-**awr**-bi-tl) Facial region located both inferior to orbital region and lateral to nasal region.

Initiation stage First stage of tooth development.

Inner enamel epithelium (IEE) (ih-**nam**-uhl ep-uh-**thee**-lee-um) Innermost cells of enamel organ that form ameloblasts.

Intercalated duct (in-**tur**-kuh-ley-ted) Duct associated with acinus or terminal part of salivary gland.

Intercellular junctions (in-ter-**sel**-yuh-ler) Mechanical attachments between cells or between cells and nearby noncellular surfaces.

Intercellular substance Transparent substance that fills in spaces between tissue cells.

Interdental gingiva (in-ter-**den**-tl jin-**jahy**-vuh) Gingival tissue between adjacent teeth adjoining attached gingiva.

Interdental ligament Principal fiber subgroup that inserts interdentally into cervical cementum of neighboring teeth.

Interdental papilla (plural, **papillae**) (puh-**pil**-uh, puh-**pil**-ee) Extension(s) of interdental gingiva between adjacent teeth adjoining attached gingiva.

Interdental septum Alveolar process between two neighboring teeth.

Interglobular dentin (in-ter-**glob**-you-ler) Dentin with only primary mineralization.

Interlabial gap (in-ter-**ley**-bee-uhl) Distance between inferior border of upper lip and superior border of lower lip when at physiologic resting position.

Intermaxillary segment (in-ter-**mak**-suh-ler-ee) Growth from paired medial nasal processes on inside of stomodeum.

Intermediate filaments (fil-uh-muhnts) Components of cytoskeleton.

Intermediate layer Layer of epithelium superficial to basal layer in nonkeratinized epithelium.

Internal basal lamina (bey-suhl **lam**-uh-nah) Basal lamina that is part of epithelial attachment to tooth surface.

International Numbering System (INS) International system for tooth designation (also quadrants) using two-digit code.

Interocclusal clearance (in-ter-uh-**kloo**-zhul) Space between dental arches when mandible is at rest.

Interphase (**in**-ter-feyz) Period when cell is between divisions but is growing and functioning.

Interproximal space (in-ter-**prok**-suh-muhl) Area between adjacent tooth surfaces.

Interradicular group (in-ter-**ra**-dik-you-ler) Alveolodental ligament subgroup on multirooted teeth inserted on cementum of one root to cementum of other root(s).

Interradicular septum Alveolar process between roots of same tooth.

Interrod enamel (ih-**nam**-uhl) Outer enamel surrounding each enamel rod core creating an interprismatic region.

Interstitial growth (in-ter-**stish**-uhl) Growth from deep within tissue or organ.

Intertubular dentin (in-ter-**too**-byuh-ler) Dentin between dentinal tubules.

Intramembranous ossification (in-trah-**mem**-bruh-nuhs os-uh-fi-**key**-shuhn) Formation of osteoid within dense connective tissue.

J

Joint capsule Two-layered connective tissue that completely encloses temporomandibular joint.

Joint disc Disc of temporomandibular joint located between temporal bone and mandibular condyle.

Junctional epithelium (JE) (**juhngk**-shuhn-uhl ep-uh-**thee**-lee-um) Deeper extension of sulcular epithelium.

K

Karyotype (**kar**-ee-uh-tahyp) Photographic analysis of chromosomes.

Keratin (**ker**-uh-tin) Intermediate protein filament found in calloused epithelium consisting of opaque waterproof substance.

Keratin layer Most superficial layer in keratinized epithelium.

Keratinocytes (ker-**raht**-uh-sahytz) Epithelial cells in oral mucosa produce keratin.

Keratohyaline granules (ker-uh-toh-**hyah**-uh-lin) Prominent granules in cytoplasm of epithelial cells that form keratin chemical precursor.

L

Labial (**ley**-bee-uhl) Structures or facial surface of teeth close to lips.

Labial commissure (**kom**-uh-shoor) Corner of mouth where upper and lower lips meet.

Labial frenum (plural, **frena**) (**free**-nuhm, **free**-nuh) Fold(s) of tissue located at midline between labial mucosa and alveolar mucosa on dental arch(es).

Labial mucosa (myoo-**koh**-suh) Mucosal lining of inner parts of lips.

Labial ridge Central ridge on labial surface of canines from greater development of middle labial developmental lobe.

Lacuna (plural, **lacunae**) (luh-**kyoo**-nuh, luh-**kyoo**-nee) Small space(s) that surrounds chondrocyte or osteocyte within cartilage matrix or bone.

Lamellae (luh-**mel**-ee) Closely apposed sheets of bone tissue in compact bone.

Lamina densa (**lam**-uh-nah **den**-suh) Dense layer of basal lamina closer to connective tissue.

Lamina dura (**door**-uh) Radiopaque line representing alveolar bone proper.

Lamina lucida (**loo**-si-duh) Clear layer of basal lamina closer to epithelium.

Lamina propria (**proh**-pree-uh) Connective tissue proper region of oral mucosa.

Laryngopharynx (luh-ring-goh-**far**-ingks) Most inferior part of pharynx close to laryngeal opening.

Larynx (**lar**-ingks) Voice box in midline of neck.

Lateral deviation of the mandible (**man**-duh-buhl) Shifting lower jaw to one side.

Lateral lingual swellings Parts of developing tongue that form on each side of tuberculum impar.

Lateral nasal process(es) Tissue on outer part of nasal pits that forms nasal alae.

Lateral occlusion (uh-**kloo**-zhuhn) Movement that occurs when mandible moves to one side until canines are in cusp-to-cusp relationship.

Lateral surface of the tongue Side of tongue.

Leeway space Space created when primary molars are shed to make room for smaller mesiodistal permanent premolars.

Lens placodes (**plak**-ohdz) Placodes forming eyes and related tissue.

Leukocyte (**loo**-kuh-sahyt) Another term for white blood cell.

Line angle Line formed by junction of two crown surfaces.

Linea alba (**lin**-ee-uh **ahl**-buh) White ridge of keratinized epithelium on buccal mucosa at level where teeth occlude.

Lines of Retzius (ret-**zee**-us) Incremental lines in mature enamel.

Lingual (**ling**-gwuhl) Structures or tooth surface closest to tongue.

Lingual frenum (**free**-nuhm) Midline fold of tissue between ventral surface of tongue and floor of the mouth.

Lingual papillae (puh-**pil**-ee) Small elevated structures of specialized mucosa on tongue.

Lingual ridge Vertically oriented and centrally placed ridge that extends from cusp tip to cingulum on lingual surface of canines.

Lingual tonsil (**ton**-suhl) Irregular mass of tonsillar tissue located posteriorly on dorsal surface of tongue.

Lining mucosa (myoo-**koh**-suh) Mucosa associated with nonkeratinized stratified squamous epithelium.

Lip incompetence Open mouth with lips apart at resting posture.

Lobes Large inner parts of glands or regions of tooth during development.

Lobules (**lob**-yoolz) Smaller inner parts of glands.

Localized resorption (ri-**sawrp**-shuhn) Resorption of bone or other hard tissue that occurs in specific area.

Loose connective tissue Superficial layer of dermis of the skin or lamina propria of oral mucosa.

Lumen (**loo**-muhn) Central opening where saliva is deposited into duct after production by secretory cells.

Lymph (**limf**) Tissue fluid that drains from surrounding region into lymphatic vessels.

Lymphadenopathy (lim-fad-n-**op**-uh-thee) Enlarged and palpable lymph nodes.

Lymphatic(s) (lim-**fat**-ik[s]) Network of lymphatic vessels that collect and transport lymph linking lymph nodes.

Lymphatic ducts Ducts that smaller lymphatic vessels containing lymph converge into and then empty into venous system.

Lymphatic nodules (**naj**-oolz) Masses of lymphocytes in lymph node.

Lymphatic vessels System of endothelium-lined channels that carry lymph.

Lymph nodes Bean-shaped filtering bodies grouped in clusters along connecting lymphatic vessels.

Lymphocyte (**lim**-fuh-sahyt) Second most common white blood cell in blood involved in immune response.

Lysosomes (**lahy**-suh-sohmz) Organelles of cell functioning in both intracellular and extracellular digestion.

M

Macrodontia (mak-ruh-**don**-shuh) Abnormally large teeth.

Macrophage (**mak**-ruh-feyj) Most common white blood cell in connective tissue proper or *monocyte* before migration from blood.

Major salivary glands (**sal**-uh-ver-ee) Large paired glands that have named associated ducts.

Malocclusion (mal-uh-**kloo**-zhuhn) Failure to have overall ideal form to dentition while in centric occlusion.

Mamelons (**mam**-uh-lons) Rounded enamel extensions on incisal ridge of anteriors.

Mandible (**man**-duh-buhl) Lower jaw.

Mandibular arch(es) (man-**dib**-yuh-ler) Lower dental arch(es) with mandibular teeth or first branchial or pharyngeal arch(es) in embryo.

Mandibular condyle (**kon**-dahyl) Bony projection off posterior and superior border of mandibular ramus.

Mandibular notch Depression between coronoid process and condyle.

Mandibular processes Processes of first branchial or pharyngeal arches that fuse at midline to form mandibular arch.

Mandibular ramus (plural, **rami**) (**rey**-muhs, **rey**-mahy) Mandibular plate(s) that extend(s) upward and backward from body on each side.

Mandibular symphysis (**sim**-fuh-sis) Midline area of mandible marking fusion of two mandibular processes.

Mandibular teeth Teeth in mandibular arch of lower jaw or mandible.

Mandibular torus (plural, **tori**) (**tohr**-uhs, **tohr**-ahy) Bone growth(s) noted on lingual aspect(s) of mandibular arch.

Mantle bundles Fasciculi located near outer surface of nerve.

Mantle dentin Outermost layer of dentin found in crown region adjacent to dentinoenamel junction.

Marginal gingiva (**mahr**-juh-nahl jin-**jahy**-vuh) Gingiva at gingival margin of each tooth.
Marginal grooves Developmental grooves that cross either marginal ridge.
Marginal ridges Rounded raised borders on mesial and distal parts of lingual surface of anteriors or occlusal table of posteriors.
Masseter muscle (mas-**seh**-ter,mas-**see**-ter) Powerful bilateral muscle of mastication.
Mast cell White blood cell similar to basophil due to involvement in allergic responses.
Mastication (mas-ti-**keyt**-shuhn) Chewing process.
Masticatory mucosa (mass-ti-**keyt**-tor-ee myoo-**koh**-suh) Mucosa associated with keratinized stratified squamous epithelium.
Masticatory surface Chewing tooth surface on crown.
Matrix (plural, **matrices**) (**mey**-triks, **mey**-tri-seez) Extracellular substance or surrounding medium; in connective tissue composed of intercellular substance and fibers; or one that is partially mineralized and serves as framework for later mineralization for hard dental tissue.
Maturation (mach-uh-**rey**-shuhn) Attainment of adult size as well as adult form and function.
Maturation stage Final stage of odontogenesis when matrices of hard dental tissue types fully mineralize.
Maxilla (mak-**sil**-uh) Upper jaw.
Maxillary arch (**mak**-suh-ler-ee) Upper dental arch with maxillary teeth.
Maxillary process Prominence from mandibular arch that grows superiorly and anteriorly on each side of stomodeum.
Maxillary sinus (**sahy**-nuhs) Paranasal sinus within maxilla.
Maxillary teeth Teeth in maxillary arch or maxilla or upper jaw.
Maxillary tuberosity (too-buh-**ros**-i-tee) Tissue-covered bony elevation just distal to last tooth of maxillary arch.
Maximum mouth opening (**MMO**) Greatest amount of interincisal opening of mouth.
Meckel cartilage (**mek**-uhl **kahr**-ti-lij) Cartilage that forms within each side of mandibular arch(es) and that disappears as bony mandible forms.
Medial nasal process(es) (**mee**-dee-uhl) Middle part of tissue growing around nasal placodes located between two nasal pits.
Median lingual sulcus (**mee**-dee-uhn **ling**-gwuhl **suhl**-kuhs) Midline depression on dorsal surface of the tongue.
Median palatine raphe (**pal**-uh-tahyn **rey**-fee) Midline ridge of tissue on palate that overlies bony fusion marked by median palatine suture.
Meiosis (mahy-**oh**-sis) Process of reproductive cell production that ensures correct number of chromosomes.
Melanin pigmentation (**mel**-uh-nin) Localized macules of pigmentation caused by presence of melanin.
Melanocytes (muh-**lan**-uh-sahtz) Cells that form pigment of melanin.
Melanosomes (muh-**lan**-uh-sohms) Cytoplasmic granules in melanocytes that store pigment.
Mental region (**men**-tl) Region of the face with chin as major feature.
Mesenchyme (**mez**-eng-kahym) Embryonic connective tissue.
Mesial (**mee**-zee-uhl) Surface of tooth closest to midline.
Mesial drift Natural movement of teeth over time toward midline of oral cavity.
Mesial step Terminal plane relationship with primary mandibular second molar is mesial to maxillary molar.
Mesiodens (**me**-zee-oh-denz) Supernumerary tooth between two permanent maxillary central incisors.
Mesoderm (**mez**-uh-durm) Embryonic layer located between ectoderm and endoderm.
Mesognathic (mez-uhg-**nath**-ik) Facial profile in centric occlusion with slightly protruded jaws with facial outline having relatively flat appearance or straight profile.
Metaphase (**met**-uh-feyz) Second phase of mitosis in which chromosomes are aligned into equatorial position.
Microdontia (mahy-kruh-**don**-shuh) Abnormally small teeth.
Microfibrils (mahy-kroh-**fahy**-bruhl) Even smaller subunits of fibrils within the collagen fibers.
Microfilaments (mahy-kruh-**fil**-uh-muhnts) Components of cytoskeleton that are delicate and threadlike.
Microplicae (**MPL**) (mahy-kroh-**plih**-kee) Ridgelike folds on surface of superficial cells of all types of oral epithelium.
Microtubules (mahy-kroh-**too**-byoolz) Components of cytoskeleton that are slender tubular microscopic structures.
Midgut (**mid**-guht) Middle part of future digestive tract.
Minor salivary glands (**sal**-uh-ver-ee) Small salivary glands with short unnamed ducts.
Mitochondria (mahy-tuh-**kon**-dree-uhn) Organelles associated with manufacture of energy for cell.
Mitosis (mahy-**toh**-sis) Cell division that occurs in phases and results in two daughter cells.
Mixed dentition (den-**tish**-uhn) Dentition with both primary and permanent teeth present.
Mixed dentition period Transitional stage involving dentition when both primary and permanent teeth are present.
Mobility Movement of tooth from loss of support by periodontium.
Molars (**moh**-lerz) Most posterior of teeth, firsts, seconds, thirds.
Monocyte (**mon**-uh-sahyt) White blood cell that becomes macrophage after migration from blood into tissue.
Morphodifferentiation (mawr-fuh-dif-uh-ren-shee-**ay**-shuhn) Development of differing form that creates specific structure.
Morphogenesis (mawr-fuh-**jen**-uh-sis) Process of development of specific tissue morphology.
Morphology (mawr-**fol**-uh-jee) Form of structure.
Mucobuccal fold (myoo-koh-**buhk**-uhl) Area within vestibule where labial mucosa or buccal mucosa meets alveolar mucosa.
Mucocele (**myoo**-koh-seel) Lesion due to retention of saliva in minor salivary gland.
Mucocutaneous junction (myoo-koh-kyoo-**tey**-nee-us) Transition zone at vermilion border outlining lips from surrounding skin.
Mucogingival junction (myoo-koh-**jin**-juh-vuhl) Line of demarcation between attached gingiva and alveolar mucosa.
Mucoperiosteum (myoo-koh-per-ee-**os**-tee-uhm) Combined structure consisting of mucous membrane involves epithelium and lamina propria of oral mucosa with periosteum of bone with oral cavity.
Mucous acini (**myoo**-kuhs **as**-uh-nahy) Group of mucous cells producing mucous secretory product.
Mucous cells Secretory cells that produce mucous secretory product.
Mulberry molars (**muhl**-ber-ee **moh**-lerz) Developmental disturbance resulting from congenital syphilis forming enamel nodules on molars' occlusal surface.
Multirooted Teeth with two or more root branches.
Muscle Fibrous tissue bundle that can contract to produce movement in or maintaining position of parts of body.
Muscles of mastication (mas-ti-**key**-shuhn) Muscles involved in mastication, masseter, temporalis, with medial/lateral pterygoid.
Myelin sheath (**mahy**-uh-lin) Cover for certain axons.
Myoepithelial cells (mahy-oh-ep-uh-**thee**-lee-uhl) Contractile epithelial cells on acini that facilitate flow of saliva out of each lumen into connecting ducts.
Myofibers (mahy-uh-**fahy**-berz) Muscle cells that compose the fascicles.
Myofibrils (**mahy**-uh-fahy-bruhlz) Smaller subunits of myofibers.
Myofilaments (mahy-uh-**fil**-uh-muhntz) Even smaller subunits of myofibrils.

N

Naris (plural, **nares**) (**nair**-is, **nair**-eez) Nostril(s) of nose.
Nasal cavity (**ney**-zuhl) Inner space of nose.
Nasal conchae (**kong**-kee) Projecting structures that extend inward from each lateral wall of nasal cavity.
Nasal pits Depressions in center of each nasal placode that evolve into nasal cavities.
Nasal placodes (**plak**-ohdz) Placodes that develop into olfactory organ for sensation of smell located in mature nose.
Nasal region Region of the face occupied by external nose.
Nasal septum (**sep**-tuhm) Midline part of nose that separates nares.

Nasmyth membrane (**nas**-mith) Residue on newly erupted teeth that may become extrinsically stained.

Nasopharynx (ney-zoh-**far**-ingks) Division of pharynx superior to level of soft palate.

Natural killer (**NK**) **cell** Large lymphocyte involved in first line of defense.

Neonatal line (nee-oh-**neyt**-l) Accentuated incremental line of Retzius in enamel or contour line of Owen in dentin from birth process.

Nerve Bundle of neural processes outside central nervous system.

Neural crest cells (**NCCs**) (**noor**-uhl) Specialized group of cells developed from neuroectoderm that migrate from crests of neural folds and disperse to specific sites within mesenchyme.

Neural folds Raised ridges in neural plate that surround deepening neural groove.

Neural groove Groove from further growth and thickening of neural plate.

Neural plate Centralized band of cells that extends length of embryo.

Neural tube Tube formed when neural folds meet and fuse superior to neural groove.

Neuroectoderm (noor-oh-**ek**-toh-durm) Specialized group of cells that differentiates from ectoderm.

Neuron (**noor**-on) Functional cellular component of nervous system.

Neutrophil (**noo**-truh-fil) Another term for polymorphonuclear leukocyte.

Nicotinic stomatitis (nik-uh-**tin**-ik stoh-muh-**tahy**-tis) Whitish lesion on hard palate caused by heat from smoking or hot liquid consumption.

Non cavitated lesion (nohn-kav-i-**tey**-ted) Initial or incipient caries lesion development before cavitation occurs.

Non invasive prenatal testing (**NIPT**) Prenatal genetic test that involves a simple blood draw from the pregnant women.

Nonkeratinized stratified squamous epithelium (nohn-**ker**-uh-tn-izd **strat**-uh-fahyd **skwey**-muhs ep-uh-**thee**-lee-um) Epithelium in superficial layers of lining mucosa.

Nonkeratinocytes (nohn-ker-**raht**-tn-uh-sahytz) Cells in oral mucosa that do not produce keratin in epithelium.

Nonsuccedaneous (nohn-suhk-si-**dey**-nee-us) Permanent teeth without primary predecessors or molars.

Nuclear envelope (**noo**-klee-er) Double membrane completely surrounding nucleus.

Nuclear pores Avenues of communication between inner nucleoplasm and outer cytoplasm.

Nucleolus (noo-**klee**-uh-luhs) Rounded nuclear organelle centrally placed in nucleoplasm.

Nucleoplasm (**noo**-klee-uh-plaz-uhm) Semifluid part within nucleus.

Nucleus (plural, **nuclei**) (**noo**-klee-uhs, **noo**-klee-ahy) Largest, densest, most conspicuous organelle(s) in cell.

O

Oblique group (oh-**bleek**) Alveolodental ligament subgroup originating in alveolar bone proper to extend apically and obliquely to insert into cementum.

Oblique ridge Transverse ridge that crosses occlusal table obliquely from mesiolingual to distobuccal on most maxillary molars.

Occlusal pits (uh-**kloo**-zuhl) Sharp pinpoint depression in fossae on occlusal table of posteriors.

Occlusal plane Imaginary curved plane formed by incisal edges of anteriors and the occlusal surfaces of posteriors.

Occlusal surface Masticatory surface of posteriors.

Occlusal table Part of occlusal surface of posteriors bordered by marginal ridges.

Occlusal trauma Trauma to periodontium from occlusal disharmony.

Occlusion (uh-**kloo**-zhuhn) Anatomic alignment of teeth and relationship to masticatory system.

Odontoblastic process (oh-**don**-tuh-blast-ik) Attached cellular extension of odontoblast within dentinal tubule.

Odontoblasts (oh-**don**-tuh-blastz) Cells that produce dentin and differentiate from outer cells of the dental papilla.

Odontoclasts (oh-**don**-tuh-klastz) Cells that resorb dentin, cementum, enamel.

Odontogenesis (oh-don-tuh-**jen**-uh-sis) Process of tooth development.

Odontoma (oh-don-**toh**-mah) Benign neoplasm of odontogenic origin.

Olfactory mucosa (ol-**fak**-tuh-ree myoo-**koh**-suh) Mucosa in roof of each part of nasal cavity that carries sense of smell receptors.

Open bite Malocclusion due to anteriors of both dental arches not occluding.

Oral cavity proper Inside of mouth.

Oral epithelium (ep-uh-**thee**-lee-um) Embryonic lining of oral cavity derived from ectoderm.

Oral mucosa (myoo-**koh**-suh) Mucosa or mucous membrane lining oral cavity.

Oral region Region of face that contains lips and oral cavity.

Orbit (**awr**-bit) Bony socket that contains eyeball.

Orbital region (**awr**-bi-tl) Facial region that includes bony orbit and eyeball.

Organ Somewhat independent body part formed from tissue that performs specific function or functions.

Organelles (awr-guh-**nels**) Specialized structures within cell that are permanent and metabolically active.

Orofacial myofunctional disorder (**OMD**) (ohr-oh-**fehy**-shuhl mahy-oh-**fuhngk**-shuh-nl) Behaviors and patterns created by inappropriate muscle function and incorrect habits involving tongue, lips, jaws, face.

Orofacial myofunctional therapy (**OMT**) Variety of exercises are involved based on individual evaluation and treatment protocols to eliminate orofacial myofunctional disorders.

Orofacial myology (**OM**) (mahy-**ol**-uh-jee) Discipline that evaluates and treats variety of orofacial muscle postural and functional disorders as well as habit patterns.

Oronasal membrane (ohr-oh-**ney**-zuhl) Embryonic membrane that disintegrates to bring nasal and oral cavities into communication.

Oropharyngeal membrane (ohr-oh-fuh-**rin**-jeez-uhl) Membrane at cephalic end of embryo.

Oropharynx (ohr-oh-**far**-ingks) Oral division of pharynx.

Orthokeratinized stratified squamous epithelium (ohr-thoh-**ker**-uh-tn-izd **strat**-uh-fahyd **skwey**-muhs ep-uh-**thee**-lee-um) Epithelium that demonstrates keratinization of epithelial cells.

Ossification (os-uh-fi-**key**-shun) Bone formation.

Osteoblasts (**os**-tee-uh-blastz) Bone-forming cells.

Osteoclast (**os**-tee-uh-klast) Cell that functions in resorption of bone.

Osteocytes (**os**-tee-uh-sahytz) Mature osteoblasts entrapped in bone matrix.

Osteoid (**os**-tee-oid) Initially formed bone matrix.

Osteons (**os**-tee-onz) Concentric layers of lamellae in compact bone.

Otic placodes (**oh**-tik **plak**-ohdz) Placodes in embryo forming future internal ear.

Outer cells of the dental papilla (puh-**pil**-uh) Cells of dental papilla tissue that differentiate into odontoblasts.

Outer enamel epithelium (**OEE**) (ih-**nam**-uhl ep-uh-**thee**-lee-um) Outer cells of enamel organ that serve as protective barrier.

Overbite Maxillary arch vertically overlaps mandibular arch.

Overeruption Physiologic movement of tooth or super-eruption from lacking opposing partner.

Overjet Maxillary arch horizontally overlaps mandibular arch.

Ovum (**oh**-vuhm) Female reproductive cell or egg that can be fertilized.

P

Palatal (**pal**-uh-tl) Lingual structures or tooth surface closest to palate.

Palatal shelves Two processes derived from maxillary processes during prenatal development.

Palatal torus (**tohr**-uhs) Normal variation of bone growth noted on midline of hard palate.

Palate (**pal**-it) Roof of mouth.

Palatine rugae (**pal**-uh-tahyn **roo**-gee/jee) Firm irregular ridges of tissue directly posterior to incisive papilla.

Palatine tonsils (**ton**-suhlsz) Tonsillar tissue located between faucial pillars.

Palmer Notation Method System of tooth designation commonly used in orthodontics; when oral cavity is divided into quadrants and each tooth is designated by a numeral 1 to 8.

Papillary layer (**pap**-uh-ler-ee) Layer of loose connective tissue of dermis or lamina propria.

Parafunctional habits (pahr-uh-**fuhngk**-shun-uhl) Mandibular movements not within motions associated with mastication, speech, respiration.

Parakeratinized stratified squamous epithelium (pahr-uh-**ker**-uh-tn-izd **strat**-uh-fahyd **skwey**-muhs ep-uh-**thee**-lee-um) Keratinized epithelium associated with masticatory mucosa of attached gingiva.

Paranasal sinuses (pahr-uh-**ney**-zuhl **sahy**-nuhs-ez) Paired air-filled cavities in bone.

Parathyroid glands (pahr-uh-**thahy**-roid) Endocrine glands along posterior aspects of thyroid.

Parotid duct (puh-**rot**-id) Duct associated with parotid.

Parotid papilla (puh-**pil**-uh) Small elevation of tissue on inner part of buccal mucosa that protects parotid duct.

Parotid salivary gland (**sal**-uh-ver-ee) Major salivary gland located from zygomatic arch to posterior border of mandible.

Passive eruption Eruption that takes place when gingiva recedes with no actual tooth movement.

Peg lateral Lateral incisor crown that is smaller from partial microdontia.

Peg molars (**moh**-lerz) Microdontia usually of third molar.

Perichondrium (per-i-**kon**-dree-uhm) Outermost connective tissue layer surrounding most cartilage.

Perikymata (per-i-**key**-maht-uh) Grooves evident on teeth associated with lines of Retzius in enamel.

Periodontal disease (per-ee-oh-**don**-tl) Inflammatory disease that affects soft and hard structures that support teeth.

Periodontal ligament (PDL) Ligament surrounding teeth that supports and attaches them to alveoli bony surface.

Periodontal ligament (PDL) space Radiolucent area representing periodontal ligament on radiographs.

Periodontal pocket Deepened gingival sulcus from periodontitis that is lined by pocket epithelium.

Periodontitis (per-ee-oh-don-**tahy**-tis) Periodontal disease involving periodontium.

Periodontium (per-ee-oh-**don**-shuhm) Supporting hard and soft dental tissue between and including parts of tooth and alveolar process.

Periosteum (per-ee-**os**-tee-uhm) Dense connective tissue layer on outer part of bone.

Peritubular dentin (per-ee-**too**-byuh-ler) Dentin that creates wall of dentinal tubule.

Permanent dentition (den-**tish**-uhn) Second and final dentition with all permanent teeth or adult teeth present; also called *permanent teeth*.

Permanent dentition period Final stage in dentition formation with all permanent teeth present.

Permanent teeth *See* Permanent dentition.

Phagocytosis (fag-uh-sahy-**toh**-sis) Engulfing and then digesting of solid waste or foreign material by cell.

Pharyngeal pouches (fuh-**rin**-jee-uhl) Four pairs of evaginations lining pharynx between branchial or pharyngeal arches.

Pharyngeal tonsils (**ton**-suhlz) Located on superior and posterior walls of nasopharynx.

Pharynx (**far**-ingks) Muscular tube of neck or throat.

Philtrum (**fil**-truhm) Vertical groove on midline of upper lip.

Pit and groove patterns Patterns formed from pits and grooves on lingual surface of permanent anteriors or occlusal surface of permanent posteriors.

Placenta (pluh-**sen**-tuh) Temporary prenatal organ that provides support to developing embryo.

Plasma (**plaz**-muh) Fluid substance in blood vessels that carries blood cells and metabolites.

Plasma cells White blood cells derived from B cell lymphocytes to form immunoglobulins or antibodies.

Platelet-rich plasma (PRP) (**pleyt**-lit) Autologous conditioned plasma derived from whole blood centrifuged to remove red blood cells.

Platelets Blood cell fragments functioning in clotting mechanism.

Plica fimbriata (plural, **plicae fimbriatae**) (**plahy**-kuh fim-bree-**ahy**-tuh, **plahy**-kee fim-bree-**ahy**-tee) Fold(s) with fringelike projections on ventral surface of the tongue.

Plunging cusps Opposing cusps allow areas of food impaction resulting in trauma to gingivosulcular area.

Pocket epithelium (PE) (ep-uh-**thee**-lee-um) Epithelium lining periodontal pocket.

Point angle Imaginary line formed by junction of three crown surfaces.

Polymorphonuclear (PMN) leukocyte (pol-ee-mawr-fuh-**noo**-klee-er **loo**-kuh-sahyt) Most common white blood cell involved in inflammatory response; also called *neutrophil*.

Posterior faucial pillar (**faw**-shuhl) Posterior lateral folds of tissue in pharynx created by underlying muscle forming structure of fauces.

Posterior teeth Molars (and premolars if present) in back of mouth.

Postglenoid process (post-**glen**-oid) Sharp ridge posterior to articular fossa.

Preameloblasts (pree-**am**-uh-loh-blastz) Cells from inner enamel epithelium of enamel organ that differentiate into ameloblasts.

Predentin Dentin matrix laid down by appositional growth by odontoblasts.

Preimplantation period (pree-im-plan-**tey**-shuhn) Period of unattached conceptus taking place during first week of prenatal development.

Premature contacts Situation in which one or two teeth initially contact before other teeth.

Premolars (pree-**moh**-luhrz) Fourth and fifth posterior teeth from midline in permanent dentition, including firsts and seconds or bicuspids.

Prenatal development (pree-**neyt**-l) Processes that occur from start of pregnancy to birth.

Prickle layer Layer that is superficial to basal layer in keratinized epithelium.

Primary bone First bone to be produced by either ossification method.

Primary dentin Dentin formed before completion of apical foramen.

Primary dentition (den-**tish**-uhn) First stage in dentition formation when all primary or deciduous teeth are present; also called *primary teeth*.

Primary dentition period Only primary teeth are present with this dentition.

Primary palate (**pal**-it) Anterior part of final palate derived from intermaxillary segment during prenatal development.

Primary teeth First teeth present or deciduous teeth; also called *primary dentition*.

Primate spaces Developmental spaces between primary teeth.

Primitive pharynx (**far**-ingks) Cranial part of foregut that forms oropharynx.

Primitive streak Furrowed rod-shaped thickening in middle of embryonic disc.

Primordium (prahy-**mawr**-dee-uhm) Earliest recognizable stage of development in an organ or tissue during prenatal development.

Principal fibers Collagen fibers organized into groups on basis of orientation to tooth and related function.

Prognathic (prog-**nath**-ik) Facial profile with rather prominent mandible and possibly usual or even retrusive maxilla or concave profile.

Proliferation (pruh-lif-uh-**rey**-shuhn) Controlled cellular growth such as that which occurs in prenatal development or tooth development.

Prophase (**proh**-feyz) First phase of mitosis with chromatin condensing into chromosomes.

Protrusion of the mandible (proh-**troo**-zhuhn) Moving lower jaw forward.

Protrusive occlusion (proh-**troo**-siv uh-**kloo**-zhuhn) Occlusion when mandible undergoes protrusion.

Proximal (**prok**-suh-muhl) Mesial and distal surface between adjacent teeth.

Pseudostratified columnar epithelium (soo-doh-**strat**-uh-fahyd) Simple epithelium that falsely appears as multiple cell layers.

Pterygomandibular fold (ter-i-goh-man-**dib**-yuh-ler) Tissue fold that extends from junction of hard and soft palates down to mandible.

Pulp Soft innermost connective tissue in both crown and root.

Pulp chamber Part of tooth containing mass of pulp.

Pulp horns Extensions of coronal pulp into cusps of posteriors.

Pulp recession Pulp cavity smaller by addition of secondary or tertiary dentin.

Pulp stones Masses of mineralized dentin in pulp.

Pulpitis (pul-**pahy**-tis) Inflammation of pulp.

Q

Quadrants (**kwod**-ruhnts) Division of each dental arch into two parts with four quadrants in oral cavity.

R

Radicular pulp (ra-**dik**-yuh-ler) Pulp located in root area of tooth.

Range of motion (ROM) Physiologic and functional reciprocal range of motion or movement for mandibular opening or closure.

Ranula (**ran**-yuh-luh) Lesion from retention of saliva usually in sublingual salivary gland.

Red blood cell (RBC) Blood cell whose cytoplasm contains hemoglobin that binds and then transports oxygen.

Reduced enamel epithelium (REE) (ih-**nam**-uhl ep-uh-**thee**-lee-um) Layers of flattened cells overlying enamel surface from compressed enamel organ.

Regeneration (ri-jen-uh-**rey**-shuhn) Renewal of a tissue and possibly even an organ.

Regions of the face Facial surface areas such as frontal, orbital, nasal, infraorbital, zygomatic, buccal, oral, mental.

Regions of the neck Areas that extend from skull and mandible inferior to clavicles and sternum.

Reichert cartilage (**ri**-kert **kahr**-ti-lij) Cartilage in second branchial or pharyngeal arch(es) that eventually disappears.
Remodeling Process by which bone is replaced over time.
Repolarization (re-poh-ler-uh-**zey**-shuhn) Process that occurs in cell with nucleus moving away from the center to a position farthest away from basement membrane.
Respiratory mucosa (**res**-per-uh-tawr-ee, **res**-per-uh-tohr-ee myoo-**koh**-suh) Mucosa that consists of pseudostratified ciliated columnar epithelium.
Resting posture Physiologic position of tongue, lips, mandible when not in function of chewing, swallowing, speech.
Retained sucking habit Parafunctional habit includes digit and pacifier use past age of 2.
Rete ridges (**ree**-tee) Interdigitation of epithelium into connective tissue.
Reticular connective tissue (reh-**tik**-yuh-ler) Delicate network of interwoven reticular fibers.
Reticular fibers Fibers in embryonic tissue.
Reticular lamina (**lam**-uh-nah) Deeper part of basement membrane.
Retraction of the mandible (reh-**trak**-shuhn) Moving lower jaw backward.
Retrognathic (reh-troh-**nath**-ik) Facial profile with protruding upper lip having recessive mandible and chin with convex profile.
Retromolar pad (reh-troh-**moh**-ler) Dense pad of tissue just distal to last tooth of mandibular arch.
Reversal lines Stained, scalloped microscopic lines caused by resorption in cartilage, bone, cementum.
Ribosomes (**rahy**-buh-sohms) Organelles of cell associated with protein production.
Ridges Linear elevations on masticatory surface of either anterior or posterior teeth.
Root(s) Part of a tooth composed of dentin covered by cementum.
Root axis line (RAL) Imaginary line representing long axis line of tooth drawn to bisect cervical line.
Root concavities Indentations on surface of root.
Root fusion Developmental disturbance that creates deep developmental grooves with root fusion.
Root of the nose Part of nose located between eyes.
Root trunk Root of multirooted teeth where root originates from crown.
Rubella (roo-**bell**-uh) Viral infection that can serve as teratogen transmitted by way of placenta to embryo.

S

Saliva (suh-**lahy**-vuh) Secretion from salivary glands that lubricates and cleanses oral cavity and helps in digestion.
Salivary glands (**sal**-uh-ver-ee) Glands that produce saliva.
Sclerotic dentin (skli-**rot**-ik) Type of tertiary dentin associated with chronic injury of caries, attrition, abrasion as well as aging tooth.
Second branchial (or pharyngeal) arch(es) (**brang**-kee-uhl/fuh-**rin**-jee-uhl) Branchial or pharyngeal arch(es) inferior to mandibular arch(es) in embryo or hyoid arch(es).
Secondary bone Mature bone tissue that replaces immature bone.
Secondary dentin Dentin that is formed after completion of apical foramen.
Secondary palate (**pal**-it) Posterior part of final palate formed by fusion of two palatal shelves.
Secretory cells (si-**kree**-tuh-ree) Epithelial cells that produce saliva.
Septum (plural, **septa**) (**sep**-tuhm, **sep**-tuh) Connective tissue divides inner part of glands.
Serous acini (**seer**-uhs **as**-uh-nahy) Group of serous cells producing serous secretory product.
Serous cells Secretory cells that produce serous secretory product.
Serous demilune (**dem**-i-loon) Serous cells superficial to mucous secretory cells in mucoserous acinus.
Sextants (**sek**-stuhnts) Dental arch division into three parts based on relationship to midline.
Sharpey fibers (**shar**-pee) Collagen fibers from periodontal ligament partially inserted into both cementum and bone.
Simple epithelium (ep-uh-**thee**-lee-um) Epithelium that consists of single layer of cells.
Sinusitis (sahy-nuh-**sahy**-tis) Inflamed mucosal tissue in paranasal sinus.
Sixth branchial (or pharyngeal) arch(es) (**brang**-kee-uhl/fuh-**rin**-jee-uhl) Branchial or pharyngeal arch(es) in embryo that fuses with fourth branchial or pharyngeal arch(es) to participate in formation of laryngeal cartilages.
Skeletal muscle Striated muscles under voluntary control of central and peripheral nervous systems.
Smear layer Production of adherent dental biofilm debris when cutting dentin during cavity preparation.
Soft palate (**pal**-it) Posterior part of palate.
Somites (**soh**-mahyts) Paired cuboidal aggregates of cells differentiated from mesoderm.
Specialized mucosa (myoo-**koh**-suh) Mucosa found on dorsal and lateral surface of tongue in the form of lingual papillae.
Sperm Cell containing male contribution of chromosomal information that fertilizes female ovum.
Spina bifida (**spahy**-nuh **bif**-i-duh) Neural tube defect affecting vertebral arches.
Squames (**skweymz**) Flattened platelike epithelial cells.
Stellate reticulum (**stel**-eyt ri-**tik**-yuh-luhm) Star-shaped cell layer between outer and inner enamel epithelium of enamel organ.
Sternocleidomastoid muscle (stur-noh-klahy-duh-**mas**-toid) Large strap muscle of neck.
Stippling Pinpoint depressions present on surface of attached gingiva.
Stomodeum (stoh-muh-**dee**-uhm) Primitive mouth in embryo.
Stratified epithelium (**strat**-uh-fahyd ep-uh-**thee**-lee-um) Epithelium consisting of two or more layers.
Stratified squamous epithelium (**skwey**-muhs) Epithelium of skin and oral mucosa.
Stratum intermedium (**strat**-uhm in-ter-**meed**-ee-uhm) Compressed layer between outer and inner enamel epithelium of enamel organ.
Striated duct (**strahy**-ey-tid) Larger duct connecting lobules of salivary gland.
Sublingual caruncle (sub-**ling**-gwuhl **kar**-uhng-uhl) Small papilla at anterior end of each sublingual fold.
Sublingual duct Short duct associated with sublingual gland.
Sublingual fold Ridge of tissue on each side of floor of the mouth.
Sublingual salivary gland (**sal**-uh-ver-ee) Major salivary gland located in neck at floor of mouth on each side.
Subluxation (sub-luhk-**say**-shuhn) Partial dislocation of both temporomandibular joints.
Submandibular duct (sub-man-**dib**-yuh-ler) Duct associated with submandibular gland.
Submandibular salivary gland (**sal**-uh-ver-ee) Major salivary gland located in neck at each side.
Submucosa (sub-myoo-**koh**-suh) Tissue deep to oral mucosa composed of loose connective tissue.
Succedaneous (suhk-si-**dey**-nee-us) Permanent teeth with primary predecessors, both anteriors and premolars.
Successional dental lamina (suhk-**sesh**-shuhn-uhl) Lingual extension of dental lamina into ectomesenchyme in relationship to primary tooth germs forming succedaneous permanent teeth.
Sulcular epithelium (SE) (**suhl**-kuh-ler ep-uh-**thee**-lee-um) Epithelium that stands away from tooth creating gingival sulcus.
Sulcus terminalis (**suhl**-kuhs tur-**muh**-nl-is) Groove located posteriorly on dorsal surface of the tongue surface.
Superficial layer Most superficial layer in nonkeratinized epithelium.
Supernumerary teeth (soo-per-**noo**-muh-rer-ee) Developmental disturbance characterized by one or more extra teeth.
Supplemental groove Secondary groove on lingual surface of anteriors and occlusal table on posteriors.
Supporting alveolar bone (SAB) Consists of both cortical bone and trabecular bone.
Supporting cusps (**kusps**) Cusps that function during centric occlusion that include lingual cusps of maxillary posteriors, buccal cusps of mandibular posteriors, incisal edges of mandibular anteriors.
Synapse (**sin**-aps) Junction between two neurons or between neuron and effector organ where neural impulses transmit.
Syndrome (**sin**-drohm) Group of specific signs and symptoms.
Synovial cavities (si-**noh**-vee-uhl) Upper and lower compartments divided by disc of temporomandibular joint.
Synovial fluid Fluid in joint capsule that fills and lubricates temporomandibular joint.
Synovial membrane Inner layer of temporomandibular joint capsule producing synovial fluid.

Syphilis (**sif**-uh-lis) Infective teratogen spirochete *Treponema pallidum* that can produce dental anomalies and other defects.

System Group of organs functioning together.

T

T cell Lymphocyte that matures in thymus working during cell-mediated immune response.

Talon cusp Sharp small extra cusp as projection from cingulum of incisor teeth.

Taste buds Barrel-shaped organs of taste associated with lingual papillae.

Taste pore Opening in taste bud.

Telophase (**tel**-uh-feyz) Final phase of mitosis with division into two daughter cells and reappearance of nuclear membrane.

Temporomandibular disorder (**TMD**) (tem-puh-roh-man-**dib**-yuh-ler) Disorder associated with one or both temporomandibular joints.

Temporomandibular joint (**TMJ**) Joint where temporal bone of skull articulates with mandible.

Teratogens (ter-**rat**-uh-juhns) Environmental agents or factors such as, infections, drugs, radiation causing malformations.

Terminal plane Ideal molar relationship in primary dentition when in centric occlusion.

Tertiary dentin Dentin formed in response to localized injury to exposed dentin.

Tetracycline stain (teh-truh-**sahy**-kleen) Intrinsic tooth stain from ingestion of antibiotic tetracycline during tooth development.

Third branchial (**or pharyngeal**) **arch**(**es**) (**brang**-kee-uhl/fuh-**rin**-jee-uhl) Branchial or pharyngeal arch(es) in embryo responsible for formation of parts of hyoid bone.

Thirds Crown surface or root division into three parts, crown horizontally and vertically and root horizontally.

Thrombocytes (**throm**-buh-sahyts) Another term for platelets.

Thyroglossal duct (thahy-roh-**gloss**-uhl) Temporary tube that connects thyroid with tongue base during prenatal development.

Thyroid cartilage (**thahy**-roid **kahr**-ti-lij) Midline prominence of larynx.

Thyroid gland Endocrine gland in neck.

Thyroxine (thahy-**rok**-sin) Hormone from thyroid gland that stimulates metabolic rate.

Tissue Structure formed by grouping of cells with similar characteristics of shape and function.

Tissue fluid Interstitial body fluid.

Tomes (**tomes**) **granular layer** Dentin beneath cementum and adjacent to dentinocemental junction that looks granular.

Tomes process Secretory surface of each ameloblast.

Tongue Oral cavity structure consisting of muscle and covered by oral mucosa.

Tongue thrust Incorrect patterning during tongue function resulting in parafunctional habit.

Tonofilaments (tohn-oh-**fil**-uh-muhnts) Intermediate filaments having major role in intercellular junctions.

Tonsillar tissue (**ton**-suh-ler) Nonencapsulated masses of lymphoid tissue.

Tooth fairy Mythological creature that takes children's shed primary teeth from under pillow and leaves sum of cash during night; helpers are always appreciated.

Tooth germ Primordium of tooth consisting of enamel organ, dental papilla, dental sac.

Trabeculae (truh-**bek**-yuh-lee) Joined matrix pieces forming lattice in cancellous bone or bands of connective tissue in lymph node that separate lymphatic nodules.

Trabecular bone (truh-**bek**-yuh-ler) Cancellous bone between alveolar bone proper and places of cortical bone.

Transverse ridge (tranz-**vurs**) Ridge formed by joining of two triangular ridges crossing occlusal table transversely or from labial to lingual outline.

Treacher Collins syndrome (**TCS**) (**tree**-chuhr **kol**-uh **sin**-drohm) Developmental disturbance with wide ranging implications due to migration failure of neural crest cells to facial region; also called *mandibulofacial dysostosis*.

Triangular fossa (**fos**-uh) Fossa that has triangular shape where triangular grooves terminate.

Triangular groove Groove that separates marginal ridge from triangular ridge of cusp and forms triangular fossae at termination of ridges.

Triangular ridge Cusp ridge that descends from cusp tips toward central part of occlusal table.

Trifurcated (trahy-**fuhr**-keyt-tuhd) Tooth having three root branches.

Trilaminar embryonic disc (trahy-**lam**-i-nahr em-bree-**on**-ik) Embryonic disc with three layers, ectoderm, mesoderm, endoderm.

Trismus (**triz**-muhs) Inability to open mouth.

Trophoblast layer (**trof**-oh-blast) Layer of peripheral cells of blastocyst.

Tubercle of the upper lip (**too**-ber-kuhl) Midline thickening of upper lip.

Tubercles Accessory cusps on cingulum of anteriors or occlusal tables of permanent molars.

Tuberculum impar (too-**ber**-kuh-luhm **im**-pahr) Initial part of developing tongue located in midline.

Turnover time Time that it takes for newly divided cells to be completely replaced throughout entire tissue.

U

Underbite When lower jaw extends forward beyond upper jaw.

Universal Numbering System (**UNS**) Numbering system for permanent teeth by using Arabic numerals #1 through #32 and for primary teeth by using capital letters *A* through *T*.

Uvula (**yoo**-vyuh-luh) Midline muscular structure hanging down from posterior margin of soft palate.

V

Vacuoles (**vak**-yoo-ohlz) Spaces or cavities within cytoplasm.

Velopharyngeal insufficiency (**VPI**) (vee-loh-fuh-**rin**-jee-uhl in-suh-**fish**-uhn-see) Failure of soft palate to close against posterior pharyngeal wall during speech.

Ventral surface of the tongue Underside of tongue.

Vermilion border (ver-**mil**-yuhn) Edge of vermilion zone.

Vermilion zone Darker appearance of lips with its outlining mucocutaneous junction at vermilion border as compared with surrounding skin.

Vertical dimension of the face Dividing face into three horizontal parts.

Vestibular fornix (ve-**stib**-yuh-ler **fawr**-niks) Deepest recess of each vestibule.

Vestibules (**ves**-tuh-byoolz) Maxillary and mandibular spaces between lips and cheeks anteriorly and laterally and also teeth and gingiva medially and posteriorly.

Volkmann canals (**fawlk**-mahn) Vascular canals in compact bone other than Haversian canals.

von Ebner salivary glands (**von eb**-nuhr **sal**-uh-ver-ee) Serous minor salivary glands associated with circumvallate lingual papillae.

W

Waldeyer tonsillar ring (val-**dahy**-er) Incomplete ring of tissue around the inner pharynx.

Wear facet With advancing attrition there is development of flat surface contact.

White blood cell (**WBC**) Blood cell from bone marrow's stem cells that matures there or in other lymphatic tissue.

Working side Side to which mandible has been moved during lateral occlusion.

X

Xerostomia (zeer-uh-**stoh**-mee-uh) Dry mouth.

Y

Yolk sac Fluid-filled cavity that faces hypoblast layer.

Z

Zygomatic arch (zahy-guh-**mat**-ik) Bony support for cheek.

Zygomatic region Facial region that overlies zygomatic arch.

Zygote (**zahy**-goht) Fertilized egg from union of ovum and sperm.

APPENDIX A

Anatomic Position

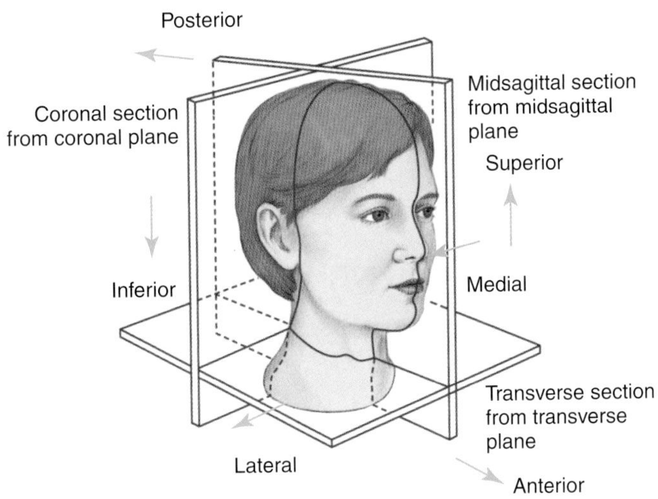

Fig. A.1 Head and Neck in Anatomic Position Showing the Midsagittal, Transverse, and Coronal Sections. (Modified from Fehrenbach MJ, Herring SW. *Illustrated Anatomy of the Head and Neck*. 5th ed. St. Louis: Elsevier; 2017.)

B APPENDIX

Units of Measure

Unit	Abbreviation	Equivalent	Measurement Application
Centimeter (**sen**-tuh-mee-ter)	cm	~0.4 inch	Naked eye: Pathologic lesions
Millimeter (**mil**-uh-mee-ter)	mm	0.1 cm	Naked eye: Extremely large body cells such as diameters of egg cell (or ovum) at 140 μm (or micrometers), largest fat cells (or adipocytes), and bone marrow cells producing blood platelets (or megakaryocytes); gingival sulcus; and periodontal pocket depth
Micrometer (previously known as micron)* (mahy-**kroh**-mee-ter)	μm	0.001 mm	Light microscopy: Most body cells, large organelles, bacteria, ameloblasts
Nanometer (**nan**-uh-mee-ter)	nm	0.001 μm	Electron microscopy: Smaller organelles, largest of macromolecules, dental tissue units

*Thickness of this paper is from 70 to 180 μm (or micrometers) and typical diameter of live body cell is 50 μm (or micrometers). In general, smallest objects the naked eye can see without aid of technology (includes microscope or other magnification device) are no smaller than 0.1 millimeters.

APPENDIX C

Tooth Measurements*

TABLE C.1 Measurements of the Permanent Incisors (in Millimeters)

	Cervicoincisal Length of Crown	Length of Root	Mesiodistal Diameter of Crown	Mesiodistal Diameter of Crown at Cervix	Labiolingual Diameter of Crown	Labiolingual Diameter of Crown at Cervix	Curvature of Cervical Line: Mesial	Curvature of Cervical Line: Distal
Maxillary central incisor	10.5	13.0	8.5	7.0	7.0	6.0	3.5	2.5
Maxillary lateral incisor	9.0	13.0	6.5	5.0	6.0	5.0	3.0	2.0
Mandibular central incisor	9.0	12.5	5.0	3.5	6.0	5.3	3.0	2.0
Mandibular lateral incisor	9.5	14.0	5.5	4.0	6.5	5.8	3.0	2.0

TABLE C.2 Measurements of the Permanent Canines (in Millimeters)

	Cervicoincisal Length of Crown	Length of Root	Mesiodistal Diameter of Crown	Mesiodistal Diameter of Crown at Cervix	Labiolingual Diameter of Crown	Labiolingual Diameter of Crown at Cervix	Curvature of Cervical Line: Mesial	Curvature of Cervical Line: Distal
Maxillary canine	10.0	17.0	7.5	5.5	8.0	7.0	2.5	1.5
Mandibular canine	11.0	16.0	7.0	5.5	7.5	7.0	2.5	1.0

TABLE C.3 Measurements of the Permanent Premolars (in Millimeters)

	Cervico-Occlusal Length of Crown	Length of Root	Mesiodistal Diameter of Crown	Mesiodistal Diameter of Crown at Cervix	Buccolingual Diameter of Crown	Buccolingual Diameter of Cervix	Curvature of Cervical Line: Mesial	Curvature of Cervical Line: Distal
Maxillary first premolar	8.5	14.0	7.0	5.0	9.0	8.0	1.0	0.0
Maxillary second premolar	8.5	14.0	7.0	5.0	9.0	8.0	1.0	0.0
Mandibular first premolar	8.5	14.0	7.0	5.0	7.5	6.5	1.0	0.0
Mandibular second premolar	8.0	14.5	7.0	5.0	8.0	7.0	1.0	0.0

*All data from Nelson S. *Wheeler's Dental Anatomy, Physiology, and Occlusion.* 10th ed. Philadelphia: Elsevier; 2015.

TABLE C.4 Measurements of the Permanent Maxillary Molars (in Millimeters)

	Cervico-Occlusal Length of Crown	Length of Root	Mesiodistal Diameter of Crown	Mesiodistal Diameter of Crown at Cervix	Buccolingual Diameter of Crown	Buccolingual Diameter at Cervix	Curvature of Cervical Line: Mesial	Curvature of Cervical Line: Distal
Maxillary first molar	7.5	Buccal = 12.0 Lingual = 13.0	10.0	8.0	11.0	10.0	1.0	0.0
Maxillary second molar	7.0	Buccal = 11.0 Lingual = 12.0	9.0	7.0	11.0	10.0	1.0	0.0
Maxillary third molar	6.5	11.0	8.5	6.5	10.0	9.5	1.0	0.0

TABLE C.5 Measurements of the Permanent Mandibular Molars (in Millimeters)

	Cervico-Occlusal Length of Crown	Length of Root	Mesiodistal Diameter of Crown	Mesiodistal Diameter of Crown at Cervix	Buccolingual Diameter of Crown	Buccolingual Diameter at Cervix	Curvature of Cervical Line: Mesial	Curvature of Cervical Line: Distal
Mandibular first molar	7.5	14.0	11.0	9.0	10.5	9.0	1.0	0.0
Mandibular second molar	7.0	13.0	10.5	8.0	10.0	9.0	1.0	0.0
Mandibular third molar	7.0	11.0	10.0	7.5	9.5	9.0	1.0	0.0

TABLE C.6 Measurements of the Primary Teeth (in Millimeters)

	Length Overall	Length of Crown	Length of Root	Mesiodistal Diameter of Crown	Mesiodistal Diameter at Cervix	Facial-Lingual Diameter of Crown	Facial-Lingual Diameter at Cervix
Maxillary Teeth							
Central incisor	16.0	6.0	10.0	6.5	4.5	5.0	4.0
Lateral incisor	15.8	5.6	11.4	5.1	3.7	4.8	3.7
Canine	19.0	6.5	13.5	7.0	5.1	7.0	5.5
First molar	15.2	5.1	10.0	7.3	5.2	8.5	6.9
Second molar	17.5	5.7	11.7	8.2	6.4	10.0	8.3
Mandibular Teeth							
Central incisor	14.0	5.0	9.0	4.2	3.0	4.0	3.5
Lateral incisor	15.0	5.2	10.0	4.1	3.0	4.0	3.5
Canine	17.0	6.0	11.5	5.0	3.7	4.8	4.0
First molar	15.8	6.0	9.8	7.7	6.5	7.0	5.3
Second molar	18.8	5.5	11.3	9.9	7.2	8.7	6.4

APPENDIX D

Tooth Development*

TABLE D.1 Development of Permanent Incisors

	Maxillary Central Incisor	Maxillary Lateral Incisor	Mandibular Central Incisor	Mandibular Lateral Incisor
Number of lobes	Four lobes			
First evidence of calcification	3–4 months	1 year	3–4 months	3–4 months
Completion of enamel	4–5 years	4–5 years	4–5 years	4–5 years
Eruption date	7–8 years	8–9 years	6–7 years	7–8 years
Completion of root	10 years	11 years	9 years	10 years

TABLE D.2 Development of Permanent Canines

	Maxillary Canine	Mandibular Canine
Number of lobes	Four lobes	
First evidence of calcification	4–5 months	4–5 months
Completion of enamel	6–7 years	6–7 years
Eruption date	11–12 years	9–10 years
Completion of root	13–15 years	12–14 years

TABLE D.3 Development of Permanent Premolars

Specific Teeth	Maxillary First Premolar	Maxillary Second Premolar	Mandibular First Premolar	Mandibular Second Premolar
Number of lobes		Four lobes		Four or five lobes
First evidence of calcification	1½–1¾ years	2–2½ years	1¾–2 years	2¼–2½ years
Completion of enamel	5–6 years	6–7 years	5–6 years	6–7 years
Eruption date	10–11 years	10–12 years	10–12 years	11–12 years
Completion of root(s)	12–13 years	12–14 years	12–13 years	13–14 years

*All data from Nelson S. *Wheeler's Dental Anatomy, Physiology, and Occlusion*. 10th ed. Philadelphia: Elsevier; 2015.

TABLE D.4 Development of Permanent Maxillary Molars

	Maxillary First Molar	Maxillary Second Molar	Maxillary Third Molar
Number of lobes	Five lobes	Four lobes	
First evidence of calcification	Birth	2½ years	7–9 years
Completion of enamel	3–4 years	7–8 years	12–16 years
Eruption date	6–7 years	12–13 years	17–21 years
Completion of root(s)	9–10 years	14–16 years	18–25 years

TABLE D.5 Development of Permanent Mandibular Molars

	Mandibular First Molar	Mandibular Second Molar	Mandibular Third Molar
Number of lobes	Five lobes	Four lobes	
First evidence of calcification	Birth	2½–3 years	8–10 years
Completion of enamel	2½–3 years	7–8 years	12–16 years
Eruption date	6–7 years	11–13 years	17–21 years
Completion of roots(s)	9–10 years	14–15 years	18–25 years

INDEX

Note: Page numbers followed by "f" indicate figures, "t" indicate tables and "b" indicate boxes.

N

O

P